T0251388

PULMONARY VASCULAR PHYSIOLOGY AND PATHOPHYSIOLOGY

LUNG BIOLOGY IN HEALTH AND DISEASE

Executive Editor: **Claude Lenfant**

Director, National Heart, Lung, and Blood Institute
National Institutes of Health
Bethesda, Maryland

Volume 1 IMMUNOLOGIC AND INFECTIOUS REACTIONS IN THE LUNG, *edited by Charles H. Kirkpatrick and Herbert Y. Reynolds*

Volume 2 THE BIOCHEMICAL BASIS OF PULMONARY FUNCTION, *edited by Ronald G. Crystal*

Volume 3 BIOENGINEERING ASPECTS OF THE LUNG, *edited by John B. West*

Volume 4 METABOLIC FUNCTIONS OF THE LUNG, *edited by Y. S. Bakhle and John R. Vane*

Volume 5 RESPIRATORY DEFENSE MECHANISMS (in two parts), *edited by Joseph D. Brain, Donald F. Proctor, and Lynne M. Reid*

Volume 6 DEVELOPMENT OF THE LUNG, *edited by W. Alan Hodson*

Volume 7 LUNG WATER AND SOLUTE EXCHANGE, *edited by Norman C. Staub*

Volume 8 EXTRAPULMONARY MANIFESTATIONS OF RESPIRATORY DISEASE, *edited by Eugene Debs Robin*

Volume 9 CHRONIC OBSTRUCTIVE PULMONARY DISEASE, *edited by Thomas L. Petty*

Volume 10 PATHOGENESIS AND THERAPY OF LUNG CANCER, *edited by Curtis C. Harris*

Volume 11 GENETIC DETERMINANTS OF PULMONARY DISEASE, *edited by Stephen D. Litwin*

Volume 12 THE LUNG IN THE TRANSITION BETWEEN HEALTH AND DISEASE, *edited by Peter T. Macklem and Solbert Permutt*

Volume 13 EVOLUTION OF RESPIRATORY PROCESSES A COMPARATIVE APPROACH, *edited by Stephen C. Wood and Claude Lenfant*

Volume 14 PULMONARY VASCULAR DISEASES, *edited by Kenneth M. Moser*

Volume 15 PHYSIOLOGY AND PHARMACOLOGY OF THE AIRWAYS, *edited by Jay A. Nadel*

Volume 16 DIAGNOSTIC TECHNIQUES IN PULMONARY DISEASE (in two parts), *edited by Marvin A. Sackner*

Volume 17 REGULATION OF BREATHING (in two parts), *edited by Thomas F. Hornbein*

Volume 18 OCCUPATIONAL LUNG DISEASES RESEARCH APPROACHES AND METHODS, *edited by Hans Weill and Margaret Turner-Warwick*

Volume 19 IMMUNOPHARMACOLOGY OF THE LUNG, *edited by Harold H. Newball*

Volume 20 SARCOIDOSIS AND OTHER GRANULOMATOUS DISEASES OF THE LUNG, *edited by Barry L. Fanburg*

Volume 21 SLEEP AND BREATHING, *edited by Nicholas A. Saunders and Colin E. Sullivan*

Volume 22 *PNEUMOCYSTIS CARINII* PNEUMONIA PATHOGENESIS, DIAGNOSIS, AND TREATMENT, *edited by Lowell S. Young*

Volume 23 PULMONARY NUCLEAR MEDICINE: TECHNIQUES IN DIAGNOSIS OF LUNG DISEASE, *edited by Harold L. Atkins*

Volume 24 ACUTE RESPIRATORY FAILURE, *edited by Warren M. Zapol and Konrad J. Falke*

Volume 25 GAS MIXING AND DISTRIBUTION IN THE LUNG, *edited by Ludwig A. Engel and Manuel Paiva*

Volume 26 HIGH-FREQUENCY VENTILATION IN INTENSIVE CARE AND DURING SURGERY, *edited by Graziano Carlon and William S. Howland*

Volume 27 PULMONARY DEVELOPMENT TRANSITION FROM INTRAUTERINE TO EXTRAUTERINE LIFE, *edited by George H. Nelson*

Volume 28 CHRONIC OBSTRUCTIVE PULMONARY DISEASE, second edition, revised and expanded,
edited by Thomas L. Petty

Volume 29 THE THORAX (in two parts),
edited by Charis Roussos and Peter T. Macklem

Volume 30 THE PLEURA IN HEALTH AND DISEASE,
edited by Jaques Chrétien, Jean Bignon, and Albert Hirsch

Volume 31 DRUG THERAPY FOR ASTHMA: RESEARCH AND CLINICAL PRACTICE,
edited by John W. Jenne and Shirley Murphy

Volume 32 PULMONARY ENDOTHELIUM IN HEALTH AND DISEASE,
edited by Una S. Ryan

Volume 33 THE AIRWAYS: NEURAL CONTROL IN HEALTH AND DISEASE,
edited by Michael A. Kaliner and Peter J. Barnes

Volume 34 PATHOPHYSIOLOGY AND TREATMENT OF INHALATION INJURIES,
edited by Jacob Loke

Volume 35 RESPIRATORY FUNCTION OF THE UPPER AIRWAY,
edited by Oommen P. Mathew and Giuseppe Sant'Ambrogio

Volume 36 CHRONIC OBSTRUCTIVE PULMONARY DISEASE: A BEHAVIORAL PERSPECTIVE,
edited by A. John McSweeny and Igor Grant

Volume 37 BIOLOGY OF LUNG CANCER: DIAGNOSIS AND TREATMENT,
edited by Steven T. Rosen, James L. Mulshine, Frank Cuttitta, and Paul G. Abrams

Volume 38 PULMONARY VASCULAR PHYSIOLOGY AND PATHOPHYSIOLOGY,
edited by E. Kenneth Weir and John T. Reeves

Volume 39 COMPARATIVE PULMONARY PHYSIOLOGY: CURRENT CONCEPTS,
edited by Stephen C. Wood

Volume 40 RESPIRATORY PHYSIOLOGY: AN ANALYTICAL APPROACH,
edited by H. K. Chang and Manuel Paiva

Volume 41 LUNG CELL BIOLOGY,
edited by Donald Massaro

Additional Volumes in Preparation

HEART-LUNG INTERACTIONS IN HEALTH AND DISEASE,
edited by Steven M. Scharf and Sharon Cassidy

PULMONARY VASCULAR PHYSIOLOGY AND PATHOPHYSIOLOGY

Edited by

E. Kenneth Weir

Department of Medicine
VA Medical Center and
University of Minnesota
Minneapolis, Minnesota

John T. Reeves

CVP Research Laboratory
University of Colorado
Health Sciences Center
Denver, Colorado

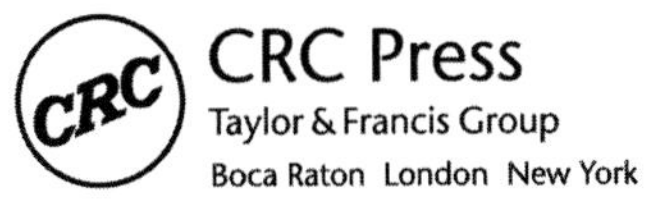
CRC Press
Taylor & Francis Group
Boca Raton London New York

CRC Press is an imprint of the
Taylor & Francis Group, an **informa** business

Library of Congress Cataloging-in-Publication Data

Pulmonary vascular physiology and pathophysiology / edited by E. Kenneth Weir, John T. Reeves.
p. cm. -- (Lung biology in health and disease ; v. 38)
Includes bibliographies and indexes.
ISBN 0-8247-7972-X
1. Pulmonary hypertension--Pathophysiology. 2. Pulmonary circulation. I. Weir, E. Kenneth. II. Reeves, John T. III. Series.
[DNLM: 1. Hypertension, Pulmonary--etiology. 2. Hypertension, Pulmonary--physiopathology. 3. Pulmonary Circulation. W1 LU62 v. 38/ WF 600 P9884].
RC776.P87P86 1988
616.2'4--dc19
DNLM/DLC
for Library of Congress 88-20423
CIP

This book is printed on acid-free paper.

MARCEL DEKKER, INC.
270 Madison Avenue, New York, New York 10016

Current printing (last digit):
10 9 8 7 6 5 4 3 2 1

PRINTED IN THE UNITED STATES OF AMERICA

INTRODUCTION

> Those therefore which I hear denying that blood, yea the whole mass of blood, may pass through the substance of the lungs, as well as the nutritive juyce through the liver, as if it were impossible and no wayes to be believed–it is to be thought that those kind of men, where they like, they easily grant, where they like not, by no means; here where need is, they are afraid, but where no need is they are not afraid to aver.
>
> William Harvey
> *De Motu Cordis*, 1628

In his Harveian Oration, William Osler wrote: "To the age of the hearer, in which men had heard and heard only, had succeeded the age of the eye in which men had seen and been content only to see. But at last came the age of the hand–the thinking, devising, planning hand, the hand as an instrument of the mind, now reintroduced into the world in a modest little monograph from which we may date the beginning of experimental medicine." He was referring to De Motu Cordis.

Ever since the pulmonary circulation was discovered by William Harvey, much work has been done on its physiology and pathophysiology. After all, the pulmonary circulation is a most important organ. What Harvey did not know is *how* the blood passed through the lungs: he thought that there was a filtration process from the arteries to the veins. Of course, the discovery of the capillary bed of the lung by Malpighi provided the anatomical basis of pulmonary physiology as we know it. Indeed, the pulmonary circulation is an important system, but it is a fragile one because of the closeness of the blood to the gaseous environment. Although anatomically simple, it is physiologically a complex system which is rich in its ability to adapt, to respond to stresses and to environmental changes.

The fourteenth volume of the series, Lung Biology in Health and Disease, titled *Pulmonary Vascular Diseases* was published in 1979. The decade that followed has seen many advances in our understanding of the pulmonary circulation in health and disease. The new methods and approaches of the 1980s have given us important tools to further increase this understanding. It is gratifying that two acknowledged experts in the investigation of the pulmonary circulation, Drs. John T. Reeves and E. Kenneth Weir, agreed to edit the new volume, *Pulmonary Vascular Physiology and Pathophysiology*. They have assembled a group of contributors who have demonstrated their expertise through years of pioneering research on the pulmonary circulation. I am grateful to all of them for their contributions to this volume, which will undoubtedly be a challenge to both current and future researchers in this field of endeavor. This new monograph in the series, Lung Biology in Health and Disease, may begin the new age of research on the pulmonary circulation.

Claude Lenfant, M.D.
Bethesda, Maryland

PREFACE

In 1912 Sir William Osler stated that there are three phases in our understanding and management of diseases. The first is "the recognition of disease and the means for its cure." The second is "the discovery of its causes," and the third is the implementation of "measures for its prevention." The various forms of pulmonary hypertension, whether primary, thromboembolic, persistent in the newborn, or secondary to chronic obstructive lung disease, pulmonary fibrosis, left to right cardiac shunts, high left heart filling pressures, and so on, are well described in a clinical sense. Unfortunately the methods of treatment that are currently available seldom restore the pulmonary vasculature to normal function. Most forms of treatment for pulmonary hypertension, such as vasodilators, oxygen, and anticoagulants, are palliative rather than curative.

Our inability to provide definitive treatment is sometimes a result of our ignorance of the primary stimulus, as in primary pulmonary hypertension or persistent pulmonary hypertension of the newborn. On other occasions it stems from our lack of understanding of the pathophysiology initiated by the primary stimulus, such as hypoxia or high flow. The study of pathophysiology is the second phase referred to by Osler: the discovery of causes. Research on the pulmonary vasculature has now reached this stage. The introduction of pulmonary arterial catheterization in humans in 1945 made possible the clinical description of different forms of pulmonary hypertension. The increasing use of the techniques of cellular and molecular biology provides the key to the understanding of pathophysiology.

This volume is divided into two parts, physiology and pathophysiology. The first describes the normal function of the pulmonary circulation under a wide variety of conditions such as exercise, pregnancy, hypoxia, hyperoxia, fetal life, hypobaria, hyperbaria, and diving. In addition it covers phylogenetic aspects of pulmonary circulatory control, pulmonary vascular hemodynamics, and right ventricular function. The second part of the volume reviews our current knowledge of the mechanisms involved in the pathophysiology of pulmonary hypertension. These mechanisms are considered in terms of the general control of cell proliferation and the interactions between smooth muscle, endothelium and leukocytes. They are also considered in relation to specific forms of pulmonary hypertension. When the cellular and molecular "causes" of pulmonary hypertension are understood, we will be able to devise better treatment and turn our attention to Osler's third phase, that of prevention.

The publication of this volume has been made possible through the support of the Pulmonary Circulation Foundation, which is gratefully acknowledged.

E. Kenneth Weir
John T. Reeves

CONTENTS

Part II PATHOPHYSIOLOGY

CONTRIBUTORS

Steven H. Abman, M.D. Assistant Professor, Department of Pediatrics, University of Colorado Health Sciences Center, Denver, Colorado

Frank J. Accurso, M.D. Associate Professor, Department of Pediatrics, University of Colorado Health Sciences Center, Denver, Colorado

Steven L. Archer, M.D. Assistant Professor of Medicine, Department of Medicine, Division of Cardiology, University of Minnesota and VA Medical Center, Minneapolis, Minnesota

T. A. Bronikowski Ph.D., Professor of Physiology, Department of Physiology, Marquette University, Milwaukee, Wisconsin

Paul Davies, Ph.D.* Assistant Professor of Pathology, Department of Pathology, Harvard Medical School, and Research Associate in Pathology, The Children's Hospital, Boston, Massachusetts

Christopher A. Dawson, Ph.D.† Professor, Department of Physiology, Medical College of Wisconsin, Milwaukee, Wisconsin

Colby W. Dempesy, Ph.D. Research Professor, Department of Neurologic Surgery, Tulane University School of Medicine, New Orleans, Louisiana

Jerome A. Dempsey, Ph.D. Department of Preventive Medicine, University of Wisconsin-Madison, Madison, Wisconsin

---

Present affiliations:

*Research Associate Professor, Department of Pharamcology and Pathology, University of Pittsburgh School of Medicine, Pittsburgh, Pennsylvania

†Research Physiologist, Department of Research Services, Clement J. Zablocki Veterans Administration Medical Center, Milwaukee, Wisconsin

Leon E. Farhi, M.D. Professor and Chairman, Department of Physiology, State University of New York at Buffalo, School of Medicine, Buffalo, New York

Charles J. Fontana Research Associate, Department of Neurologic Surgery, Tulane University School of Medicine, New Orleans, Louisiana

Robert F. Grover, M.D., Ph.D.* Professor Emeritus of Medicine, Department of Medicine, University of Colorado School of Medicine, Denver, Colorado

Bertron M. Groves, M.D. Director, Cardiac Catheterization Laboratory, Division of Cardiology, University of Colorado Health Sciences Center, Denver, Colorado

Michael A. Heymann, M.D. Professor, Departments of Pediatrics, Obstetrics, Gynecology, and Reproductive Services, University of California, San Francisco, San Francisco, California

James C. Hogg, M.D., Ph.D., F.R.C.P.(C) Professor, Department of Pathology, University of British Columbia, Vancouver, British Columbia, Canada

Albert L. Hyman, M.D. Professor, Departments of Surgery, Medicine and Pharmacology and Director, Cardiopulmonary Research Laboratory, Tulane University School of Medicine, New Orleans, Louisiana

Roger A. Johns, M.D. Assistant Professor of Anesthesiology, Department of Anesthesiology, University of Virginia School of Medicine, Charlottesville, Virginia

Arnold Johnson, Ph.D.+ Assistant Professor of Physiology, Department of Physiology, Albany Medical College, Albany, New York

Philip J. Kadowitz, Ph.D. Professor of Pharmacology, Department of Pharmacology, Tulane University School of Medicine, New Orleans, Louisiana

J. H. Linehan, Ph.D. Professor of Mechanical and Biomedical Engineering, Marquette University, Milwaukee, Wisconsin

---

Present affiliations:
*Retired
+Research Scientist, Department of Research Service, Veterans Administration Medical Center, Albany, New York

Howard L. Lippton, B.S., M.D. Fellow, Department of Pulmonary/Critical Care Medicine, Tulane University School of Medicine, New Orleans, Louisiana

Claes E. G. Lundgren, M.D. Professor of Physiology, Department of Physiology, and Director for the Center for Research in Special Environment, State University of New York at Buffalo, School of Medicine, Buffalo, New York

Asrar B. Malik, M.D. Professor of Physiology, Department of Physiology, Albany Medical College, Albany, New York

Ivan F. McMurtry, Ph.D. Associate Professor, Department of Medicine, University of Colorado Health Sciences Center, Denver, Colorado

Lorna Grindlay Moore, M.D. Professor, Department of Anthropology, University of Colorado, and Professor, Department of Medicine, University of Colorado Health Sciences Center, Denver, Colorado

Douglass A. Morrison, M.D. Assistant Professor, Department of Internal Medicine and Radiology, University of Colorado Health Sciences Center, and Director, Cardiac Catheterization Laboratory, Denver VA Medical Center, Denver, Colorado

Michael J. Peach, B.S., M.S., Ph.D. Professor and Associate Dean for Research, Department of Pharmacology, University of Virginia School of Medicine, Charlottesville, Virginia

Marlene Rabinovitch, M.D. Associate Professor, Departments of Pediatrics and Pathology, University of Toronto, and Associate, Departments of Cardiology and Pathology, The Hospital for Sick Children, Toronto, Ontario, Canada

John T. Reeves, M.D. Professor of Medicine, and Associate Director, CVP Research Laboratory, University of Colorado Health Sciences Center, Denver, Colorado

Lynne M. Reid, M.D. S. Burt Wolbach Professor of Pathology, Department of Pathology, Harvard Medical School, and Pathologist-in-Chief, Department of Pathology, The Children's Hospital, Boston, Massachusetts

Donald E. Richardson, M.D., F.A.C.S. Professor and Chairman, Department of Neurological Surgery, Tulane University School of Medicine, New Orleans, Louisiana

Richard W. Rieck, Ph.D. Assistant Professor of Anatomy, Department of Anatomy, Tulane University School of Medicine, New Orleans, Louisiana

C. Edward Rose, Jr., M.D. Associate Professor of Medicine, Department of Internal Medicine, University of Virginia School of Medicine, Charlottesville, Virginia

Sharon I.S. Rounds, M.D.* Associate Professor of Medicine, Evans Memorial Department of Clinical Research and Medicine, Boston University School of Medicine, Boston, Massachusetts

Scott J. Soifer, M.D. Assistant Professor of Pediatrics, and Director, Division of Pediatric Critical Care Medicine, Department of Pediatrics, University of California, San Francisco, San Francisco, California

Kurt R. Stenmark, M.D. Assistant Professor of Pediatrics, Cardiovascular and Pulmonary Research Laboratory, University of Colorado Health Sciences Center, Denver, Colorado

S. Marsh Tenney, M.D. Nathan Smith Professor of Physiology, Department of Physiology, Dartmouth Medical School, Hanover, New Hampshire

John A. Trapp, Ph.D. (Mech. Eng.) Associate Professor, Mechanical Engineering Department, University of Colorado College of Engineering and Applied Science, Denver, Colorado

Darya Turkevich, M.D. Clinical Assistant Professor, Department of Medicine (Cardiology), University of Colorado School of Medicine, Denver, Colorado

Norbert F. Voelkel, M.D. Associate Professor of Medicine, Cardiovascular Pulmonary Research Laboratory, University of Colorado Health Sciences Center and Webb-Waring Lung Institute, Denver, Colorado

Peter D. Wagner, M.D. Professor of Medicine, Department of Medicine, University of California, San Diego, La Jolla, California

E. Kenneth Weir, M.D. Professor of Medicine, Department of Medicine, VA Medical Center and University of Minnesota School of Medicine, Minneapolis, Minnesota

---

Present affiliation:

*Associate Professor of Medicine, Department of Medicine, Brown University, Providence VA Medical Center, Providence, Rhode Island

PULMONARY VASCULAR PHYSIOLOGY AND PATHOPHYSIOLOGY

Part I

PHYSIOLOGY

1

A Phylogenetic Perspective of Control of the Pulmonary Circulation

S. MARSH TENNEY

Dartmouth Medical School
Hanover, New Hampshire

I. Prologue

Lungs were undoubtedly existent in many primitive fishes as long ago as the Devonian period, and their available service for respiratory gas exchange was a crucial feature for survival when the oxygen supply from the water became limited due to rising temperature and widespread organic decay. Only those species in possession of a mechanism to respire air could survive, either by waiting out a temporary adversity or possibly by migrating over land to a new aquatic habitat. The impetus for colonization of the land that followed in late Devonian times was not really the attractiveness of air as a more favorable respiratory medium than water; rather, it was the pressure to escape the increasingly diminishing oxygen content of water, a problem made more urgent by the fact that the freshwater lakes and swamps had begun to dry up altogether. It is no coincidence that of the three genera of lung fishes surviving today all are found in swamps and shallow lakes low in oxygen content and subject to seasonal drought.

Any organ designed for exchange of gas with the environment must also reckon with the need for a blood supply properly matched with the air (or water) supply in order to achieve optimal effectiveness. Vascular arrangements in varying degrees of complexity that serve this purpose can be traced phylogenetically, and to a considerable extent they are reproduced developmentally. The steady progress of the respiratory apparatus to the stage of lungs of mammals and birds was always in advance of the comparable vascular circuitry, but the evolution of the latter was toward a clear separation of the pulmonary and systemic branches. The discussion that follows treats the comparative anatomical features of the pulmonary circulation very slightly and emphasizes the phylogeny of control of pulmonary blood flow. The central question asked is: How are we to interpret global pulmonary vasoconstriction, as it occurs in most mammals in response to hypoxia, when the consequences can have no benefit for gas exchange and merely place an added burden on the heart? In short, the response must be judged maladaptive, yet perhaps in tracing its evolutionary origins a once useful purpose will be found, one that is still carried as a piece of archaic baggage but is ill suited now for mammalian cardiorespiratory design and hence has become a handicap.

The thesis advanced [no claim for originality is intended; the idea has been clearly expressed by Reeves et al. (1979) and can be regarded as implicit in Johansen (1982)] is that the global increase in pulmonary vascular resistance elicited by hypoxia and CO_2 in mammals is a carryover of a premammalian ancestral response designed to divert blood flow from the lung if the respired air became asphyxic (or was not replenished, as in a dive) to another exchange surface (gills or skin). The effective operation of such a control plan depends on a parallel arrangement of pulmonary and systemic circuits, a design still found in the mammalian fetus; when that is lost in the adult, the once useful response of generalized pulmonary vasoconstriction becomes inappropriate and harmful.

II. Fish

In water-breathing fish, all of the systemic venous return is pumped to the gills, and the gill efferents carry the oxygenated blood to the systemic circulation. The single ventricle thus supplies the energy for both circuits, but since they are arranged in series, and the gill circuit is proximal, blood pressure in the gills must be higher than in the systemic beds. There are anatomical shunts around the secondary lamellas, but bypassing this region of gas exchange, even if the water is asphyxic, can serve no useful purpose unless it is to reduce the energy demand on the ventricle; gill flow and systemic flow still remain equal. However, if there is an alternative region of gas exchange, one that would be more favorable than the one dependent on poorly oxygenated water, then the utility of a bypass mechanism becomes obvious. The principle of controlled parallel circuitry is of supreme importance in effecting the transition from water to air breathing (and vice versa) in bimodal systems.

The lungs of Dipnoi and the air bladder of teleosts are considered to be homologous organs, and although the air bladder evolved to become an organ of buoyancy, it still also serves, in many species, as a supplementary organ of respiration. In those instances the gills and the circulation to the gills are reduced, and the remaining circuit through the branchial arches is characterized by large channels that can serve as a shunt that bypasses the gills if gas exchange switches predominantly to the "lungs" (Johansen et al., 1968). In those fish that employ the air bladder for gas exchange, new vessels have developed from the branchial circulation (sixth aortic arch) and are homologous with the pulmonary artery in higher vertebrates (Johansen, 1970). Further, the lungfish possesses a pulmonary vein that drains directly into the atrium.

One of the first regulatory requirements for efficient gas exchange in a system that offers gills and/or lungs as the site for exchange is to provide a blood supply to each appropriate for its share of the total ventilation. The Australian lungfish, *Neoceratodus*, is primarily a water breather with well-developed gills, and its branchial vascular resistance is about the same as in teleosts and elasmobranchs (Johansen et al., 1968). *Neoceratodus* does have lungs, but they are not often needed, because the aquatic habitat of this fish is always sufficiently oxygenated. In Figure 1 the anatomy of heart and blood vessels in *Neoceratodus* is portrayed. In the African lungfish, *Protopterus*, and the South American lungfish, *Lepidosiren*, aerial respiration is obligatory and the gills are degenerate. The shallow lakes and swamps in which they live dry up periodically and force prolonged estivation, during which time there is no alternative to air breathing (Delaney et al., 1974). Clearly, in this circumstance of obligatory air breathing, blood flow to the lungs should be strongly favored over that to the gills, and in the lungfish, in contrast to other fishes that breathe air, there is a partial interatrial septum, and the beginnings of a two-circuit system – pulmonary and systemic – can be discerned (Lahiri et al., 1970; Fishman et al., 1985). It is also notable that pulmonary vascular resistance in lungfish is less than systemic vascular resistance, a feature not found in any other fish.

An indication of the close matching of blood flow to the lung and ventilation of the lung can be observed in *Protopterus*. Like all lungfish, *Protopterus* is a periodic breather. During the breathing phase the cardiac output, heart rate, and systemic blood pressure all increase, and about 95% of the blood that returns to the heart from the pulmonary veins is distributed to the systemic circulation (Johansen and Hol, 1968). During the apneic phase the fraction declines to 65%. In most fish, exposure to air increases branchial vascular resistance because the small vessels in the gills collapse, but in *Protopterus* branchial vascular resistance decreases due to an increase of shunt flow.

Close coupling of ventilation and blood flow (see Fig. 2) in lungfish is thought to be reflex in origin, probably dependent on pulmonary stretch receptors. The lungs of dipnoans are supplied by pulmonary branches of the vagus

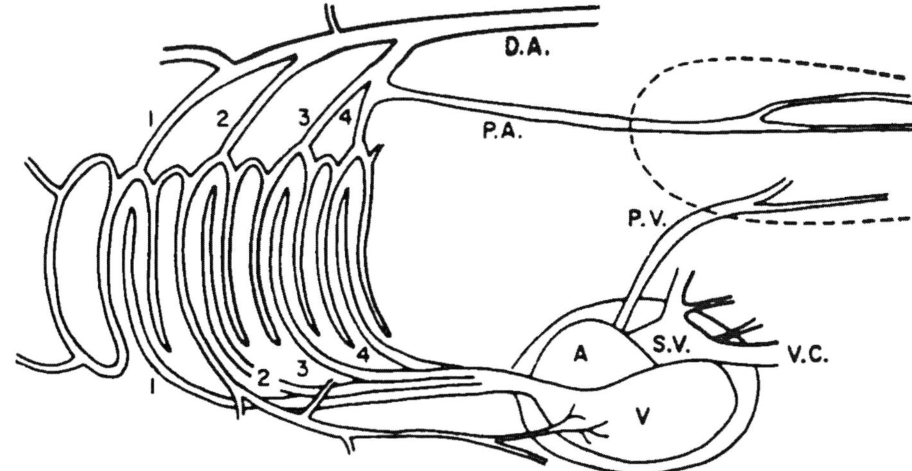

Figure 1 Schematic drawing of heart and major blood vessels in *Neoceratodus forsteri*. A, atrium; V, ventricle; SV, sinus venosus. Numbers refer to afferent and efferent blood vessels. DA, dorsal aorta; PA, pulmonary artery; PV, pulmonary vein; VC, vena cava. (Reproduced with permission from Johansen, et al., 1967.)

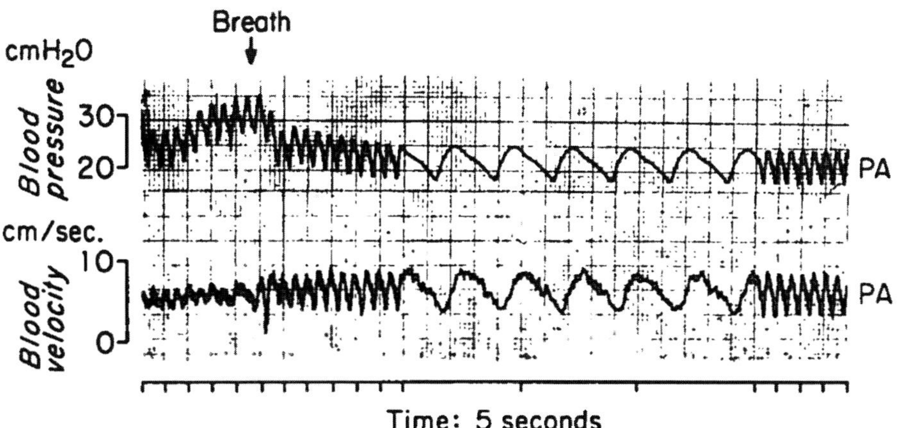

Figure 2 Blood flow through the lungs and pressure in the pulmonary artery of *Protopterus* increase just after a breath and then decrease slightly until the next breath is taken. (Reproduced with permission from Johansen et al., 1968.)

(Nicol, 1951); acetylcholine is a branchial vasoconstrictor, and adrenalin relaxes branchial vessels in lungfish (Johansen et al., 1968). Hypoxic water initiates an increase of cardiac output and an increase in the proportion of blood circulated to the lungs, a response dependent on chemoreceptors in the gill region that face the ambient water, or perhaps they are located in the efferent branchial vessels (Johansen et al., 1967). Increase of CO_2 in the ambient water increases pulmonary ventilation and decreases branchial respiration, with blood flow appropriately adjusted to the two sites. In the longnose gar there is good experimental evidence for the existence of chemoreceptors in two loci: one, internal, sensing PO_2 in the air bladder and driving lung ventilation; the other external, sensing PO_2 of water and depressing gill ventilation in hypoxia (Smatresk et al., 1986).

Protopterus also employs a mechanism for apportioning flow between the pulmonary and systemic circuits that heralds a comparable regulatory device in the mammalian fetus. The ductus arteriosus of lungfish is a short channel that connects the efferent vessels of the posterior arches and the dorsal aorta. Its wall is muscular and is innervated by myelinated and unmyelinated fibers (Fishman et al., 1985). Acetylcholine exerts a weak dilatory action on the ductus; norepinephrine, a powerful constriction; under hypoxic conditions the ductal lumen is patent, but in hyperoxia it is nearly obliterated (Fishman et al., 1985). Since the ductus originates just before the origin of the pulmonary arteries, its degree of patency provides a highly effective means for distributing flow between the pulmonary and systemic circuits.

Control of the pulmonary vascular resistance would be a further means for regulating pulmonary blood flow, but that service resides in a thickened segment of the extrapulmonary pulmonary artery; further, unlike the ductus arteriosus, its smooth muscle is sparsely innervated (Fishman et al., 1985). This extrapulmonary pulmonary artery vasomotor segment constricts under the influence of acetylcholine, but it is unresponsive to hyperoxia and norepinephrine (Fishman et al., 1985). Norepinephrine does, however, constrict the intrinsic pulmonary vessels.

The responses of the pulmonary artery vasomotor segment in lungfish are certainly subject to the influence of local PO_2 and to reflexes with a vagal efferent path – a system that will be seen to carry forward to amphibians and reptiles.

III. Amphibians

The current accepted view is that amphibians (and therefore, all tetrapod vertebrates) arose about 300 million years ago from the rhipidistian Crossopterygii, ancient bottom-dwelling carnivorous fishes with paired, lobed fins well suited to evolve into limbs; and, most probably, they possessed an air bladder that was employed as an accessory respiratory organ. The near certainty of a functional "lung" in these fishes is qualified only because knowledge was limited to what could be read in the fossil record until the discovery in 1938 of a living coelacanth, *Latimeria*, off the coast of South Africa. This mid-Paleozoic fish came quickly to be known as a "living fossil," and although its one lung is filled with fat, in its freshwater ancestors the lung undoubtedly was a hollow, air-filled viscus that served as an accessory organ of gas exchange. However, after migration to the ocean the lung became an organ of buoyancy, and now *Latimeria* never surfaces to breathe.

It remains a puzzle how exactly the air bladder came to be located dorsally while the lung is always a ventral organ (Goodrich, 1930). The original location of the air bladder (lung) was probably ventral, but migration dorsally was essential when its function became primarily concerned with buoyancy (a ventral air bladder would tend to flip the fish upside down), and consequently the left pulmonary vessels are found to course around the esophagus ventrally, together with the duct, to reach the now dorsally located air bladder in Dipnoi. The stages in the transition of the pulmonary circulation from that of air-breathing fishes to modern amphibians is incomplete because of lack of information regarding extinct amphibian species. However, with the gradual loss of branchial respiration there is a stage-by-stage fusion of the afferent branchial arteries (Das and Saxena, 1958) and by the stage of a modern adult amphibian the fifth aortic arch has disappeared, and the sixth has become the pulmocutaneous artery (see Fig. 3). Much more so than in fish, cutaneous gas exchange is an important option in amphibians (Krogh, 1904), and in them there are two sets of valves at the distal end of the bulbus cordis that serve to separate ventricular outflow into systemic and pulmocutaneous directions (Johansen and Hanson, 1968). The pulmocutaneous arch divides into a pulmonary and a cutaneous vessel, and there are control mechanisms that can direct flow preferentially to one or the other region. In water-breathing fish, where the gill and systemic circulations are in series, change of flow to one region must have a similar effect on the other, a situation like that in mammals where the ventricles are completely separate. In amphibians the circuit design allows regulation of flow between the pulmonary and cutaneous gas-exchange surfaces by changes of regional vascular impedance (Shelton, 1976, 1986). In this scheme the dominant regulatory mechanism appears to reside in the pulmonary circulation, and probably the vasodilation during ventilation is dependent on mechanical, local reflex, chemical, and possibly, central influences. Control of cutaneous flow is subsidiary but is not always a strictly passive follower.

The expectation, following the phylogenetic progression, would be to find regulatory responses comparable with those of the lungfish. The first and most elementary stimulus in any list of factors that promote pulmonary blood flow

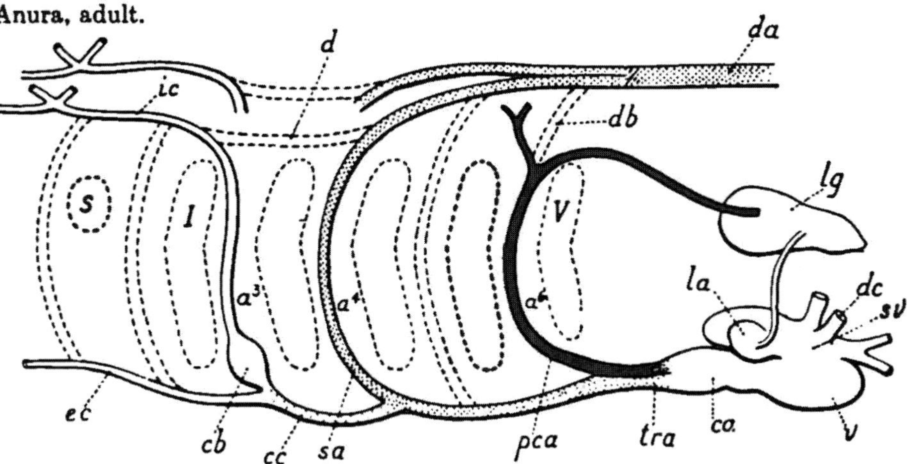

Figure 3 Schematic drawing of anatomy of heart and blood vessels in an adult anuran. Vessels carrying venous blood are black, those that are stippled carry mixed blood, and the white vessels are the most arterial. The structures of major interest are: v, ventricle; la, left auricle; lg, lung; ca, conus arteriosus; tra, truncus arteriosus (ventral aorta); A^{1-6}, primary arterial arches; da, median dorsal aorta; db, ductus Botalli (ductus arteriosus); pca, pulmonary artery. (Reproduced from Goodrich, 1930.)

is pulmonary ventilation, and, as is the case for lungfish, in amphibians also there is a close relationship between the two (Shelton, 1970; Emilio and Shelton, 1972; West and Burggren, 1984). (See Fig. 4.) When the lungs are ventilated, pulmonary vascular resistance decreases and pulmonary blood flow increases with reciprocal changes in cutaneous blood flow, but cutaneous vascular resistance does not seem to change. The response is the same with either spontaneous or assisted ventilation. The reduced pulmonary blood flow during apnea (it makes no difference whether the apneic period is in air or during submergence) constitutes an important part of the diving response, which also includes slowing of the heart rate and decreases in cardiac output and blood pressure (Shelton and Jones, 1965; Hoffman and Cordeira de Sousa, 1982). In this condition the lungs are an important store of oxygen, which is made available to the rest of the body in proportion to the extent of pulmonary blood flow ("oxygen conservation"), and the shift of emphasis to the skin, preferentially distributing deoxygenated blood to the body surface for oxygen uptake from the environment, is an advantageous response (Poczopko, 1959) for which the central circulatory design of amphibians is uniquely suited (Feder and Burggren, 1985).

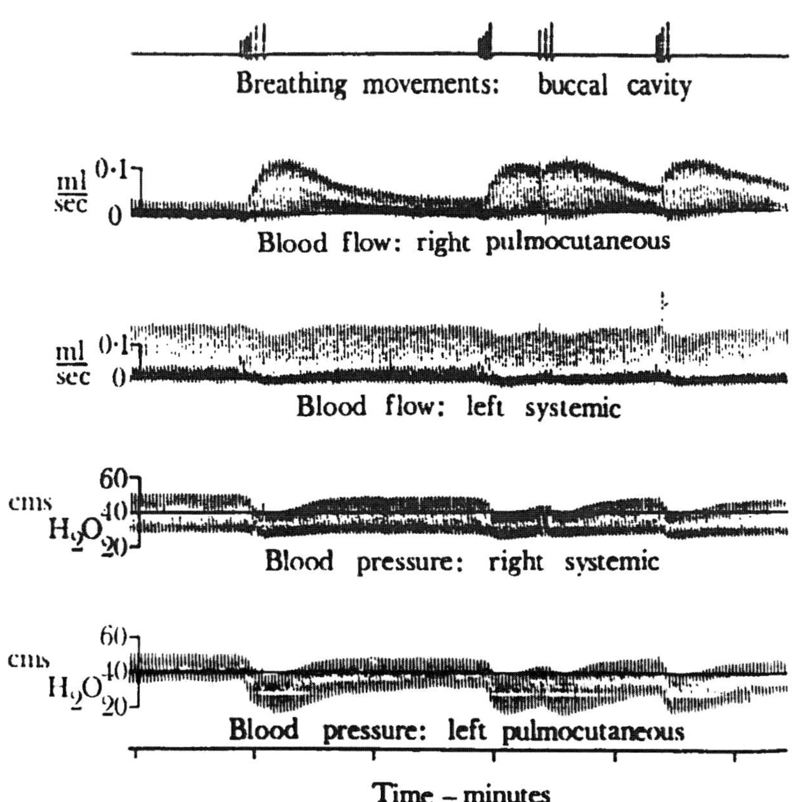

Figure 4 Pressures and flow in the arterial arches of *Xenopus*. Breathing movements shown in the top trace are indicative of lung ventilation; their effect on flow in the several vessels is illustrated. (Reproduced with permission from Shelton, 1970.)

Pulmonary stretch receptors and chemoreceptors are both involved in the afferent limb of this reflex, and the vagus is the efferent pathway. There is evidence of central integration of the reflex, since it is abolished if the whole brain, or just the medulla, is destroyed (Bastert, 1929), but no more precise localization has been determined. The effector mechanism controlling pulmonary blood flow is a sphincter in the pulmonary artery (De Saint-Aubain and Wingstrand, 1979) – already anticipated in the constrictor segment of lungfish – that contracts actively when the lungs are collapsed. Acetylcholine, as would be expected, constricts the sphincter and decreases pulmonary blood flow, but epinephrine has no effect although there is adrenergic innervation (Malvin and Dail,

1986). The catecholamines are more active in controlling gill vascular resistance, as in the salamander, where α-adrenergic receptors are vasoconstrictor and β receptors are dilator (Malvin, 1985).

The influences of oxygen and carbon dioxide are always of particular interest, and in bimodal breathers the location of stimulus application is an important consideration. In normoxia, about 80% of the cardiac output is distributed to the lungs of unanesthetized bullfrogs; if they are in water and the aqueous PO_2 is reduced to 40 torr, pulmonary flow rises to 96% of the cardiac output; but if a similar reduction of PO_2 is made in air inspired by the lungs, pulmonary flow falls to 75% of the cardiac output (Boutilier et al., 1986). The combined effects of lung ventilation and the oxygen content of inspired air on pulmonary blood flow are apparent from the descending order of effectiveness of ventilation to increase flow, dependent on inspired O_2 concentration: 100% O_2, most effective; room air, somewhat less; 0% O_2 (N_2), least effective (Emilio and Shelton, 1972). Five percent CO_2 at constant lung volume acts to decrease pulmonary blood flow in toads (West and Burggren, 1984), and the effect is potentiated by hypoxia. There are also direct, local chemical effects of hypoxia on the pulmonary microvasculature (Koyama and Morimoto, 1983), nicely demonstrated by exposing only 0.2% of lung surface area to hypoxia. Such a minimal contact ensures that whole-body blood gas composition will not be affected. Direct observation of the exposed vessels indicated a 21% reduction in arteriolar flow.

Respiratory gas composition also affects cutaneous blood flow, and that response is complementary with pulmonary vascular responses in the total control scheme. Cutaneous gas exchange can be used to infer cutaneous blood flow, and in such a study Malvin and Hlastala (1986) found that inflation of the lungs of *Rana pipiens* with oxygen decreased cutaneous flow to a greater extent than when the lungs were inflated with room air, but 4.8% CO_2 in the inspired air had no effect, a conclusion consistent with the observation that CO_2 into the lungs had no effect on cutaneous conductance (Jackson and Braun, 1979). Direct exposure of the skin to increased concentration of O_2 increased cutaneous blood flow, the effect achieving a perfusion matching comparable to the ventilation: perfusion matching in the lung (Malvin and Hlastala, 1986). Exposure to CO_2 through the skin increases pulmonary ventilation and opens cutaneous capillaries (Poczopko, 1959).

It has already been remarked that the pulmonary artery pressure in lower vertebrates is higher than in mammals and may be as much as two or three times as high. This fact, taken together with the further information that colloid osmotic pressure of the plasma is usually lower, leads to a prediction from the Starling principle governing transcapillary fluid exchange that the lungs of amphibians ought to be edematous and therefore compromised in their effectiveness as a gas-exchange organ. A study of fluid balance in the amphibian lung

(Smits et al., 1986) confirms the precarious state of this organ but also discloses the design of a control system that acts protectively. The pulmonary arterial branches have a muscular coat (Smith and Campbell, 1976) whose tone is reflexly adjusted (in part) by activity of a baroreceptor located in the pulmocutaneous artery (Ishii and Ishii, 1978; West and van Vliet, 1983). Afferent fibers from this receptor travel in the recurrent laryngeal nerve and become part of the vagal trunk; if the central end of the cut vagosympathetic trunk is electrically stimulated or, in an intact preparation, if the reflexogenic region of the pulmonary artery is distended, there is a fall in heart rate and a decrease of both pulmonary and systemic blood pressures. Cutting of the recurrent laryngeal nerve is followed by a threefold increase of pulmonary blood flow, a doubling of the pressure drop from pulmonary artery to pulmonary vein, and a tenfold increase of net transcapillary fluid flux (Smits et al., 1986). This dramatic effect leads to the conclusion that a tonic neural input from the baroreceptor maintains sufficient tone in the pulmonary artery to check pulmonary blood flow and prevent pulmonary edema. Although earlier studies claimed that 50-70% of the pulmonary vascular resistance in amphibians resided in the pulmonary venous segment (Maloney and Castle, 1970), this may have been an artifact of their pithed preparation, and, more likely, the effect of the pulmonary baroreceptor mechanism is on precapillary resistance, thus serving to bias capillary pressure away from outward fluid filtration.

IV. Reptiles

Most of the notable features of the pulmonary circulation of reptiles are not different in any important way from those of amphibians, but it is relevant that the situation differs in the absence of significant cutaneous gas exchange. There is, in fact, no remnant of the amphibian pulmocutaneous circuit in reptiles. The skin is supplied by intersegmental arteries. Although some distinction must be made for the crocodilian reptiles, the remarks apply generally to the whole class.

At the start, a phenomenon equally apparent in amphibians (Johansen et al,, 1970) but not taken up in that section concerns the temporal relations of pressure development and flow in the pulmonary artery and aortic arches of reptiles. The rise of pressure in the pulmonary artery precedes that in the systemic arches, the peak flow occurs almost 0.2 sec before ejection begins into the aortas (White, 1976). (See Fig. 5.) Hence, the first blood to leave the ventricle is delivered to the lungs, and only subsequently is there ejection into the systemic circuit. This sequence creates the functional behavior of two ventricles. During air breathing the pressure in the pulmonary artery and its calculated resistance are both lower than in the systemic circulation. The low afterload imposed on the ventricle by the low-resistance pulmonary circuit

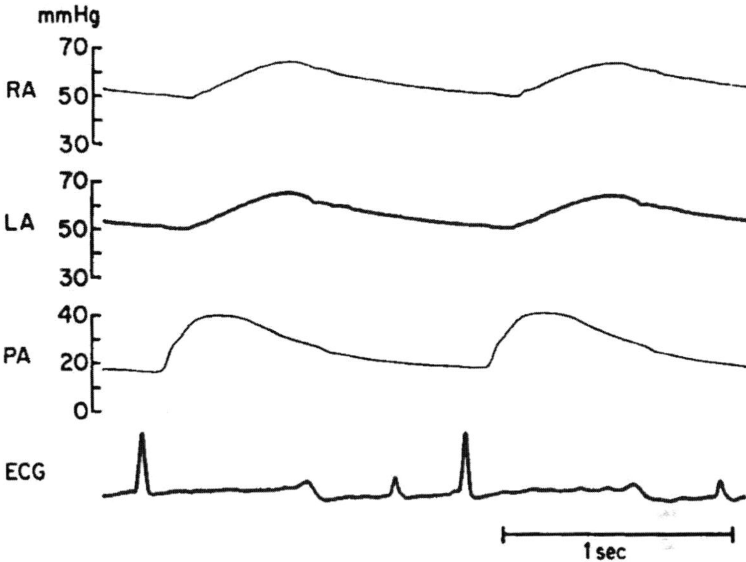

Figure 5 Pressure pulses recorded in an anesthetized iguana. RA, right aortic arch; LA, left aortic arch; PA, pulmonary artery. Bottom trace is electrocardiogram (ECG). Note early rise in pulmonary arterial pressure. (Reproduced from White, 1968.)

favors higher initial velocities of ejection, higher dP/dt, and there is consequently an effective left-to-right shunt of blood. When breathing is arrested, as in a dive, the situation changes, principally because pulmonary vascular resistance increases. That event and the associated phenomena have been well documented, as in the following.

In a study of unanesthetized turtles, White and Ross (1966) recorded pressures in the pulmonary artery that were lower than in the systemic circuit, and 60% of the cardiac output was delivered to the lung. Those predive values changed abruptly with diving, at which time systemic vascular resistance fell, pulmonary vascular resistance rose, a bradycardia developed, and the cardiac output shrank to 5% of its predive value (see Fig. 6). Blood flow shifted away from the lungs and to the systemic circuit; in effect, diving converted a left-to-right shunt to a right-to-left shunt.

The nature of pulmonary vascular resistance in the reptilian lung, and its control, require close examination of its major components and a brief consideration of the mechanical properties of the pulmonary circuit (Burggren, 1977). The common pulmonary artery and proximal extrinsic arteries are almost devoid of smooth muscle, the wall being made up largely of elastic fibers. Consequently,

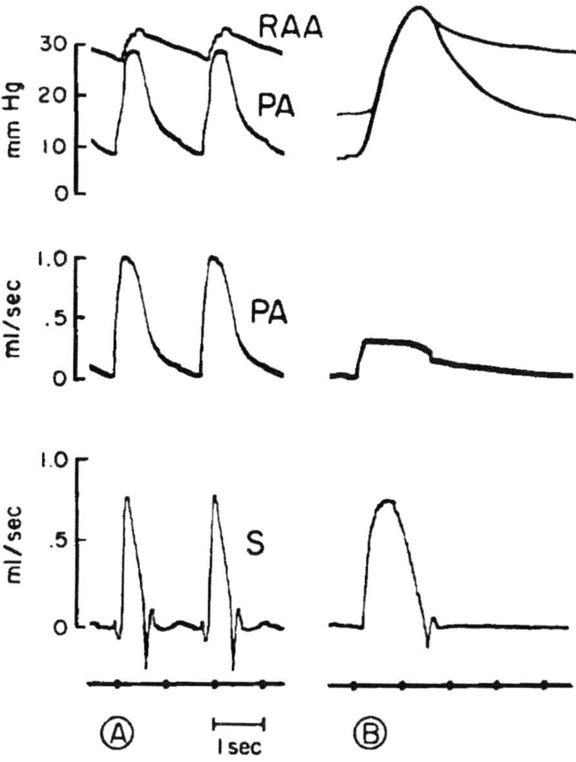

Figure 6 Pressures and flows in an unanesthetized turtle. RAA, right aortic arch; PA, pulmonary artery; S, subclavian artery. Traces in left-hand array were taken during breathing of room air; those in right-hand array were made during diving bradycardia. (Reproduced with permission from White and Ross, 1966.)

these vessels are highly compliant and cannot be expected to show much active development of wall tension. The distal pulmonary arteries, on the contrary, are much less distensible, and their walls are highly muscular. The major regulation of resistance must reside at this site. However, there is a complex interrelationship between the proximal and distal vessels, the former serving as a vascular reservoir that functions as a windkessel that maintains flow in diastole by virtue of the energy stored in its walls during systole (Burggren, 1977), and the latter constituting a component in the total resistance for pulmonary blood flow.

These distal pulmonary arteries constrict under the influence of acetylcholine or vagal stimulation. They are unresponsive to epinephrine, but if the bed is constricted under parasympathetic influence, then the administration of epinephrine has a relaxing effect. There is a demonstrable adrenergic innervation (McLean and Burnstock, 1967).

Although vascular resistance in the lung is regulated, in part, by this usual scheme of contraction and relaxation of vascular smooth muscle, an important mechanism regulating pulmonary blood flow is located at the pulmonary outflow tract, and its function is based on two distinct groups of musculature. Vascular smooth muscle lining the tract under the bulbus cordis undergoes changes of tone that influence the diameter of the outflow tract and, therefore, inflow resistance to the pulmonary circuit; but the bulbus cordis itself undergoes a contraction-relaxation cycle with each systole, exerting a transient effect on inflow resistance in phase with myocardial contraction. These two muscular components in the outflow tract regulate filling of the slightly more distal elastic reservoir and also constitute a resistance in series with that of the distal pulmonary vasculature. Whether resistance of the outflow tract increases in apnea and contributes to the redistribution of blood flow to the systemic circuit is controversial (Burggren, 1977), but it is probable that for the response to occur there must be a period of prolonged apnea. Mechanoreceptors are located in the bulbus cordis and the proximal pulmonary artery of the pond turtle (Faraci et al., 1982).

Considering all components together in an integrated system, the chelonian pulmonary circulation appears to be under close control, with participation of muscular units in the outflow tract and in the distal pulmonary arteries, with an intervening passive elastic blood reservoir. The muscles are all excited by parasympathetic influence and, in a tonically contracted state, are subject to dilatory action of adrenergic influences.

The parasympathetic mechanisms for these changes that induce a right-to-left shunt were first elucidated in a classic study of amphibian and reptilian pulmonary vascular control by Luckhardt and Carlson (1921), who demonstrated in both frogs and turtles that sectioning the vagus led to dilatation of the pulmonary artery. Stimulating the vagus caused constriction of the pulmonary artery, as did the administration of histamine or pituitary extract. Cutting the sympathetics in the turtle had no effect on the pulmonary artery, but epinephrine relaxed it. Constriction could also be induced by irritating the nares or stimulating the sciatic nerve.

In general, there is common agreement that cholinergic innervation is excitatory to pulmonary vascular smooth muscle and that adrenergic actions are either weakly inhibitory (as in lizards) or may not exist (in tortoises) (Berger, 1972).

There appears to be some comparative difference between terrestrial and aquatic chelonian reptiles, the former generating a substantially higher pulmonary artery pressure, but in both species under the influence of 5% O_2 in inspired air there was an increase of ventilation and pulmonary blood flow but a decrease of the ventilation/perfusion ratio (Burggren et al., 1977). Pulmonary arterial pressure rose only slightly, indicating a fall in resistance.

Crocodilian reptiles are the first vertebrates that do not have a right-to-left communication in the heart, and they have the mammalian characteristics of a low pulmonary and high systemic blood pressure. In spite of a complete anatomical separation of both atria and ventricles, the crocodilians retain the capacity to distribute the cardiac output preferentially to either the pulmonary or systemic circuit by virtue of a shunt between the two aortas, which bypasses the pulmonary circulation. In normal breathing, systemic pressure is high, the entire right ventricular output flows through the lung, and right and left ventricular outputs are equivalent. However, during apnea, pulmonary vascular resistance rises and so too does right ventricular pressure, the result being a diversion of right ventricular output to the left aorta and a shunt flow around the lung. To a possibly greater extent than in the chelonians, an important controller function is served by activity of the muscular band at the junction of the ventricular outflow tract and the pulmonary artery (White, 1969). The contribution of this site to the hindrance of pulmonary flow that occurs with apena in a diving alligator is apparent from the appearance of a striking increase in the pressure difference between the right ventricle and the pulmonary artery, a phenomenon equally apparent with the right ventricular hypertension brought about by hypoxia (Fig. 7). Analysis of the pattern of "runoff" during diastole confirms the difference in location of the resistance change in chelonian and crocodilian reptiles, but in both instances the efferent control remains via the vagus and nitrogen breathing intensifies the response. The effect of the constriction on flow distribution is likewise the same in both: the creation of a right-to-left shunt.

There is a curious and provocative finding related to the spread of the electrical impulse through the reptilian heart. The last region of the myocardium to be depolarized is at the base of the pulmonary artery (White, 1968; Burggren, 1978) and is presumably near, or at, the muscular band that is so important in the regulation of pulmonary blood flow. The spread of the wave of ventricular depolarization is from left to right at a velocity of 0.15 m/sec in apneic turtles, but during breathing the spread is from right to left at a velocity of 0.09 m/sec. Although the reptilian ventricle, like the mammalian ventricle, is said to be devoid of parasympathetic innervation, vagal stimulation shifts the pattern from the apneic to the breathing type (Burggren, 1978). The effect may be due to vagal endings in the conduction pathway, but it is not clear what unique contribution the activity of the muscular band in the outflow tract makes to the ECG contour when parasympathetic influence is introduced, nor is it obvious what the mechanical consequences of the different patterns of electrical activation would be.

The problem of "wet lung" in reptiles was introduced by Burggren (1982), who showed that red blood cell concentration in pulmonary venous

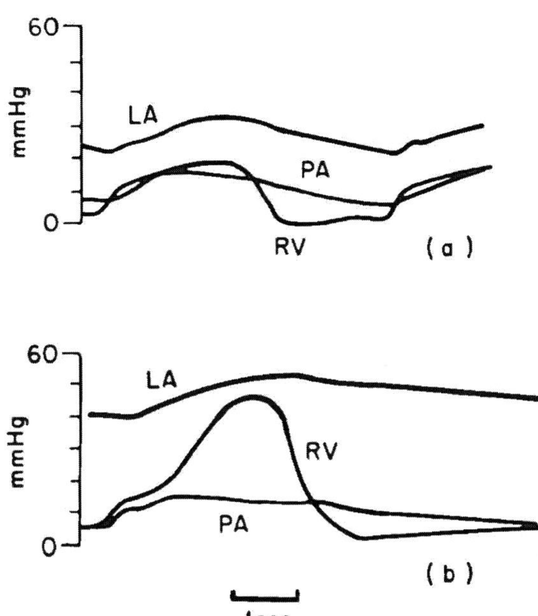

Figure 7 Pressures recorded in an unanesthetized alligator. LA, left aortic arch; PA, pulmonary artery; RV, right ventricle. Top trace (a) was made during air breathing; bottom trace (b) was made after 5 min exposure to N_2. Note rise of RV pressure when anoxic and large pressure drop from RV to PA. (Reproduced with permission from White, 1969.)

blood of turtles was 10-40% higher than in a sample taken from the pulmonary artery, from which it can be inferred that there has been a net loss of fluid from the vascular space into the lung. When the turtle is breathing, that loss is 10-20 times what is normally found in a mammalian lung. During the apneic period the fluid is reabsorbed, owing to the fact that pulmonary blood flow and pulmonary artery pressure are reduced at that time. The efflux of fluid seems to be more dependent on pulmonary blood flow than on pulmonary artery pressure, but in either case the need for precapillary mechanisms to regulate resistance is apparent.

V. Mammals

Pulmonary vasomotor reactivity in mammals was known in the last century, but the 1946 publication of von Euler and Liljestrand reporting on the vasoconstrictive action of hypoxia in cats also advanced the idea that this response, when local, would have the important effect of normalizing *regional* ventilation/perfusion ratio distributions throughout the lung. This is an attractive proposition and has received wide currency, seemingly satisfying the need to find some underlying "purposefulness," but it fails utterly to come to grips with the problems created by the increase of pulmonary vascular resistance *throughout* the lung when there is alveolar hypoxia.

On the premise that natural selection tends to eliminate features in a living system that are unfavorable for survival, the most reasonable prediction would be that hypoxic pulmonary vasoconstriction should no longer be apparent in mammals unless it represents a residual response that served a useful purpose at one time but is yet to be discarded. Of course, the implied question is rhetorical, and the answer has been fully anticipated by all of the preceding discussion: The mammalian fetus lives in a watery environment and, being unable to use its lungs for gas exchange, has little use for perfusing them; the immature circulatory design includes shunt pathways that make pulmonary bypass possible. The remarkable similarity of response to PO_2 by the ductus arteriosus of lungfish (Fishman et al., 1985) and the ductus arteriosus of the human fetus (Oberhansli-Weiss, et al., 1972) – relax with hypoxia, constrict with hyperoxia – which serves the same useful purpose in each case, is a fine instance of carry-through on a wide evolutionary scale. It is often said that the respiratory system is a poor choice in defense of the dictum that ontogeny recapitulates phylogeny, but this example belies that reservation.

The questions that must be asked next concern whether there is evidence for some loss of pulmonary vascular reactivity with maturation and aging – to suggest discarding a once useful but now useless phenomenon – and also whether animals living naturally in a hypoxic environment (high altitude) have less pulmonary vascular reactivity to PO_2 than do normal sea-level residents – to suggest improved fitness for survival by selecting those species that react least to a stimulus that evokes an adverse response. These problems are amenable to the approach of comparative mammalian respiratory physiology.

As for the developmental aspect, it is well known that newborns and young children characteristically have a more pronounced pulmonary vasoconstrictor response than do adults (Dawes, 1968), but the rabbit may be exceptional in that the newborn of this species has no hypertensive response to hypoxia, and the adult only a weak one (Owen-Thomas and Reeves, 1969). What exactly accounts for these changes in reactivity might be identified more readily if the fundamental mechanisms responsible for the vascular smooth muscle response to PO_2 were better known.

A provocative case arises with the marsupials, because they have only the briefest intrauterine life and must at a very early stage of their development depend on breathing for their oxygen supply. The North American opossum spends only 13 days in the womb and must start pulmonary ventilation with a primitive lung and minimal control apparatus (Farber et al., 1972) in a pouch environment that is mildly asphyxic (Farber and Tenney, 1971). There is virtually no need for the developing opossum to bypass the lung [the embryo has no foramen ovale, and the interatrial perforations are nearly obliterated at birth (McCrady, 1938); a 5-day-old newborn opossum dissected by J. P. Farber and W. W. Ballard (personal communication) showed no evidence of a ductus arteriosus, nor can I find any mention of a ductus arteriosus in the literature on the anatomy of the opossum] – indeed, there is almost immediately, at a very early stage of development, an urgent need to supply the lung generously with blood. It would be a reasonable conjecture, therefore, that marsupials have little or no pulmonary vasoconstrictor response to hypoxia. As far as I am aware, no experiment has been performed to test this possibility, but the result would be instructive.

Diving mammals present a different question of adaptation, one related to asphyxic state that prevails with prolonged apnea. The diving response, which includes bradycardia (wholly vagal in origin) and a much reduced cardiac output, would undoubtedly lead to a low pulmonary arterial pressure even if there were some pulmonary vasoconstriction, but the question of the reactivity of these vessels to hypoxia remains of interest. Nonetheless, I find no study of this subject. A similar question arises with fossorial mammals, because they too spend a good deal of time in a mildly asphyxic environment but without the apneic factor of diving mammals. The limited evidence available is divided on the point of whether there is an environmental influence. The ferret is a brisk responder, but the hamster (Walker et al., 1982) is weak.

Both vagal stimulation and acetylcholine have a relaxing effect on pulmonary vessels (Nandiwada et al., 1983), and sympathetic stimulation is mildly constrictor (Daly and Daly, 1959; Daly et al., 1975), although the greater effect of sympathetic stimulation is to stiffen the vessel wall (Ingram et al., 1968). There is morphological evidence for autonomic innervation throughout the pulmonary vascular bed, but these influences are predominatly on the small muscular arteries. Autonomic stimuli are distinctly opposite in their effects from those found in cold-blooded vertebrates [it should be noted that stimulation of vagal efferents may exert a weak constrictor action if the vessel wall has no tone (Nandiwada et al. 1983)] and, in fact, the neuroreflex control of the mammalian pulmonary vascular resistance in mammals is subsidiary to chemical and humoral agents that seem to act locally. A trivial parasympathetic influence is expected due to the well-known evolutionary trend of cardiovascular control away from cholinergic systems (Bagshaw, 1985), but the usual shift is toward a greater influence of adrenergic systems, which is not the case for the pulmonary circulation. The turnabout of parasympathetic effect in

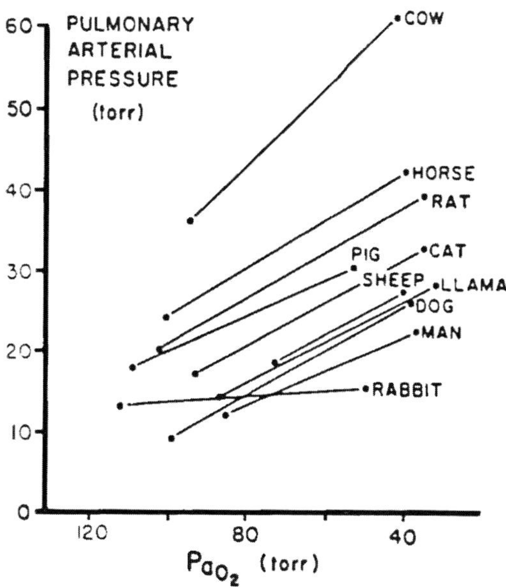

Figure 8 Interspecific differences in pulmonary arterial pressor responses to *acute* alveolar hypoxia in a group of mammals. Reproduced with permission from Reeves et al., 1979.

mammals from that in all premammalian vertebrates is a puzzling change, although the absence in mammals of a muscular mechanism in the right ventricular outflow tract that functions like the truncus arteriosus is significant.

The circulatory phenomena associated with the breathing cycle also merit comment. In premammalian vertebrates, the act of breathing increases heart rate and cardiac output and decreases pulmonary vascular resistance, all dependent on vagal afferents; in mammals, breathing quickens the heart rate and increases cardiac output, but the effect on pulmonary vascular resistance is scarcely noticeable. There is no need to manipulate pulmonary vascular resistance, since, in the absence of a shunt circuit, the lung must receive the entire cardiac output. Vagal afferents continue to play a role in mammals as in their ancestors, operating chiefly when excited in inspiration to participate with the mechanisms causing sinus arrhythmia and increasing the heart rate in that phase of the respiratory cycle. Slowing of the heart rate with each expiration is akin to the bradycardia associated with diving apnea in this view.

The interspecific variation in the pulmonary hypertensive response of mammals to *acute hypoxia* is not great (Reeves et al., 1979), although the rabbit is a notorious nonresponder (see Fig. 8). In a study employing isolated lungs, the dog showed no response; rabbits and cats, an intermediate response; and the ferret and pig, the largest response (Peake et al., 1981).

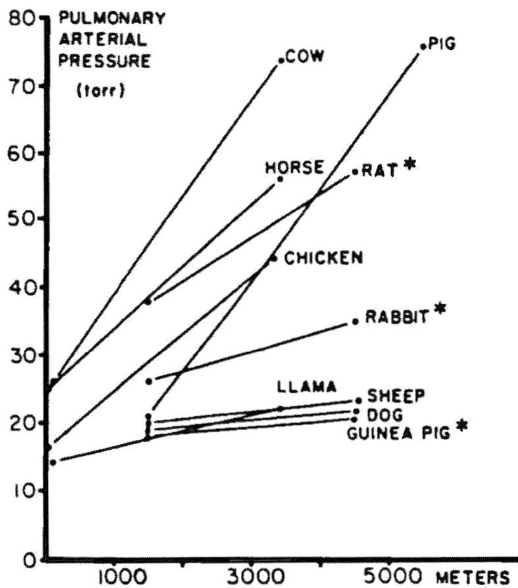

Figure 9 Interspecific differences in pulmonary pressor responses to chronic residence at high altitude. (Reproduced with permission from Reeves et al., 1979.)

It is plausible hypothesis that the chronic response ought to be at least in those species that have had a long evolutionary history at high altitude and have adapted to *chronic hypoxia* (see Fig. 9) for many generations. Much effort has been devoted by the group at the University of Colorado to documenting such a distinction (e.g., Reeves et al. 1979), and the pattern that emerges is strongly suggestive, although other factors [such as age and sex (Moore et al., 1978; McMurtry et al., 1973)] sometimes complicate reaching a firm conclusion. However, there is clearly a more impressive separation of strong responders and weak responders under chronic than under acute conditions. The weak responders are guinea pig (Reeves et al., 1979), hamster (Walker et al., 1982), rabbit (Owen-Thomas and Reeves, 1969), dog (Vogel et al., 1971), sheep (Reeves et al., 1963), and llama (Branchero et al., 1971). The brisk responders are rat (Moore et al., 1978), cow (Will et al., 1975; Reeves et al., 1962; Ruiz et al., 1973), cat (Weidman et al., 1965), pig (McMurtry et al., 1973), and pony (Bisgard et al., 1975). In the former group, all but the dog are animals native to high altitude, and the dog acclimatizes well. The latter group are not normally resident at high altitudes and, in general, do not acclimatize well, but it is important to note that there may be significant strain differences within a species.

Animals normally resident at high altitudes – llama (Heath et al., 1968, 1974) and vizcacha (Heath et al., 1981) show the expected structural correlates of mild pulmonary hypertension: thin-walled pulmonary vessels and slight right ventricular hypertrophy. Species that normally reside at sea level and develop a severe pulmonary hypertension at high altitude, e.g. cattle, develop hypertrophy of vascular smooth muscle and the right ventricle (Heath et al., 1968; Weir et al., 1979). A comprehensive listing comparing many more species has been prepared by Tucker et al. (1975) and Kay (1983).

Cattle are in the more responsive group, and, at high altitude, severe pulmonary hypertension is a feature of brisket disease. This disabling syndrome is a serious threat for high-altitude grazing, and the economic incentive spurred breeding of a resistant stock. The availability of closely related animals with quantitatively different responses to hypoxia is a boon that complements the opportunity provided by interspecific differences in the search for mechanisms. A similar example of strain differences is to be found in the Madison and Hilltop strains of Sprague-Dawley rats studied by Ou et al. (1986). Although a correspondence in magnitude of acute and chronic response to hypoxia would seem highly probable – a prediction confirmed in cattle (Will et al., 1975) – the aforementioned rat strains demonstrate just the opposite, which leads, in that instance, to the conclusion that chronic hypoxia in resistant animals (those that acclimatize well) evokes an inhibitory response (probably humoral) that causes relaxation of vascular smooth muscle and "blunts" the acute vasoconstriction. The magnitude of the pulmonary hypertension is thus reduced from that measured in the early phase of hypoxic exposure; the susceptible animals, on the contrary, continue to develop an increasing pulmonary hypertension as the hypoxic exposure is prolonged.

An imaginative hypothesis advanced to account for species differences in the pulmonary vascular response to hypoxia is based on the observation that there are associated differences in collateral ventilation (Kuriyama and Wagner, 1981). Cattle and swine are brisk responders and have no collateral ventilation; dogs and sheep are weak responders and have an extensive collateral ventilation. The idea is that the collaterals serve to maintain an even distribution of PO_2 throughout the lung and thus tend to reduce the intense vasoconstriction that would normally occur in regions of very low ventilation.

Although it is not the purpose of this chapter to analyze the evidence for and against the postulated mechanisms that participate in the regulation of the pulmonary circulation, some of the comparative features call attention to directions for study. Interspecific structural correlates are significant. An anatomical finding likely to be directly related to vascular reactivity is the amount of smooth muscle in the pulmonary vessels (Kay, 1983). There is a significant correlation between the amount of smooth muscle in the small pulmonary arteries and arterioles and the pulmonary hypertensive response to hypoxia (Tucker et al., 1975; Peake et al., 1981). This is a reasonable and intuitively satisfying relationship, but it is not a comprehensive answer. The pig, a sea-level animal, has a thick, muscular pulmonary artery and is a brisk responder to hypoxia, while the vizcacha (Heath et al., 1981) and the llama (Heath et al.,

1968), both native dwellers at high altitude, are not very responsive, and their pulmonary arteries are thin-walled. This is the expected pattern, but that tidy consistency is shattered by the ferret, which has a pronounced vasoconstrictive response to hypoxia but thin-walled pulmonary arteries (Kay, 1983).

Of course, muscular thickening in the vessel walls of a species maintained at high altitude will be the expected response to prolonged pulmonary hypertension, and indeed, sea-level animals studied after a prolonged period at high altitude invariably have more muscular pulmonary arteries than are found in the same species at sea level, a finding of no help in the search for mechanism, because it puts cause and effect in the wrong order.

The intensive search for transmitter and other humoral agents active in promoting constriction or relaxation of pulmonary vascular smooth muscle continues without resolution, although the list of possibly contributing mechanisms has grown steadily. This aspect of control of the pulmonary circulation has been thoroughly reviewed in recent publications (Fishman, 1984; Grover et al., 1985) and chapters in the present volume. The comparative approach to elucidating cellular and humoral mechanisms involved in pulmonary vascular control has yet to receive much attention.

VI. Birds

The structure of the lungs of birds is so different from that of mammals, and cardiovascular control so little studied in comparison, that little further contribution can be made by this class of vertebrates to the theme developed so far. The cardiovascular circuitry is, as in mammals, a series arrangement, and therefore general increases in pulmonary vascular resistance would lead to consequences similar to those in mammals. The diving response in birds appears in most respects to resemble the mammalian response (Johansen and Aakhus, 1963; Langille and Jones, 1975), but the pulmonary hemodynamic response has not been fully reported, although Johansen and Aakhus (1963) quote the work of Eliasson (1960), who recorded a rise in the pulmonary artery pressure of ducks during a dive.

The unique aspect of avian environmental stress is the requirement to fly at high altitudes and, in some species, at extreme altitudes. Although most of the time is not spent at extreme elevations, the breeding grounds of many species are fairly high, and the ability to sustain high oxygen demands during migration, which, in the case of the bar-headed goose, may be at altitudes over 30,000 ft, puts an extraordinary demand on the cardiorespiratory system. There can be little doubt that, as with mammals, there are important interspecific characteristics that make possible such remarkable performance in hypobaric hypoxia. The chicken is not well adapted to life at high altitudes; this species is known to develop pulmonary hypertension, right ventricular hypertrophy, and right heart failure (Burton et al., 1968; Cueva et al., 1974; Sillau et al., 1980). On the other hand, the bar-headed goose develops very little rise in right ventricular (Black and Tenney, 1980a) or pulmonary artery pressure (Faraci et al., 1984; Faraci and Fedde, 1986) in comparison with ducks exposed to a comparable degree of hypoxia. The fact that the rise in pressure is nearly proportional with the rise in cardiac output (Black and Tenney, 1980b) suggests that there has been little or no change in pulmonary vascular resistance in this species. On the other hand, an increase in the pulmonary vascular resistance in ducks has been inferred from the decrease in flow to one lung if it is made hypoxic (Holle et al., 1976) and from the increase in transit time through the lungs in asphyxia (Johansen and Aakhus, 1963).

VII. Epilogue and Recapitulation

The strategy of comparative physiology points up similarities in differences and differences in similarities that lead to an overview illuminated by highlights, but less often to revelation of a fundamental mechanism. Such is the weakness, but such too is the merit of a phylogenetic "story" whose theme is discovered by touching briefly on a salient feature in each vertebrate class and deliberately avoiding detailed descriptions, even interspecific characteristics within a class, lest they serve more to distract than to contribute. The aim is to identify a unifying principle. Focusing on control of the pulmonary circulation, the unifying theme appears to be achievement of a proper balance between blood flow and air flow (or, more specifically, oxygen supply) in the lung. To that end a linked chain of operative mechanisms, stretching from early vertebrates to contemporary mammals, can be discerned.

In some ancient fishes, and in the lungfish living today, the lung is a respiratory organ accessory to the gills.

Depending on whether an air-breathing mode or a water-breathing mode offers the better oxygen supply, organisms endowed with bimodal gas-exchange systems have the potential for using the one that carries the greater advantage. However, the option of selectivity requires a parallel arrangement of the cardiovascular circuit design so that flow diverted from one region can be taken up by the other.

Pulmonary ventilation, probably by a stretch reflex, and high oxygen content of air or low oxygen content of water favor blood flow to the lungs by decreasing pulmonary vascular resistance and increasing the resistance in channels of shunt flow around the lung. These responses in lungfish are apparent in amphibians, where the bulbus cordis also regulates pulmonary inflow resistance, under vagal control and operating in concert with regulation of flow to the skin under control of the O_2 and CO_2 content of the aqueous environment. The PO_2 of lung air has a mild direct effect on pulmonary vascular resistance.

In reptiles the orifice of the outflow tract from the ventricle is under vagal control as in amphibians, and this region, together with pulmonary vascular resistance, controls pulmonary blood flow, to make proper adjustments during the apnea during diving, or if there is altered gaseous composition of the environment. There is no site serving as an alternative to the lungs for gas exchange, but the single ventricle continues the principle of parallel circuitry and, by regulating its contractile pattern, can bypass the lung.

Mammals are also restricted to their lungs as a site for gas exchange, and their cardiovascular design puts the lungs in series with the systemic circuit, except in the embryo and fetus. The dominant premammalian response depended on vagal influence, but in the mammal, hypoxia and CO_2 take on the dominant role and autonomic influences become minor.

In the mammalian fetus, hypoxic vascoconstriction serves the useful purpose of bypassing the nonventilated lungs in utero, shunt flow made possible by the ductus arteriosus and interatrial and interventricular windows.

In the mammalian adult, when the shunts have closed, the design leaves the lungs in series with the systemic circulation, and global pulmonary vasoconstriction (as with ambient hypoxia) must be considered maladaptive – a now useless residuum of the developmental and, ultimately, phylogenetic past. Regional pulmonary vasoconstriction, on the other hand, is still an advantageous response in normalizing ventilation/perfusion ratio distribution in the lung.

The disadvantage of global vasoconstriction to hypoxia is apparent in the broad biological context of evolution. Resident species at high altitude have less pulmonary vasoconstrictor response to chronic hypoxia than do sea-level native species.

References

Bagshaw, R. M. (1985). Evolution of cardiovascular baroreceptor control. *Biol. Rev. 60*:121-162.

Banchero, N., Grover, R. F., and Will, J. A. (1971). Altitude-induced pulmonary arterial hypertension in the llama (*Llama glama*). *Am. J. Physiol. 220*: 422-427.

Bastert, C. (1929). Uber die Regulierung des Sauerstoff-verbranches aus der Lunge der Froshe. *Z. vergleich. Physiol. 9*:212-258.

Berger, P. J. (1972). The vagal and sympathetic innervation of the isolated pulmonary artery of a lizard and a tortoise. *Comp. Gen. Pharmacol. 3*:113-124.

Bisgard, G. E., Orr, J. A., and Will, J. A. (1975). Hypoxic pulmonary hypertension in the pony. *Am. J. Vet. Res. 36*:49-52.

Black, C. P., and Tenney, S. M. (1980a). Pulmonary hemodynamic responses to acute and chronic hypoxia in two waterfowl species. *Comp. Biochem. Physiol. 67A*:291-293.

Black, C. P., and Tenney, S. M. (1980b). Oxygen transport during progressive hypoxia in high altitude and sea level waterfowl. *Resp. Physiol. 39*:217-239.

Boutilier, R. G., Glass, M. L., and Heisler, N. (1986). The relative distribution of pulmocutaneous blood flow in *Rana catesbeiana*: effect of pulmonary or cutaneous hypoxia. *J. Exp. Biol. 126*:33-40.

Burggren, W. (1977). The pulmonary circulation of the chelonian reptile: morphology, hemodynamics and pharmacology. *J. Comp. Physiol. 116*:303-323.

Burggren, W. W. (1978). Influence of intermittent breathing on ventricular depolarization patterns in chelonian reptiles. *J. Physiol. (Lond.) 278*:349-364.

Burggren, W. W. (1982). Pulmonary blood plasma filtration in reptiles: a "wet" vertebrate lung? *Science 215*:77-78.

Burggren, W. W., Glass, M. L., and Johansen, K. (1977). Pulmonary ventilation: perfusion relationships in terrestrial and aquatic chelonian reptiles. *Can. J. Zool. 55*:2024-2034.

Burton, R. R., Besch, E. L., and Smith, A. H. (1968). Effect of chronic hypoxia on the pulmonary arterial blood pressure of the chicken. *Am. J. Physiol. 214*:1438-1442.

Cueva, S., Sillow, H., Valenzuela, A., and Plooz, H. (1974). High altitude-induced pulmonary hypertension and right heart failure in broiler chickens. *Res. Vet. Sci. 16*:370-374.

Daly, I. deB., and Daly, M. deB. (1959). The effects of stimulation of the carotid body chemoreceptors on the pulmonary vascular bed in the dog: the vasosensory controlled perfused living animal preparation. *J. Physiol. (Lond.) 148*:201-219.

Daly, I. deB., Ramsay, D. J., and Waaler, B. A. (1975). Pulmonary vasomotor responses in isolated perfused lungs of *Macaca mulatta* and *Papio* species. *J. Physiol. (Lond.) 250*:463-473.

Das, S. M., and Saxena, D. (1958). Stages of transition in the afferent branchial arteries from fish to amphibian stage: a case of parallel evolution. *Proc. Natl. Acad. Sci. (India) 28(B)*:108-115.

Dawes, G. S. (1968). *Fetal and Neonatal Physiology*. Year Book Publishers, Chicago.

Delaney, R. G., Lahiri, S., and Fishman, A. P. (1974). Aestivation of the African lungfish, *Protopterus aethiopicus*: cardiovascular and respiratory functions. *J. Exp. Biol. 61*:111-128.

DeSaint-Aubain, M. L., and Wingstrand, K. (1979). A sphincter in the pulmonary artery of the frog *Rana temporaria* and its influence on blood flow in skin and lungs. *Acta Zool. (Stockh.) 60*:163-172.

Eliassen, E. (1960). *Arbok for universitetet i Bergen*. Mat.-Naturo. Serie No. 2. Norwegian Univ. Press, Bergen, Oslo

Emilio, M. G., and Shelton, G. (1972). Factors affecting blood flow to the lungs in the amphibian *Xenopis laevis. J. Exp. Biol. 56*:67-77.

Euler, U. S. von, and Liljestrand, G. (1946). Observations on the pulmonary arterial pressure in the cat. *Acta Physiol. Scand. 12*:301-320.

Faraci, F. M., and Fedde, M. R. (1986). Regional circulatory responses to hypocapnia and hypercapnia in bar-headed geese. *Am. J. Physiol. 250*:R499-R504.

Faraci, F. M., Shirer, H. W., Orr, J. A., and Trank, J. W. (1982). Circulatory mechanoreceptors in the pond turtle *Pseudomys scriptans. Am. J. Physiol. 242*:R216-R219.

Faraci, F. M., Kilgore, D. L., Jr., and Fedde, M. R. (1984). Attenuated pulmonary pressor response to hypoxia in bar-headed geese. *Am. J. Physiol. 247*: R402-R403.

Farber, J. P., and Tenney, S. M. (1971). The pouch gas of the Virginia opossum (*Didelphis virginiana*). *Resp. Physiol. 11*:335-345.

Farber, J. P., Hultgren, H. N., and Tenney, S. M. (1972). Development of the chemical control of breathing in the Virginia opossum. *Resp. Physiol. 14*: 267-277.

Feder, M. E., and Burggren, W. M. (1985). Cutaneous gas exchange in vertebrates: design, pattern, control and implications. *Biol. Rev. 60*:1-45.

Fishman, A. P. (1985). Pulmonary circulation. In *The Handbook of Physiology.* Sect. 3, *The Respiratory System*. Vol. I. Edited by A. P. Fishman and A. B. Fisher. American Physiological Society, Bethesda, MD, Chap. 3, pp. 93-166.

Fishman, A. P., Delaney, R. G., and Laurent, P. (1985). Circulatory adaptation to bimodal respiration in the dipnoan lungfish. *J. Appl. Physiol. 59*:285-294.

Goodrich, E. S. (1930). *Studies on Structure and Development of Vertebrates.* MacMillan, London.

Grover, R. F., Wagner, W. W., Jr., McMurtry, E. F., and Reeves, J. T. (1983). Pulmonary circulation. In *The Handbook of Physiology.* Sect. 2, *The Cardiovascular System*. Vol. III. Edited by J. T. Shepherd and F. M. Abboud. American Physiological Society, Bethesda, MD., pp. 103-136.

Heath, D., Harris, P., Castillo, Y., Aries-Stella, J. (1968). Histology, distensibility and chemical composition of the pulmonary trunk of dogs, sheep cattle and llamas living at high altitude. *J. Pathol. Bacteriol. 96*:161-167.

Heath, D., Smith, P., Williams, D., Harris, P., Arias-Stella, J., and Kruger, H. (1974). The heart and pulmonary vasculature of the llama (*Llama glama*). *Thorax 29*:462-471.

Heath, D., Williams, D., Harris, P., Smith, P., Kruger, H., and Ramiriz, A. (1981). The pulmonary vasculature of the mountain vizcacha (*Lagidium peruanum*). The concept of acclimatized and adapted vascular smooth muscle. *J. Comp. Pathol. 91*:293-301.

Hoffman, A., and Cordeiro de Sousa, M. B. (182). Cardiovascular reflexes in conscious toads. *J. Auton. Nerv. Syst. 5*:345-355.

Holle, J. P., Heisler, N., Scheid, P., (1976). Effects of O_2 and CO_2 on regional pulmonary blood flow in ducks. *Pfleugers Arch. 365* (suppl.):R20.

Ingram, R. H., Szidon, J. F., Skalak, R., and Fishman, A. P. (1968). Effects of sympathetic nerve stimulation of the pulmonary arterial tree of the isolated lobe perfused in situ. *Circ. Res. 22*:801-815.

Ishii, K., and Ishii, K. (1978). A reflexogenic area for controlling blood pressure in the toad. *Jap. J. Physiol. 28*:423-431.

Jackson, D. C., and Braun, B. A. (1979). Respiratory control in the bullfrog: cutaneous vs. pulmonary response to CO_2 exposure. *J. Comp. Physiol. 129*:339-342.

Johansen, K. (1970). Air breathing in fishes. In *Fish Physiology*. Vol. IV. Edited by W. S. Hoar and D. J. Randall. Academic, New York, Chap. 9, pp. 361-441.

Johansen, K. (1982). Blood, circulation, and the rise of air breathing: passes and bypasses. In *A Companion to Animal Physiology*. Edited by C. R. Taylor, K. Johansen, and L. Bolis. Cambridge University Press, Cambridge, Chap. 7, pp. 91-105.

Johansen, K., and Aakhus, T. (1963). Central cardiovascular responses to submersion asphyxia in the duck. *Am. J. Physiol. 205*:1167-1171.

Johansen, K., and Hanson, D. (1968). Functional anatomy of the hearts of lung fishes and amphibians. *Am. Zool. 8*:191-210.

Johansen, K., and Hol, D. (1968). A radiological study of the central circulation in the African lungfish, *Protopterus aethiopicus. J. Morphol. 126*:333-348.

Johansen, K., Lenfant, C., and Grigg, G. C. (1967). Respiratory control in the lungfish, *Neoceratodus fosteri* (Krefft). *Comp. Biochem. Physiol. 20*:835-854.

Johansen, K., Lenfant, C., and Hanson, D. (1968). Cardiovascular dynamics in lungfishes. *Z. vergleich. Physiol. 59*:157-186.

Johansen, K., Lenfant, C., and Hanson, D. (1970). Phylogenetic development of pulmonary circulation. *Fed. Proc. 29*:1135-1140.

Kay, J. M. (1983). Comparative morphological features of pulmonary vasculature of mammals. *Am. Rev. Resp. Dis. 128*:S53-S57.

Koyama, T., and Morimoto, M. (1983). Blood flow reduction in local pulmonary microvessels during acute hypoxia imposed on a small fraction of the lung. Resp. Physiol. 52:181-189.

Krogh, A. (1904). On the cutaneous and pulmonary respiration of the frog. *Skand. Arch. f. Physiol. 15*:328-419.

Kuriyama, T., and Wagner, W. W., Jr. (1981). Collateral ventilation may protect against high altitude pulmonary hypertension. *J. Appl. Physiol. 51*:1251-1256.

Lahiri, S., Szidon, J. P., and Fishman, A. P. (1970). Potential respiratory and circulatory adjustments to hypoxia in the African lungfish. *Fed. Proc. 29*: 1141-1148.

Langille, B. L., and Jones, D. R. (1975). Central cardiovascular dynamics of ducks. *Am. J. Physiol. 228*:1856-1861.

Luckhardt, A. B., and Carlson, A. J. (1921). Studies on the visceral sensory nervous system. VIII. On the presence of vasomotor fibers in the vagus nerve to the pulmonary vessels of the amphibian and reptilian lung. *Am. J. Physiol. 56*:72-112.

McCrady, E. (1938). The embryology of the opossum. *Am. Anat. Mem.* No. 16.

McLean, J. R., and Burnstock, G. (1967). Innervation of the lungs of the sleepy lizard (*Trachysaurus rugosus*). I. Fluorescent histochemistry of catecholamines. *Comp. Biochem. Physiol. 22*:809-813.

McMurtry, J. F., Frith, C. H., and Will, D. H. (1973). Cardiopulmonary responses of male and female swine to simulated high altitude. *J. Appl. Physiol. 35*: 459-462.

Maloney, J. E., and Castle, B. L. (1970). Dynamic intravascular pressures in the microvessels of the frog lung. *Resp. Physiol. 10*:51-63.

Malvin, G. M. (1985a). Vascular resistance and vasoactivity of gills and pulmonary artery of the salamander, *Ambystoma tigrinum. J. Comp. Physiol. 155*: 241-249.

Malvin, G. M. (1985b). Adrenoceptor types in the respiratory vasculature of the salamander gill. *J. Comp. Physiol. 155*:591-596.

Malvin, G. M., and Dail, W. G. (186). Adrenergic innervation of the gills, pulmonary artery and dorsal aorta of a salamander, *Ambystoma tigrinum. J. Morphol. 189*:67-70.

Malvin, G. M., and Hlastala, M. P. (1986a). Regulation of cutaneous gas exchange by environmental oxygen and carbon dioxide in the frog. *Resp. Physiol. 65*:99-111.

Malvin, G. M., and Hlastala, M. P. (1986b). Effects of lung volume and O_2 and CO_2 content on cutaneous gas exchange in frogs. *Am. J. Physiol. 251*: R941-R946.

Moore, L. G., McMurtry, I. F., and Reeves, J. T. (1978). Effects of sex hormones on cardiovascular and hematologic responses to chronic hypoxia in rats. *Proc. Soc. Exp. Biol. Med. 158*:658-662.

Nandiwada, P. A., Hyman, A. L., and Kadowitz, P. J. (1983). Pulmonary vasodilator responses to vagal stimulation and acetylcholine in the cat. *Circ. Res. 53*:86-95.

Nicol, J. A. C. (1951). Autonomic nervous system in lower Chordates. *Biol. Rev. 21*:1-49.

Oberhansli-Weiss, I. M., Heymann, A., Rudolph, A. M., and Melmon, K. L. (1972). The pattern and mechanism of response to oxygen by the ductus arteriosus and umbilical artery. *Pediatr. Res. 6*:693-700.

Ou, L. C., Sardella, G. L., Hill, N. S., and Tenney, S. M. (1986). Acute and chronic pulmonary depressor responses to hypoxia: the role of blunting in acclimatization. *Resp. Physiol. 64*:81-91.

Owen-Thomas, J. B., and Reeves, T. J. (1969). Hypoxia and pulmonary arterial pressure in the rabbit. *J. Physiol. (Lond.) 201*:665-672.

Peake, M. D., Harabin, A. L., Brennan, N. J., and Sylvester, J. T. (1981). Steady-state vascular responses to graded hypoxia in isolated lungs of five species. *J. Appl. Physiol. 51*:1214-1219.

Poczopko, P. (1959). Changes in blood circulation in *Rana esculenta L.* while diving. *Zool. Polon. 10*:29-43.

Reeves, J. T., Grover, R. F., Will, D. H., and Alexander, A. F. (1962). Hemodynamics in normal cattle. *Circ. Res. 10*:166-170.

Reeves, J. T., Grover, E. G., and Grover, R. F. (1963). Pulmonary circulation and oxygen transport in lambs at high altitude. *J. Appl. Physiol. 18*: 560-566.

Reeves, J. T., Wagner, W. W., Jr., McMurtry, I. F., and Grover, R. F. (1979). Physiological effects of high altitude on the pulmonary circulation. In *International Review of Physiology. Environmental Physiology III.* Vol. 20. Edited by D. Robertshaw. University Park Press, Baltimore, Chap. 6, pp. 289-310.

Ruiz, A. V., Bisgard, G. E., and Will, J. A. (1973). Hemodynamic responses to hypoxia in calves at sea level and altitude. *Pfluegers Arch. 344*:275-286.

Shelton, G. (1970). The effect of lung ventilation on blood flow in the lungs and body of the amphibian, *Xenopus laevis. Resp. Physiol. 9*:183-196.

Shelton, G. (1976). Gas exchange, pulmonary blood supply, and the partially divided amphibian heart. In *Perspectives in Experimental Biology*. Vol. 1, *Zoology.* Edited by P. Spencer Davis. Pergamon, New York, pp. 247-259.

Shelton, G. (1986). Functional and evolutionary significance of cardiovascular shunts in the Amphibia. In *Cardio-Vascular Shunts*. Alfred Benzon Symposium 21. Edited by K. Johansen and W. W. Burggren. Munksgaard, Copenhagen, pp. 100-120.

Shelton, G., and Jones, D. R. (1965). Central blood pressure and heat output in surfaced and submerged frogs. *J. Exp. Biol. 42*:339-357.

Sillau, A. H., Cueva, S., and Morales, P. (1980). Pulmonary arterial hypertension in male and female chickens at 3300 m. *Pfleugers Arch. 386*: 269-275.

Smatresk, N. J., Burleson, M. L., and Azizi, S. Q. (1986). Chemoreflex responses to hypoxia and NaCN in longnose gar: Evidence for two chemoreceptor loci. *Am. J. Physiol. 251*:R116-R125.

Smith, D. G., and Campbell, G. (1976). The anatomy of the pulmonary vascular bed in the toad *Bufo marinus. Cell Tiss. Res. 165*:199-215.

Smits, A. W., West, N. H., and Burggren, W. W. (1986). Pulmonary fluid balance following pulmo-cutaneous baroreceptor denervation in the toad. *J. Appl. Physiol. 61*:331-337.

Tucker, A., McMurtry, I. F., Reeves, J. T., Alexander, A. F., Will, D. H., and Grover, R. F. (1975). Lung vascular smooth muscle as a determinant of pulmonary hypertension at high altitude. *Am. J. Physiol. 228*:762-767.

Vogel, J. A., Genovese, R. L., Powell, T. L., Bishop, G. W., Bucci, T. J., and Harris, C. W. (1971). Cardiac size and pulmonary hypertension in dogs exposed to high altitude. *Am. J. Vet. Res. 32*:2059-2065.

Walker, B. R., Voelkel, N. F., McMurtry, I. F., and Adams, E. M. (1982). Evidence for diminished sensitivity of the hamster pulmonary vasculature to hypoxia. *J. Appl. Physiol. 52*:1571-1574.

Weidman, W. H., Titus, J. L., and Shepherd, J. T. (1965). Effect of chronic hypoxia on the pulmonary circulation of cats. *Proc. Soc. Exp. Biol. Med. 118*:1158-1164.

Weir, E. K., Will, D. H., Alexander, A. F., McMurtry, I. F., Looga, R., Reeves, J. T., and Grover, R. F. (1979). Vascular hypertrophy in cattle susceptible to hypoxic pulmonary hypertension. *J. Appl. Physiol. 46*:517-521.

West, N. H., and Burggren, W. W. (1984). Factors influencing pulmonary and cutaneous arterial blood flow in the toad *Bufo marinus*. *Am. J. Physiol. 247*:R884-R894.

West, N. H., and Van Vliet, B. N. (1983). Open-loop analysis of the pulmocutaneous reflex in the toad *Bufo marinus*. *Am. J. Physiol. 245*:R642-R650.

White, F. N. (1968). Functional anatomy of the heart of reptiles. *Am. Zool. 8*: 211-219.

White, F. N. (1969). Redistribution of cardiac output in the diving alligator. *Copeia 1969*(3):567-570.

White, F. N. (1976). Circulation. In *Biology of the Reptilia*. Vol. 5. Edited by C. Gans and W. R. Dawson, Academic Press, New York, Chap. 5, pp. 275-334.

White, F. N., and Ross, G. (1966). Circulatory changes during experimental diving in the turtle. *Am. J. Physiol. 211*:15-18.

Will, D. H., Hicks, J. L., Card, C. S., Reeves, J. T., and Alexander, A. F. (1975). Correlation of acute with chronic hypoxic pulmonary hypertension in cattle. *J. Appl. Physiol. 38*:495-498.

2

Control of Fetal and Neonatal Pulmonary Circulation

MICHAEL A. HEYMANN and SCOTT J. SOIFER

University of California, San Francisco
San Francisco, California

I. Introduction

A. Fetal Pulmonary Circulation

In the fetus, O_2 and CO_2 exchange occur in the placenta, and pulmonary blood flow therefore is quite low, supplying only some of the nutritional requirements for lung growth and perhaps, as in the adult, serving some metabolic or "para-endocrine" function. Pulmonary blood flow in undisturbed, near-term fetal lambs (term is about 145 days gestation) is about 100 ml/min per 100 g lung tissue (Clozel et al., 1985; Soifer et al., 1985; LeBidois et al., 1987), representing between 8 and 10% of the total (combined left and right ventricular) output of the heart (Heymann et al., 1973; Rudolph and Heymann, 1967, 1970). This low pulmonary flow occurs despite the dominance of the right ventricle, which in the fetus ejects about two-thirds of the total cardiac output of 450-500 ml/min per kilogram (Heymann et al., 1973) and is brought about by the high fetal pulmonary vascular resistance. Most of the flow from the right ventricle thus is diverted away from the lungs, through the widely patent ductus arteriosus, to the descending thoracic aorta from which the major proportion (about 45% of total cardiac output) reaches the placenta for gas exchange. In the younger fetus (at about 0.5 of gestation) only about 3-4% of total cardiac output passes through the lungs; there is an increase to about 6% at about 0.8 gestation, corresponding temporally with the onset of the release of surface-active material into lung fluid, with a further progressive slow rise thereafter to about 8-10% near term (Rudolph and Heymann, 1970). Fetal pulmonary arterial blood pressure increases progressively with advancing gestation; at term, mean pulmonary arterial blood pressure is about 50 mmHg (Lewis et al., 1976) and this generally exceeds mean aortic blood pressure by about 1-2 mmHg (Heymann and Rudolph, 1976). Baseline or resting pulmonary vascular resistance, relative to that in the infant or adult, is extremely high early in gestation, probably due to the small number of vessels present. Pulmonary vascular resistance falls progressively over the last half of gestation (Rudolph, 1979), due most likely to rapid new vessel growth and a large increase in cross-sectional area (Levin et al., 1976; Reid, 1982); however, baseline pulmonary vascular resistance still is very much higher than in the adult.

B. Transitional Circulation

After birth and initiation of pulmonary ventilation, pulmonary vascular resistance falls rapidly, associated with an eight- to tenfold increase in pulmonary blood flow, which shortly after birth is about 400 ml/min per kilogram in lambs born at term (Kuipers et al., 1982). In normal full-term lambs, pulmonary arterial blood pressure falls to near adult levels within 2-4 hr; in the human this takes considerably longer, and by 24 hr of age, mean pulmonary arterial blood pressure may be only half of systemic arterial blood pressure (Moss et al., 1963). After the initial rapid fall in pulmonary vascular resistance and pulmonary arterial blood pressure, there is a slow progressive fall, with adult levels reached within 2-6 weeks after birth (Rudolph et al., 1961; Krovetz and Goldbloom, 1972). With the large increase in pulmonary blood flow, the increased pulmonary venous return to the left atrium leads to an increase in left atrial pressure and closure of the valve of the foramen ovale, thereby preventing any significant amount of right-to-left shunting of blood. In addition, the ductus arteriosus constricts and closes functionally within several hours (Clyman and Heymann, 1981), thereby effectively separating the pulmonary and systemic circulations.

II. Morphologic Development of the Pulmonary Circulation

In the fetus and newborn, small pulmonary arteries of all sizes have a significantly thicker muscular wall relative to the external diameter than equivalent arteries in the adult. It is thought that this greater muscularity is responsible, at least in part, for the vasoreactivity and for the high pulmonary vascular resistance found in the fetus. In fetal lamb lungs, perfusion fixed at pressures similar to those found normally in utero, the medial smooth muscle was most prominent in the smallest arteries (fifth and sixth generation arteries, external diameter

20-50 μm); over the latter half of gestation, the medial smooth muscle thickness remained relatively constant with respect to the external diameter of the artery (Levin et al., 1976). Similar observations utilizing slightly different techniques have been made in human lungs (Hislop and Reid, 1972; Reid, 1979, 1982).

After birth, particularly within the first 1-2 weeks, there is a progressive reduction in the thickness of the walls of the small pulmonary arteries with thinning of the muscle and an increase in external diameter (Davies and Reid, 1970; Hislop and Reid, 1973; Rendas et al., 1978; Wagenvoort et al., 1961). By 4-6 weeks, the adult medial thickness/external diameter pattern with only a very thin, usually single-cell thick, layer of medial smooth muscle is established (Reid, 1982).

In any given pulmonary artery traced longitudinally toward the periphery of the lung, a level is reached where the completely encircling medial smooth muscle coat gives way to a region of incomplete muscularization; in these partially muscularized arteries, the smooth muscle is arranged in a spiral or helix. The muscle then disappears from the arteries that are still larger than capillaries (nonmuscularized small pulmonary arteries) (Reid, 1979, 1982). In the nonmuscular small pulmonary arteries, an incomplete pericyte layer is found within the endothelial basement membrane; in the nonmuscular portions of the partially muscular small pulmonary arteries, intermediate cells, i.e., cells intermediate in position and structure between pericytes and mature smooth muscle cells, are found (Meyrick and Reid, 1979). These cells are precursor smooth muscle cells, and under certain conditions, such as hypoxia, they may rapidly differentiate into mature smooth muscle cells (Meyrick and Reid, 1978).

In humans, small pulmonary arteries have been identified by their relationship to the airways (Reid, 1982). Preacinar pulmonary arteries are those lying proximal to or with the terminal bronchiolus, and intraacinar pulmonary arteries are those found associated with respiratory bronchioli or alveolar ducts or within the alveolar walls. In the fetus during the last 20% of gestation, only about half the pulmonary arteries running with respiratory bronchioli are muscularized or partially muscularized, and the alveoli are free of muscular arteries (Hislop and Reid, 1972). In the adult, circumferential muscularization extends peripherally along the intraacinar arteries so that the majority of small pulmonary arteries in relationship to alveoli are muscularized. Between birth and teenage, there is a progressive peripheral muscularization of the arteries so that the adultlike pattern is reached at about puberty.

During fetal growth in lambs, there is a large increase in the number of small arteries, not only in absolute terms but also per unit volume of lung (Levin et al., 1976). Halfway through gestation, there are about 7000 arteries per milliliter of lung; at term, this has increased almost tenfold.

The main preacinar pulmonary arterial branches that accompany the larger airways are developed by 16 weeks gestation in the human (Hislop and Reid,

1972); however, the intraacinar circulation more closely follows alveolar development, which occurs late in gestation and perhaps even mainly after birth (Reid, 1977, 1982). As alveoli multiply, so do arteries, a process generally complete by 10 years of age (Davies and Reid, 1970; Hislop and Reid, 1973).

III. Normal Physiology of the Perinatal Pulmonary Circulation

A. Mechanical Factors Affecting Pulmonary Vascular Resistance

The fetal lung is fluid filled, and under normal conditions spontaneous fetal breathing movements do not appear to affect pulmonary vascular resistance. However, rhythmic ventilation of fetal lungs with a gas, but not a liquid, even without changing arterial blood PO_2, produces a fall in pulmonary vascular resistance of varying degrees (Cassin et al., 1964a; Colebatch et al., 1965; Dawes and Mott, 1962; Dawes et al., 1953). This fall is most likely related to two phenomena. The first, surface tension factors acting at the alveolar air–liquid interface tending to reduce perivascular tissue pressure (Cassin et al., 1964a; Enhorning et al., 1966) probably contributes only slightly to the postnatal fall in pulmonary vascular resistance. Secondly, and more important in this event, are the effects of the movement or mechanical distortion and distention of the lung tissue leading to the secondary release of vasoactive substances (see below).

B. Oxygen

Under normal resting conditions in the fetal lamb, femoral arterial blood PO_2 is about 22-24 torr and pulmonary arterial blood PO_2 is about 17-20 torr. Because reduction of PaO_2 to almost the same levels in newborn animals produces a marked increase in pulmonary vascular resistance (Rudolph and Yuan, 1966; Soifer et al., 1982; Stahlman et al., 1964), it is most probable that the low PaO_2 found normally in the fetus is involved in maintaining pulmonary vasoconstriction and thereby an increased pulmonary vascular resistance. Further reducing fetal PaO_2 below normal baseline levels by inducing maternal hypoxemia (Cohn et al., 1974; Lewis et al., 1976) produces an even further and significant increase in pulmonary vascular resistance. This response is most marked close to term, while at about 0.6 gestation, very little pulmonary vasoconstriction occurs. The reason for this gestational difference is not yet known.

The exact mechanisms responsible for hypoxemic vasoconstriction are not clearly established. Both reflex-mediated chemoreceptor stimulation and direct local effects have been considered. Because hypoxia in fetal lambs produces significant adrenal secretion of catecholamines (Comline and Silver, 1961), it initially was thought that norepinephrine might be responsible, at least in part, for hypoxemia-induced fetal pulmonary vasoconstriction. In exteriorized immature fetal lambs, bilateral adrenalectomy did not alter the pulmonary vasoconstrictor response to asphyxia produced by umbilical cord constriction, suggesting that catecholamine release by the adrenals was not involved (Cassin et al., 1964b); however, alpha-adrenergic blockade prevented the pulmonary vasoconstriction induced by asphyxia. Asphyxia-induced pulmonary vasoconstriction therefore could have been due either to an extraadrenal release of catecholamines or to their local release at sympathetic nervous endings. When asphyxia was induced in fetal lambs in which one lung was perfused with blood either from a reservoir or from a normal nonasphyxiated donor twin fetus, pulmonary vasoconstriction developed (reflex mediated); this was abolished by cutting the sympathetic nerve to the lung. This pulmonary vasoconstriction occurred in mature but not in immature fetal lambs, suggesting that the reflex role of the sympathetic nervous system in producing hypoxic pulmonary vasoconstriction was related to fetal gestational age (Campbell et al., 1967a, b). In more physiologic conditions in chronically instrumented lambs in utero (Lewis et al., 1976), the fetal pulmonary vasoconstriction produced by maternal hypoxemia was not prevented by pharmacologic blockade of alpha- or beta-adrenergic or chrolinergic receptor function. Silove and Grover (1968) also concluded that the sympathetic nervous system did not contribute to hypoxic vasoconstriction because pretreatment of neonatal calves with reserpine did not affect the pulmonary vascular response to hypoxia.

There is some evidence to indicate that the pulmonary vascular responses to reduced oxygen are due rather to local effects, either direct or, as will be discussed later, more probably mediated by the local secondary release of locally acting vasoactive substances. In several studies where one fetal lung was either ventilated or perfused independently in situ without changing the oxygen environment of the other lung, oxygen-related vascular changes could be produced in the perfused or ventilated lung only (Campbell et al., 1967a, b; Cook et al., 1963). These studies thereby suggested that resistance changes in the isolated lung were locally mediated but could not distinguish between direct oxygen effects or those mediated by an oxygen-induced secondary release of a vasoactive substance.

Although gaseous expansion or ventilation of fetal lungs without increasing PaO_2 leads to a fall in pulmonary vascular resistance, a greater fall occurs with the addition to the gas mixture of oxygen, thereby increasing the PO_2 to which the resistance vessels are exposed (Born et al., 1955; Cassin et al., 1964a; Cook et al., 1963; Dawes and Mott, 1962). This effect of oxygen has been further substantiated without expanding or ventilating the lungs by exposing fetal lambs to hyperbaric oxygenation (Assali et al., 1968; Heymann et al., 1969). It also is not known whether increased oxygen directly affects the pulmonary vascular smooth muscle or whether a rise in oxygen environment results in the release of an intermediary substance that either actively dilates the pulmonary circulation or inhibits vasoconstriction.

C. Autonomic Nervous System

In acute studies in exteriorized fetal lambs or in newborn lambs, bilateral cervical or thoracic sympathectomy had no significant effect on resting pulmonary vascular resistance (Colebatch et al., 1965), suggesting that sympathetic nervous tone plays little or no role in the maintenance of normal resting pulmonary vascular tone. In the same study, bilateral cervical vagotomy also did not affect pulmonary vascular resistance, and therefore the parasympathetic nervous system as well was believed to play no role in maintenance of normal pulmonary vascular tone. Later studies in chronically prepared mature fetal lambs used selective pharmacologic blockade rather than nerve section to evaluate the role of the autonomic nervous system. Alpha-adrenergic blockade with phentolamine or parasympathetic blockade with atropine did not change resting pulmonary vascular tone (Rudolph et al., 1977). In addition, alpha- and beta-adrenergic as well as parasympathetic blockade had no effect on the vasoconstrictor response to hypoxemia in mature fetal lambs (Lewis et al., 1976), thus suggesting that at least during hypoxemic stress in the fetus, pulmonary vascular changes are not mediated directly by these autonomic nervous pathways. Similar observations have been made in newborn calves with alpha-adrenergic blockade (Silove and Grover, 1968); however, in young postnatal lambs, beta-adrenergic blockade accentuates hypoxic pulmonary vasoconstriction (Lock et al., 1981).

On the other hand, electrical stimulation of the distal end of the cut vagus nerve or the peripheral end of the cut thoracic sympathetic nervous chain in fetal lambs produced pulmonary vasodilatation or vasoconstriction, respectively (Colebatch et al., 1965). Pharmacologic stimulation of cholinergic or adrenergic receptors also has a significant effect on vasomotor tone. In perfused fetal lamb lungs or in acute preparations in fetal lambs, acetylcholine produces vasodilatation (Cassin et al., 1964; Cassin et al., 1964; Dawes and Mott, 1962). In intact fetal lambs studied chronically in utero, acetylcholine infused into the pulmonary circulation also produced significant vasodilatation close to term but had little or no effect in the immature fetal lambs (Lewis et al., 1976). After ventilation of the lungs, the dramatic pulmonary vasodilatation produced by acetylcholine in the fetus was no longer observed (Dawes et al., 1953). Alpha-adrenergic stimulation by methoxamine (Barrett et al., 1972; Cassin et al., 1964a, b) increases pulmonary vascular resistance, and beta-adrenergic stimulation by isoproterenol (Cassin et al., 1964b; Smith et al., 1964) reduces pulmonary vascular resistance.

It appears, therefore, that the autonomic nervous system plays no role in normal resting control of the fetal pulmonary vascular resistance but, when stimulated, could alter pulmonary vascular resistance. The increased pulmonary vasomotor tone found in the fetus accentuates the responses to various stimuli. Whether or not these mechanisms are invoked during fetal stress or are involved in perinatal changes is not clear.

D. Vasoactive Substances and Hormones

Several vasoactive substances have been shown to affect the fetal pulmonary circulation, producing either pulmonary vasoconstriction or vasodilatation. Which, if any, play a physiologic role in the maintenance of the normally high pulmonary vascular resistance in the fetus, in prenatal responses to stress, or in postnatal changes associated with the onset of ventilation is not clearly established.

Fetal Pulmonary Vasoconstriction

Several studies have suggested that histamine release somehow is involved in the pulmonary vasoconstrictor response to hypoxia in adults (Hauge and Melmon, 1968; Hauge and Staub, 1969) and therefore might be involved in regulation of the fetal pulmonary circulation in the normally low oxygen environment in the fetus. However, in the fetus and newborn, histamine is a pulmonary vasodilator and not a constrictor (Cassin et al., 1964b; Goetzman and Milstein, 1980). Similarly, angiotensin II had been considered to play a role in the pulmonary vasoconstrictor response to hypoxemia in adults (Berkov, 1974) and therefore possibly in maintenance of the high pulmonary vascular resistance in the fetus. In the fetus, however, blockade of angiotensin II activity with saralasin had no effect on baseline pulmonary vascular resistance or on the response to further induced hypoxemia (Hyman et al., 1975). The more likely role of angiotensin II in perinatal pulmonary vasodilatation and the possible role of histamine are discussed later.

One class of substances, the leukotrienes, (LTs), which are derived from arachidonic acid via the lipoxygenase pathway, have generated considerable interest as possible mediators of pulmonary vasoconstriction in view of their constricting effect on smooth muscle. The leukotrienes may be responsible, at least in part, for mediating hypoxic pulmonary vasoconstriction in adult animals (Ahmed and Oliver, 1983; Morganroth et al., 1984a, b) and in newborn lambs (Schreiber et al., 1985). We therefore considered that leukotrienes could be involved in regulating the normal degree of pulmonary vasoconstriction in the fetus. End organ antagonism (with the putative LT receptor blocker FPL57231) of leukotriene effect in late gestation fetal lambs reduced pulmonary vascular resistance and increased pulmonary blood flow to the levels expected with normal ventilation after birth (Soifer et al., 1985). Because of the possible nonspecific effects of FPL57231, we also evaluated LT synthesis inhibition (with U60257) in the same preparation and found a similar dramatic fall in pulmonary vascular resistance and increase in pulmonary blood flow (LeBidois et al., 1987). Our studies in newborn lambs indicate that LTD_4 is the active component. (Schrieber et al., 1987), and in the fetus we have shown that the LT effect is not mediated by LT stimulation of thromboxane production (Clozel et al., 1985). All these studies strongly suggest a physiologic role for LTs in maintaining pulmonary vasoconstriction and thereby a low pulmonary blood flow in the normal fetus.

Postnatal Vasodilatation

As with the maintenance of pulmonary vasoconstriction in the fetus, several vasoactive substances have been implicated in postnatal pulmonary vasodilatation. One such substance is bradykinin, a potent vasoactive peptide that produces marked pulmonary vasodilatation when infused into fetal lambs (Assali et al., 1971; Campbell et al., 1968; Gilbert et al., 1973) and that is released from fetal lungs either by ventilation with air or during hyperbaric oxygenation without ventilation (Heymann et al., 1969). Bradykinin could effect these pulmonary vascular changes by several mechanisms (Fig. 1). It could act directly by B_1 or B_2 receptor stimulation, or through the stimulation of production of a second vasoactive substance such as endothelial-dependent relaxing factor (EDRF), platelet activating factor (PAF), or, more particularly, PGI_2 (see below).

Because prostaglandins (PGs), another group of arachidonic acid metabolites, but in this case, cyclooxygenase mediated, are potent vasoactive substances, their potential role in perinatal pulmonary vascular changes has now been studied quite extensively. In fetal goats and lambs, exogenous prostaglandin E_1 (PGE_1) and prostaglandin E_2 (PGE_2) are both modest pulmonary vasodilators (Cassin et al., 1975, 1979; Tyler et al., 1977). Exogenous prostaglandin I_2 (PGI_2) is also a pulmonary vasodilator (Cassin et al., 1981b; Leffler and Hessler, 1979; Lock et al., 1980; Starling et al., 1981) and is somewhat more potent than both PGE_1 and PGE_2. It is possible that the production and release of these substances may modulate the constrictor effects of, for example, the normally low fetal PaO_2, but this has not been definitely established. Prostaglandin F_{2a} (PGF_{2a}) produces only pulmonary vasoconstriction in fetal goats (Tyler et al., 1977) and therefore could play some role in the active production of pulmonary vasoconstriction.

As prostaglandins have been shown to dilate the fetal pulmonary circulation, these substances have received attention as possible mediators of the postnatal fall in pulmonary vascular resistance. PGI_2 is the dominant prostaglandin produced by the fetal and neonatal vasculature as well as by endothelial cells (Remuzzi et al., 1979; Skidgel et al., 1983; Terragno and Terragno, 1979; Terragno et al., 1977). None of the prostaglandins is truly specific for the pulmonary circulation, and all affect the systemic circulation to a similar degree, particularly during hypoxemia (Cassin et al. 1981b; Tripp et al., 1978, 1980). However, the nonspecific systemic effects do not exclude the possibility that endogenous local production and rapid metabolism occur in the perinatal period, and there is quite strong evidence that PGI_2 does play an important physiologic role in causing postnatal pulmonary vasodilatation. Several very different mechanisms could be responsible for the production of PGI_2.

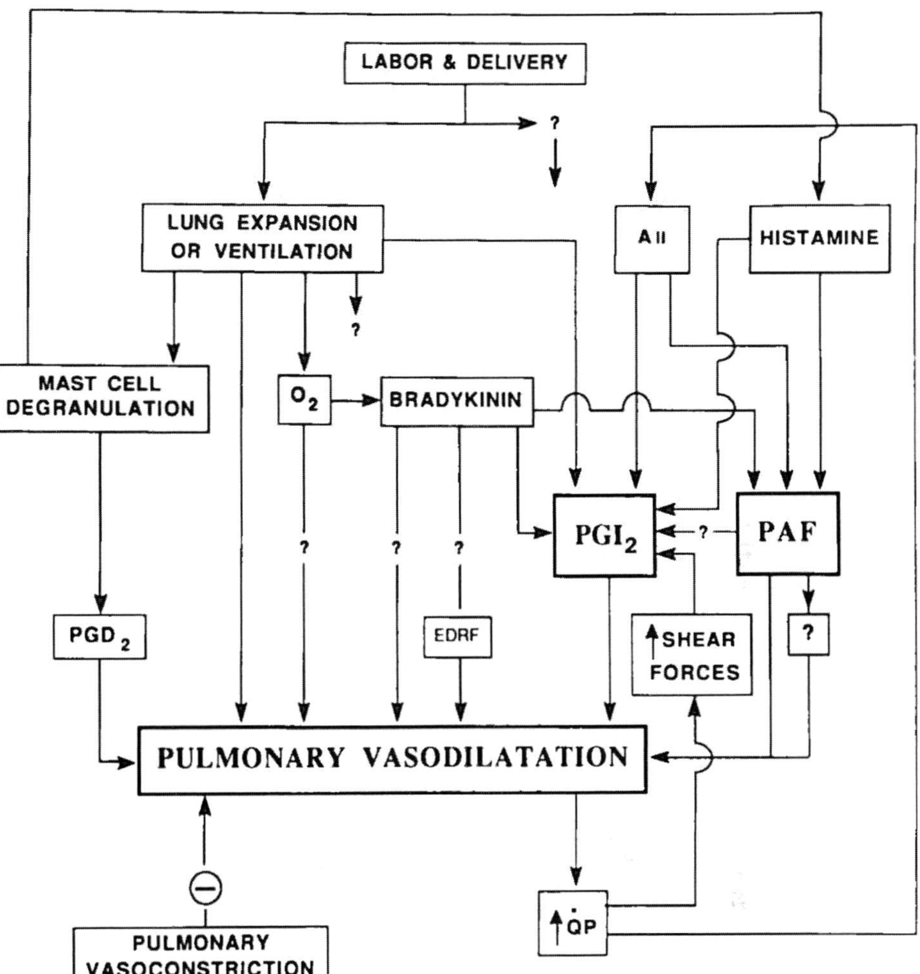

Figure 1 Hypothetical scheme of factors involved in postnatal pulmonary vasodilatation (see text for abbreviations).

Lung distention and distortion or mechanical stimulation of lungs leads to PG production (Edmonds et al., 1969; Gryglewski, 1980; Gryglewski et al., 1978), and spontaneous or mechanical ventilation of fetal lungs, even without changing PaO_2, is associated with the net production and release into left atrial blood of small amounts of the stable metabolite of PGI_2 (6-keto-PGF_{1a}) by the lungs (Leffler and Hessler, 1981; Leffler et al., 1980, 1984a, b). Concentrations of the metabolite fell rapidly over several hours, further suggesting a role for PGI_2 in the immediate postnatal period.

The exact mechanisms responsible for the stimulation of endogenous PGI_2 production are not yet known but probably involve a complex interaction of several factors (Fig. 1). As indicated previously, bradykinin is produced by the lung in response to oxygenation (Heymann et al., 1969). Bradykinin induces PGI_2 production by the lung (Gryglewski, 1980; Leffler et al., 1984a). Addition of bradykinin to cultures of endothelial cells increases the concentration of 6-keto-$PGF_{1\alpha}$, the stable metabolite of PGI_2 (Clark et al., 1986; Hong, 1980; McIntyre et al., 1985). In isolated perfused guinea pig lungs, bradykinin stimulates the release of prostaglandins (Palmer et al., 1973). Thus bradykinin-induced PGI_2 production is clearly a potential mechanism for perinatal pulmonary vasodilatation.

Another possible mechanism for PGI_2 stimulation involves the role of angiotensin II (AII), which increases in concentration with the establishment of the pulmonary circulation at birth and is known to stimulate PGI_2 production by the lung (Dusting, 1981). Further supporting this possibility are the data indicating that the stimulation of PGI_2 production by the neonatal lung is far more sensitive to AII induction than in the fetal or adult lung (Omini et al., 1983). If, as is discussed below, mast cell degranulation occurs at birth, the resultant release of histamine could stimulate the production of PGI_2 as has been shown to occur with endothelial cells in culture (McIntyre et al., 1985). A further possible mechanism for PGI_2 release involves the physical effects of increased blood flow and resultant increase in shear forces that induces pulmonary vascular endothelial cell PGI_2 production (Van Grondelle et al., 1984). If pulmonary blood flow (QP) increases due to any other cause (e.g., in response to O_2 or bradykinin directly), then a subsequent shear-induced PGI_2 production could produce further or sustained pulmonary vascular dilatation.

Very recent information suggests that perhaps not only PGI_2 but also a second lipid mediator, PAF, may be involved in regulation of the postnatal pulmonary circulation. Voeklel and co-workers (1986) have shown that small doses of PAF produce pulmonary vasodilatation in isolated rat lungs. Because PAF is not a circulating substance and probably acts only very close to the endothelial cell from which it is derived (McIntyre et al., 1985), the fact that pulmonary vasodilatation was found only with small amounts (? physiologic) of PAF whereas large, probably pharmacologic, amounts produced pulmonary vasoconstriction supports the possible role of PAF in pulmonary vascular regulation. Accurso et al. (1986) presented preliminary evidence in fetal sheep that PAF produced pulmonary vasodilatation in that model as well. Endothelial cell PAF production can be stimulated by the same agonists as PGI_2 production. (McIntyre et al., 1985): bradykinin (B_2 receptor) and histamine (H_1 receptor). Furthermore, AII apparently also stimulates PAF production in endothelial cell culture. The possibility therefore arises that both PGI_2 and PAF, independently or together with varying dominance, subserve the major role of producing and maintaining a dilated pulmonary circulation after birth. Production of each or both could be stimulated by bradykinin, AII, histamine, or perhaps some other mediator.

Prostaglandin D_2 (PGD_2) also has been shown to be a pulmonary vasodilator in perfused fetal lungs (Cassin et al., 1981a). In intact, newly delivered, term lambs with hypoxia-induced pulmonary hypertension, PGD_2 produced a significant and specific fall in pulmonary arterial pressure and calculated pulmonary vascular resistance with an increase in both pulmonary and systemic blood flows and no change in systemic arterial blood pressure (Soifer et al., 1982). This response disappears by 1-2 weeks of age (Soifer et al., 1983); thereafter, PGD_2 produces pulmonary vasoconstriction. These changes of effect during this part of development are very similar to those that occur with histamine (Goetzman and Milstein, 1980). The fairly specific effects of PGD_2 in the immediate newborn period suggest a physiologic role for PGD_2. This is further supported by studies in rhesus monkeys, which showed an increase in the number of mast cells in the fetal lungs toward the end of gestation and significantly fewer mast cells found in the lungs after birth (Schwartz et al., 1974). Because PGD_2 is released from mast cells, degranulation of these cells with the release of PGD_2 may play some role in the regulation of the perinatal vascular changes. However, unlike PGI_2, there currently are no known specific mechanisms that could initiate this chain of events.

The positive role of vasodilating prostaglandins in the immediate postnatal period has been further substantiated by studies using inhibition of cyclooxygenase activity (Cassin, 1980, 1982; Leffler et al., 1978). The fall in calculated pulmonary vascular resistance that normally occurs when close to term fetal lungs perfused in situ are ventilated was shown to have two separate phases: an initial rapid fall within 30-60 sec after the onset of ventilation, followed by a slower fall that occurred over about 15 min. In fetal goats, this latter, second phase was inhibited or attenuated by pretreatment with indomethacin. These latter studies do not indicate which prostaglandin is responsible or which is more important, but they confirm the role of a cyclooxygenase product of arachidonic acid metabolism. However, these are important observations that support the hypothesis that perhaps two (at least) quite different mechanisms are involved in the establishment of the pulmonary circulation. PAF could be responsible for the early changes, and PGI_2 for the later.

It therefore is probable that control of the perinatal pulmonary circulation reflects a balance between factors producing active pulmonary vasoconstriction in the fetus and those leading to pulmonary vasodilation with the onset of pulmonary ventilation. The dramatic increase in pulmonary blood flow after birth most likely reflects a shift from active pulmonary vasoconstriction to active pulmonary vasodilatation. It is possible that arachidonic acid metabolism shifts from lipoxygenase products (LTs) in the fetus toward cyclooxygenase products

(PGs) due either to mechanical stimulation with lung expansion or to the higher oxygen environment after birth. Some support exists for this latter hypothesis as cyclooxygenase activity seems to increase with increasing O_2 environment (Lands, 1979) and hypoxia reduces bovine pulmonary arterial endothelial cell PGI_2 production (Madden et al., 1986).

Acknowledgements

This work was supported in part by U.S. Public Health Service Program Project grant HL 24056, by grant HL 35518, and by BRSG grant S07 RR05355 awarded by the Biomedical Research Support Program, Division of Research Resources, National Institutes of Health.

References

Accurso, F., Abman, S., Wilkening, R. B., Worthen, S., and Henson P. M. (1986). Exogenous PAF produces pulmonary vasodilation in the ovine fetus. *Am. Rev. Resp. Dis. 133*:11 (abstract).

Ahmed, T., and Oliver, W., Jr. (1983). Does slow-reacting substance of anaphylaxis mediate hypoxic pulmonary vasoconstriction? *Am. Rev. Resp. Dis. 127*:566-571.

Assali, N. S., Kirschbaum, T. M., and Dilts, P. V., Jr. (1968). Effects of hyperbaric oxygen on uteroplacental and fetal circulation. *Circ. Res. 22*:573-588.

Assali, N. S., Johnson, G. H., Brinkman, C. R., and Huntsman, D. J., (1971). Effects of bradykinin on the fetal circulation. *Am. J. Physiol. 221*:1375-1382.

Barrett, C. T., Heymann, M. A., and Rudolph, A. M. (1972). Alpha- and beta-adrenergic function in fetal sheep. *Am. J. Obstet. Gynecol. 112*:1114-1121.

Berkov, S. (1974). Hypoxic pulmonary vasoconstriction in the rat: the necessary role of angiotensin II. *Circ. Res. 35*:256-261.

Born, G. V. R., Dawes, G. S., and Mott, J. C. (1955). The viability of premature lambs. *J. Physiol. (Lond.) 130*:191-212.

Campbell, A. G. M., Cockburn, F., Dawes, G. S., and Milligan, J. E. (1967a). Pulmonary vasoconstriction in asphyxia during cross-circulation between twin foetal lambs. *J. Physiol. (Lond.) 192*:111-121.

Campbell, A. G. M., Dawes, G. S., Fishman, A. P., and Hyman, A. I. (1967b). Pulmonary vasoconstriction and changes in heart rate during asphyxia in immature foetal lambs. *J. Physiol. (Lond.) 192*:93-110.

Campbell, A. G. M., Dawes, G. S., Fishman, A. P., Hyman, A. I., and Perks, A. M. (1968). The release of a bradykinin-like pulmonary vasodilator substance in foetal and newborn lambs. *J. Physiol. (Lond.) 195*:83-96.

Cassin, S. (1980). Role of prostaglandins and thromboxanes in the control of the pulmonary circulation in the fetus and newborn. *Semin. Perinatol.* *4*:101-107.

Cassin, S. (1982). Humoral factors affecting pulmonary blood flow in the fetus and newborn infant. In *Cardiovascular Sequelae of Asphyxia in the Newborn.* Edited by G. Peckham and M. A. Heymann. Ross Laboratories, Columbus, Ohio, pp. 10-18.

Cassin, S., Dawes, G. S., Mott, J. C., Ross, B. B., and Strang, L. B. (1964a). The vascular resistance of the foetal and newly ventilated lung of the lamb. *J. Physiol. (Lond.)* *171*:61-79.

Cassin, S., Dawes, G. S., and Ross, B. B. (1964b). Pulmonary blood flow and vascular resistance in immature foetal lambs. *J. Physiol. (Lond.)* *171*:80-89.

Cassin, S., Tyler, T. L., and Wallis, R. (1975). The effects of prostaglandin E_1 on fetal pulmonary vascular resistance (38588). *Proc. Soc. Exp. Biol. Med.* *148*:584-587.

Cassin, S., Tyler, T. L., Leffler, C., and Wallis, R. (1979). Pulmonary and systemic vascular responses of perinatal goats to prostaglandin E_2 and E_2. *Am. J. Physiol.* *236*:H828-H32.

Cassin, S., Tod, M., Philips, J., Frisinger, J., Jordan, J., and Gibbs, C. (1981a). Effects of prostaglandin D_2 in perinatal circulation. *Am. J. Physiol.* *240*:H755-H760.

Cassin, S., Winikor, I., Tod, M., Philips, J., Frisinger, S., Jordan, J., and Gibbs, C. (1981b). Effects of prostacyclin on the fetal pulmonary circulation. *Pediatr. Pharmacol.* *1*:197-207.

Clark, M. A., Littlejohn, D., Mong, S., and Crooke, S. T. (1986). Effect of leukotrienes, bradykinin and calcium ionophore (A 23187) on bovine endothelial cells: release of prostacyclin. *Prostaglandins* *31*:157-166.

Clozel, M., Clyman, R. I., Soifer, S. J., and Heymann, M. A. (1985). Thromboxane is not responsible for the high pulmonary vascular resistance in fetal lambs. *Pediatr. Res.* *19*:1254-1257.

Clyman, R. I., and Heymann, M. A. (1981). Pharmacology of the ductus arteriosus. *Pediatr. Clin. N. Am.* *28*:77-93.

Cohn, H. E., Sacks, E. J., Heymann, M. A., and Rudolph, A. M. (1974). Cardiovascular responses to hypoxemia and acidemia in fetal lambs. *Am. J. Obstet. Gynecol.* *120*:817-824.

Colebatch, H. J. H., Dawes, G. S., Goodwin, J. W., and Nadeau, R. A. (1965). The nervous control of the circulation in the foetal and newly expanded lungs of the lamb. *J. Physiol. (Lond.)* *178*:544-562.

Comline, R. S., and Silver, M. (1961). The release of adrenaline and noradrenaline from the adrenal glands of the foetal sheep. *J. Physiol. (Lond.)* *156*:424-444.

Cook, C. D., Drinker, P. A., Jacobson, N. H., Levison, H., and Strang, L. B. (1963). Control of pulmonary blood flow in the foetal and newly born lamb. *J. Physiol. (Lond.) 169*:10-29.

Davies, G., and Reid, L. (1970). Growth of the alveoli and pulmonary arteries in childhood. *Thorax 25*:669-681.

Dawes, G. S., and Mott, J. C. (1962). The vascular tone of the foetal lung. *J. Physiol. (Lond.) 164*:465-477.

Dawes, G. S., Mott, J. C., Widdicombe, J. C., and Wyatt, D. G. (1953). Changes in the lungs of the newborn lamb. *J. Physiol. (Lond.) 121*:141-162.

Dusting, A. J. (1981). Angiotensin-induced release of a prostacyclin-like substance from the lungs. *J. Cardiovasc. Pharmacol. 3*:197-206.

Edmonds, J. F., Berry, E., and Wyllie, J. H. (1969). Release of prostaglandins by distension of the lungs. *Brit. J. Surg. 56*:622-623.

Enhorning, G., Adams, F. H., and Norman, A. (1966). Effect of lung expansion on the fetal lamb circulation. *Acta Paediatr. Scand. 55*:441-451.

Gilbert, R. D., Hessler, J. R., Eitzman, D. V., and Cassin, S. (1973). Effect of bradykinin and alterations of blood gases on fetal pulmonary vascular resistance. *Am. J. Physiol. 225*:1486-1489.

Goetzman, B. W., and Milstein, J. M. (1980). Pulmonary vascular histamine receptors in newborn and young lambs. *J. Appl. Physiol. 49*:380-385.

Gryglewski, R. J. (1980). The lung as a generator of prostacyclin. *Ciba Found. Symp. 78*:147-164.

Gryglewski, R. J., Korbut, R., and Ocetkiewicz, A. (1978). Generation of prostacyclin by lungs in vivo and its release into the arterial circulation. *Nature 273*:765-767.

Hauge, A., and Melmon, K. L. (1968). Role of histamine in hypoxic pulmonary hypertension in the rat. II. Depletion of histamine, serotonin and catecholamines. *Circ. Res. 22*:385-392.

Hauge, A., and Staub, N. C. (1969). Prevention of hypoxic vasoconstriction in cat lung by histamine-releasing agent 48/80. *J. Appl. Physiol. 26*:693-699.

Heymann, M. A., and Rudolph, A. M. (1976). Effects of acetylsalicylic acid on the ductus arteriosus and circulation in fetal lambs in utero. *Circ. Res. 38*:418-422.

Heymann, M. A., Rudolph, A. M., Nies, A. S., and Melmon, K. L. (1969). Bradykinin production associated with oxygenation of the fetal lamb. *Circ. Res. 25*:521-534.

Heymann, M. A., Creasy, R. K., and Rudolph, A. M. (1973). Quantitation of blood flow patterns in the foetal lamb in utero. In *Proceedings of the Sir Joseph Barcroft Centenary Symposium. Foetal and Neonatal Physiology.* Edited by K. S. Comline, K. W. Cross, G. S. Dawes, and P. W. Nathanielsz. Cambridge University Press, Cambridge, pp. 129-135.

Hislop, A., and Reid, L. M. (1972). Intra-pulmonary arterial development during fetal life-branching pattern and structure. *J. Anat. 113*:35-48.

Hislop, A., and Reid, L. (1973). Pulmonary arterial development during childhood: branching pattern and structure. *Thorax 28*:129-135.

Hong, S. L. (1980). Effect of bradykinin and thrombin on prostacyclin synthesis in endothelial cells from calf and pig aorta and human umbilical cord vein. *Thromb. Res. 18*:787-795.

Hyman, A., Heymann, M. A., Levin, D. L., and Rudolph, A. M. (1975). Angiotensin is not the mediator of hypoxia-induced pulmonary vasoconstriction in fetal lambs. *Circulation 52*:11-132 (abstract).

Krovetz, L. J., and Goldbloom, J. (1972). Normal standards for cardiovascular data II pressure and vascular resistances. *Johns Hopkins Med. J. 130*:187-195.

Kuipers, J. R. G., Sidi, D., Heymann, M. A., and Rudolph, A. M. (1982). Comparison of methods of measuring cardiac output in newborn lambs. *Pediatr. Res. 16*:594-598.

Lands, W. E. M. (1979). The biosynthesis and metabolism of prostaglandins. *Ann. Rev. Physiol. 49*:633-652.

LeBidois, J., Soifer, S. J., Clyman, R. I., and Heymann, M. A. (1987). Piriprost, a putative leukotriene inhibitor, increases pulmonary blood flow in fetal lambs. *Pediatr. Res. 22*:350-354 (in press).

Leffler, C. W., and Hessler, J. R. (1979). Pulmonary and systemic vascular effects of exogenous prostaglandin I_2 in fetal lambs. *Eur. J. Pharmaccol. 54*: 37-42.

Leffler, C. W., and Hessler, J. R. (1981). Perinatal pulmonary prostaglandin production. *Am. J. Physiol. 241*:H756-H759.

Leffler, C. W., Tyler, T. L., and Cassin, S. (1978). Effect of indomethacin on pulmonary vascular response to ventilation of fetal goats. *Am. J. Physiol. 234*:H346-H351.

Leffler, C. W., Hessler, J. R., and Terragno, N. A. (1980). Ventilation-induced release of prostaglandin-like material from fetal lungs. *Am. J. Physiol. 238*:H282-H286.

Leffler, C. W., Hessler, J. R., and Green, R. S. (1984a). Mechanism of stimulation of pulmonary prostaglandin synthesis at birth. *Prostaglandins 28*:877-887.

Leffler, C. W., Hessler, J. R., and Green, R. S. (1984b). The onset of breathing at birth stimulates pulmonary vascular prostacyclin synthesis. *Pediatr. Res. 18*:938-942.

Levin, D. L., Rudolph, A. M., Heymann, M. A., and Phibbs, R. H. (1976). Morphological development of the pulmonary vascular bed in fetal lambs. *Circulation 53*:144-151.

Lewis, A. B., Heymann, M. A., and Rudolph, A. M. (1976). Gestational changes in pulmonary vascular responses in fetal lambs in utero. *Circ. Res. 39*:536-541.

Lock, J. E., Olley, P. M., and Coceani, F. (1980). Direct pulmonary vascular responses to the prostaglandins in the conscious newborn lamb. *Am. J. Physiol. 238*:H631-H638.

Lock, J. E., Olley, P. M., and Coceani, F. (1981). Enhanced beta-adrenergic receptor responsiveness in the hypoxic neonatal pulmonary circulation. *Am. J. Physiol. 240*:H697-H703.

McIntyre, T. M., Zimmerman, G. A., Satoh, K., and Prescott, S. M. (1985). Cultured endothelial cells synthesize both platelet-activating factor and prostacyclin in response to histamine, bradykinin, and adenosine triphosphate. *J. Clin. Invest. 76*:271-280.

Madden, M. C., Vender, R. L., and Friedman, M. (1986). Effect of hypoxia or prostacyclin production in cultured pulmonary artery endothelium. *Prostaglandins 31*:1049-1062.

Meyrick, B., and Reid, L. (1978). The effect of continued hypoxia on rat pulmonary arterial circulation: an ultrastructural study. *Lab Invest. 38*:188-200.

Meyrick, B., and Reid, L. (1979). Ultrastructural features of the distended pulmonary arteries of the normal rat. *Anat. Rec. 193*:71-97.

Morganroth, M. L., Reeves, J. T., Murphy, R. C., and Voelkel, N. F. (1984a). Leukotriene synthesis and receptor blockers block hypoxic pulmonary vasoconstriction. *J. Appl. Physiol. 56*:1340-1346.

Morganroth, M. L., Stenmark, K. R., Zonole, J. A., Mauldrin, R. Mathias, M., Reeves, J. T., Murphy, R. C., and Voelkel, N. F. (1984b). Leukotriene C_4 production during hypoxic pulmonary vasoconstriction in isolated rat lungs. *Prostaglandins 28*:867-875.

Moss, A. J., Emmanouilides, G., and Duffie, E. R., Jr. (1963). Closure of the ductus arteriosus in the newborn infant. *Pediatrics 32*:25-30.

Omini, C., Vigano, T., Marini, A., Pasargiklian, R., Fano, M., and Maselli, M. A. (1983). Angiotensin II: a releaser of PGI_2 from fetal and newborn rabbit lungs. *Prostaglandins 25*:901-910.

Palmer, M. A., Piper, J. J., and Vane, J. R. (1973). Release of rabbit aorta contracting substance (RCS) and prostaglandins induced by chemical or mechanical stimulation of guinea pig lungs. *Brit. J. Pharmacol. 49*:226-242.

Reid, L. (1977). The lung: its growth and remodeling in health and disease. *Am. J. Roentgenol. 129*:777-788.

Reid, L. (1979). The pulmonary circulation: remodeling in growth and disease. *Am. Rev. Respir. Dis. 119*:531-546.

Reid, L. (1982). The development of the pulmonary circulation. In *Cardiovascular Sequelae of Asphyxia in the Newborn. Report of the Eighty-Third Ross Conference on Pediatric Research.* Edited by G. J. Peckham and M. A. Heymann. Ross Laboratories, Columbus, Ohio, pp. 2-10.

Remuzzi, G., Misiani, R., and Muratore, D. (1979). Prostacyclin and human fetal circulation. *Prostaglandins 18*:341-348.

Rendas, A., Branthwaite, M., and Reid, L. (1978). Growth of the pulmonary circulation in normal pig: structural analysis and aspects of cardiopulmonary function. *J. Appl. Physiol. 45*:806-817.

Rudolph, A. M. (1979). Fetal and neonatal pulmonary circulation. *Ann. Rev. Physiol. 41*:383-395.

Rudolph, A. M., and Heymann, M. A. (1967). The circulation of the fetus in utero. Methods for studying distribution of blood flow, cardiac output and organ blood flow. *Circ. Res. 21*:163-184.

Rudolph, A. M., and Heymann, M. A. (1970). Circulatory changes during growth in the fetal lamb. *Circ. Res. 26*:289-299.

Rudolph, A. M., and Yuan, S. (1966). Response of the pulmonary vasculature to hypoxia and H^+ ion concentration changes. *J. Clin. Invest. 45*:399-411.

Rudolph, A. M., Auld, P. A. M., Golkino, R. J., and Paul, M. H. (1961). Pulmonary vascular adjustments in the neonatal period. *Pediatrics 28*:28-34.

Rudolph, A. M., Heymann, M. A., and Lewis, A. B. (1977). Physiology and pharmacology of the pulmonary circulation in the fetus and newborn. In *Lung Biology in Health and Disease. Development of the Lung.* Edited by W. A. Hodson. Marcel Dekker, New York, pp. 497-523.

Schreiber, M. D., Heymann, M. A., and Soifer, S. J. (1985). Leukotriene inhibition prevents and reverses hypoxic pulmonary vasoconstriction in newborn lambs. *Pediatr. Res. 19*:437-441.

Schreiber, M. D., Heymann, M. A., and Soifer, S. J. (1987). The differential effects of leukotriene C4 and D4 on the pulmonary and systemic circulations in newborn lambs. *Pediatr. Res. 21*:176-182.

Schwartz, L. W., Osburn, B. I. and Frick, O. L. (1974). An ontogenic study of histamine and mast cells in the fetal rhesus monkey. *J. Allergy Clin. Immunol. 56*:381-386.

Silove, E. D., and Grover, R. F. (1968). Effects of alpha-adrenergic blockade and tissue catecholamine depletion on pulmonary vascular responses to hypoxia. *J. Clin. Invest. 47*:274-285.

Skidgel, R. A., Friedman, W. F., and Printz, M. P. (1983). Prostaglandin biosynthetic activities of isolated fetal lamb ductus arteriosus, other blood vessels and lung tissue. *Pediatr. Res. 18*:12-18.

Smith, R. W., Morris, J. A., and Assali, N. S. (1964). Effects of chemical mediators on the pulmonary and ductus arteriosus circulation in the fetal lamb. *Am. J. Obstet. Gynecol. 89*:252-260.

Soifer, S. J., Morin, F. C., III, and Heymann, M. A. (1982). Prostaglandin D_2 reverses induced pulmonary hypertension in the newborn lamb. *J. Pediatr. 100*:458-463.

Soifer, S. J., Morin, F. C., III, Kaslow, D. C., and Heymann, M. A. (1983). The developmental effects of PGD_2 on the pulmonary and systemic circulations in the newborn lamb. *J. Dev. Physiol. 5*:237-250.

Soifer, S. J., Loitz, R. D., Roman, C., and Heymann, M. A. (1985). Leukotriene end organ antagonists increase pulmonary blood flow in fetal lambs. *Am. J. Physiol. 249*:H570-H576.

Stahlman, M., Shepard, F., Gray, J., Jr., Young, W. (1964). The effects of hypoxia and hypercapnia on the circulation in newborn lambs. *J. Pediatr. 65*: 1091-1092.

Starling, M. B., Neutzee, J. M., Elliott, R. L., and Elliott, R. B. (1981). Comparative studies of hemodynamic effects of prostaglandin E_1, prostacyclin, and tolazoline upon elevated pulmonary vascular resistance in neonatal swine. *Prostaglandins Med. 7*:349-361.

Terragno, N. A., and Terragno, A. (1979). Prostaglandin metabolism in fetal and maternal vasculature. *Fed. Proc. 38*:75-77.

Terragno, N. A., Terragno, A., McGiff, J. C., and Rodriguez, D. J. (1977). Synthesis of prostaglandins by the ductus arteriosus of the bovine fetus. *Prostaglandins 14*:721-727.

Tripp, M. E., Heymann, M. A., and Rudolph, A. M. (1978). Hemodynamic effects of prostaglandin E_1 on lambs *in utero* In *Advances in Prostaglandin and Thromboxane Research.* Vol. 4. Edited by F. Coceani and P. M. Olley. Raven Press, New York, pp. 221-229.

Tripp, M. E., Drummond, W. H., Heymann, M. A., and Rudolph, A. M. (1980). Hemodynamic effects of pulmonary arterial infusion of vasodilators in newborn lambs. *Pediatr. Res. 14*:1311-1315.

Tyler, T. L., Leffler, C. W., and Cassin, S. (1977). Effects of prostaglandin precursors, prostaglandins, and prostaglandin metabolites on pulmonary circulation in perinatal goats. *Chest 71S*:271S-273S.

Vangrondelle, A., Worthen, S., Ellis, D., Mathias, M. M., Murphy, R. C., Murphy, R. J. Strife, J., Reeves, J. T., and Voelkel, N. F. (1984). Altering hydrodynamic variables influences PGI_2 production by isolated lungs and endothelial cells. *J. Appl. Physiol. 57*:388-395.

Voelkel, N. F., Chang, S. W., Pfeffer, K. D., Worthen, S. G., McMurtry, I. F., and Henson, P. M. (1986). PAF antagonists: different effects on platelets, neutrophils, guinea pig ileum and PAF-induced vasodilation in isolated rat lung. *Prostaglandins 32*:359-372.

Wagnenvoort, C. A., Neufeld, H. N., and Edwards, J. E. (1961). The structure of the pulmonary arterial tree in fetal and early postnatal life. *Lab. Invest. 10*:751-761.

3

Pressure and Flow in the Pulmonary Vascular Bed

CHRISTOPHER A. DAWSON*

Medical College of Wisconsin
Milwaukee, Wisconsin

J. H. LINEHAN and T. A. BRONIKOWSKI

Marquette University
Milwaukee, Wisconsin

I. Introduction

The geometry and physical properties of the pulmonary vessels that determine the relationship between pressure and flow in the pulmonary circulation are important determinants of cardiac and pulmonary function. The pulmonary input impedance determines the work of the right ventricle (McDonald, 1974; Milnor, 1982; O'Rourke, 1982; Piene, 1986), and the longitudinal (artery to vein) distribution of vascular pressures is a key factor in lung fluid balance (Bhattacharya, 1986; Effros, 1984; Fishman, 1985; Staub, 1978; Taylor and Parker, 1985). The parallel distribution of vascular resistance is an important determinant of the local ventilation/perfusion ratios and, therefore, of pulmonary gas exchange (Grover et al., 1983; West and Wagner, 1977). The vessel geometry and viscoelasticity of the vessel wall can be altered both actively and passively (Cox, 1982, 1984; Patel et al., 1960, 1962). We will refer to an active response as one that produces a change in the relationship between diameter and transmural pressure of the individual vessels. This is in contrast to a passive response in which vessel diameters and compliance change as a result of a change in vessel transmural pressure. This distinction between active and passive responses is shown diagrammatically in Figure 1. The vessel diameter and the slope of the

**Present affiliation*: Clement J. Zablocki Veterans Administration Medical Center, Milwaukee, Wisconsin

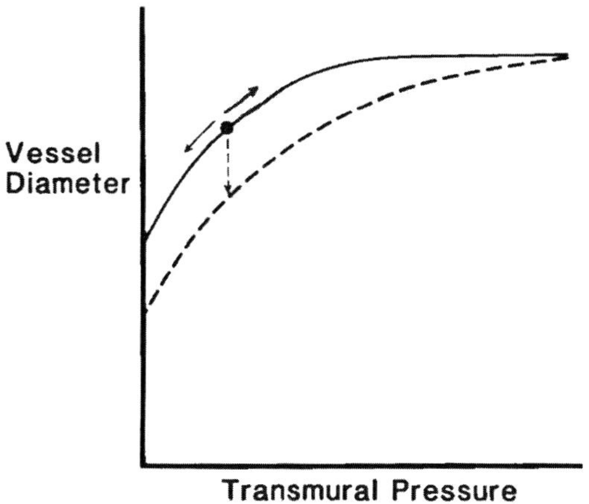

Figure 1 Hypothetical diameter versus pressure curves for a small pulmonary artery. The solid line represents a relaxed vessel with no vasomotor tone. The solid arrows indicate passive changes in diameter and compliance of the relaxed vessel as transmural pressure is changed. The dashed line represents a curve for the same vessel when the smooth muscle is activated. The dashed arrow then represents a purely active change in vessel diameter and compliance.

diameter versus pressure relationship can be altered passively by changing transmural pressure (the solid arrows) or actively by changing to a new diameter versus transmural curve (the dashed arrow). According to this classification, passive responses are the result of local forces generated by forces external to the vessel such as those controlling cardiac output, lung volume (i.e., pleural and alveolar pressure), and left atrial pressure, or those due to airway muscle contraction, gravity, and so on. Active responses occur within the vessels themselves, as the result of activation or relaxation of vascular smooth muscle in response to various vasomotor stimuli or as the result of changes in vessel wall thickness and composition in response to developmental changes and certain chronic stimuli. In addition to changes in the individual vessels, the geometry of the entire vascular bed can be altered by changing the number of parallel vessels. This might be the result of active remodeling of the vascular bed such as occurs during growth and development (Reid, 1979) and in response to various pathophysiologic conditions (Moser, 1979; Rabinovitch et al., 1979; Reid, 1979), or of passive obstruction, for example, from pulmonary thrombosis or embolism (Malik, 1983; Moser, 1979).

While the distinction between active and passive responses can be made conceptually, such responses usually do not occur independently. For example, active responses in a particular order of vessels can result in a change in the transmural pressures of the upstream vessels and in the transmission of pressure and flow pulsations to downstream vessels. Commonly, pulmonary vasomotor responses are also associated with cardiovascular and respiratory reflexes that change cardiac output, the pattern of transpulmonary pressure oscillations, and so on, thereby further complicating the picture. Since these passive effects can be substantial (Culver and Butler, 1980; Feeley et al., 1963), it can be difficult to determine the relative roles of active and passive mechanical responses when changes in pulmonary pressure-flow relations are observed. In this chapter we will examine the pressure-flow relations in the pulmonary vascular bed, giving particular attention to the detection and localization of active responses of the pulmonary vessels.

The site of action for a given acute pulmonary vasoactive stimulus is determined by the interaction of a potentially complex set of factors. The muscularity (Reid, 1979; Reid and Meyrick, 1982; Simons and Reid, 1969), innervation (Downing and Lee, 1980; Hebb, 1969; Richardson, 1979), and membrane electrical properties (Suzuki and Twarog, 1982a, b), and the locations and concentrations of receptors for various mediators vary along the pulmonary vascular tree (Altura and Chand, 1981; Greenberg et al., 1981; Gruetter et al., 1981; Holl et al., 1980; Joiner et al., 1975a, b). A given vasoactive stimulus can often influence the synthesis and release of other vasoactive mediators from endothelial cells and other cells within the lungs (Bakhle and Vane, 1977; Chand and Altura, 1981; Furchgott, 1984; Vanhoutte et al., 1981). These mediators can have additive, synergistic, or antagonistic effects. The endothelium can also influence the ability of certain mediators to reach their receptor sites by controlling local mediator concentrations (Bakhle and Vane, 1977; Dawson and Linehan, 1988; Rickaby et al., 1980). In addition, the sites of chronic changes in the vessel walls are probably dependent on conditions that influence the local concentrations of various growth factors (Benitz et al., 1986; Vender et al., 1987; Humphries et al., 1986). A number of methods have been used to evaluate pressure-flow relations in the pulmonary circulation to detect and to locate the longitudinal (from pulmonary artery to vein) sites of active responses within the intact organ. In addition to providing the means for calculating various parameters descriptive of pulmonary vascular function, each of these methods involves a set of hypotheses that not only are the basis for interpretation of data but also represent current concepts about how the pulmonary vascular bed works. Thus, an examination of the methods for evaluating pressure flow relations is one way to examine these concepts as well. Since we will focus on methods based on the measurement of pressures and flows at the inlet to and/or outlet from the pulmonary vascular bed, or at individual locations within the bed, the emphasis will be on the longitudinal or serial distribution of vascular pressures. The important topic of regional or parallel variations in pressure-flow relations (Greenleaf et al., 1974; Hakim et al., 1986, 1987; West and Dollery, 1965), which generally requires regional measurements, will not be emphasized.

II. Pressure-Flow Relations

A. Pulmonary Vascular Resistance

The pulmonary vascular resistance is probably the least invasive and least technically difficult hemodynamic parameter to obtain from measurements of pressure and flow in vivo. The pulmonary vascular resistance, R, in the normal postnatal circulation is the ratio of the mean pulmonary arterial – left atrial pressure difference to the cardiac output $\dot{Q}$:

$$R = (P_a - P_{la})/\dot{Q} \tag{1}$$

where P_a is the mean pulmonary artery pressure and P_{la} is the left atrial pressure. In practice, P_{la} is generally replaced in Eq. (1) by the pulmonary arterial wedge pressure, P_w. The P_w is obtained by measuring the pressure at the tip of a catheter passed into a pulmonary branch artery. The catheter is then used to occlude the artery in which the catheter tip resides. The occlusion is accomplished by inflating a balloon located just upstream from the catheter tip (O'Quin and Marini, 1983) or by advancing the catheter tip until it is wedged in an artery whose diameter is the same as the catheter tip diameter (Connolly et al., 1954; Luchsinger et al., 1962; Walston and Kendall, 1973). Thus, the flow in the smaller arteries, the capillaries, and the veins subtended by the occluded artery ceases. The tip of the wedged catheter is then open downstream through the resulting stagnant column of blood extending from the catheter tip through the microvascular bed to a vein of about the same diameter as the occluded artery. As long as this stagnant fluid column is continuous, the catheter tip pressure will be equal to the venous pressure at the confluence of this vein with the next larger vein carrying flowing blood. If the occluded artery is fairly large (on the order of 3 mm or larger), as is usually the case when a balloon-tipped catheter is used, the confluence will also be in a large vein, and the wedge pressure will normally be virtually identical to left atrial pressure. The mean pulmonary artery pressure and the thermal dilution cardiac output can be measured using the same catheter. Thus, the mean pressures and flow in Eq. (1) can be obtained using a single percutaneous venous catheter.

One problem in obtaining the left atrial pressure from the wedge pressure is that the alveolar capillaries are collapsible. Thus, if the hydrostatic pressure at the relevant venous confluence is less than alveolar pressure, the catheter tip can be facing a blind termination in capillaries collapsed by the alveolar pressure. Under these conditions P_w will no longer be a useful estimate of left atrial pressure (Hasan et al., 1985; Hotchkiss et al., 1986; O'Quin and Marini, 1983). Figure 2 represents the effect of catheter tip position diagrammatically. This problem is normally avoided by wedging the catheter in arteries that are below the level of the left atrium. However, during positive pressure ventilation even

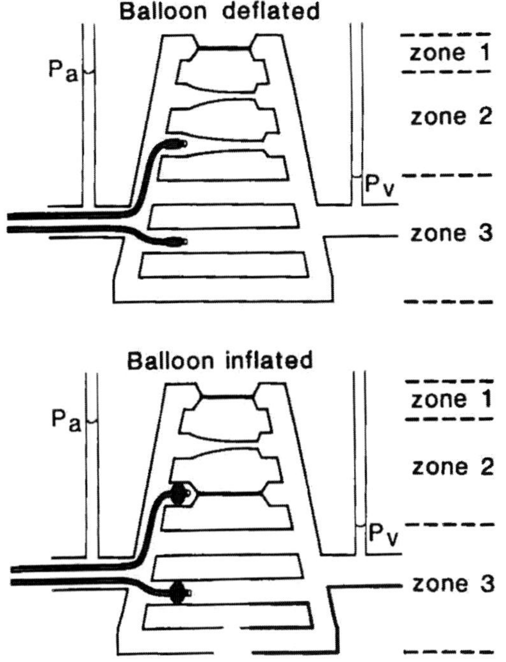

Figure 2 A diagrammatic representation of the effect of catheter tip position on pulmonary arterial wedge pressure. The vessels are arranged at different vertical levels such that the uppermost alveolar vessel is completely collapsed because the arterial pressure, P_a, is not as high as the alveolar pressure surrounding the vessel. This condition is referred to as zone 1 (West and Dollery, 1965). Moving down the lung, a region is encountered in which the arterial pressure exceeds alveolar pressure, but alveolar pressure exceeds the pressure at the venous end of the alveolar vessels. This is the zone 2 condition. In zone 2, stable flow occurs, but the alveolar vessels are compressed, particularly toward their venous ends, where the alveolar pressure exceeds the vascular pressure. This is the Starling resistance behavior referred to in the text. Further down, both Pa and venous pressure Pv exceed alveolar pressure, in what is referred to as zone 3. The bottom panel shows the effect of inflating the catheter tip balloon. When the balloon is inflated in zone 2, the pressure at the catheter tip will fall toward venous pressure until the pressure in the collapsible alveolar vessel reaches alveolar pressure. At that point the alveolar vessels will collapse and the column of blood connecting the catheter tip to the veins will be broken. In zone 3, the catheter tip pressure will fall all the way to the venous pressure when the balloon is inflated, and the continuous column of blood will remain.

this precaution does not guarantee equivalence of P_w and P_a (O'Quin and Marini, 1983). A potential, but rare, problem is that of large vein obstruction in which a significant wedge pressure-left atrial pressure gradient could develop and go undetected without a measure of the pressure in the left atrium (O'Quin and Marini, 1983). The pulmonary arterial wedge pressure has also been referred to by alternative names (O'Quin and Marini, 1983). The term "pulmonary capillary wedge pressure" should probably be avoided, since in zone 3 the P_w is generally a pressure downstream from the capillaries close to P_{la} (Wiedemann, 1986).

Given that the pressures in Eq. (1) are referenced to the same vertical level and the difference in kinetic energy between pulmonary artery and left atrium is small, the pulmonary vascular resistance calculated from Eq. (1) is a measure of the mechanical energy dissipated to overcome the viscous work resulting from the blood flow through the lungs. The vascular resistance is a function of the vessel geometry and the blood viscosity. For Poiseuille flow (long, straight, unbranched tubes with steady flow of a Newtonian fluid), the relationship between resistance, geometry, and viscosity is

$$R = 8\mu L/\pi r^4 \qquad (2)$$

where L is vessel length, r is vessel radius, and μ is the viscosity of the fluid. Under these conditions $8L/\pi r^4$, referred to as the geometric factor, comes from the parabolic velocity profile that results. There are alternative forms for the dependence of resistance on geometry for the different geometries and conditions actually extant in blood vessels (Fung, 1977, 1984; Fung and Sobin, 1969; Milnor, 1982). However, given a constant blood viscosity, a change in pulmonary vascular resistance generally implies a change in the geometry of the vascular bed. The problem in interpretation is that a change in resistance does not reveal the mechanism responsible for the change in geometry. The vessel transmural pressures are profoundly influenced by pleural pressure (Friedman and Wanner, 1977; Quebbeman and Dawson, 1977; Smith and Mitzner, 1980; Wanner et al., 1975), alveolar pressure (Fung, 1977; Fung and Yen, 1986; Hakim et al., 1982a, 1985; Permutt et al., 1962; Roos et al., 1961; West and Dollery, 1965), alveolar surface tension (Bruderman et al., 1964; Lloyd and Wright, 1960; Pain and West, 1966; Sun et al., 1987), lung volume (Dawson et al., 1977, 1979; Hakim et al., 1982a; Howell et al., 1961; Permutt et al., 1961; Quebbeman and Dawson, 1977; Smith and Mitzner, 1980), and the properties of the lung parenchyma (Fung et. al., 1983; Lai-Fook, 1979; Smith and Mitzner, 1980), as well as by intravascular pressure. The impact of active changes in the vessel walls may or may not be detectable or recognizable as changes in vascular resistance (i.e., in vascular geometry) given concurrent passively generated changes in transmural pressures. This does not mean that the pulmonary vascular resistance is not a useful parameter for evaluating active pulmonary vascular responses. In fact, it has been very useful, and, given some insight into the magnitude of the effects of the various passive influences, changes in vascular resistance can unambiguously reveal active responses. Generally, the other methods for evaluating pulmonary pressure-flow relations, to be discussed below, require more invasive measurements and/or more complicated approaches to data analysis and are therefore primarily research tools, whereas the measurements required to calculate pulmonary vascular resistance are clinically quite practical.

One issue that has been the source of some confusion is the fact that the arterial-venous pressure drop in Eq. (1), which represents the mechanical energy loss due to flow through the lungs, is not necessarily the driving pressure controlling the flow rate. This is exemplified by the effect of alveolar pressure on pulmonary blood flow. Since the capillaries situated within the alveolar septa [referred to as alveolar vessels (Mead and Whittenberger, 1964)] are thin-walled collapsible vessels, the effective extravascular pressure is alveolar pressure [or alveolar pressure attenuated by the effect of alveolar surface tension (Bruderman et al., 1964; Lloyd and Wright, 1960; Pain and West, 1966; Sun et al., 1987)]. When alveolar pressure exceeds the intravascular pressure at the venous end of these collapsible vessels, the vessels narrow, and the alveolar pressure becomes the effective back pressure for the flow. The arterial-alveolar pressure difference, rather than the arterial-left atrial pressure difference, is then the driving pressure for the flow. Under these conditions, referred to as zone 2 conditions (West and Dollery, 1965), the flow through the alveolar vessels has been likened to the flow over a waterfall or sluice gate, in which case the height of the waterfall, analogous with the difference between alveolar and left atrial pressures, does not influence the flow (Permutt et al., 1962). Changes in the alveolar-left atrial pressure difference occurring under zone 2 conditions are not necessarily accompanied by change in flow, but they reflect the changes in mechanical energy dissipated as the geometry of the alveolar vessels changes. The added resistance associated with the narrowing of the alveolar vessels is commonly referred to as the *Starling resistance* after a device used by Knowlton and Starling (1912) to control arterial pressure in an isolated heart-lung preparation. The influence of this behavior of the alveolar vessels on pressure-flow relations in the lungs is used to help explain the normal gravity-dependent vertical gradient in pulmonary blood flow (West and Dollery, 1965). The mechanical phenomenon involved for the low Reynolds number flow in the alveolar vessels has been discussed by Fung and co-workers (Fung and Sobin, 1972; Fung and Yen, 1986; Fung and Zhuang, 1986). The concept that active tension can act in a manner similar to alveolar pressure in producing a Starling resistor-like phenomenon in pulmonary vessels even when vascular pressures exceed alveolar pressure (Lopez-Muniz et al., 1968; Permutt and Riley, 1963) has also been used to interpret pulmonary vascular pressure-flow relations as discussed below.

B. The Pulmonary Mean Pressure-Flow Curve

In an attempt to improve on measurements of pulmonary vascular resistance as a means of detecting active pulmonary vascular changes, the arterial-venous pressure difference has been measured over a range of flow rates (Boiteau et al., 1986; Even et al., 1971; Goll et al., 1986; Graham et al., 1982, 1983; Grand

and Downing, 1970; Janicki et al., 1985; Lategola, 1958; Lodato et al., 1985; Murray et al., 1986; Nyhan et al., 1986; Williams, 1954). The resulting pressure-flow curve typically has a hyperbolic appearance, concave to the flow axis (Fig. 3). The curve appears to approach an asymptote such that it appears nearly linear over the higher portion of the range of physiological flow rates. The slope of the cord connecting the origin at zero flow with any point on the curve is the pulmonary vascular resistance at that flow rate as defined by Eq. (1). Thus, it is clear that the vascular resistance falls with increasing flow. One advantage of measuring the pressure-flow curve is that changes in vasomotor tone are commonly associated with changes in cardiac output. Because of the shape of the pressure-flow curve, if cardiac output and the arterial-venous pressure difference change in the same direction an associated change in vasomotor tone would be difficult to recognize if only the vascular resistance were measured. On the other hand, a change in vasomotor tone could be detected as a shift in the pressure-flow curve if the arterial-venous pressure difference were measured over a range of flows.

To obtain additional insights from changes in the shape of the pressure-flow curve, attempts have been made to explain the curve in terms of the vessel mechanics that might be responsible for its shape. One popular view is that the pulmonary vascular bed is made up of parallel pathways of essentially nondistensible vessels, with the flow through each pathway controlled by the pulmonary artery pressure and a critical closing pressure for the pathway (Graham et al., 1982, 1983; Lodato et al., 1985; McGregor and Sniderman, 1985; Mitzner, 1983; Mitzner and Sylvester, 1981; Murray et al., 1986; Rock et al., 1985; Soohoo et al., 1987). According to this view the resistance in each pathway can be conceptually divided into two series components, one a constant resistance, which is the resistance of the open rigid pathway, and the other a Starling resistance. The constant resistance has been referred to as an Ohmic resistance, by analogy with an electrical resistor in which the resistance is constant and independent of voltage or current (Rock et al., 1985). We will use the term *ohmic resistance* in this way to distinguish between the constant resistance and the variable Starling resistance, although some authors have used the term ohmic resistance for the resistance defined by Eq. (1) (Soohoo et al., 1987). When venous pressure exceeds alveolar pressure (zone 3), the Starling resistance would be viewed as the narrowing of collapsible vessels that results when the collapsing force due to the perivascular pressure or active tension in muscule vessel walls exceeds the vascular pressure within some flow-limiting segment of the vasculature (e.g., in muscular arteries or veins). According to this concept, this collapsing force is the effective closing pressure. When downstream pressures within a given pathway are low relative to this closing pressure, flow is determined by the arterial pressure-closing pressure difference. When arterial pressure is below the closing pressure, the pathway is closed. The shape of the pressure-flow curve

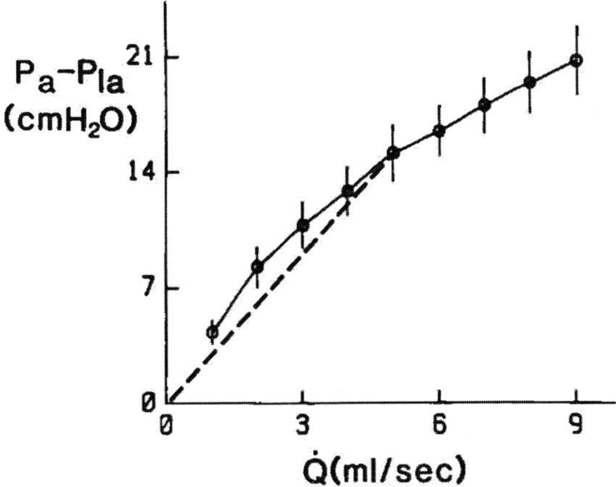

Figure 3 An average pressure versus flow curve obtained from isolated cat lungs (From Krishnan et al., 1986). The curve shows the typical hyperbolic shape. The slope of the dashed line is the pulmonary vascular resistance defined in Eq. (1) for one particular value of flow. The pressure flow curves are often graphed with $\dot{Q}$ as the dependent variable. However, we tend to favor pressure as the dependent variable, as in this graph, because under normal conditions the right ventricle acts more like a flow pump than a pressure source.

is then explained by assuming that there is a distribution of closing pressures among parallel pathways. Near the origin of the pressure-flow curve, pressure rises rapidly with increasing flow, but the resistance falls as the closing pressures of increasing numbers of vessels are exceeded. When the pressure is high enough, all vessels are open, and the slope of the pressure-flow curve becomes constant. When this constant slope is extrapolated back to zero flow, it intercepts the pressure axis at a pressure equal to the conductive-weighted mean of the closing pressures for the entire pulmonary vascular bed. In some (Graham et al., 1982; Soohoo et al., 1987) but not all (Fowler et al., 1966; Lloyd and Wright, 1960; West and Dollery, 1965) studies an arterial-venous pressure difference or arterial-alveolar pressure difference has remained even when flow is decreased to zero, and such pressure differences have been referred to as the *minimum* of the closing pressures in the pulmonary vascular bed. The arterial pressure-mean closure pressure difference is then considered to be the driving pressure for flow through the pulmonary vascular bed, and the slope of the linear portion of the pressure-flow curve is the harmonic mean of the parallel ohmic resistances upstream from the locus of the closing pressure (Mitzner, 1983). This view is appealing because it provides a conceptualization for a two-parameter description of the pressure-flow curve fitted with a linear line. The slope of the line is the upstream ohmic resistance, and the intercept is the mean closing pressure.

One problem with this view is that the information in the pressure-flow curve itself is not sufficient to demonstrate the uniqueness of this explanation for the zone 3 pressure-flow curve. This hypothesis also ignores the potential influence of the distensibility of the small vessels (Cox, 1982; Maloney et al., 1970, 1976; Sobin et al., 1972, 1978; Yen and Foppiano, 1981; Yen et al., 1980) and the increase in blood viscosity at low shear rates (Benis et al., 1968; Lockhart and Benis, 1970). Recently, Zhuang et al. (1983) have demonstrated that a pressure-flow curve with a shape that appears to be experimentally indistinguishable from that typical for the lungs can be obtained using a model in which there are no closing pressures but the vessels are distensible. Since this model is based on actual measurements of vessel distensibility, it would appear that the nearly linear portion of the pulmonary pressure-flow curve does involve some distension of the resistance vessels. Thus, the description of the pressure-flow curve strictly in terms of closing pressures and nondistensible vessels probably overstates the importance of the ohmic and Starling resistance dichotomy. This dichotomy also has the consequence that as long as the slope of the pressure-flow curve continues to be constant with increasing flow, any pressure downstream from the locus of the critical closing pressure is less than the critical closing pressure. The implication of this is that the downstream pressure drop is a very small fraction of the total arterial-venous pressure difference (Fowler et al., 1966). If one assumes that the capillaries (Bhattacharya and Staub, 1980; Fowler et al., 1966; Zhuang et al., 1983) and/or veins (Feeley et al., 1963; Gilbert et al., 1958; Hyman, 1969; Hyman et al., 1963; Kadowitz et al., 1975; Kuida et al., 1958; Kuramoto et al., 1962; Zhuang et al., 1983; Zidulka and Hakim, 1985) contribute substantially to the total resistance in the zone 3 lung, the anatomical location for the closing pressure must be close to the venous outflow from the vascular bed, and it is not clear how the closing pressure would be generated in these vessels (Fung et al., 1983).

The slope-intercept description of the pulmonary pressure-flow curve has been used to evaluate the effects of pulmonary vasoconstriction in terms of its effect on the mean closing pressure and vessel diameters (Boiteau et al., 1986; Goll et al., 1986; Graham et al., 1983; Mitzner and Sylvester, 1981; Murray et al., 1986; Nyhan et al., 1986). According to this model a parallel upward shift in the pressure-flow curve indicates an increase in closing pressures, resulting in an increase in Starling resistance, while an increase in slope indicates a narrowing of vessels, resulting in an increase in ohmic resistance. A parallel shift, such as has been observed with hypoxic vasoconstriction (see Fig. 4) (Gregory et al., 1982; Hakim et al, 1983; Mitzner and Sylvester, 1981; Sylvester et al., 1983), has been used as evidence in favor of this dichotomy of effects. However, recently Mitzner and Huang (1987) have shown how a parallel shift in the pressure-flow curve

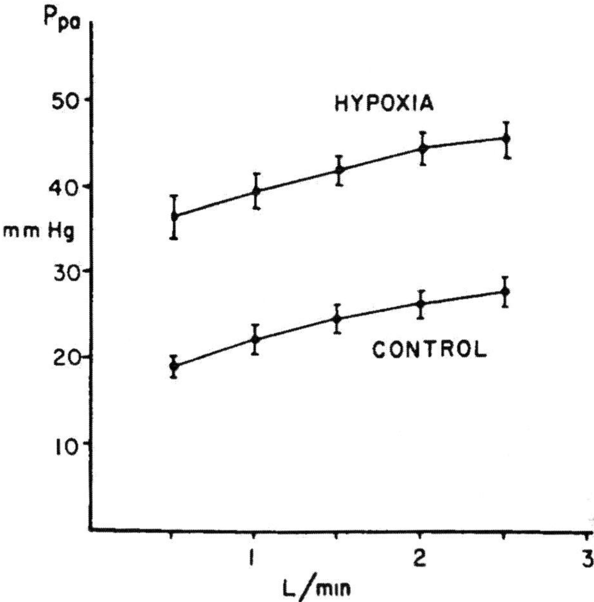

Figure 4 The effect of hypoxic vasoconstriction on the pulmonary artery pressure, P_{pa}, versus flow curve from isolated pig lungs. (From Mitzner and Sylvester, 1981).

can result if vessel constriction increases both the compliance and the resistance of the constricted vessels. In general, active narrowing of pulmonary vessels results in a decrease in the elastic modulus (Cox, 1982), and this is associated with an increase in the slope over at least some portion of the diameter-pressure curve (Cox, 1982). This behavior of the vessels is consistent with the model of Mitzner and Haung (1987). The distensible vessel model appears to account for the response to vasoconstriction equally as well as the ohmic-Starling resistor model, but on closer examination the two concepts may not be as divergent as they seem. In fact, the compliance of a vessel under Starling resistor conditions is very large when compared to the compliance that obtains when the transmural pressure is positive over the entire length of the vessel (Shapiro, 1977). Thus, increasing closing pressures to the extent that fully open vessels develop a Starling resistance would cause a large increase in vessel compliance. The model of Mitzner and Huang (1987) may simply be a demonstration that the all-or none Starling resistor model is a conceptual oversimplification that does incorporate certain aspects of the relevant physics. However, the previous interpretations of the slope and intercept are obscured so that, while these parameters may be useful empirical descriptors of the pressure-flow curve, their physical meaning is not so clear. Their utility then comes from the fact that a shift in the pressure-curve in the absence of substantial changes in lung volume or pleural or left atrial pressure is convincing evidence for a change in pulmonary vasomotor tone. On the other hand, it is clear that, for example, when vasoconstriction in response to one stimulus produces an increase in the slope while the vasoconstriction in response to another stimulus increases the intercept of the pressure-flow curve, there is a difference in the mechanical effects of the two stimuli. Such differences in the effects of different stimuli on the shape of the pressure-flow curve may reflect differences in site of action. Interpretation of changes in pressure-flow curves in terms of sites of action have received relatively little attention (Fowler et al., 1966; Mitzner and Sylvester, 1981), and the data are probably less sensitive to changes in the longitudinal resistance and compliance distribution than are the pressure and flow data obtained during other kinds of experimental manipulations (Fowler et al., 1966; Krishnan et al., 1986).

C. Oscillatory Pressure-Flow Relations and Input Impedance

The pulmonary arterial input impedance can be calculated from measurements of pulsatile pressure and flow near the entrance of the pulmonary artery (Bergel and Milnor, 1965; Bos et al., 1982; Caro and McDonald, 1961; Dujardin et al., 1982; Elkins and Milnor, 1971; Elkins et al., 1974; Grant and Paradowski, 1987; Hammon et al., 1981; Hopkins et al., 1979, 1980; Lefevre, 1983; Lucas et al., 1975; Maloney et al., 1968; Mills et al., 1970; Milnor, 1972, 1982; Milnor et al., 1969; Pace, 1971; Patel et al., 1963; Piene, 1976, 1986; Piene and Hauge, 1976; Pollack et al., 1968; Radke et al., 1985; Reuben and Kitchin, 1975; Reuben et al., 1971). An advantage of pulsatile pressure-flow data over mean pressure and flow is that they contain information about the elastic properties as well as the geometry of the pulmonary arterial tree. The input impedance, defined as the ratio of the amplitude of oscillatory pressure to that of oscillatory flow at a given frequency, can be determined from the measured phasic pressure-flow curves when they are decomposed into their sinusoidal components. A disadvantage of the input impedance method is that the data are technically more difficult to obtain than the mean pressures and flow. Accurate measurements of the oscillating pressure and flow in the pulmonary artery must be obtained using methods that do not distort the relatively high frequency components of the curves. In addition, the data analysis is somewhat complicated.

To calculate the input impedance, the measured pulsatile pressure and flow must be expressed as the sum of sinusoidal waves of various amplitudes, frequencies, and phase angles. The data analysis is based on the Fourier theorem that any periodic function such as a pressure wave, P(t), or flow wave, $\dot{Q}(t)$ can be produced by an infinite series, namely,

$$P(t) = \bar{P} + \sum_{k=1}^{\infty} (A_k \cos(k\omega t) + B_k \sin(k\omega t)) \tag{3}$$

and

$$\dot{Q}(t) = \bar{\dot{Q}} + \sum_{k=1}^{\infty} [C_k \cos(k\omega t) + D_k \sin(k\omega t)] \tag{4}$$

where k represents successive positive integer multiples (harmonics) of the fundamental angular frequency ω, in radians ($\omega = 2\pi f$, where f is the heart rate); $\bar{P}$ and $\bar{\dot{Q}}$ are, respectively, the mean pulmonary artery pressure and flow found from the areas of the respective curves. For example,

$$\bar{P} = \frac{1}{T} \int_0^T P(t)\, dt$$

where T is the period of the pulsations. Commonly the data are analyzed by Fourier analysis in which the pressure and flow waveforms are approximated by a finite sum, with the maximum harmonic k_{max} generally ranging from 10 to less than 30. The Fourier coefficients A_k and B_k for the time-varying pressure can be calculated from

$$A_k = \frac{2}{n} \sum_{i=0}^{n} P_i \cos(k\omega t_i) \tag{5}$$

$$B_k = \frac{2}{n} \sum_{i=0}^{n} P_i \sin(k\omega t_i) \tag{6}$$

where n is the number of equal finite time divisions Δt subdividing the period T of each pulse. (For a pulse wave that is fit exactly by harmonics 1 through

k_{max}, the minimum value of n would be $2k_{max}$; however, in practice n is usually chosen to be around 100 to avoid aliasing.) i is the number of Δt increments from t = 0 to t_i (thus, $t_i = i\Delta t$ for i ranging from 0 to n), and P_i is the pressure at t_i. C_k and D_k can be obtained in similar fashion by equations analogous to Eqs. (5) and (6), respectively, in which P_i is replaced by $\dot{Q}_i$. With the Fourier coefficients so determined, it is convenient to express Eqs (3) and (4) in an alternative form for purposes of computing the input impedance:

$$P(t) = \overline{P} + \sum_{k=1}^{k_{max}} P_k \cos(k\omega t - \beta_k) \tag{7}$$

and

$$\dot{Q}(t) = \overline{\dot{Q}} + \sum_{k=1}^{k_{max}} \dot{Q}_k \cos(k\omega t - \alpha_k) \tag{8}$$

where the amplitudes of the pressure and flow oscillations are, respectively,

$$P_k = (A_k + B_k)^{1/2} \quad \text{and} \quad \dot{Q}_k = (C_k + D_k)^{1/2} \tag{9a,b}$$

The phase angles β_k and α_k are, respectively,

$$\beta_k = \tan^{-1}(B_k/A_k) \quad \text{and} \quad \alpha_k = \tan^{-1}(D_k/C_k) \tag{10a,b}$$

To calculate the input impedance, each harmonic of the above series can be written in terms of a complex number according to

$$p_k = P_k \ \exp[j(k\omega t - \beta_k)] \tag{11}$$

and

$$q_k = \dot{Q}_k \ \exp[j(k\omega t - \alpha_k)] \tag{12}$$

where $j = \sqrt{-1}$. The input impedance is than a complex number defined as

$$Z(k\omega) = \frac{p_k}{q_k} = \frac{P_k}{\dot{Q}_k} \exp[j(\alpha_k - \beta_k)] \tag{13}$$

which is characterized by a modulus, $Z_k = P_k/\dot{Q}_k$, and a phase angle, $\phi_k = (\alpha_k - \beta_k)$. The pressure and flow amplitudes, and the phase angle between them for frequency $k\omega$, are depicted graphically in Figure 5.

An assumption underlying the concept of the input impedance is that the pulmonary arterial tree behaves as a linear system; that is, the pressure and flow waves of a given frequency are independent of the magnitude of the pressure, and the pressure and flow waves of each frequency are independent of those of other frequencies. The assumption of linearity can be only an approximation in real blood vessels, but it appears to be consistent enough with the behavior of the pulmonary arterial bed that nonlinearities do not appear to confuse the interpretation of the calculated impedance (Frasher and Sobin, 1965; Hammon et al., 1981; Milnor, 1982).

The impendence spectrum, in terms of modulus and phase angle, is dependent on both the geometry and compliance of the pulmonary arterial tree. In the normal lung the pulmonary arterial input impedance modulus first decreases from the zero frequency value and then fluctuates between relative maxima and minima with increasing frequency. The phase angle is negative (flow leading pressure) for low frequencies and then becomes positive near the first minimum in the modulus (Fig. 6). The modulus at zero frequency represents the input resistance, that is, the mean arterial pressure divided by mean flow as distinct from the pulmonary vascular resistance defined by Eq.

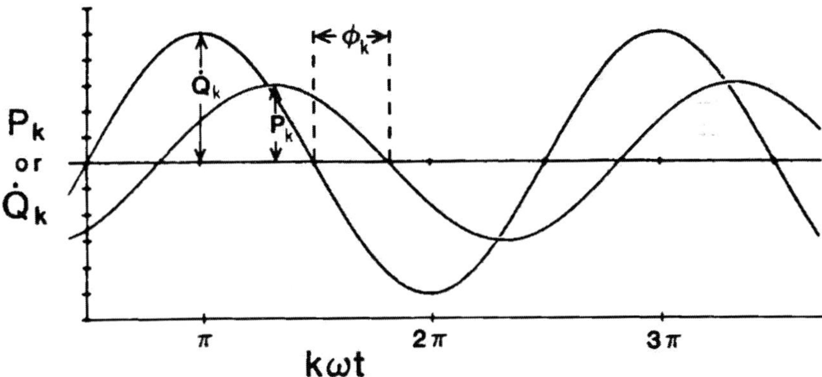

Figure 5 A hypothetical example of the pressure and flow oscillations for the kth harmonic of the pulsatile pulmonary arterial pressure and flow. $\dot{Q}_k$ and P_k are the amplitudes of the flow and pressure oscillations, respectively. The ratio $P_k/\dot{Q}_k$ is the input impedance modulus Z_k, and the impedance phase angle is ϕ_k.

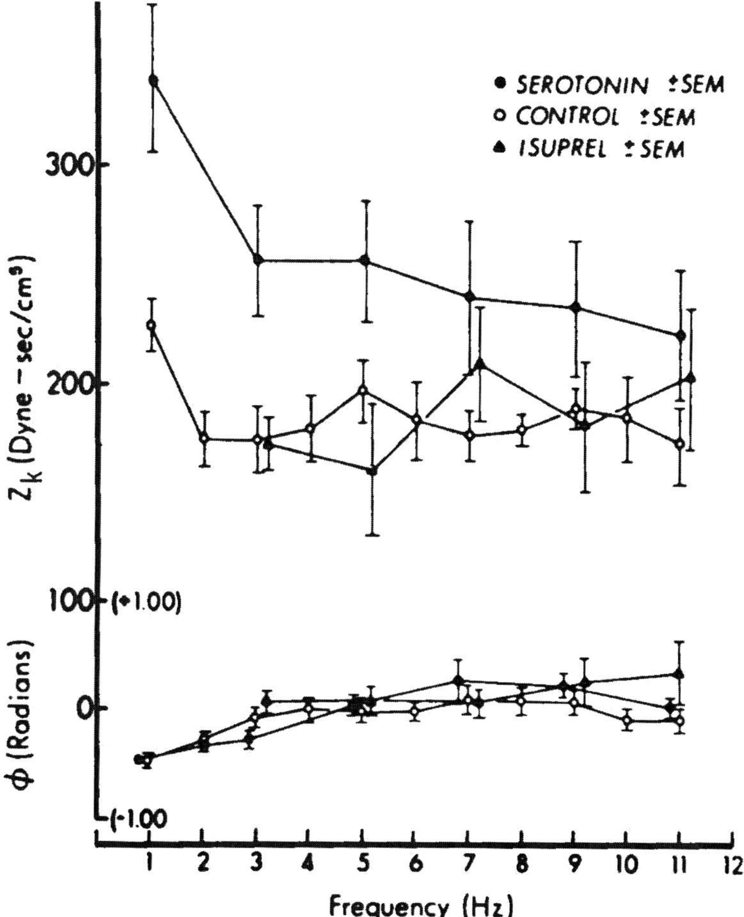

Figure 6 An example of the average input impedance spectra obtained from unanesthetized dogs under normal conditions (control) and during serotonin or isoproterenol infusion. Z_k is the impedance modulus, and ϕ the impedance phase angle. (From Hammon et al., 1981.)

(1). The fluctuations in the impedance modulus with frequency are due to reflections from regions within the vascular bed in which there is a change in the characteristic impedance. Such changes are essentially continuous through the vascular bed, but relatively sharp changes occur in the distal arterial tree. This results in fairly consistent fluctuations in the normal impedance spectrum. Much of the data on pulmonary input impedance has been obtained in studies on dogs. In the normal dog of about 20 kg, the spectrum is characterized by a minimum around 2-4 Hz and a maximum around 5-8 Hz with additional smaller fluctuations. These frequencies are dependent on the distance between measuring site and sites of major reflections as well as compliance and wave velocity in the arteries. Thus, they are quite dependent on animal size. The negative phase angle at low frequencies indicates the dominance of the arterial compliance, while the positive phase angle at higher frequencies reveals the dominance of inertial effects including reflections. The characteristic impedance of the pulmonary artery is the value of the input impedance had there been no reflections. Thus, the characteristic impedance cannot be measured directly in vivo. An estimate is generally obtained by averaging the impedance moduli for frequencies equal to or greater than the frequency of the first minimum (Milnor, 1982). Thus, the fluctuations due to reflections are essentially averaged out.

The characteristic impedance, the frequency of the first minimum and maximum, and other specific features of the input impedance spectrum then provide objective means of characterizing changes in the input impedance spectrum. Narrowing or dilation of the small arteries changes the input resistance and the wave reflection and thus the magnitudes of the maxima and the frequencies at which they occur. A decrease in compliance of the large arteries shifts the maxima and minima to higher frequencies. The characteristics impedance is increased by stiffening and/or narrowing of the arteries. As in the case of the vascular resistance, interpretation of the measured input impedance in terms of active responses of the pulmonary arterial tree is complicated by the fact that the vessel elastic properties and geometry are influenced by both active and passive factors. Thus, evaluation of the contribution of active and passive phenomenon can be problematic. In general, an increase in characteristic impedance is evidence for a decrease in compliance of the large arteries, whereas an increase in the input resistance is consistent with increased resistance in small vessels or elevated left atrial pressure.

Figure 6 shows the influence of serotonin infusion on the input impedance in the dog pulmonary artery. The interpretation of the response to serotonin in this study was that serotonin increased vascular resistance by constriction of small vessels and that the large pulmonary arteries were actively stiffened. This is reflected in the increase in the impedance modulus over the entire range of frequencies. The higher frequency of the zero crossing of the phase angle under the influence of serotonin suggests an increase in wave velocity and possibly a movement of reflection sites toward the pulmonary artery. In this study the impedance spectrum during isoproterenol infusion was not significantly different from control. The authors suggest that in the normal awake dog the pulmonary vasculature has so little tone that the vasodilating action of isoproterenol is of little consequence (Hammon et al., 1981).

A number of models of the pulmonary vascular bed have been proposed to assist in the interpretation of the input impedance. These models vary in the amount of detail they consider, ranging from the two-element windkessel model to models with representations of the individual vessel lengths, numbers, diameters, and viscoelastic wall properties (Attinger, 1963; Collins and Maccario, 1979; Engelberg and DuBois, 1959; Grant and Paradowski, 1987; Lucas, 1984; Milnor, 1982; Pollack et al., 1968; Radke et al., 1985; Rideout and Katra, 1969; Wiener et al., 1966). The detailed models have been particularly useful in revealing the potential sensitivity of the impedance spectrum to specific changes in geometry and wall properties within the vascular bed. From the standpoint of obtaining parameters descriptive of the pulmonary arterial tree from the phasic pressure-flow data, lumped element models having the minimum number of elements required to fit the data have been useful (Grant and Pardowski, 1987; Lucas, 1984).

Pulsatile pressure and flow measurments have also been used in alternative approaches for evaluating the influence of pulmonary vasomotion (Ingram et al., 1968; Milnor, 1972). The use of the nitrous oxide uptake method for measuring pulsatile pulmonary capillary flow has been particularly useful (Lee and DuBois, 1955; Morkin et al., 1964; Reuben, 1971; Reuben et al., 1970; Wasserman et al., 1966).

III. The Longitudinal Distribution of Pulmonary Vascular Resistance and Pressure

Attempts at evaluation of the arterial and venous sites of active changes in the intact lung have involved a variety of approaches. Commonly, these approaches have tended to be more invasive than those discussed above. In some cases this is because of the need for more direct access to the vessels, but control over passive influences to facilitate detection of active responses has also been important in these experimental approaches. This control is most easily accomplished in isolated lungs, and therefore, isolated lung preparations have been used extensively in these studies.

A. Direct Observation of Vessel Dimensions

Measurements of vessel diameters using dimension transducers (Dawson et al., 1978; Morgan et al., 1968; Patel et al., 1960, 1962) and microscopic (Capen and Wagner, 1982; Glazier and Murray, 1971; Kind and Gallemore, 1956; Wagner and Latham, 1975; Wearn et al., 1934) and angiographic (Allison and Stanbrook, 1980; Hirschman and Boucek, 1963; Lazaris et al., 1969; Sada et al., 1985, 1987; Shirai et al., 1986, 1987) methods have made possible observations of the action of vasoconstrictor and vasodilator stimuli on the smallest pulmonary vessels as well as on the large pulmonary arteries and veins. Using time-sequenced digital subtraction angiography, Sada et al. (1985, 1987, and Shirai et al., (1986, 1987) have measured the changes in small (about 500 to 100 μm in diameter) arterial and venous vessel diameters and local flows under a variety of conditions in cat lungs (Fig. 7). These vessels are in the size range of vessels identified as muscular vessels by Reid and co-workers (Reid, 1979; Reid and Meyrick, 1982; Simons and Reid, 1969) and are thus important sites of active vasomotion in the lungs.

B. Direct Measurements of Pressures

Direct measurements of vascular pressures in vessels within the lungs have also been used to determine sites of pulmonary vascular responses. Small venous catheters have been used extensively for studying the effects of vasomotion on pressure drops downstream from veins larger than about 400 μm in diameter (Aviado, 1960; Feeley et al., 1963; Gilbert et al., 1958; Hyman, 1968, 1969; Hyman et al., 1963; Kadowitz et al., 1975; Kuida et al., 1958; Kuramoto et al., 1962; Michel et al., 1984). Small wedge catheters have also been used to obtain pressures in small veins as a means of estimating microvascular pressures (Aviado, 1960; Gilbert et al., 1958; Kudia et al., 1958; Zidulka and Hakim, 1985). Bhattacharya and Staub (1980) introduced the subpleural vessel micropuncture method to measure pressures in vessels as small as 10 μm in diameter, and this method has been used to study the sites of vasoconstriction as well (Bhattacharya and Staub, 1980; Bhattacharya et al., 1982a, b; Nagasaka et al., 1984; Raj and Chen, 1986a, b; Raj et al., 1986a, b; 1987). A comparison of the pressures measured with small catheters and micropuncture of subpleural vessels in the normal lung is somewhat confusing. Bhattacharya and Staub (1980) found that about 46% of the total arterial-venous pressure drop was measured across subpleural vessels of dog lungs less than 10 μm in diameter and that 80% of the pressure drop was in vessels whose diameters were less than 20 μm. The pressure in veins larger than about 20 μm was virtually equal to left atrial pressure. These results are typical of those obtained using this technique. On the other hand, studies using small-catheter measurements have consistently reported pressure drops of 20-50% of the total arterial-venous pressure difference in much larger veins (Aviado, 1960; Feeley et al., 1963; Gilbert et al., 1958; Hyman, 1968, 1969; Hyman et al., 1963; Kadowitz et al., 1975; Kuida et al., 1958. Kuramato et al., 1962; Michel et al., 1984). The reasons for these apparent inconsistencies are not entirely clear. However, with respect to the latter method, obstruction due to a small vein catheter might decrease flow upstream from the site of the cathether tip. This might result in a pressure at the catheter tip which is closer to pulmonary arterial pressure than if the catheter were not there. In some cases the pres-

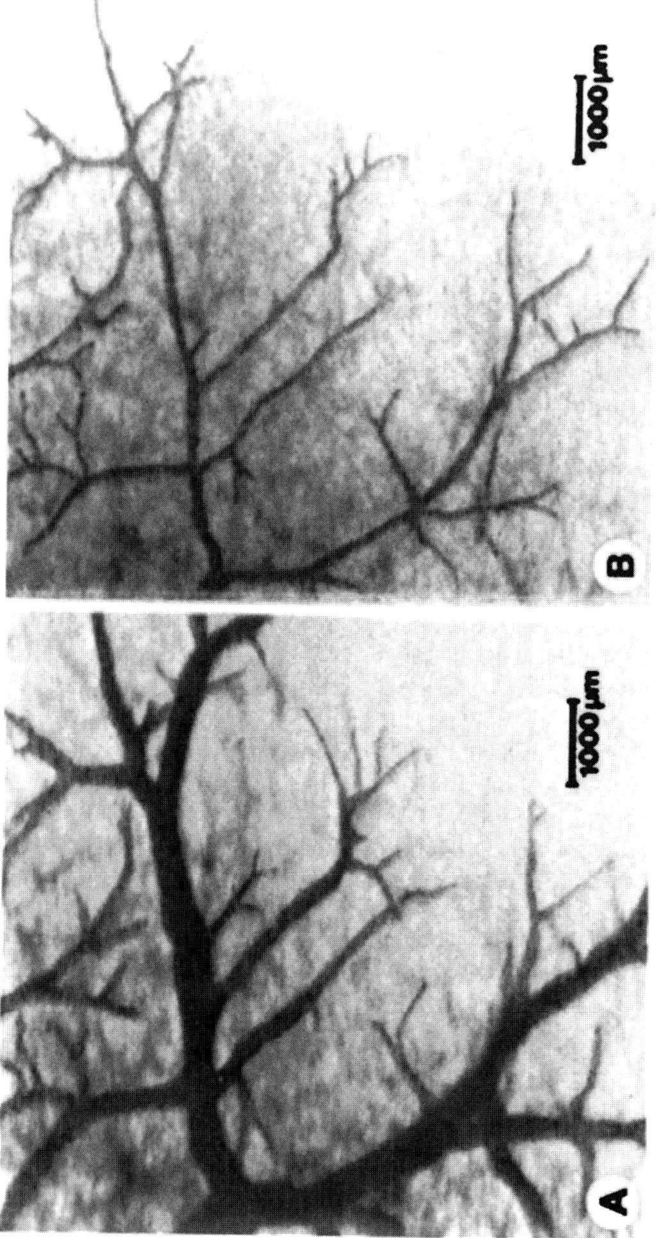

Figure 7 Angiograms of small pulmonary arteries of the cat (A) under control conditions and (B) during intravenous infusion of serotonin. (From Sada et al., 1985.)

sure drops attributed to large veins by the small-catheter method do appear to be rather large compared to estimates based on the morphometry of such large veins measured in human (Horsfield and Gordon, 1981) and (Zhuang et al., 1983) lungs. The interpretation of the subpleural vessel pressure data is complicated by the fact that geometry of the subpleural vessels is different from that of the intraparenchymal vessels. For example, the subpleural surface has less than half the intraparenchymal capillary density (Guntheroth et al., 1982). In addition, the transit times from main pulmonary artery to subpleural arterioles, and from subpleural arterioles to subpleural veins, are longer than normally assumed for mean pulmonary arterial (Dawson et al., 1987) and mean pulmonary capillary (Wagner et al., 1982) transit times, respectively, suggesting that the local flows are relatively low. Although flow continues through the impaled microvessels (Bhattacharya and Staub, 1980), some disruption of flow probably occurs in micropunctured vessels as well as in large catheterized vessels. How these considerations specifically influence the relationship between subpleural vessel pressures and pressure in vessels of similar size deeper in the lung parenchyma have not been clarified quantitatively. As with the small-catheter measurements, it is not clear whether the longitudinal pressure gradients suggested by the micropuncture data are consistent with the available morphometric data (Overholser et al., 1982; Zhuang et al., 1983). In regard to the present topic, it is not clear to what degree these questions regarding the direct measurement of pressures within the intrapulmonary vessels might interfere with interpretation of the data in terms of sites of active responses.

C. Indirect Methods

As a result of some questions regarding the interpretation of the direct measurements, and because the direct measurements can be difficult to obtain under certain conditions, indirect approaches have been used as well. For example, sites of vasomotion have been inferred from changes in capillary volume measured using the DL_{CO} method (Hyde et al., 1964; Lewis et al., 1960; Wanner et al., 1978; Young et al., 1963) and from the changes in arterial volume using the ether transit time method (Dawson et al., 1975; Friedman and Wanner, 1977; Quebbeman and Dawson, 1977; Reuben et al., 1970; Sackner et al., 1966; Wanner et al., 1978). Several indirect approaches to the calculation of longitudinal segmental resistances have also been carried out.

Low-Viscosity Bolus

Piiper (1970) conceived of a method for evaluating the longitudinal distribution of vascular resistance by observing the time-varying changes in arterial pressure that occur when a bolus having a viscosity different from that of blood passes through the lung vasculature from artery to veins. Modified versions of this method have been used to evaluate the sites of both passive and active pulmonary vascular responses (Brody and Stemmler, 1968; Dawson et al., 1977, 1978, 1979; Grimm et al., 1977; Hakim et al., 1983). When an injected bolus has viscosity lower than that of blood, its passage through the vascular bed will produce a decrease in the arterial to venous pressure gradient (Pa–Pv). The magnitude of this decrease will follow a time course that depends on the longitudinal location of the bolus within the vascular bed at a given time and the preinjection resistance at that location. Thus, the decrease in Pa–Pv will be largest when the bolus is located in regions of highest preinjection resistance. Figure 8 shows an example of the time variation in the arterial–venous pressure gradient as a saline bolus passed through a dog lung lobe. Representing the instantaneous longitudinal resistance distribution as a finite sum of individual serial resistances, the arterial-venous pressure gradient is related to flow and the time-varying resistance distribution by

$$P_a(t) - P_v(t) = \dot{Q} \sum_{k=1}^{N} R_k(t) \tag{14}$$

where $\dot{Q}$ is the steady flow through the lung and R_k is the resistance of the *k*th serial segment. R_k changes with time as the viscosity μ within segment k changes with time during the bolus passage. Thus, the change in resistance $\Delta R_k(t)$ due to the bolus passage is

$$\Delta R_k(t) = \alpha_k \Delta\mu_k(t) \tag{15}$$

and

$$\Delta(P_a(t) - P_v(t)) = \dot{Q} \sum_{k=1}^{N} \alpha_k \Delta\mu_k(t) \tag{16}$$

where α_k is the segmental geometric factor, $\Delta\mu_k(t)$ is the change in viscosity due to the mixture of bolus and blood in the segment, and $\Delta(P_a(t)–P_v(t))$ is the change in the arterial-venous pressure gradient from its preinjection value. Given the measured values of $\Delta(P_a(t)–P_v(t))$ and $\dot{Q}$, the α_k's could be calculated directly from a system of *N* simultaneous algebraic equations if the $\Delta\mu_k(t)$ values were known. The $\Delta\mu(t)$ at the arterial inlet, $\Delta\mu_a(t)$, and venous outlet, $\Delta\mu_v(t)$, can be measured (Dawson et al., 1988; Grimm et al., 1977), but the bolus disperses as it passes through the vascular bed (Fig. 8). Thus, some assumption about the dispersion of the bolus must be made to obtain the $\Delta\mu_k(t)$ values for each segment. We have assumed that the dispersion of the bolus from the arterial inlet to the end of the *k*th segment occurs with a relative dispersion

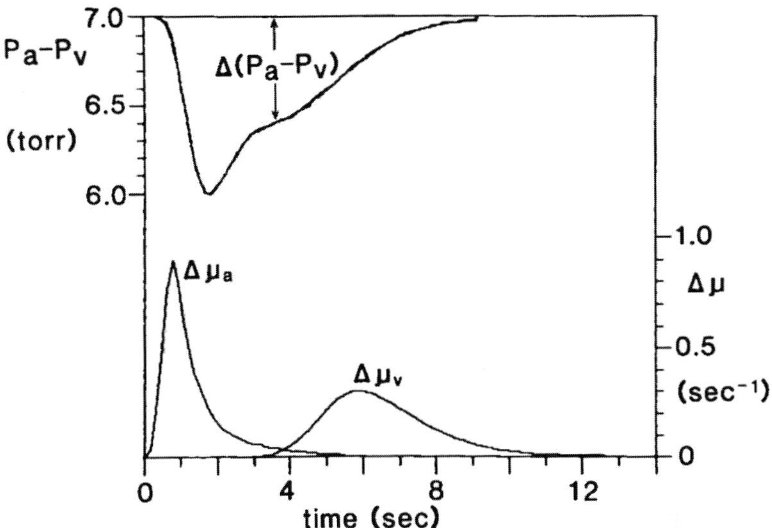

Figure 8 The change in the arterial venous pressure difference, $\Delta(P_a - P_v)$, that was observed when a bolus of saline passed through an isolated dog lung lobe. $\Delta\mu_a$ and $\Delta\mu_v$ are the changes in blood viscosity at the lobar artery and lobar vein. The $\Delta\mu$ curves are normalized to unit area, and an increase in the normalized $\Delta\mu$ values represents a decrease in viscosity. The dispersion of the bolus as it passes through the vascular bed is indicated by the decrease in the height of the peak and the increase in the spread of the $\Delta\mu_v$ curve compared to the $\Delta\mu_a$ curve.

equal to the relative dispersion of the whole lung (Dawson et al., 1988). This assumption results in a smooth transition of the bolus from inlet to outlet and allows the $\Delta\mu_k(t)$'s to be estimated from the probability density function of bolus transit times through the lung. This bolus transit time distribution, referred to as the *organ transport function* (Bassinghwaighte, 1970), can be obtained by numerical deconvolution of $\Delta\mu_a(t)$ and $\Delta\mu_v(t)$, given that

$$\Delta\mu_v(t) = \int_0^t \Delta\mu_a(\lambda)h(t-\lambda)\,d\lambda \tag{17}$$

where h(t) is the organ transport function. The $h_k(t)$'s (the distribution of transit times from arterial inlet to the outlet of the *k*th segment) are then obtained from

$$h_k(t) = \frac{N}{k}\,h\left(\frac{N}{k}\,t\right) \tag{18}$$

and the $\Delta\mu_k$'s are calculated from the convolution integral

$$\Delta\mu_k(t) = \int_0^t \Delta\mu_a(\lambda) h_k(t-\lambda)\, d\lambda \tag{19}$$

Thus, the measured $\Delta\mu_a(t)$ and $\Delta\mu_v(t)$ curves can be used to obtain the $\Delta\mu_k(t)$ values required to solve system (16) for the α_k's. Figure 9 shows an example of the calculated $\Delta\mu_k(t)$ curves as a bolus passed through a dog lung lobe.

System (16) tends to be ill conditioned in the presence of even a small degree of noise in the experimental data. This problem has been dealt with by various methods (Brody et al., 1968; Grimm et al., 1977). Recently, we have found that the damped least squares method for solving system (16) for the unknown α_k's is an improvement on previous methods (Dawson et al., 1988). Using this method to solve the for α_k's, the segmental R_k's can then be obtained from

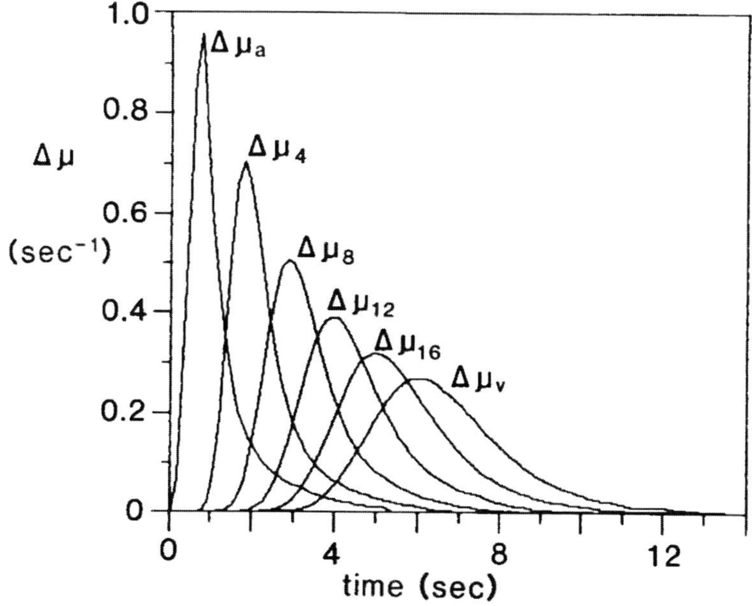

Figure 9 An example of the measured $\Delta\mu_a$ and $\Delta\mu_v$ curves and four of the $\Delta\mu_k$ curves calculated according to Eqs. (13)-(15). The $\Delta\mu$ curves are normalized to unit area, and an increase in the normalized $\Delta\mu$ values represents a decrease in viscosity. For clarity, only four of the many $\Delta\mu_k$ curves are shown.

$$R_k(0) = \alpha_k \mu(0) \tag{20}$$

where $\mu(0)$ is the steady-state viscosity.

These serial $R_k(0)$'s are located on a cumulative volume scale from arterial inlet to venous outlet. The cumulative volume from the arterial inlet to the end of the *k*th segment is obtained from the product of $\dot{Q}$ and the mean transit time $\bar{t}_k$ of $h_k(t)$, where

$$\bar{t}_k = \int_0^\infty t h_k(t)\, dt \tag{21}$$

An example of a resulting resistance-cumulative volume profile for a dog lung lobe is shown in Figure 10.

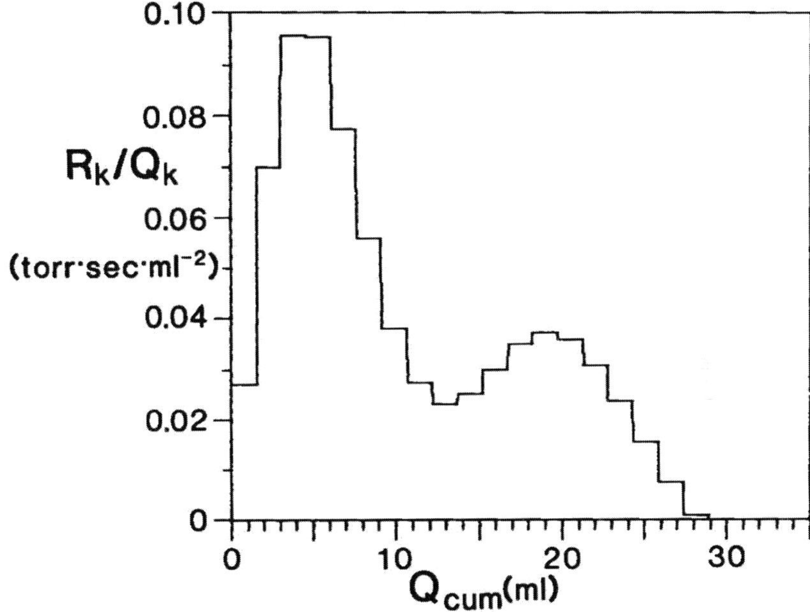

Figure 10 An example of the distribution resistance per unit volume, R_k/Q_k, versus cumulative vascular volume Q_{cum} from a dog lung lobe obtained using the low-viscosity bolus method. The cumulative volume begins at zero at the arterial inlet and ends at the venous outlet, which in this example gives a total volume of about 29 ml. The area under the graph is the total lobar vascular resistance.

The interpretation of the resistance distribution obtained using this low-viscosity bolus method is also potentially complicated. The model represents the vascular bed as series volume elements, and the volume segments are defined in terms of the transit time from the arterial inlet. Since the lung is made up of parallel paths having different flow rates, lengths, and volumes, each of the series volume elements that are identified in terms of increasing values of t_k potentially includes a mix of vessels of different sizes and types. For example, the first volume element closest to the arterial inlet includes only or mostly arteries. However, proceeding from the arterial inlet to the venous outlet, the volume elements become a mix of large and small arteries, then small arteries and capillaries, capillaries and small veins, and so on. The fact that a bimodal distribution is obtained suggests that, on the average, the various parallel pathways are sufficiently homogenous that the relatively high resistance per unit volume in the small arteries and veins along each pathway is reflected by the upstream and downstream modes, respectively, in the distribution. This allows for detection of changes in the arterial and venous resistances and an estimate of the mean capillary pressure from the sum of the resistances downstream from the centrally located relative minimum of the distribution and the steady flow rate. However, the probable heterogeneity of vessel types within each volume segment precludes the assignment of specific values of resistance to the arterial, capillary, and venous segments. In addition, since vessel constriction or relaxation can change local volumes either actively or passively, the anatomical composition of the *k*th volume segment is not necessarily the same from one condition to another. Figures 11 and 12 show how the resistance distribution can be altered by vasoconstriction in an isolated dog lung lobe. These figures suggest that serotonin constricted the intralobar arteries while norepinephrine constricted both the arteries and veins.

Vascular Occlusion

The transient pressure data obtained immediately following rapid occlusion of the venous outflow, the arterial inflow, or both contain information about the longitudinal distribution of vascular resistance versus compliance in the pulmonary vascular bed (Bronikowski et al., 1984, 1985; Cope et al., 1986; Dawson et al., 1986; Hakim et al., 1979, 1982a, b, 1983; Holloway et al., 1983; Linehan and Dawson, 1983; Linehan et al., 1982, 1986; Parker et al., 1983; Rock et al., 1985). The data provide for an approach to the evaluation of sites of action by taking advantage of the fact that the muscular pulmonary arteries and veins are located upstream and downstream, respectively, from the compliant capillary bed. The result of this configuration of the pulmonary vascular bed is that the occlusion data can provide information as to anatomical sites of action as well as the resistance-compliance distribution (Dawson et al., 1982; Hakim et al., 1979, 1983; Linehan and Dawson, 1983; Linehan et al., 1982). Of the methods used to

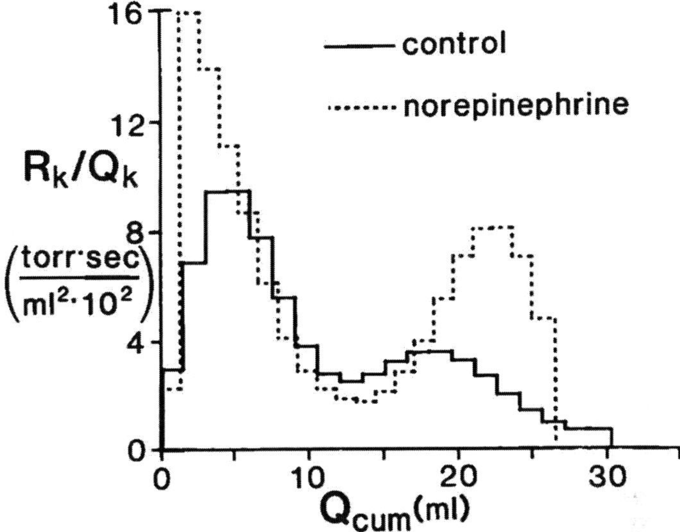

Figure 11 The effect of norepinephrine infusion on the resistance versus volume distribution in an isolated dog lung lobe. See Figure 10 for explanation.

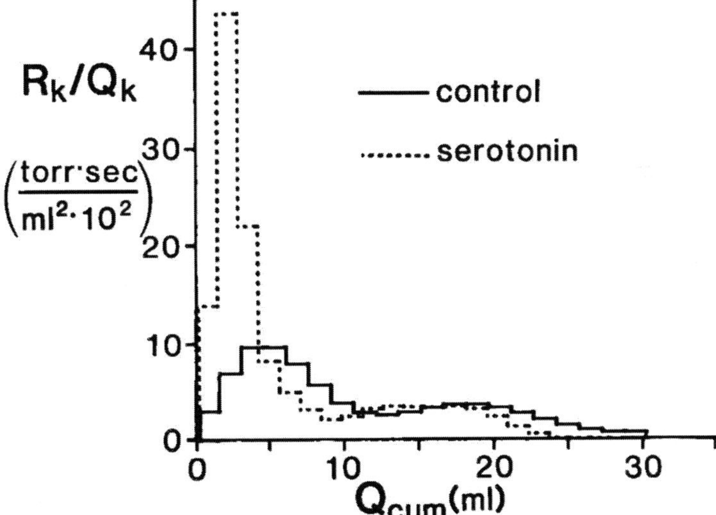

Figure 12 The effect of serotonin infusion on the resistance versus volume distribution in an isolated dog lung lobe. See Figure 10 for explanation.

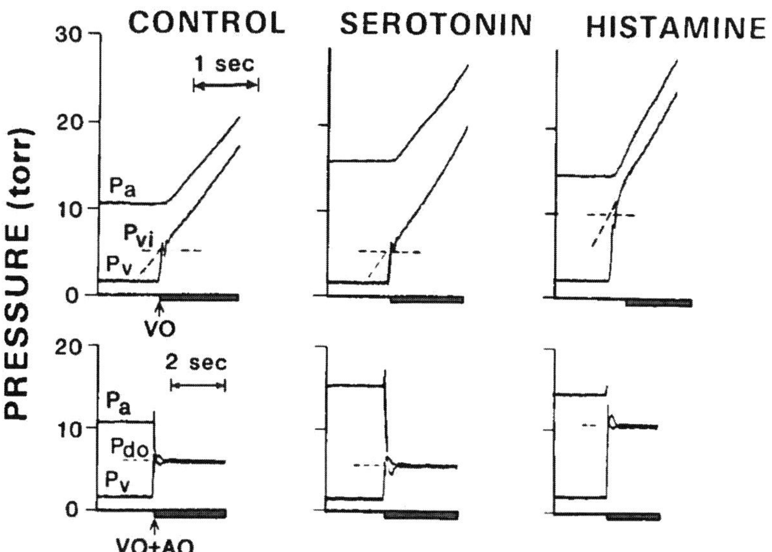

Figure 13 The arterial P_a and venous P_v pressure responses following venous occlusion, VO (top row), or simultaneous venous and arterial occlusion, VO+AO (bottom row), in an isolated dog lung lobe. The horizontal dashed line designated P_{vi} is the pressure obtained by extrapolating the nearly linear portion of the P_v curve back to the instant of venous occlusion. The horizontal dashed line designated P_{do} is the equilibrium pressure reached by both P_a and P_v following simultaneous arterial and venous occlusion. The relationships between P_a, P_v, P_{vi}, and P_{do} are altered by vasoconstriction induced by serotonin and histamine infusion. (From Dawson, 1984, and Dawson et al., 1982.)

determine the arterial and venous sites of action, the rapid flow occlusion methods described below are probably the easiest to perform.

When the venous outflow from a lung lobe is rapidly occluded, the venous pressure undergoes a rapid jump, which is followed by a slower, almost linear and parallel, increase in both arterial and venous pressures (Fig. 13). The magnitude of the rapid jump in relation to the total arterial-venous pressure difference varies depending on the distribution of the vascular resistance relative to the distribution of vascular compliance. A simple hemodynamic model that can explain these most obvious features of the pressure curves is shown as an electrical analog T section in Figure 14. In this model, when flow through the downstream resistance (R_v) stops as the result of opening the switch just downstream from P_v (venous occlusion), the venous pressure jumps immediately to the preocclusion pressure P_{vi} at the central compliance C_L. Since the flow $\dot{Q}$ through

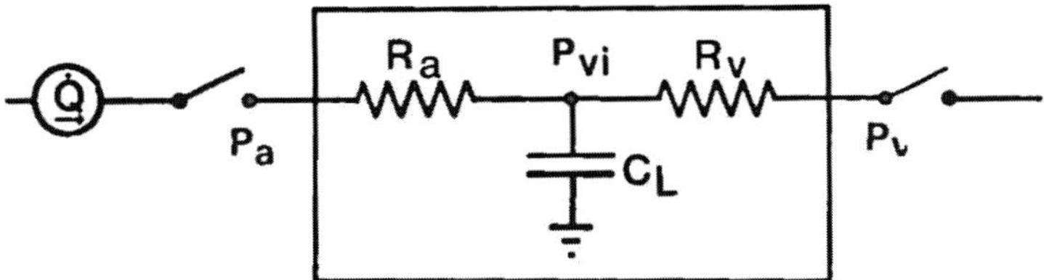

Figure 14 A model representing the pulmonary vascular bed as an electrical analog single T section. P_a is the arterial pressure, P_v is the venous pressure; and R_a and R_v are resistances upstream and downstream, respectively from the vascular compliance C_L. In this model the switches upstream from P_a and downstream from P_v would be closed during normal steady flow. When the downstream switch is opened (venous occlusion), the venous pressure will jump to P_{vi} and the P_a and P_v will rise in parallel as C_L is filled by the constant inflow Q. (From Dawson et al., 1984.)

R_a remains constant following the occlusion, the pressure P_{vi} of the volume storage element will equal P_v, which will increase linearly with time, $dP_v/dt = \dot{Q}/C_L$. The pressure, P_a, upstream of R_a will rise in parallel with P_v according to $P_a = P_v + R_a\dot{Q}$. This model can also explain the rapid fall and subsequent exponential decay in arterial pressure following rapid occlusion of the arterial inflow to a lung lobe (Fig. 15) and the rapid convergence of arterial and venous pres-

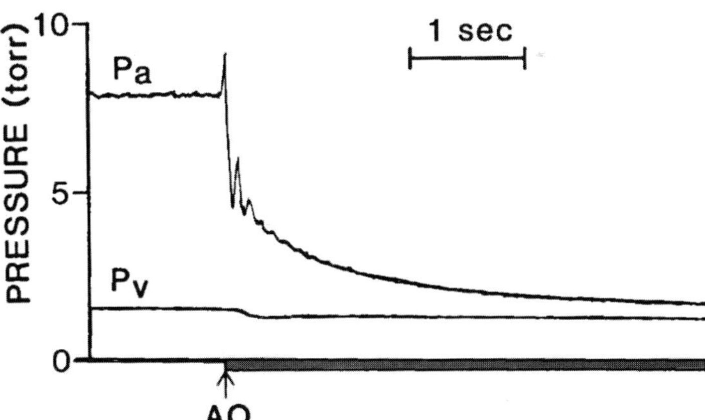

Figure 15 The arterial P_a and venous P_v pressures following occlusion of the arterial inflow to an isolated dog lung lobe at AO. The arterial pressure curve is characterized by a rapid fall and then a slower exponential decrease with time. (From Dawson, 1984.)

sures when both arterial inflow and venous outflow are rapidly occluded (Fig. 13). The magnitude of the rapid jumps observed following these occlusion maneuvers are quite sensitive to the arterial or venous site of changes in pulmonary vascular resistance (Dawson et al., 1982; Hakim et al., 1979, 1983; Linehan and Dawson, 1983; Linehan et al., 1982), and estimates of the changes in arterial and venous resistances can be made using the simple model in Figure 14 (Dawson et al., 1982; Hakim et al., 1979).

Although the model in Figure 14 accounts for the dominant characteristics of the experimental data following the occlusions, there are some less obvious features of the data that suggest the applicability of more distributed models. A feature not predicted by the model is the short time delay following venous occlusion before the arterial pressure begins to rise (Fig. 16). In addition, following double occlusion the equilibrium pressure P_{do} is a little larger than P_{vi} obtained from venous occlusion, and following arterial occlusion the rapid fall in arterial pressure doesn't quite reach the value of P_{vi} obtained during venous

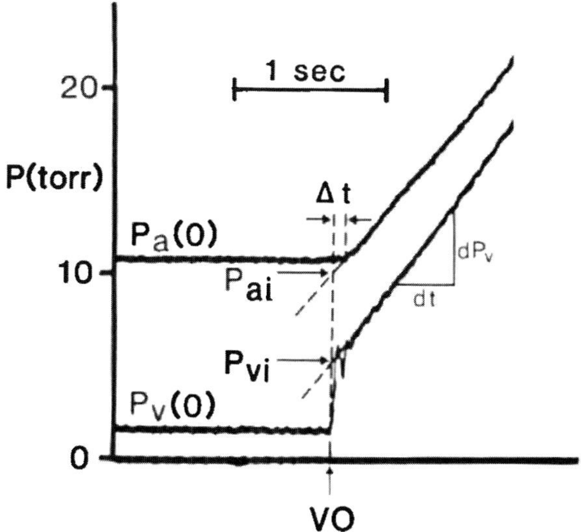

Figure 16 An example of the response of the arterial P_a and venous P_v pressures when the venous outflow from a dog lung lobe was suddenly occluded at VO. P_{ai} and P_{vi} are pressures obtained by extrapolating the nearly linear portions of $P_a(t)$ and $P_v(t)$ back to the time of occlusion. The slope of the nearly linear portion of the venous pressures curves is dP_v/dt. There is a small time delay Δt following venous occlusion before $P_a(t)$ begins to rise in parallel with $P_a(t)$.

occlusion. These differences between the data and simple model predictions appear to be due to the fact that, contrary to the compartmental model in Figure 14, the resistance and compliance are actually continuously distributed from artery to vein. For the venous occlusion data there are two more distributed RC networks that contain the largest number of symmetrically arranged compartmental resistances and compliances that can be assigned unique values using the pressure intercepts P_{ai} and P_{vi} obtained by extrapolating the arterial and venous pressure curve back to the instant of occlusion as in Figure 16 (Linehan et al., 1982). These more distributed models are depicted in Figure 17.

For model 1, the slope of the nearly linear, slowly rising portion of the venous pressure curve in Figure 16 can be used to calculate a vascular compliance, C_1, according to

$$C_L = C_u + C_d = \frac{\dot{Q}}{dP_v/dt} \tag{22}$$

In the model, the symmetry comes from setting $C_u = C_d$, so that the analysis of model 1 yields algebraic equations that can be used to determine the serial hemodynamic resistances R_a, R_c, and R_v, from the flow rate, $\dot{Q}$, the preoc-

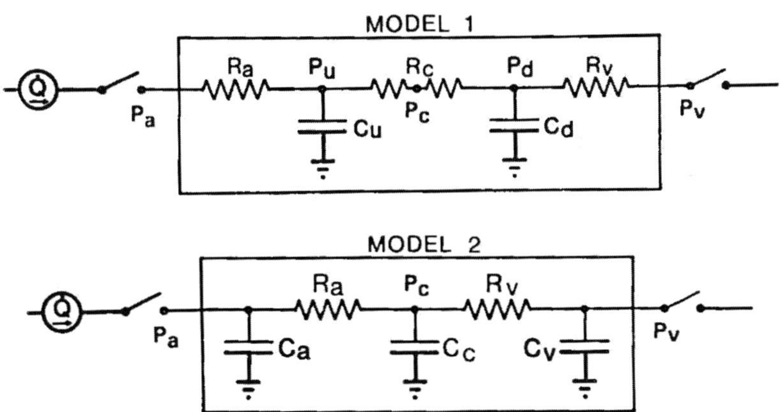

Figure 17 Two compartmental RC models that can account for both P_{vi} and P_{ai} obtained from the venous occlusion experiment. P_v is the venous pressure and P_a the arterial pressure. The switches upstream from P_a and downstream from P_v would be closed during normal steady flow. The downstream switches would be opened to simulate venous occlusion. The relationships between the R's, C's, and internal pressures following occlusion are indicated in the text. (From Dawson et al., 1984.)

clusion arterial and venous pressures, $P_a(0)$ and $P_v(0)$, and P_{ai} and P_{vi} (Linehan et al., 1982). The total vascular resistance, R_L, can be subdivided into the segmental resistances using these data as follows:

$$R_v = [P_{vi} - P_v(0) - P_a(0) + P_{ai}]/\dot{Q} \tag{23}$$

$$R_c = 4[P_a(0) - P_{ai}]/\dot{Q} \tag{24}$$

and

$$R_a = R_L - R_c - R_v \tag{25}$$

where

$$R_L = [P_a(0) - P_v(0)]/\dot{Q} \tag{26}$$

The preocclusion pressure at the midpoint of R_c, referred to as $P_c(0)$, is also theoretically equal to the equilibrium arterial and venous pressure following double occlusion, P_{do}, but it can also be calculated from the venous occlusion data according to

$$P_c(0) = P_a(0) - P_{ai} + P_{vi} \tag{27}$$

For model 2 the vascular compliance is

$$C_L = C_a + C_c + C_v = \frac{\dot{Q}}{dP_v/dt} \tag{28}$$

Setting $C_a = C_v$, the central compliance C_c and the upstream and downstream resistances, R_u and R_d, respectively, can be calculated from

$$C_c = C_L \left[\frac{4P_{ai} - 3P_a(0) - P_v(0)}{P_a(0) - P_v(0)}\right]^{1/2} \tag{29}$$

$$R_d = R_L \left[\frac{P_{vi} - P_v(0)}{P_a(0) - P_v(0)} - 0.25\left(1 - \frac{C_c}{C_L}\right)^2\right]\frac{C_L}{C_c} \tag{30}$$

$$R_u = R_L - R_d \tag{31}$$

For model 2 the preocclusion pressure at C_c is $P_c(0)$, and

$$P_c(0) = [P_a(0) - P_v(0)](R_d/R_L) + P_v(0) \tag{32}$$

These two alternative models can represent the key features of the data in the time period shortly after venous occlusion and provide an estimate of the microvascular pressure $P_c(0)$. The arterial occlusion data, such as shown in Figure 15, can theoretically provide an additional piece of information that allows for the individual compartmental compliances to vary independently (Dawson et al., 1984). For example, if in model 1, C_u and C_d are allowed to vary independently, then for venous occlusion,

$$\left(\frac{R_c}{R_L}\right)\left(\frac{C_u C_d}{C_L{}^2}\right) = \frac{P_a(0) - P_{ai}}{P_a(0) - P_v(0)} \tag{33}$$

and

$$\left(\frac{R_c}{R_L}\right)\left(\frac{C_u{}^2}{C_L{}^2}\right) + R_v/R_L = \frac{P_{vi} - P_v(0)}{P_a(0) - P_v(0)} \tag{34}$$

Equations (22), (26), (33), and (34) are four equations in the five unknowns R_a/R_L, $R_c/R_v/R_L$, C_u/C_L, and C_d/C_L. To obtain a fifth independent equation, P_u and P_d are defined to be the pressures of the compliances C_u and C_d, respectively. The steady state is described by the pressures $P_a(0)$, $P_u(0)$, $P_d(0)$, and $P_v(0)$ and the flow $\dot{Q}$. For arterial occlusion, the arterial switch is opened while P_v is held constant at $P_v(0)$. From the analysis of this model, the arterial pressure P_a undergoes a jump discontinuity from $P_a(0)$ to $P_u(0)$ the instant the arterial switch is opened, and thus

$$P_a(0) = P_u(0) + R_a\dot{Q} \tag{35}$$

For times $t>0$, $P_a(t)$ is the sum of two decreasing expontials of the form

$$P_a(t) = a_1\, e^{(-k_1 t)} + a_2\, e^{(-k_2 t)} + P_v(0) \tag{36}$$

This suggests fitting the $P_a(t)$ data with two exponentials using a multiexpoential curve-fitting technique to determine the zero time intercept, $P_u(0)=a_1+a_2+P_v(0)$. Thus, R_a/R_L can be calculated by combining Eqs. (26) and (35) to give

$$\frac{R_a}{R_L} = \frac{P_a(0) - P_u(0)}{P_a(0) - P_v(0)} \tag{37}$$

Using Eqs. (22), (25), (33), (34), and (37), C_u/C_L and R_c/R_L in terms of the measured pressures are

$$\frac{C_u}{C_L} = \frac{P_a(0) - P_{ai}}{P_u(0) - P_{vi} - P_a(0) + P_{ai}} \tag{38}$$

and

$$\frac{R_c}{R_L} = \frac{[P_u(0) - P_{vi} - P_a(0) + P_{ai}]^2}{[P_a(0) - P_v(0)]\,[P_u(0) - P_{vi} - 2P_a(0) + 2P_{ai}]} \tag{39}$$

Then C_d/C_L and R_v/R_L can be calculated directly from Eqs. (22) and (25) respectively. Since C_L and R_L can be determined from Eqs. (22) and (26), respectively, R_a, R_c, R_v, C_u, and C_d can be calculated from the combined data obtained from a venous occlusion and an arterial occlusion. The use of the arterial occlusion data as described above is, however, subject to the vagaries of multi-exponential curve fitting and other considerations that make it more difficult to apply in practice than the venous and double occlusion approaches (Dawson et al., 1984).

These compartmental approaches allow for the calculation of specific compartmental parameters. The behavior of the compartmental parameters in response to pulmonary vasoconstriction suggests that, even though the resistance and compliance are actually continuously distributed, they are distributed in such a way that the arterial and venous sites of changes in resistance can be identified using the compartmental models. This is despite the fact that the compartmental parameter values do not correspond precisely to anatomical compartments such as arteries, capillaries, and veins.

To further evaluate the relationship between the compartmental models and the actual continuous distribution producing the venous occlusion data, we have examined the theoretical bounds that can be placed on the continuous distribution of resistance and compliance by $P_a(0)$, $P_v(0)$, P_{ai}, and P_{vi} obtained from the venous occlusion data (Bronikowski et al., 1984, 1985). The results of the analysis, which give specific boundaries for the continuous distribution compatible with the venous occlusion data, are most easily visualized by representing the resistance versus compliance distribution as a graph of cumulative resistance versus cumulative compliance. All cumulative R versus C graphs that are compatible with the steady-state pressures $P_a(0)$ and $P_v(0)$ and pressures P_{ai} and P_{vi} are continuously increasing functions within the hatched region defined in Figure 18. In other words, they all have a shape similar to the shape of the region itself. If P_c is now defined as the pressure at the midpoint of the cumulative vascular compliance, one important result of this analysis of the continuous model is that the measurable pressure data can be thought of as placing

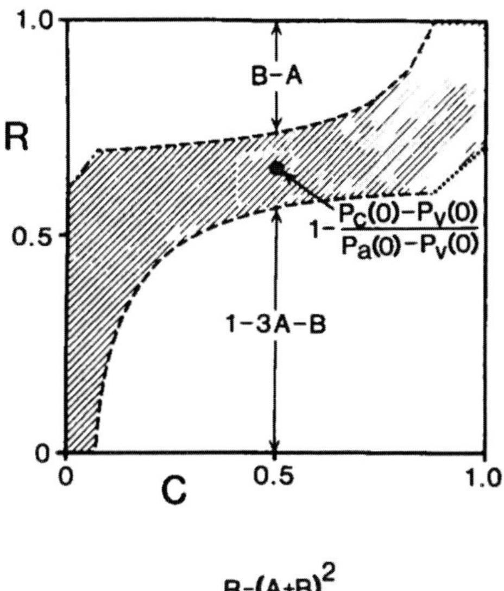

-·-·-·-·- $R = \dfrac{B-(A+B)^2}{C^2-2(A+B)C+B}$

------ $R = 1-A-B+\dfrac{A}{1-C}$

----- $R = 1-A-B-\dfrac{A}{C}$

·········· $R = \dfrac{(C-A-B)^2}{C^2-2(A+B)C+B}$

Figure 18 The shaded region contains all possible cmululative resistance versus compliance dis-butions that can fit P_{ai} and P_{vi}. On this graph R is the cumulative vascular resistance beginning from the arterial inlet at R = 0, divided by the total vascular resistance R_L; C is the cumulative vascular compliance beginning from the arterial inlet at C = 0, divided by the total vascular compliance C_L. Thus, 1.0 on the vertical and horizontal axes represents the total vascular resistance and compliance, respectively, accumulated from arterial inlet to venous outlet. The lower bounds on the fractions of the total vascular resistance upstream and downstream from the midpoint of the cumulative compliance (c = 0.5) and $1-3\,A-B$ and $B-A$, respectively, where $A = [P_a(0)-P_{ai}]/[P_a(0)-P_v(0)]$ and $B = [P_{vi} - P_v(0)]\ /\ P_a(0)-P_v(0)]$. B+A is the fraction of the total resistance downstream from $P_c(0)$ as defined by Eq. (23) and located by the dot in the middle of the shaded region. However, if P_c is defined specifically as the pressure at the compliance midpoint, it could fall anywhere between the upper and lower boundaries of the shaded region at C = 0.5. Thus, $(B-A) \leqslant [P_c-P_v(0)]/[P_a(0)] \leqslant B+3A$. (From Bronikowski et al., 1984, 1985.)

secure bounds on the value of P_c regardless of the actual continuous distribution of resistance versus compliance as shown in Figure 18. Figure 19 shows the influence of vasoconstriction in dog lung lobes on the location of P_c along the intravascular pressure drop from lobar artery to lobar vein. The fact that with vasoconstriction the shaded sections of the horizontal bars change relatively little in comparison to the change in the total pressure drop is consistent with the concept that these vasoconstrictor stimuli act primarily upstream and/or downstream from a centrally located relatively compliant region.

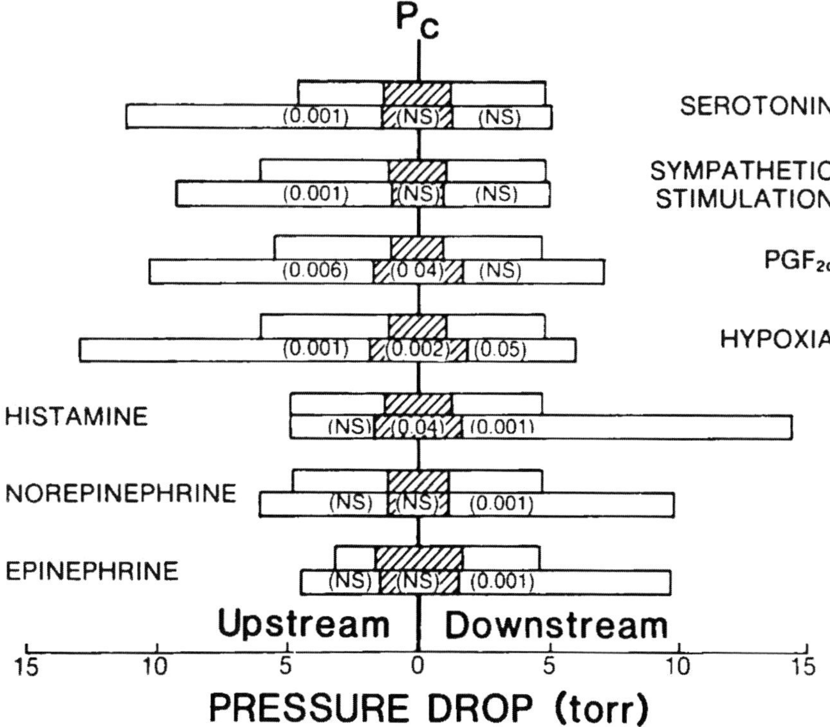

Figure 19 The influence of vasoconstriction with various stimuli on the pressure drops upstream (arterial) and downstream (venous) to P_c as determined from venous occlusion on in situ perfused dog lung lobes. The upper bar of each pair of horizontal bars is for the control or vasodilated state. The lower bar represents the result after vasoconstriction with the designated stimulus. Sympathetic stimulation refers to electrical stimulation of the stellate ganglion. The hatched section of each bar is 4 $[P_a(0) - P_{ai}]$ centered at P_c defined by Eq. (27). The unshaded bar to the left (upstream) is the lower bound on the pressure drop upstream from the midpoint of the vascular compliance, and the unshaded bar on the right (downstream) is the lower bound on the pressure drop downstream from the compliance midpoint. (From Dawson et al., 1984.)

If a balloon-tipped catheter is placed in a lobar artery and then inflated to obtain a wedge pressure, the time course of the fall in pressure at the catheter tip contains information about the resistance versus compliance distribution between the catheter tip and the left atrium. Holloway et al. (1983) and Cope et al. (1986) have investigated the use of this arterial occlusion approach for evaluating capillary pressure in vivo. When the balloon was inflated they observed a fairly rapid fall followed by slower decay, reminiscent of the response of the simple RC model. This approach has the promise of being useful for estimating pulmonary capillary pressure in vivo. However, it can be difficult to identify a clear break in the decay curve, and back extrapolation of the exponential decay can be equivocal. On the other hand, pulmonary vasoconstriction with arterial or venous constrictors shows clear differences in the exponential decay of the catheter tip pressure to the steady wedge pressure (Cope et al., 1986). When pulmonary diastolic pressure is high relative to left arterial pressure, a rapid fall in the catheter tip pressure to the steady wedge pressure suggests that capillary pressure is close to left atrial pressure, whereas a slow fall in pressure suggests that capillary pressure is closer to arterial pressure. Thus, methods for objectively evaluating these pressure curves should prove useful for evaluating the site of elevated resistance in vivo.

Some conclusions regarding the occlusion data are as follows. The occlusion data contain information about the longitudinal distribution of resistance versus compliance in the pulmonary vascular bed and the sites of resistance changes. The venous occlusion data allow one to determine the value of an intravascular pressure, P_c, from Eq. (27) that can be thought of as a pressure at a point located along the arterial-to-venous distribution of cumulative vascular compliance where half the compliance is upstream and half is downstream. P_c can be found in the sense that an upper and lower bound on its value can be calculated in a simple manner using the venous occlusion data. When the upper and lower bounds are narrow, the vascular compliance is concentrated near P_c. This configuration of the resistance versus compliance distribution in the lung lobe results in a situation wherein P_c and the double occlusion pressure P_{do} are essentially equal. Although the double occlusion procedure alone does not allow bounds to be determined, it is particularly useful for obtaining microvascular pressure in studies of lung fluid balance (Selig et al., 1986) because it can be obtained without the transient increase or decrease in microvascular pressure produced during arterial or venous occlusion, respectively. It is also useful for studying the lung in situ (Dawson et al., 1982). The addition of the other occlusion maneuvers such as arterial occlusion may provide additional information that can specify parameters in more complex models and thus provide a more detailed analysis of the mechanics of the pulmonary circulation. The venous occlusion method has the advantage that the data used in the analysis are obtained during a quasi steady state after the effects of the inertance of the blood have essentially died out (Bronikowski et al., 1984; Linehan et al., 1982). Since no such steady state exists in the time frame of interest following arterial occlusion, the influence of inertial effects, manifest by pressure oscillations immediately following the occlusion, are more difficult to deal with. The simple models discussed here ignore the viscous wall properties and nonlinear behavior of the resistances and compliances of the vessels as functions of vascular volume. These aspects of the occlusion data have also been evaluated to some extent using more complex models (Linehan et al., 1986).

Isogravimetric Method

Another approach to evaluating pressure-flow relations in terms of the site of active pulmonary vascular responses is the isogravimetric method of Pappenheimer and Soto-Rivera (1948) originally applied to the lungs by Gaar et al. (1967). In this method, the total vascular resistance is conceptualized as two series segments, one located upstream and one downstream from a pressure equal to the mean pressure controlling fluid filtration. This pressure is a virtual capillary pressure P_{ci}. The rate of change in lung weight measured under conditions of constant vascular pressure and vascular volume is assumed to be equal to the net rate of fluid transport across the vessel walls between vascular and interstitial spaces. When the weight does not change with time, the lung is defined as being isogravimetric. When the lungs are isogravimetric, the flow rate $\dot{Q}_i$ through the upstream resistance R_a equals the flow rate through the downstream resistance R_v. That is,

$$\dot{Q}_i = \frac{P_a - P_{ci}}{R_a} = \frac{P_{ci} - P_v}{R_v} \tag{40}$$

Thus,

$$P_v = -\dot{Q}_i R_v + P_{ci} \tag{41}$$

and

$$P_a = \dot{Q}_i R_a + P_{ci} \tag{42}$$

In addition, for the isogravimetric state to obtain,

$$P_{ci} = P_{is} + \pi_c - \pi_{is} \tag{43}$$

where P_{is} is the interstitial pressure, and π_c and π_{is} are the intracapillary and interstitial oncotic pressures, respectively.

The goal of the experimental protocol is to quantify P_{ci}. To this end P_a and P_v are measured at two or more values of $\dot{Q}_i$. The value of P_{ci} and R_v or R_a can then be calculated from Eqs. (41) or (42), respectively, assuming that π_c, π_{is}, and P_{is} do not vary from one value of $\dot{Q}_i$ to the next. In practice, several values of $\dot{Q}_i$ are usually obtained by adjusting P_a and P_v to several different levels, and then P_{ci}, R_a, and R_v are calculated by linear regression analysis of the

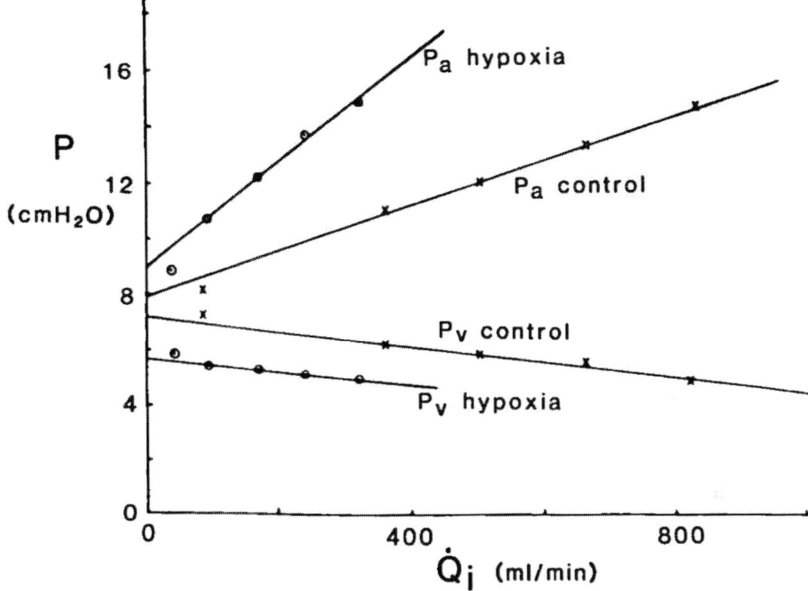

Figure 20 Graph of pulmonary arterial, P_a, and venous, P_v, pressures is isogravimetric flow $\dot{Q}_i$ was reduced in a dog lung. (X) values obtained when lung was ventilated with 95% O_2-5% CO_2 (control); (O) values obtained while the lung was ventilated with 95% N_2-5% CO_2 (hypoxia). The linear extrapolations of the arterial and venous cruves do not always converge at the ordinate, and thus the average of the intercepts is often taken as P_{ci}. The slopes are related to the resistances upstream (R_a) and downstream (R_v) from P_{ci} according to Eqs. (41) and (42). (Data from Parker et al., 1981.)

P_v or P_a and $\dot{Q}_i$ data to fit Eqs. (41) and (42), respectively. Typically P_a and P_v are initially set at particular levels until a $\dot{Q}_i$ is established. Then P_a and P_v are adjusted to new values, and, following any rapid transient change in weight due to a change in blood volume, the lung weight is monitored for some period of time. If during this period the weight change per unit time is smaller than some arbitrarily prescribed value, the lung is considered to be isogravimetric at the new values of P_a and P_v. If during this period the rate of weight change is too large, another smaller change in P_a and P_v is made, and the rate of change in weight is reassessed after the rapid blood volume transient. This tuning procedure is repeated until a new isogravimetric condition is established. When several isogravimetric flows have been obtained in this way, P_{ci}, R_a, and R_v can be estimated as shown in Figure 20 (Parker et al., 1981). This approach has not been used as often as some of the others for evaluating sites of vasomotion (Parker et al., 1981; Rippe et al., 1984) because each measurement of P_{ci}, R_a, and R_v requires considerable time and it can be difficult to maintain constant stimulus strength for bloodborne agents when $\dot{Q}_i$ is changed from one value to another. The example in Figure 20 shows the effect of hypoxic vasoconstriction on the arterial and venous pressure versus isogravimetric flow relation in an isolated dog lung (Parker et al., 1981).

In studies on lung lobes, P_{ci} obtained by the isogravimetric method has been found to be equal or very nearly equal to P_c or P_{do} obtained by the venous or double occlusion methods (Dawson et al., 1982 Parker et al., 1983; Rippe et al., 1987). This indicates that nearly the same mean vascular pressure controls both fluid filtration and lobar vascular volume. In fact, it may be that the near equivalence of these pressures is also important to the successful implementation of the isogravimetric method. It appears that it would be difficult to develop a stable servomechanism to adjust P_a and P_v while maintaining constant values of P_{is} and π_{is} during the transition from one value of $\dot{Q}_i$ to another if the vascular pressures controlling interstitial and vascular volumes were not nearly the same. This is because, given a finite interstitial compliance, a change in interstitial volume will change P_{is} and π_{is}. Since changes in interstitial volume are indistinguishable from changes in blood volume during the microvascular pressure transients that occur while homing in on a particular value of $\dot{Q}_i$, if P_{ci} and P_c are not nearly equal, it would be difficult to move from one $\dot{Q}_i$ to another in a short time to prevent a change in P_{is}.

IV. Conclusions

Each of the methods discussed in this chapter involves assumptions that can be subjected to closer scrutiny. Fortunately, in most of the methods, the observable pattern of the data obtained clearly reveal when changes in the geometry and properties of the vessels have occurred from one condition to another. The models used to evaluate the data have utility for quantitative comparisons by yielding parameters that are conceptually meaningful, even though the details may be subject to reevaluation in light of new information regarding their underlying assumptions. From the nature of the data it appears that model refinements will not grossly change the interpretation of the data. On the other hand, an inevitable result of using simplifying assumptions in an attempt to conceptualize complicated data is that some of the hypotheses used in the evaluation of different types of data appear contradictory at times. Often the reasons for apparent contradictions can be explained in terms of the recognizable consequences of the simplifying assumptions. However, there are instances in which it is clear that we do not understand the pulmonary vascular bed well enough to estimate the quantitative impact of all of the simplifying assumptions, or even to recognize what all of the important implicit assumptions are. The main objective of this review is to indicate some approaches that have been used to detect and to locate active responses within the intact pulmonary vascular bed from measurable pressure-flow relations. Even the present superficial examination reveals some examples of situations in which the hypotheses upon which the approaches are based lead to apparent contradictions. These apparent contradictions then indicate questions about the pulmonary vascular mechanics that remain to be answered, particularly to the end of extracting more physiological understanding from the pressure and flow data.

Acknowledgments

The authors thank Linda Hoffman for her assistance in preparing the manuscript. Work from our laboratory included in this chapter was supported by Research Grant HL-19298 from the National Heart, Lung and Blood Institute and by the Medical Research Service of the Veterans Administration.

References

Allison, D. J., and Stanbrook, H. S. (1980). A radiologic and physiologic investigation into hypoxic pulmonary vasoconstriction in the dog. *Invest. Radiol. 15*:178-190.

Altura, B. M., and Chand, N. (1981). Differential effects of prostaglandins on canine intrapulmonary arteries and veins. *Brit. J. Pharmacol. 73*:819-827.

Attinger, E. O. (1963). Pressure transmission in pulmonary arteries related to frequency and geometry. *Cir. Res. 12*:623-641.

Aviado, D. M. (1960). Pulmonary venular responses to anoxia, 5-hydroxytrptamine and histamine. *Am. J. Physiol. 198*:1032-1036.

Bakhle, Y. S., and Vane, J. R., editors (1977). *Lung Biology in Health and Disease.* Vol. 4, *Metabolic Functions of the Lung.* Marcel Dekker, New York.

Bassingthwaighte, J. B. (1970). Blood flow and diffusion through mammalian organs. *Science 167*:1347-1353.

Benis, A. M., Peslin, R., Mortara, F., and Lockhart, A. (1968). Rheological aspects of pressure-flow relations studied on perfused isolated lobes of the canine lung. *Bull. Physio-Pathol. Resp. 4*:417-441.

Benitz, W. E., Lessler, D. S., Coulson, J. D., and Bernfield, M. (1986). Heparin inhibits proliferation of fetal vascular smooth muscle cells in the absence of platelet-derived growth factor. *J. Cell Physiol. 127*:1-7.

Bergel, D. H., and Milnor, W. R. (1965). Pulmonary vascular impedance in the dog. *Circ. Res. 16*:401-415.

Bhattacharya, J. (1986). The lung microvascular pressure profile. *Am. Rev. Resp. Dis. 134*:854-855.

Bhattacharya, J., and Staub, N. C. (1980). Direct measurement of microvascular pressures in isolated perfused dog lung. *Science 210*:327-328.

Bhattacharya, J., Nanjo, S., and Staub, N. C. (1982a). Micropuncture measurement of lung microvascular pressure during 5-HT infusion. *J. Appl. Physiol. 52*:634-637.

Bhattacharya, J., Nanjo, S., and Staub, N. C. (1982b). Factors affecting lung microvascular pressure. *Ann. NY Acad. Sci. 384*:107-114.

Boiteau, P., Ducas, J., Schick, U., Girling, L., and Prewitt, R. M. (1986). Pulmonary vascular pressure-flow relationship in canine oleic acid pulmonary edema. *Am. J. Physiol. 251 (Heart Circ. Physiol. 20)*:H1163-H1170.

Bos, G. C. van den, Westerhof, N., and Randall, O. S. (1982). Pulse wave reflection: can it explain the differences between systemic and pulmonary pressure and flow waves? *Circ. Res. 51*:479-485.

Brody, J. S., and Stemmler, E. J. (1968). Differential reactivity in the pulmonary circulation. *J. Clin. Invest. 47*:800-808.

Brody, J. S., Stemmler, E. J., and DuBois, A. B. (1968). Longitidunal distribution of vascular resistance in pulmonary arteries, capillaries and veins. *J. Clin. Invest. 47*:783-799.

Bronikowski, T. A., Linehan, J. H., and Dawson, C. A. (1984). A model of the vascular resistance and compliance distribution in a lung lobe. *Microvasc. Res. 28*:289-310.

Bronikowski, T. A., Dawson, C. A., and Linehan, J. H. (1985). Limits on the continuous distribution of pulmonary vascular resistance versus compliance from outflow occlusion. *Microvasc. Res. 30*:306-313.

Bruderman, I., Somers, K., Hamilton, W. K., Tooley, W. H., and Butler, J. (1964). Effect of surface tension on circulation in the excised lungs of dogs. *J. Appl. Physiol. 19*:707-712.

Capen, R. L., and Wagner, W. W., Jr. (1982). Intrapulmonary blood flow redistribution during hypoxia increases gas exchange surface area. *J. Appl. Physiol. 52*:1575-1581.

Caro, C. G., and McDonald, D. A. (1961). The relation of pulsatile pressure and flow in the pulmonary vascular bed. *J. Physiol. (London) 157*:426-453.

Chand, N., and Altura, B. M. (1981). Acetylcholine and bradykinin relax intrapulmonary arteries by acting on endothelial cells: role in lung vascular diseases. *Science 213*:1376-1379.

Collins, R., and Maccario, J. A. (1979). Blood flow in the lung. *J. Biomech. 12*: 373-395.

Connolly, D. C., Kirklin, J. W., and Wood, E. H. (1954). The relationship between pulmonary artery wedge pressure and left atrial pressure in man. *Circ. Res. 2*:434-440.

Cope, D. K., Allison, R. C., Parmentier, J. L., Miller, J. N., and Taylor, A. E. (1986). Measurement of effective pulmonary capillary pressure using the pressure profile after pulmonary artery occlusion. *Crit. Care Med. 14*:16-22.

Cox, R. H. (1984). Visoelastic properties of canine pulmonary arteries. *Am. J. Physiol. 246 (Heart Circ. Physiol. 15)*:90-96.

Cox, R. H. (1982). Comparsion of mechanical and chemical properties of extra- and intralobar canine pulmonary arteries. *Am. J. Physiol. 242 (Heart Circ. Physiol. 11)*:H245-H253.

Culver, B. H., and Butler, J. (1980). Mechanical influences on the pulmonary microcirculation. *Ann. Rev. Physiol. 42*:187-198.

Dawson, C. A. (1984). Role of pulmonary vasomotion in physiology of the lung. *Physiol. Rev. 64*:544-616.

Dawson, C. A., and Linehan, J. H. (1988). Biogenic amines, In: *Lung Cell Biology.* Edited by D. Massaro. Marcel Dekker, New York.

Dawson, C. A., Forrester, T. E., and Hamilton, L. H. (1975). Effects of hypoxia and histamine infusion on lung blood volume. *J. Appl. Physiol. 38*:811-816.

Dawson, C. A., Grimm, D. J., and Linehan, J. H. (1977). Effects of lung inflation on longitudinal distribution of pulmonary vascular resistance. *J. Appl. Physiol. 43*:1089-1092.

Dawson, C. A., Grimm, D. J., and Linehan, J. H. (1978). Influence of hypoxia on the longitudinal distribution of pulmonary vascular resistance. *J. Appl. Physiol. 44*:493-498.

Dawson, C. A., Grimm, D. J. and Linehan, J. H. (1979). Lung inflation and longitudinal distribution of pulmonary vascular resistance during hypoxia. *J. Appl. Physiol. 47*:532-536.

Dawson, C. A., Linehan, J. H. and Rickaby, D. A. (1982). Pulmonary microcirculatory hemodynamics. *Ann. NY Acad. Sci. 384*:90-106.

Dawson, C. A., Linehan, J. H., Bronikowski, T. A., and Rickaby, D. A. (1987). Pulmonary microvascular hemodynamics: occlusion methods. In *The Pulmonary Circulation in Health and Disease.* Edited by J. A. Will, C. A. Dawson, E. K. Weir, and C. K. Buckner. Academic Press, Orlando, FL.

Dawson, C. A., Rickaby, D. A., and Linehan, J. H. (1986). Location and mechanisms of pulmonary vascular volume changes. *J. Appl. Physiol. 60*:402-409.

Dawson, C. A., Bronikowski, T. A., Linehan, J. H., and Rickaby, D. A. (1988) Distribution of vascular resistance and pressure in the lung. *J. Appl. Physiol. 64*:274-284.

Dawson, C. A., Capen, R. L., Latham, L. P., Hanson, W. L., Hofmeister, S. E., Bronikowski, T. A., Rickaby, D. A., and Wagner, W. W. (1987). Pulmonary arterial transit times. *J. Appl. Physiol. 63*:770-777.

Downing, S. E., and Lee, J. C. (1980). Nervous control of the pulmonary circulation. *Annu. Rev. Physiol. 42*:199-210.

Dujardin, J. P. L., Stone, D. N., Forcino, C. D., Paul, L. T., and Pieper, H. P. (1982). Effects of blood volume changes on characteristic impedance of the pulmonary artery. *Am. J. Physiol. 242 (Heart Circ. Physiol. 11)*:H197-H202.

Effros, R. M. (1984). Pulmonary microcirculation and exchange. In *Handbook of Physiology Sect. 2, The Cardiovascular System, Microcirculation*, Vol. IV, Part 2. Edited by E. M. Renkin and C. C. Michel. Am. Physiol. Soc., Bethesda, MD, Chap. 18, pp. 865-915.

Elkins, R. C., and Milnor, W. R. (1971). Pulmonary vascular response to exercise in the dog. *Circ. Res. 29*:591-599.

Elkins, R. C., Peyton, M. D., and Greenfield, L. J. (1974). Pulmonary vascular impedance in chronic pulmonary hypertension. *Surgery 76*:57-64.

Engelberg, J., and DuBois, A. B. (1959). Mechanics of pulmonary circulation in isolated rabbit lungs. *Am. J. Physiol. 196*:401-414.

Even, P., Duroux, P., Ruff, F., Caubarrere, I., Vernejoul, P. de, and Brouet, G. (1971). The pressure-flow relationship of the pulmonary circulation in normal man and in chronic obstructive pulmonary diseases. Effects of muscular exercise. *Scand. J. Resp. Dis. 52 (Suppl. 77)*:72-76.

Feeley, J. W., Lee, T. D., and Milnor, W. R. (1963). Active and passive components of the pulmonary vascular response to vasoactive drugs in the dog. *Am. J. Physiol. 205*:1193-1199.

Fishman, A. P. (1985). Pulmonary circulation. In *Handbook of Physiology*. Sect. 3, *The Respiratory System*. Vol. I, *Circulation and Nonrespiratory Functions*. Edited by A. P. Fishman and A. B. Fisher. Am. Physiol. Soc., Bethesda, MD, pp. 93-165.

Fowler, K. T., West, J. B., and Pain, M. C. F. (1966). Pressure-flow characteristics of horizontal lung preparation of minimal height. *Resp. Physiol. 1*: 88-98.

Frasher, W. G., and Sobin, S. S. (1965). Pressure-volume response of isolated living main pulmonary artery in dogs. *J. Appl. Physiol. 20*:675-682.

Friedman, M., and Wanner, A. (1977). Volume characteristics of extra- and intraparenchymal segments of the canine pulmonary artery. *J. Appl. Physiol. 42*:519-524.

Fung, Y. C. (1977). Pulmonary alveolar blood flow. In *Bioengineering Aspects of the Lung*. Edited by J. B. West. Marcel Dekker, New York, pp. 267-359.

Fung, Y. C. (1984). *Biodynamics: Circulation*. Springer-Verlag, New York.

Fung, Y. C., and Sobin, S. S (1969). Theory of sheet flow in lung alveoli. *J. Appl. Physiol. 26*:472-488.

Fung, Y. C., and Sobin, S. S. (1972). Pulmonary alveolar blood flow. *Circ. Res. 30*:470-490.

Fung, Y. C. and Yen, R. T. (1986). A new theory of pulmonary blood flow in zone 2 condition. *J. Appl. Physiol. 60*:1638-1650.

Fung, Y. C., and Zhuang, F. Y. (1986). An analysis of the sluicing gate in pulmonary blood flow. *J. Biomech. Eng. 108*:175-182.

Fung, Y. C., Sobin, S. S., Tremer, H., Yen, M. R. T., and Ho, H. H. (1983). Patency and compliance of pulmonary veins when airway pressure exceeds blood pressure. *J. Appl. Physiol. 54*:1538-1549.

Furchgott, R. F. (1984). Role of endothelium in the responses of vascular smooth muscle to drugs. *Ann. Rev. Pharmacol. 24*:175-197.

Gaar, K. A., Taylor, A. E., Owens, L. J., and Guyton, A. C. (1967). Pulmonary capillary pressure and filtration coefficient in the isolated perfused lung. *Am. J. Physiol. 213*:910-914.

Gilbert, R. P., Hinshaw, L. B., Kuida, H., and Visscher, M. B. (1958). Effects of histamine, 5-hydroxytrptamine, and epinephrine on pulmonary hemodynamics with particular reference to arterial and venous segment resistances. *Am. J. Physiol. 194*:165-170.

Glazier, J. B., and Murray, J. F. (1971). Sites of pulmonary vasomotor reactivity in the dog during alveolar hypoxia and serotonin and histamine infusion. *J. Clin. Invest. 50*:2550-2558.

Goll, H. M., Nyhan, D. P., Geller, H. S., and Murray, P. A. (1986). Pulmonary vascular responses to angiotensin II and captopril in conscious dogs. *J. Appl. Physiol. 61*:1552-1559.

Graham, R., Skoog, C., Oppenheimer, L., Rabson, J., and Goldberg, H. S. (1982). Critical closure in the canine pulmonary vasculature. *Circ. Res. 50*: 566-572.

Graham, R., Skoog, C., Macedo, W., Carter, J., Oppenheimer, L., Rabson, J., and Goldberg, H. S. (1983). Dopamine, dobutamine, and phentolamine effects on pulmonary vascular mechanics. *J. Appl. Physiol. 54*:1277-1283.

Grand, G. M., and Downing, S. E. (1970). Metabolic and reflex influences on pulmonary vasomotion. *Am. J. Physiol. 218*:654-661.

Grant, B. J. B., and Paradowski, L. J. (1987). Characterization of pulmonary arterial input impedance with lumped parameter models. *Am. J. Physiol. 252 (Heart Circ. Physiol. 21)*:H585-H593.

Greenberg, S., Kadowitz, P. J., Hyman, A., and Curro, F. A. (1981). Adrenergic mechanisms in canine intralobar pulmonary arteries and veins. *Am. J. Physiol. 240 (Heart Circ. Physiol. 9)*:H274-H285.

Greenleaf, J. F., Ritman, E. L., Sass, D. J., and Wood, E. H. (1974). Spartial distribution of pulmonary blood flow in dogs in the left decubitus position. *Am. J. Physiol. 227*:230-244.

Gregory, T. J., Newell, J. C., Hakim, T. S., Levitzky, M. G., and Sedransk, N., (1982). Attenuation of hypoxic pulmonary vasoconstriction by pulsatile flow in dog lungs. *J. Appl. Physiol. 53*:1583-1588.

Grimm, D. J., Linehan, J. H., and Dawson, C. A. (1977). Longitudinal distribution of vascular resistance in the lung. *J. Appl. Physiol. 43*:1093-1101.

Grimm, D. J., Dawson, C. A., Hakim, T. S., and Linehan, J. H. (1978). Pulmonary vasomotion and the distribution of vascular resistance in a dog lung lobe. *J. Appl. Physiol. 45*:545-550.

Grover, R. F., Wagner, W. W., McMurtry, I. F., and Reeves, J. T. (1983). Pulmonary circulation. In *Handbook of Physiology.* Sect. 2, *The Cardiovascular System.* Vol. III, *Peripheral Circulation and Organ blood Flow.* Part 1. Edited by J. T. Shepherd and F. M. Abboud. Am. Physiol. Soc. Bethesda, MD, pp. 103-136.

Gruetter, C. A., Ignarro, L. J., Hyman, A. L., and Kadowitz, P. J. (1981). Contractile effects of 5-hydroxytryptamine in isolated intrapulmonary arteries and veins. *Can. J. Physiol. Pharmacol. 59*:157-162.

Guntheroth, W. G., Luchtel, D. L., and Kawabori, I. (1982). Pulmonary microcirculation: tubules rather than sheet and post. *J. Appl. Physiol. 53*:510-515.

Hakim, T. S., Dawson, C. A., and Linehan, J. H. (1979). Hemodynamic responses of a dog lung lobe to lobar venous occlusion. *J. Appl. Physiol. 47*:145-152.

Hakim, T. S., Michel, R. P., and Chang, H. K. (1982a). Effect of lung inflation on pulmonary vascular resistance by arterial and venous occlusion. *J. Appl. Physiol. 53*:1110-1115.

Hakim, T. S., Michel, R. P., and Chang, H. K. (1982b). Partitioning of pulmonary vascular resistance in dogs by arterial and venous occlusion. *J. Appl. Physiol. 52*:710-715.

Hakim, T. S., Michel, R. P., Minami, H., and Chang, H. K. (1983). Site of pulmonary hypoxic vasoconstriction studied with arterial and venous occlusion. *J. Appl. Physiol. 54*:1298-1302.

Hakim, T. S., Chang, H. K., and Michel, R. P. (1985). The rectilinear pressure-flow relationship in the pulmonary vasculature: zones 2 and 3. *Resp. Physiol. 61*:115-123.

Hakim, T. S., Lisbona, R., and Dean, G. W. (1986). Central-peripheral gradient in pulmonary blood flow in humans. *Prog. Resp. Res. 21*:233-235.

Hakim, T. S. Lisbona, R., and Dean, G. W. (1987). Gravity nondependent distribution of pulmonary blood flow. In *The Pulmonary Circulation in Health and Disease.* Edited by J. A. Will, C. A. Dawson, E. K. Weir, and C. K. Buckner. Academic Press, Orlando, FL, pp. 231-248.

Hammon, J. W., Jr., Smith, P. K., McHale, P. A., Vanbenthuysen, K. M., and Anderson, R. W. (1981). Analysis of pulsatile pulmonary artery blood flow in the unanesthetized dog. *J. Appl. Physiol. 50*:805-813.

Hasan, F. M., Weiss, W. B., Braman, S. S., and Hoppin, F. G., Jr. (1985). Influence of lung injury on pulmonary wedge-left atrial pressure correlation during positive end-expiratory pressure ventilation. *Am. Rev. Resp. Dis. 131*:246-250.

Hirschman, J. C., and Boucek, R. J. (1963). Angiographic evidence of pulmonary vasomotion in the dog. *Brit. Heart J. 25*:375-381.

Hebb, C. (1969). Motor innervation of the pulmonary blood vessels of mammals. In *The Pulmonary Circulation and Interstitial Space*. Edited by A. P. Fishman and H. H. Hecht. Univer. of Chicago Press, Chicago, Il, pp. 195-222.

Holl, J. E., Kolbeck, R. C., and Speir, W. A., Jr. (1980). Pulmonary vascular responsiveness to histamine exquisite sensitivity of small intrapulmonary arteries. *Am. Rev. Resp. Dis. 122*:909-913.

Holloway, H., Perry, M., Downey, J., Parker, J., and Taylor, A. (1983). Estimation of effective pulmonary capillary pressure in intact lungs. *J. Appl. Physiol. 54*:846-851.

Hopkins, R. A., Hammon, J. W., Jr., McHale, P. A., Smith, P. K., and Anderson, R. W. (1979). Pulmonary vascular impedance analysis of adaptation to chronically elevated blood flow in the awake dog. *Circ. Res. 45*:267-274.

Hopkins, R. A., Hammon, J. W., Jr., McHale, P. A., Smith, P. K., and Anderson, R. W. (1980). An analysis of the pulsatile hemodynamic responses of the pulmonary circulation to acute and chronic pulmonary venous hypertension in the awake dog. *Circ. Res. 47*:902-910.

Horsfield, K., and Gordon, W. I. (1981). Morphometry of pulmonary veins in man. *Lung 159*:211-218.

Hotchkiss, R. S., Katsamouris, A. N., Lappas, D. G., Mihelakos, P. T., Wilson, R. S., Long, M., Coyle, J., Brewster, D., and Greene, R. (1986). Interpretation of pulmonary artery wedge pressure and pullback blood gas determinations during positive end-expiratory pressure ventilation and after exclusion of the bronchial circulation in the dog. *Am. Rev. Resp. Dis. 133*: 1019-1023.

Howell, J. B. L., Permutt, S., Proctor, D. F., and Riley, R. L. (1961). Effect of inflation of the lung on different parts of pulmonary vascular bed. *J. Appl. Physiol. 16*:71-76.

Humphries, D. E., Lee, S.-L., Fanburg, B. L., and Silbert, J. E. (1986). Effects of hypoxia and hyperoxia on proteoglycan production by bovine pulmonary artery endothelial cells. *J. Cell. Physiol. 126*:249-253.

Hyde, R. W., Lawson, W. H., and Forrester, R. E. (1964). Influence of carbon dioxide on pulmonary vasculature. *J. Appl. Physiol. 19*:734-744.

Hyman, A. L. (1968). The effects of bradykinin on the pulmonary veins. *J. Pharmacol. Exp. Ther. 161*:78-87.

Hyman, A. L. (1969). Effects of large increases in pulmonary blood flow on pulmonary venous pressure. *J. Appl. Physiol. 27*:179-185.

Hyman, A. L., Burch, G. E., DePasquale, N. P., and Tyler, J. M. (1963). Spontaneous variations in pulmonary venous pressure in intact dogs. *Proc. Soc. Exp. Biol. Med. 112*:1032-1037.

Ingram, R. H., Szidon, J. P., Skalak, R., and Fishman, A. P. (1968). Effects of sympathetic nerve stimulation on the pulmonary arterial tree of the isolated lobe perfused in situ. *Circ. Res. 22*:801-815.

Janicki, J. S., Weber, K. T., Likoff, M. J., and Fishman, A. P. (1985). The pressure-flow response of the pulmonary circulation in patients with heart failure and pulmonary vascular disease. *Circulation 72*:1270-1278.

Joiner, P. D., Kadowitz, P. J., Hughes, J. P., and Hyman, A. L. (1975a). NE and ACh responses of intrapulmonary vessels from dog, swine, and man. *Am. J. Physiol. 228*:1821-1827.

Joiner, P. D., Kadowitz, P. J., Davis, L. B., and Hyman, A. L. (1975b). Contractile responses of canine isolated pulmonary lobar arteries and veins to norepinephrine, serotonin, and tyramine. *Can. J. Physiol. Pharmacol. 53*: 830-838.

Kadowitz, P. J., Joiner, P. D., and Hyman, A. L. (1975). Influences of sympathetic stimulation and vasoactive substances on the canine pulmonary veins. *J. Clin. Invest. 56*:354-365.

Kind, L. S., and Gallemore, J. I. (1956). Pulmonary vascular changes in the mouse during anaphylactic shock. *Proc. Soc. Exp. Biol. Med. 92*:345-347.

Knowlton, F. P., and Starling, E. H. (1912). The influence of variations in temperature and blood-pressure on the performance of the isolated mammalian heart. *J. Physiol. London 44*:206-219.

Krishnan, A., Linehan, J. H., Rickaby, D. A., and Dawson, C. A. (1986). Cat lung hemodynamics: comparison of experimental results and model predictions. *J. Appl. Physiol. 61*:2023-2034.

Kuida, H., Hinshaw, L. B., Gilbert, R. P., and Visscher, M. B. (1958). Effect of gram-negative endotoxin on pulmonary circulation. *Am. J. Physiol. 192*:335-344.

Kuramoto, K., Med, D., and Rodbard, S. (1962). Effects of blood flow and left atrial pressure on pulmonary venous resistance. *Circ. Res. 11*:240-246.

Lai-Fook, S. J. (1979). A continuum mechanics analysis of pulmonary vascular interdependence in isolated dog lobes. *J. Appl. Physiol. 46*:419-429.

Lategola, M. T. (1958). Pressure flow relations in the dog lung during acute subtotal pulmonary vascular occlusion. *Am. J. Physiol. 192*:613-619.

Lazaris, Y. A., Serebrovskaya, I. A., and Cherepanova, A. G. (1969). Study of reaction of pulmonary vascular bed to some vasoactive agents using serial contrast reoentgenovasography. *Cor Vasa 11*:21-28.

Lee, G. de J., and DuBois, A. B. (1955). Pulmonary capillary blood flow in man. *J. Clin. Invest. 34*:1380-1390.

Lefevre, J. (1983). Teleonomical optimization of a fractal model of the pulmonary arterial bed. *J. Theor. Biol. 102*:225-248.

Lewis, B. M., McElroy, W. T., Hayford-Welsing, E. J., and Samberg, L. C. (1960). The effects of body position, ganglionic blockade and norepinephrine on the pulmonary capillary bed. *J. Clin. Invest. 39*:1345-1352.

Linehan, J. H., and Dawson, C. A. (1983). A three-compartment model of the pulmonary vasculature: effects of vasoconstriction. *J. Appl. Physiol. 55*: 923-928.

Linehan, J. H., Dawson, C. A., and Rickaby, D. A. (1982). Distribution of vascular resistance and compliance in a dog lung lobe. *J. Appl. Physiol. 53*: 158-168.

Linehan, J. H., Dawson, C. A., Rickaby, D. A., and Bronikowski, T. A. (1986). Pulmonary vascular compliance and visoelasticity. *J. Appl. Physiol. 61*: 1802-1814.

Lloyd, T. C., Jr. and Wright, G. W. (1960). Pulmonary vascular resistance and vascular transmural gradient. *J. Appl. Physiol. 15*:241-245.

Lockhart, A., and Benis, A. M. (1970). Influence of rheology of perfusate on pressure-flow curves in isolated lung lobe of the dog. *Prog. Resp. Res. 5*: 61-75.

Lodato, R. F., Michael, J. R., and Murray, P. A. (1985). Multipoint pulmonary vascular pressure-cardiac output plots in conscious dogs. *Am. J. Physiol. 249 (Heart Circ. Physiol 18)*:H351-H357.

Lopez-Muniz, R., Stephens, N. L., Bromberger-Barnea, B., Permutt, S., and Riley, R. L. (1968). Critical closure of pulmonary vessels analyzed in terms of Starling resistor model. *J. Appl. Physiol. 24*:625-635.

Lucas, C. L. (1984). Fluid mechanics of the pulmonary circulation. *CRC Crit. Rev. Biomed. Eng. 10*:317-392.

Lucas, C. L., Wilcox, B. R., and Coulter, N. A., Jr. (1975). Pulmonary vascular response to atrial septal defect closure in children. *J. Surg. Res. 18*:571-586.

Luchsinger, P. C., Seipp, H. W., and Patel, D. J. (1962). Relationship of pulmonary artery-wedge pressure to left atrial pressure in man. *Circ. Res. 11*:315-318.

McDonald, D. A. (1974). *Blood Flow in Arteries.* Williams and Wilkins, Baltimore, MD.

McGregor, M., and Sniderman, A. (1985). On pulmonary vascular resistance: the need for more precise definition. *Am. J. Cardiol. 55*:217-221.

Malik, A. B. (1983). Pulmonary microembolism. *Physiol. Rev. 63*:1114-1207.

Maloney, J. E., Bergel, D. H., Glazier, J. B., Hughes, J. M. B., and West, J. B. (1968). Transmission of pulsatile blood pressure and flow through the isolated lung. *Circ. Res. 23*:11-24.

Maloney, J. C., Rooholamini, S. A., and Wexler, L. (1970). Pressure-diameter relations of small blood vessels in isolated dog lung. *Microvasc. Res. 2*:1-12.

Maloney, J. E., Cannata, J., and Ritchie, B. C. (1976). The influence of transpulmonary pressure on the diameter of small arterial blood vessels in the lung. *Microvasc. Res. 11*:57-66.

Mead, J., and Whittenberger, J. L. (1964). Lung inflation and hemodynamics. In *Handbook of Physiology*. Sect. 3, Vol. 1. Edited by W. O. Fenn and H. Rahn. Am. Phys. Soc., Washington, DC, Chap. 18, pp. 477-486.

Michel, R. P., Hakim, T. S., and Chang, H. K. (1984). Pulmonary arterial and venous pressures measured with small catheters in dogs. *J. Appl. Physiol. 57*:309-314.

Mills, C. J., Gabe, I. T., Gault, J. H., Mason, D. T., Ross, J., Jr., Braunwald, E., and Shillingford, J. P. (1970). Pressure-flow relationships and vascular impedance in man. *Cardiovasc. Res. 4*:405-417.

Milnor, W. R. (1972). Pulmonary hemodynamics. In *Cardiovascular Fluid Dynamics*. Vol. 2. Edited by D. H. Bergel. Academic Press, New York, pp. 299-340.

Milnor, W. R. (1982). *Hemodynamics*. Williams and Wilkens, Baltimore, MD.

Milnor, W. R., Conti, C. R., Lewis, K. B., and O'Rourke, M. F. (1969). Pulmonary arterial pulse wave velocity and impedance in man. *Circ. Res. 25*:637-649.

Mitzner, W. (1983). Resistance of the pulmonary circulation. *Clin. Chest Med. 4*: 127-137.

Mitzner, W., and Huang, I. (1987). Interpretation of pressure-flow curves in the pulmonary vascular bed. In *The Pulmonary Circulation in Health and Disease*. Edited by J. A. Will, C. A. Dawson, E. K. Weir, and C. K. Buckner. Academic Press, Orlando, FL, pp. 215-230.

Mitzner, W., and Sylvester, J. T. (1981). Hypoxic vasoconstriction and fluid filtration in pig lungs. *J. Appl. Physiol. 51*:1065-1071.

Morgan, B. C., Church, S. C., and Guntheroth, W. G. (1968). Hypoxic constriction of pulmonary artery and vein in intact dogs. *J. Appl. Physiol. 25*: 356-361.

Morkin, E., Levine, O. R., and Fishman, A. P. (1964). Pulmonary capillary flow pulse and the site of pulmonary vasoconstriction in the dog. *Circ. Res. 15*: 146-160.

Moser, K. M., editor (1979). *Lung Biology in Health and Disease*. Vol. 14. *Pulmonary Vascular Disease*. Marcel Dekker, New York.

Murray, P. A., Lodato, R. F., and Michael, J. R. (1986). Neural antagonists modulate pulmonary vascular pressure-flow plots in conscious dogs. *J. Appl. Physiol. 60*:1900-1907.

Nagasaka, Y., Bhattacharya, J., Nanjo, S., Gropper, M. A., and Staub, N. C. (1984). Micropuncture measurement of lung microvascular pressure profile during hypoxia in cats. *Circ. Res. 54*:90-95.

Nyhan, D. P., Geller, H. S., Goll, H. M., and Murray, P. A. (1986). Pulmonary vasoactive effects of exogenous and endogenous AVP in conscious dogs. *Am. J. Physiol. 251 (Heart Circ. Physiol. 20)*:H1009-H1016.

O'Quin, R., and Marini, J. J. (1983). Pulmonary artery occlusion pressure: clinical physiology, measurement, and interpretation. *Am. Rev. Resp. Dis. 128*:319-326.

O'Rourke, M. F. (1982). Vascular impedance in studies of arterial and cardiac function. *Physiol. Rev. 62*:570-623.

Overholser, K. A., Bhattacharya, J., and Staub, N. C. (1982). Microvascular pressures in the isolated, perfused dog lung: comparison between theory and measurement. *Microvasc. Res. 23*:67-76.

Pace, J. B. (1971). Sympathetic control of pulmonary vascular impedance in anesthetized dogs. *Circ. Res. 29*:555-568.

Pain, M. C. F., and West, J. B. (1966). Effect of the volume history of the isolated lung on distribution of blood flow. *J. Appl. Physiol. 21*:1545-1550.

Pappenheimer, J. R., and Soto-Rivera, X. (1948). Effective osmotic pressure of the plasma proteins and other quantities associated with the capillary circulation in the hindlimbs of cats and dogs. *Am. J. Physiol. 152*:471-491.

Parker, R. E., Granger, D. N., and Taylor, A. E. (1981). Estimates of isogravimetric capillary pressures during alveolar hypoxia. *Am. J. Physiol. 241 (Heart Circ. Physiol. 10)*:H732-H739.

Parker, J. C., Kvietys, P. R., Ryan, K. P., and Taylor, A. E. (1983). Comparison of isogravimetric and venous occlusion capillary pressures in isolated dog lungs. *J. Appl. Physiol. 55*:964-968.

Patel, D. J., Schilder, D. P., and Mallos, A. J. (1960). Mechanical properties and dimensions of the major pulmonary arteries. *J. Appl. Physiol. 15*: 92-96.

Patel, D. J., DeFreitas, F. M., and Mallos, A. J. (1962). Mechanical function of the main pulmonary artery. *J. Appl. Physiol. 17*:205-208.

Patel, D. J., DeFreitas, F. M., and Fry, D. L. (1963). Hydraulic input impedance in aorta and pulmonary artery in dog. *J. Appl. Physiol. 18*:134-140.

Permutt, S., and Riley, R. L. (1963). Hemodynamics of collapsible vessels with tone: the vascular waterfall. *J. Appl. Physiol. 18*:924-932.

Permutt, S., Howell, J. B. L., Proctor, D. F., and Riley, R. L. (1961). Effect of lung inflation on static pressure-volume characteristics of pulmonary vessels. *J. Appl. Physiol. 16*:64-70.

Permutt, S., Bromberger-Barnea, B., and Bane, H. N. (1962). Alveolar pressure, pulmonary venous pressure, and vascular water fall. *Med. Thorac. 19*:239-260.

Piene, H. (1976). The influence of pulmonary blood flow rate on vascular input impedance and hydraulic power: the sympathetically and noradrenaline stimulated cat lung. *Acta Physiol. Scand. 98*:44-53.

Piene, H. (1986). Pulmonary arterial impedance and right ventricular function. *Physiol. Rev. 66*:606-652.

Piene, H., and Hauge, A. (1976). Reduction of pulsatile hydraulic power in the pulmonary circulation caused by caused by moderate vasoconstriction. *Cardiovasc. Res. 10*:503-513.

Piiper, J. (1970). Attempts to determine volume, compliance and resistance to flow of pulmonary vascular compartments. *Prog. Resp. Res. 5*:40-52.

Pollack, G. H., Reddy, R. V., and Noordergraff, A. (1968). Input impedance, wave travel, and reflection in the human pulmonary arterial tree: studies using an electrical analog. *IEEE Trans. Biomed. Eng. 15*:151-164.

Quebbeman, E. J., and Dawson, C. A. (1977). Effect of lung inflation and hypoxia on pulmonary arterial blood volume. *J. Appl. Physiol. 43*:8-13.

Rabinovitch, M., Gamble, W., Nadas, A. S., Miettinen, O. S., and Reid, L. (1979). Rat pulmonary circulation after chronic hypoxia: hemodynamics and structural features. *Am. J. Physiol. 236 (Heart Circ. Physiol. 5)*: H818-H827.

Radke, N. F., Lucas, C. L., Wilcox, B. R., and Keagy, B. A. (1985). Infant pulmonary vascular model based on the pulmonary input impedance spectrum. *Ann. Biomed. Eng. 13*:531-550.

Raj, J. U., and Chen, P. (1986a). Microvascular pressures measured by micropuncture in isolated perfused lamb lungs. *J. Appl. Physiol. 61*:2194-2201.

Raj, J. U., and Chen, P. (1986b). Micropuncture measurement of microvascular pressures in isolated lamb lungs during hypoxia. *Circ. Res. 59*:398-404.

Raj, J. U., Bland, R. D., and Lai-Fook, S. J. (1986a). Microvascular pressures measured by micropipettes in isolated edematous rabbit lungs. *J. Appl. Physiol. 60*:539-545.

Raj, J. U., Chen, P., and Navazo, L. (1986b). Micropuncture measurement of lung microvascular pressure profile in 3- to 4-week-old rabbits. *Pediatr. Res. 20*:1107-1111.

Raj, J. J., Chen, P., and Navazo, L. (1987). Effect of inflation on microvascular pressures in lungs of young rabbits. *Am. J. Physiol. 252 (Heart Circ. Physiol. 21)*:H80-H84.

Reid, L. M. (1979). The pulmonary circulation: remodeling in growth and disease. *Am. Rev. Resp. Dis. 119*:531-546.

Reid, L., and Meyrick, B. (1982). Microcirculation definition and organization at tissue level. *Ann. NY Acad. Sci. 384*:3-20.

Reuben, S. R. (1971). Compliance of the human pulmonary arterial system in disease. *Circ. Res. 29*:40-50.

Reuben, S. R., and Kitchin, A. H. (1975). Pulmonary artery input impedance in pulmonary hypertension. *Prog. Resp. Res. 9*:261-266.

Reuben, S. R., Gersh, B. J., Swadling, J. P., and De J. Lee, G. (1970). Measurement of pulmonary arterial distensibility in the dog. *Cardiovasc. Res 4*: 473-481.

Reuben, S. R., Swadling, J. P., Gersh, B. J., and Lee, G. De J. (1971). Impedance and transmission properties of the pulmonary arterial system. *Cardiovasc. Res.* *5*:1-9.

Richardson, J. B. (1979). Nerve supply to the lungs. *Am. Rev. Resp. Dis.* *119*: 785-802.

Rickaby, D. A., Dawson, C. A., and Maron, M. B. (1980). Pulmonary inactivation of serotonin and site of serotonin pulmonary vasoconstriction. *J. Appl. Physiol.* *48*:606-612.

Rideout, V. C., and Katra, J. A. (1969). Computer simulation study of the pulmonary circulation. *Simulation* *12*:239-245.

Rippe, B., Allison, R. C., Parker, J. C., and Taylor, A. E. (1984). Effects of histamine, serotonin and norepinephrine on circulation of dog lungs. *J. Appl. Physiol.* *57*:223-232.

Rippe, B., Parker, J. C., Townsley, M. I., Mortillaro, N. A., and Taylor, A. E. (1987). Segmental vascular resistances and compliances in dog lung. *J. Appl. Physiol.* *62*:1206-1215.

Rock, P., Patterson, G. A., Permutt, S., and Sylvester, J. T. (1985). Nature and distribution of vascular resistance in hypoxic pig lungs. *J. Appl. Physiol.* *59*:1891-1901.

Roos, A., Thomas, L. J., Nagel, E. L., and Prommas, D. C. (1961). Pulmonary vascular resistance as determined by lung inflation and vascular pressures. *J. Appl. Physiol.* *16*:77-84.

Sackner, M. A., Will, D. H., and DuBois, A. B. (1966). The site of pulmonary vasomotor activity during hypoxia or serotonin administration. *J. Clin. Invest.* *45*:112-121

Sada, K., Shirai, M., and Ninomiya, I. (1985). X-ray TV system for measuring microcirculation in small pulmonary vessels. *J. Appl. Physiol.* *59*:1013-1018.

Sada, K., Shirai, M., and Ninomiya, I. (1987). Effects of prostaglandin $F_{2\alpha}$ and prostacyclin on pulmonary microcirculation in the cat. *J. Appl. Physiol.* *62*:1124-1132.

Selig, W. M., Noonan, T. C., Kern, D. F., and Malik, A. B. (1986). Pulmonary microvascular responses to arachidonic acid in isolated perfused guinea pig lung. *J. Appl. Physiol.* *60*:1972-1979.

Shapiro, A. H. (1977). Steady flow in collapsible tubes. *J. Biomech. Eng.* *99*: 126-147.

Shirai, M., Sada, K., and Ninomiya, I. (1986). Effects of regional alveolar hypoxia and hypercapnia on small pulmonary vessels in cats. *J. Appl. Physiol.* *61*:440-448.

Shirai, M., Sada, K., and Ninomiya, I. (1987). Nonuniform effects of histamine on small pulmonary vessels in cats. *J. Appl. Physiol.* *62*:451-458.

Simons, P., and Reid, L. (1969). Muscularity of pulmonary artery branches in the upper and lower lobes of the normal young and aged lung. *Brit. J. Dis. Chest. 63*:38-44.

Smith, J. C., and Mitzner, W. (1980). Analysis of pulmonary vascular interdependence in excised dog lobes. *J. Appl. Physiol. 48*:450-467.

Sobin, S. S., Fung, Y. C., Tremer, H. M., and Rosenquist, T. H. (1972). Elasticity of the pulmonary alveolar microvascular sheet in the cat. *Circ. Res. 30*:440-450.

Sobin, S. S., Lindal, R. G., Fung, Y. C., and Tremer, H. M. (1978). Elasticity of the smallest noncapillary pulmonary blood vessels in the cat. *Microvasc. Res. 15*:57-68.

Soohoo, S. L., Goldberg, H. S., Graham, R., and Jasper, A. C. (1987). Zone 2 and zone 3 pulmonary blood flow. *J. Appl. Physiol. 62*:1982-1988.

Staub, N. C., editor (1978). *Lung Biology in Health and Disease.* Vol. 7, *Lung Water and Solute Exchange.* Marcel Dekker, New York.

Sun, R. Y., Nieman, G. F., Hakim, T. S., and Chang, H. K. (1987). Effects of lung volume and alveolar surface tension on pulmonary vascular resistance. *J. Appl. Physiol. 62*:1622-1626.

Suzuki, H., and Twarog, B. M. (1982a). Membrane properties of smooth muscle cells in pulmonary arteries of the rat. *Am. J. Physiol. 242 (Heart Circ. Physiol. 11)*:H900-H906.

Suzuki, H., and Twarog, B. M. (1982b). Membrane properties of smooth muscle cells in pulmonary hypertensive rats. *Am. J. Physiol. 242 (Heart Circ. Physiol. 11)*:H907-H915.

Sylvester, J. T., Mitzner, W., Ngeow, Y., and Permutt, S. (1983). Hypoxic constriction of alveolar and extra-alveolar vessels in isolated pig lungs. *J. Appl. Physiol. 54*:1660-1666.

Taylor, A. E., and Parker, J. C. (1985). Pulmonary interstitial spaces and lymphatics. In *Handbook of Physiology.* Sect. 3, *The Respiratory System.* Vol. I, *Circulation and Nonrespiratory Functions.* Edited by A. P. Fishman and A. B. Fisher. Am. Physiol. Soc., Bethesda, MD, pp. 167-230.

Vanhoutte, P. M., Verbeuren, T. J., and Webb, R. C. (1981). Local modulation of adrenergic neuroeffector interaction in the blood vessel wall. *Physiol. Rev. 61*:151-247.

Vender, R. L., Clemmons, D. R., Kwock, L., and Friedman, M. (1987). Reduced oxygen tension induces pulmonary endothelium to release a pulmonary smooth muscle cell mitogen(s). *Am. Rev. Resp. Dis. 135*:622-627, 1987.

Wagner, W. W., Jr. and Latham, L. P. (1975). Pulmonary capillary recruitment during airway hypoxia in the dog.*J. App. Physiol. 39*:900-905.

Wagner, W. W., Jr., Latham, L. P., Gillespie, M. N., Guenther, J. P., and Capen, R. L. (1982). Direct measurement of pulmonary capillary transit times. *Science 218*:379-381.

Walston, A., and Kendall, M. E. (1973). Comparison of pulmonary wedge and left atrial pressure in man. *Am. Heart J. 86*:159-164.

Wanner, A., Zarzecki, S., and Sackner, M. A. (1975). Effects of lung inflation on pulmonary arterial blood volume in intact dogs. *J. Appl. Physiol. 38*:675-680.

Wanner, A., Begin, R., Conn, M., and Sackner, M. A. (1978). Vascular volumes of the pulmonary circulation in intact dogs. *J. Appl. Physiol. 44*:956-963.

Wasserman, K., Butler, J., and Van Kessel, A. (1966). Factors affecting the pulmonary capillary blood flow pulse in man. *J. Appl. Physiol. 21*:890-900.

Wearn, J. T., Ernstene, A. C., Bromer, A. W., Barr, J. S., German, W. J., and Zschiesche, L. J. (1934). The normal behavior of the pulmonary blood vessels with observations on the intermittence of the flow of blood in the arterioles and capillaries. *Am. J. Physiol. 109*:236-256.

West, J. B., and Dollery, C. T. (1965). Distribtuion of blood flow and the pressure-flow relations of the whole lung. *J. Appl. Physiol. 20*:175-183.

West, J. B., and Wagner, P. D. (1977). Pulmonary gas exchange. In *Lung Biology in Health and Disease.* Vol. 3, *Bioenginnering Aspects of the Lung.* Edited by J. B. West. Marcel Dekker, New York, pp. 361-457.

Wiedemann, H. P. (1986). Wedge pressure in pulmonary veno-occlusive disease. *New Engl. J. Med. 315*:1233.

Wiener, F., Morkin, E., Skalak, R., and Fishman, A. P. (1966). Wave propagation in the pulmonary circulation. *Circ. Res. 19*:834-850.

Williams, M. H. (1954). Relationships between pulmonary artery pressure and blood flow in the dog lung. *Am. J. Physiol. 179*:243-245.

Yen, R. T., and Foppiano, L. (1981). Elasticity of small pulmonary veins in the cat. *J. Biomed. Eng. 103*:38-42.

Yen, R. T., Fung, Y. C., and Bingham, N. (1980). Elasticity of small pulmonary arteries in the cat. *J. Biomed. Eng. 102*:170-177.

Young, R. C., Jr., Nagano, H., Vaughan, T. R., Jr., and Staub, N. C. (1963). Pulmonary capillary blood volume in dog: effects of 5-hydroxytryptamine. *J. Appl. Physiol. 18*:264-268.

Zhuang, F. Y., Fung, Y. C., and Yen, R. T. (1983). Analysis of blood flow in cat's lung with detailed anatomical and elasticity data. *J. Appl. Physiol. 55*:1341-1348.

Zidulka, A., and Hakim, T. S. (1985). Wedge pressure in large vs. small pulmonary arteries to detect pulmonary venoconstriction. *J. Appl. Physiol. 59*: 1329-1332.

4

Pulmonary Circulation During Exercise

JOHN T. REEVES

University of Colorado
Health Sciences Center
Denver, Colorado

JEROME A. DEMPSEY

University of Wisconsin-Madison
Madison, Wisconsin

ROBERT F. GROVER *

University of Colorado School of Medicine
Denver, Colorado

I. Introduction

As the drama of exercise unfolds, ever-increasing demands for oxygenated blood require the full resources of the lung. Ventilation is driven to bring greater quantities of oxygen to the pulmonary capillaries, while cardiac output rises to increase blood flow through an expanded pulmonary capillary bed. A fascinating interplay between ventilation and lung perfusion is called upon in an effort to preserve the efficiency of blood oxygenation. The increases in capillary perfusion Q should be distributed to match the increases in alveolar ventilation VA so that the distribution of their ratio, VA/Q, remains as uniform as possible. How well the participants in this drama realize their respective objectives will be discussed in this chapter.

To increase blood flow through the lung, you must increase the vascular driving pressure from the pulmonary artery to the left atrium. The resistance to blood flow presented by the pulmonary vascular bed during this process may or may not change. We will examine this in some detail, since we have found many misconceptions on this subject. We will present evidence that increasing cardiac output is associated with a consistent rise in wedge pressure to remarkable levels during heavy exercise. This appears to be a major factor in capillary recruitment,

*Retired

particularly in the upright posture. However, it may also contribute to the more imperfect matching of perfusion to ventilation during exercise. This, plus a significant diffusion limitation, contributes to some loss of efficiency in pulmonary gas exchange. These considerations raise the possibility that limitations of adaptability of the pulmonary circulation to heavy exercise may constitute a handicap to the trained athlete although not to the healthy untrained individual.

II. Pulmonary Hemodynamics

A. Approach and Methods

We have reviewed published hemodynamic data to examine the behavior of the pulmonary circulation during exercise and to examine in particular the effect of posture. Because pulmonary circulatory measurements that include wedge pressure in both the supine and the upright posture in the same subjects are not available, it was necessary to examine postural effects between different groups of subjects. In the supine posture, a total of 196 measurements in 91 subjects (63 mean, 28 women) were analyzed by class of oxygen uptake in steps of 500 or 1000 ml/min as work load increased (Bevegard, 1963; Bevegard et al., 1960, 1963; Dexter et al., 1951; Gurtner et al., 1975; Holmgren et al., 1960; Varnauskas, 1955); see Table 1. For each class of oxygen uptake, measurements in the women were found to be similar to those in the men, and so the data were combined. For subjects in the upright posture, a total of 104 measurements in 24 subjects (23 men, 1 woman) were examined (Bevegard et al., 1963; Groves et al., 1987; Reeves et al., 1987; Moon, unpublished); see Table 1. These subjects tended to be more fit, and they achieved higher oxygen uptakes than the supine subjects. The body sizes and ages were similar in the two groups (Fig. 1). Hence we considered that the upright and supine groups were similar enough that comparisons could reasonably be made.

To ensure the quality of the data collected for the present analysis, we included only healthy subjects with normal pulmonary arterial pressures. The combined pulmonary arterial pressures for 106 normal subjects 6-83 years old were 14±3 (SD) mmHg (Reeves and Groves, 1984). Hence we selected only subjects whose resting pulmonary arterial pressures were within less than two standard deviations of normal, in the range of 9-20 mmHg. Because of ambiguities in some of the wedged catheter measurements, they were included only if the wedge pressure was at least 3 mmHg less than the mean pulmonary arterial pressure. The methods for each study involved direct measurements of pressure at cardiac catheterization, with a similar choice of zero reference. Cardiac output was by the Fick method using oxygen or multiple inert gases. For each set of data analyzed, the coefficients of variation (SD/mean value) were small and were similar to those previously reported, indicating agreement within and between

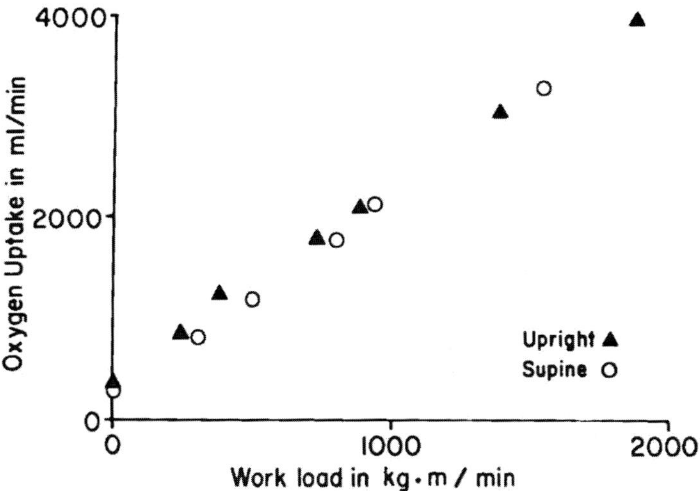

Figure 1 As work load is increased, the resulting increase in oxygen uptake is similar whether exercise is performed in the upright (△) or the supine (○) posture. Mean data from Table 1.

laboratories. The large number of measurements for most classes of oxygen uptake resulted in a small standard error of the mean. Therefore, because the subjects in the upright and supine groups were comparable and the data were collected by comparable methods and were determined to be of high quality, it seemed reasonable to proceed with the analysis.

B. Supine Exercise

Group Data

Hemodynamic measurements in supine subjects were available at rest and during exercise up to work loads of 1600 kg-m/min, which required oxygen uptakes of more than 3000 ml/min (Table 1). Pulmonary arterial pressure, wedge pressure, and cardiac output increased with increasing effort. With mild supine exercise at the lowest work load that increased oxygen uptake two- to threefold, there was no change in the pulmonary vascular resistance (Table 1). With higher work loads, the calculated resistances decreased slightly. It should be noted that for the highest work load (oxygen uptake of 3300 ml/min) there were measurements in only seven subjects (Bevegard et al., 1963; Holmgren et al., 1960), and in them the resistances of 0.4±0.1 unit constitute a very small decrease from their resting resistances of 0.5±0.2 unit. The combined group data illustrated graphically in Figure 2 suggest a relatively small decrease in the calculated pul-

Table 1 Pulmonary Hemodynamics at Rest and During Exercise in Normal Young Men and Women[a,b]

	Supine Measurements						Sitting Measurements					
	VO_2 ml/min	Work, kg-m/min	Ppa, mmHg	Pwedge, mmHg	Q, liters/min	PVR, units	VO_2 ml/min	Work, kg-m/min	Ppa, mmHg	Pwedge, mmHg	Q, liters/min	PVR, units
Mean	273	0	14	8	7.6	0.8	371	0	14	5	6.5	1.5
SD	53	0	3	3	1.8	0.3	57	0	3	2	1.5	0.5
n	70	70	70	62	70	62	21	21	21	15	21	15
Mean	811	307	19	10	11.5	0.8	871	234	18	9	10.7	0.8
SD	106	62	4	3	2.0	0.4	87	72	2	2	1.8	0.3
n	31	31	31	26	31	26	5	5	5	5	5	5
Mean	1182	501	21	10	13.6	0.7	1235	383	21	11	13.3	0.8
SD	138	97	4	3	1.6	0.2	134	60	5	4	1.8	0.2
n	46	46	46	39	46	39	16	16	16	16	16	16

Mean	1765	802	23	12	17.5	0.6	1792	727	22	12	16.6	0.7
SD	137	110	5	5	1.7	0.2	117	75	5	5	1.5	0.2
n	27	27	27	25	27	25	18	18	18	12	18	12
Mean	2126	943	23	12	18.4	0.6	2093	879	25	14	18.2	0.6
SD	85	27	5	5	2.0	0.2	67	126	6	7	1.4	0.1
n	14	14	14	14	14	14	9	9	9	8	9	8
Mean	3292	1550	29	16	25.9	0.4	3036	1386	31	18	22.6	0.6
SD	234	132	5	5	1.6	0.1	345	279	7	6	1.9	0.2
n	8	8	8	7	8	7	29	29	29	22	29	22
Mean							3980	1887	35	24	25.4	0.5
SD							309	292	7	7	2.2	0.1
n							6	6	6	5	6	5

[a]Group data arranged by class of oxygen uptake.
[b]VO_2, oxygen uptake; work, work load; Ppa, pulmonary arterial pressure; Pwedge, wedge pressure; Q, cardiac output; PVR, pulmonary vascular resistance; n, number of subjects. Data presented as mean ± standard deviation (SD).

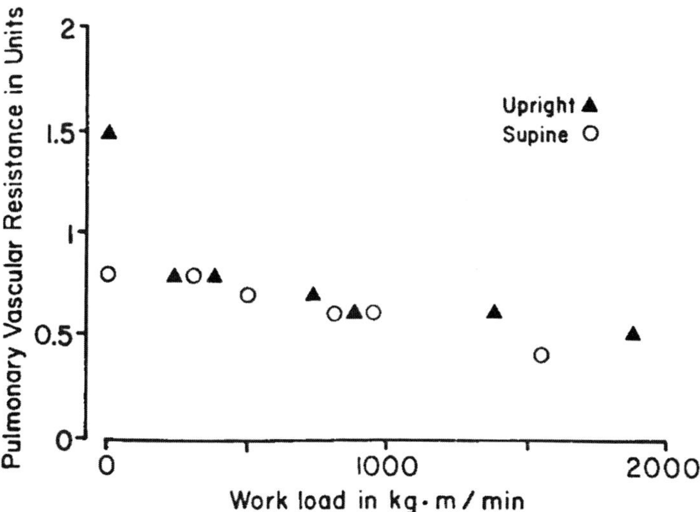

Figure 2 Pulmonary vascular resistance during exercise is similar in both upright (Δ) and supine (O) subjects. Only at rest is resistance higher upright than supine. Group mean data from Table 1.

monary vascular resistance on going from rest to heavy exercise in the supine posture.

Individual Data

A difficulty with the data in Table 1 and Figure 2 was that there were different subjects in the various classes of oxygen uptake examined, and it is important to know how the lung circulation behaved in a given individual. In the supine data examined, pulmonary arterial pressure and flow measurements were available at rest and for at least two levels of exercise of increasing severity in 63 persons, including 21 women. Hence it was possible in each person to obtain a regression line relating pulmonary arterial pressure to flow. Because the lines were similar in men and women, the data have been combined to give a mean regression line (Table 2) for all the data (Fig. 3A). On average, each liter increase of cardiac output was accompanied by a 1 mmHg increase in pulmonary arterial pressure.

The wedge pressure was available in 53 supine persons having one resting and at least two exercise measurements. The wedge pressure did not remain constant but showed a consistent increase with increasing cardiac output (Table 2, Figure 4A).

The net driving force for blood flow through the lung is the pulmonary arterial minus the wedge pressure. We noted that the regression lines for the

Table 2 Slope and Intercept of Regression Lines for Pulmonary Pressure–Flow Relationships Based on Individual Data[a,b]

	Supine Measurements			Upright Measurements		
Variables	n	Slope	Intercept	n	Slope	Intercept
			Normal Young Men and Women			
Q, Ppa	63	1.00	8.2	21	1.01	6.7
SD		0.94	7.9		0.43	4.3
Q, Pw	53	0.30	6.3	16	0.84	–0.7
SD		0.35	4.2		0.39	5.2
Q, Ppa-Pw	53	0.53	2.0			
SD		0.44	4.2			
			Normal Old Man			
Q, Ppa	14	2.54	2.3			
SD		0.77	5.4			
Q, Pw	14	1.93	–0.76			
SD		0.94	6.7			
Q, Ppa-Pw	14	0.64	3.1			
SD		0.57	3.2			

[a]For each individual, a regression line was calculated, based on at least three sets of data at rest and exercise. From these individual lines, the mean regression line was determined. Both supine and upright data were available for young men and women, but complete data in the old men were available only in the supine posture.
[b]Q, Ppa, pulmonary arterial pressure (ordinate) vs. cardiac output (abscissa); Q, Pw, wedge pressure (ordinate) vs. cardiac output (abscissa); Q, Ppa-Pw, pulmonary arterial pressure minus wedge pressure, i.e., pressure gradient (ordinate) vs. cardiac output (abscissa); n, number of subjects. Data presented as mean ± standard deviation (SD).

wedge and pulmonary arterial pressures had similar intercepts on the Y axis (Table 2). Consequently, the regression line for the pressure difference – the pulmonary arterial minus wedge pressure gradient – had an intercept of only 2 mmHg, which is very close to the origin (Table 2). Recall that lines that do pass

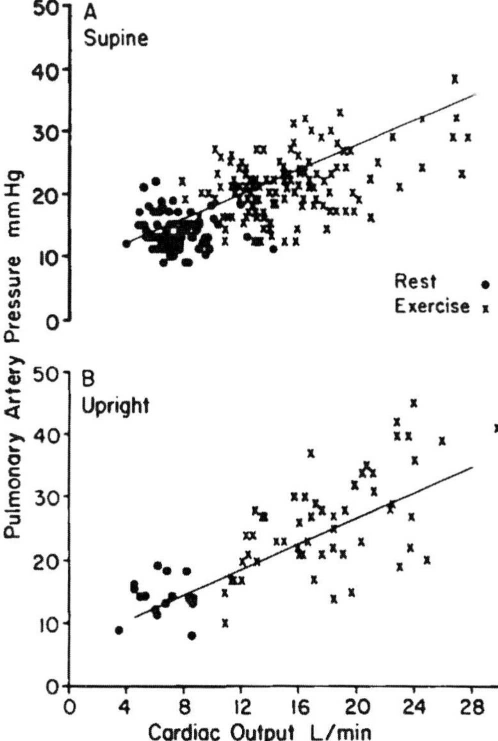

Figure 3 Rise in pulmonary arterial pressure with increase in cardiac output from rest (●) to exercise (x) in normal young men and women. In panel A (upper) are shown 211 supine measurements in 63 persons, with the mean regression line from Table 2. Panel B (lower) shows 121 upright measurements in 21 persons, with the mean regression line from Table 2. The lines have identical slopes and similar intercepts.

through the origin of the pressure-flow diagram are lines of constant resistance. Hence, as illustrated in Figure 5A, increasing flow was associated with very little decrease in resistance. In fact, the regression line through all the data differs little from a line based just on the exercise data and forced through the origin (Fig. 5A). This latter line corresponds to a constant resistance of 0.61 unit. Thus, this pressure-flow analysis of individual data supported that from group data in Figure 2: that supine exercise induced very little decrease in the pulmonary vascular resistance.

C. Upright Exercise

Group Data

A complete set of measurements upright at rest and during exercise was available in only 21 normal young subjects (Table 1) indicating the relative paucity of up-

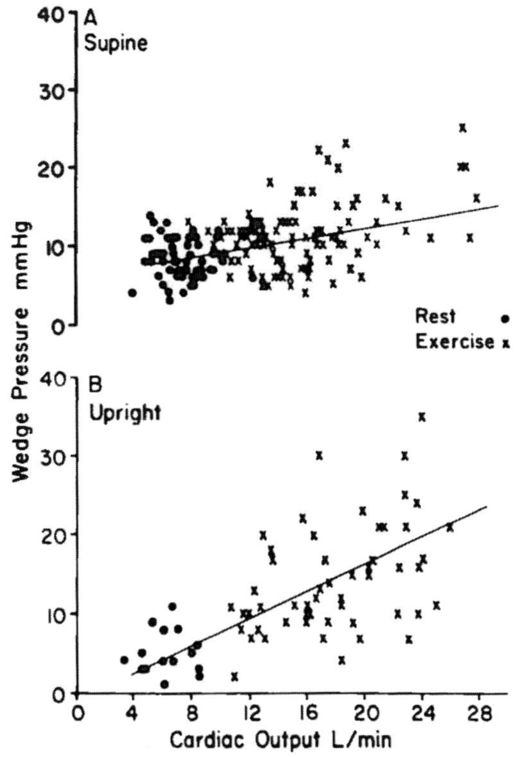

Figure 4 Change in wedge pressure with increase in cardiac output from rest (•) to exercise (x) in normal young men and women. Panel A (upper) shows 162 supine measurements in 53 persons; the mean regression line is from Table 2. In panel B (lower) are shown 100 upright measurements in 16 persons and their line of regression from Table 2. The two lines are clearly different in both slope and intercept.

right compared to supine data. They accomplished work loads up to nearly 1900 kg-m/min yielding oxygen uptakes of approximately 4000 ml/min. With increasing oxygen uptake, pulmonary arterial and wedge pressure and cardiac output increased. In all five subjects performing the mildest exercise, which merely doubled the oxygen uptake, the wedge pressure increased significantly to 9±2 mmHg from the resting value of 5±3 mmHg, and the calculated pulmonary vascular resistance fell to 0.8±0.3 unit from the resting value of 1.5±0.5 unit (Table 1). With subsequent heavier exercise there was only a small further fall in the calculated pulmonary vascular resistance. The subjects performing exercise at the heaviest work load, which increased the oxygen uptake to tenfold the resting value, decreased their pulmonary vascular resistance from 2.1±0.6 units at rest to 0.8±0.2 unit with mild exercise, but only decreased further to 0.5±0.1 unit with the heaviest exercise. This *nonlinear* fall in resistance is particularly noteworthy. The resitance measurements illustrated graphically in Figure 2 demonstrated this same pattern – a large fall from rest to mild exercise, with a much smaller further decrease with heavier exercise to work loads approaching maximum effort.

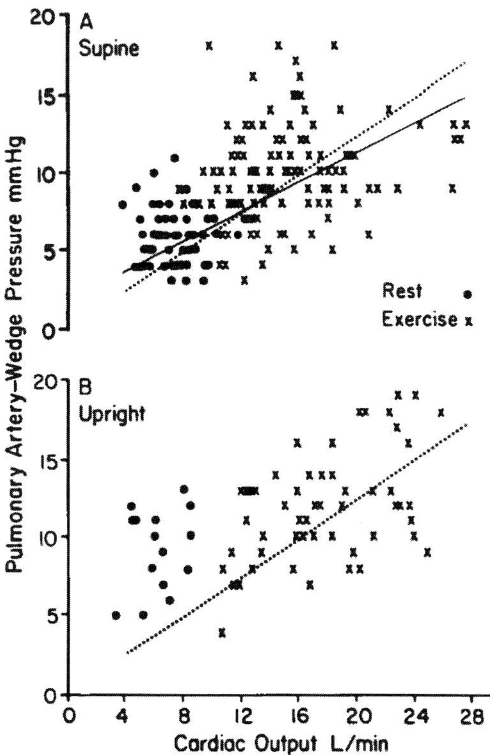

Figure 5 Relationship of the pulmonary vascular pressure gradient (pulmonary arterial minus wedge pressure) to increasing flow (cardiac output) from rest (●) to exercise (x) in normal young men and women. The upper panel (A) shows 162 supine measurements in 53 persons. The solid line is the regression line from Table 2 based on both the resting and exercise data. The dotted regression line was calculated using only the exercise data, excluding the resting data, and forced through the origin; it is therefore a line of constant resistance. Note that the dotted line passes through much of the resting data and does not differ from the solid line. In the lower panel (B) are shown 100 upright measurements in 16 persons. Since the data are clearly *nonlinear*, a regression line based on all the data is not justified. Rather, a regression line (dotted) has been calculated based only on the exercise data, excluding the resting data, and again forced through the origin. Note that while this line fits the exercise data very well, it passes below all the resting points. This reflects the higher resting resistance in the upright posture and the prompt fall with the onset of exercise. The two dotted lines supine (A) and upright (B) have almost identical slopes, indicating the same constant resistance during exercise in both postures.

Individual Data

In the upright data examined, pulmonary arterial pressure and flow measurements were available at rest and for at least two levels of exercise of increasing severity in 21 persons, including 1 woman. The pulmonary arterial pressure-flow relationship was established for each person, and the average slope and intercept of the lines for the 21 persons are given in Table 2. All data points are shown in

Figure 3B. Since the overall pressure-flow relationship appeared to be linear, a mean regression line including both rest and exercise was calculated. From this it can be seen that on average, each liter of cardiac output increase was accompanied by a 1 mmHg increase in pulmonary arterial pressure, i.e., the same as in the supine posture.

Measurements of wedge pressure and blood flow were available in only 16 persons performing multiple levels of exercise. As before, the wedge pressure increased significantly with increasing cardiac output. All data points are shown in Figure 4B. Again, the overall wedge pressure-flow relationship appeared to be approximately linear, and so a mean regression line was calculated including both rest and exercise. The intercept of this line on the pressure axis was not different from zero.

Although the relation of flow to pulmonary arterial pressure and its relation to wedge pressure were each approximately linear (Figs. 3B and 4B), the relation of flow to the pressure gradient, that is, pulmonary artery minus wedge pressure, was clearly *not linear* (Fig. 5B). With the transition from rest to mild exercise in the upright posture, the increase in flow was associated with virtually no increase in the pressure gradient. This finding implies that with the onset of mild exercise there is a relatively large decrease in overall pulmonary vascular resistance.

From mild to heavy exercise, increasing cardiac output is now clearly associated with a progressive increase in the pulmonary arterial-wedge pressure gradient (Fig. 5B). A regression line based only on these exercise data, excluding the resting data, and forced through the origin fits these exercise data very well but falls outside all of the resting data (Fig. 5B). This line corresponds to a constant resistance of 0.63 unit, which is remarkably close to the value of 0.61 unit for supine exercise. Thus, the pressure-flow analysis based on individual data supported that for group data in Figure 2 – namely, that upright exercise induced a decrease in the pulmonary vascular resistance – and the overall decrease was relatively large. However, this decrease was *nonlinear*. Virtually all of the decrease occurred as lung perfusion increased with the transition from rest to mild exercise. With further increase in pulmonary blood flow as the work load increased, pulmonary vascular resistance remained almost constant and at the same low levels present during supine exercise.

D. Upright versus Supine Exercise: Effect of Posture

The main effect of posture on the pulmonary circulation appeared to be at rest. Once the transition from rest to mild exercise had been made, both the resistance calculations and the pressure-flow relationships indicated that posture had virtually no further influence with increasing exercise intensity. Higher resting resistances in upright compared to supine subjects seemed valid in that the subjects had both higher pressure gradients and lower flows. The higher pressure gradient cannot be ascribed to an error in the placement of the transducer zero relative to the heart, because subtracting wedge from pulmonary arterial pressure would cancel any such error. Furthermore, it is known that the upright posture is associated with a redistribution of the blood volume to the dependent body, resulting in reduced cardiac filling (Bevegard et al., 1960; Reeves et al., 1961). The present data confirmed that wedge pressures were lower in the resting upright subjects. The possibility that wedge measurements reflected airway rather than left atrial pressures would not invalidate the conclusion that the gradient was higher upright than supine.

Topographical Distribution of Perfusion

In the upright posture, the vertical distance from lung base to apex combined with the normal low pulmonary arterial pressure causes preferential perfusion of the lower lung segments (Harf et al., 1978; West, 1979). In the supine posture, the vertical distance is less, such that the whole lung can be perfused rather evenly with the same low pulmonary arterial pressure. Thus, one likely explanation for the higher vascular resistances observed in the upright subjects was preferential perfusion of only a portion of the lung – the lower segments – whereas the supine subjects perfused the entire lung. The higher resting wedge (left atrial) pressures supine versus upright would also allow perfusion of more lung vasculature supine, since pulmonary venous pressure is an important factor favoring vascular recruitment (Permutt et al., 1963; Wagner et al., 1979). The perfusion of a smaller lung vascular bed would account for a higher pulmonary vascular resistance in the upright subjects and would also be compatible with the concept that the normal pulmonary arterial pressure (which is the same supine and upright) is too low to cause evenly distributed perfusion of the lung in the upright posture (West, 1979).

The finding that even mild upright exercise abolished postural differences in the lung circulation suggested that even a small increase in cardiac output abolished uneven lung perfusion by recruiting upper lobe vessels (Harf et al., 1978). Increased ventilation, which has been reported to recruit the upper lung segments (Bake et al., 1974), may have been an additional factor. However, an increase in vascular pressure is more likely the primary factor causing recruitment. Increases in flow per se in the absence of increased pressure have failed to produce lung vascular recruitment (Wagner et al., 1979). In the upright subjects, increased wedge pressure with exercise may have been the dominant factor, because upon going from rest to the mildest exercise the increase in pulmonary arterial pressure equaled the increase in wedge pressure and no increase in pressure gradient occurred (Table 1). An important factor in the decrease in pulmonary vascular resistance with the onset of mild upright exercise may therefore be the increase in wedge pressure.

Increased Wedge Pressure

The increase in the wedge pressure during both supine and upright exercise has a large influence on the lung circulation, but its importance has not been emphasized in the physiological literature. The importance of this is illustrated by measurements in healthy older men aged 60-83 years (Granath et al., 1964; Table 2). The increase in wedge pressure with exercise was remarkable compared to that in younger persons (Fig. 6A). The increase in pulmonary arterial pressure with exercise was also greater than was found in younger subjects (Fig. 6B). However, the pressure *gradient* from pulmonary artery to wedge was not clearly different (Table 2). The high wedge pressures during exercise were responsible for pulmonary arterial pressures higher than 40 mmHg in three subjects having oxygen uptakes less than 1500 ml/min. The authors considered that age-related myocardial stiffness causing decreased diastolic compliance of the ventricular wall contributed to higher ventricular filling pressures. (Granath et al., 1964). Hence, the resulting increases in wedge pressures were the major contributor to exercise-induced pulmonary hypertension.

In young men, similar levels of pulmonary hypertension were achieved during upright exercise, but at much higher work loads and with higher lung blood flows than in the older men. Six subjects had mean pulmonary arterial pressures of 40 mmHg or more associated with cardiac outputs of 24.4±2.7 liters/min (Groves et al., 1987; Moon, personal communication). Their wedge pressures averaged 27±5 mmHg, implying substantial left atrial hypertension. Thus, in normal subjects, both old and young, exercise-induced pulmonary hypertension was due more to increased wedge pressure than to an increased pressure gradient from pulmonary artery to wedge.

The data we employed in the foregoing analyses show consistent elevations in wedge pressure during exercise. Some readers may question their validity. Obviously we would like to have direct measurements of left atrial pressure under these conditions, but we are not likely to see such data from humans performing heavy exercise. Consequently, we must work with what we do have – the wedge pressures published in the literature by a number of different workers. Concern over accuracy could be based on the uncertain influence of large swings in intrathoracic pressure hyperventilation. Presumably the concern is that the reported wedge pressures are erroneously high. If the true left atrial pressure were actually lower, then the pressure gradient across the pulmonary vascular bed would be greater, that is, the pulmonary vascular resistance would actually be *higher* than we have calculated. The implication of such calculations would be that during exercise pulmonary vascular resistance would decrease even less than the small amount we have indicated, and might even *increase*. This, too, would be a surprising conclusion. Certainly the evidence is provocative. Echocardiographic measurements of the dimensions of the left atrium during exercise would help resolve these concerns.

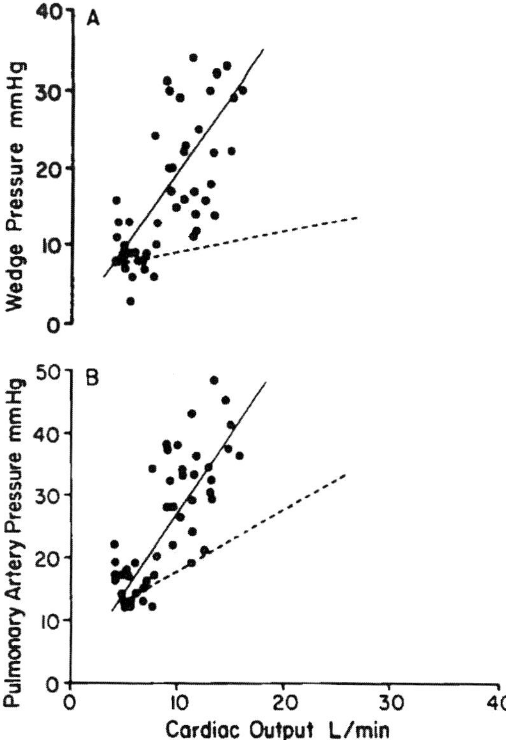

Figure 6 The effect of age on pulmonary hemodynamics in 14 health men 61-83 years old. Shown here are 52 measurements of wedge pressure (upper panel A) and of pulmonary arterial pressure (lower panel B) with increasing cardiac output from rest to exercise supine. The solid regression lines for these data are compared with the dotted regression lines for young men and women, from Table 2. The more rapid rise in wedge pressure in the older men is reflected by the steeper rise in pulmonary arterial pressure during exercise.

E. Pulmonary Circulatory Control During Exercise

Passive Factors

The apparent dependence of pulmonary vascular resistance and lung vessel recruitment on vascular pressures, in particular venous pressures, as reviewed above, suggests that the lung resistance vessels behave in a largely passive manner during exercise. The higher resistance upright than supine at rest, the decrease in resistance with small increases in wedge pressure at the onset of exercise in upright subjects, and the parallel large increments in pulmonary arterial pressure with large increments in wedge pressure all support the concept of a largely passive microcirculation. The small pulmonary arteries and veins have little medial smooth muscle and little resting tone. If in a resting supine subject most of the arteries are already recruited, perhaps it is not surprising that a three- to fourfold increase in flow with exercise is accompanied by only a small fall in resistance. Similar conclusions were reached by Harris et al. (1968) using exercise during unilateral pulmonary artery occlusion in normal supine subjects. When one major pulmonary arterial branch was occluded, flow through the contralateral branch was nearly doubled, even though the subject was still at rest. Superimposing exercise then increased flow through that one lung even more.

Some vasodilation does occur during either supine or upright exercise. Widimski et al. (1963) found that for up to an hour following supine exercise of moderate intensity pulmonary vascular resistance remained 20% below that observed before the exercise. Ekelund (1967) found that pulmonary vascular resistance at 60 min of upright cycle exercise had fallen below the value observed at 10 min of exercise. Authors of both reports speculated that time-dependent stress relaxation had occurred in the medial smooth muscle of the pulmonary vascular bed. If so, then there is some vascular tone that can be overcome by the increased pressures during exercise.

Vasomotor Factors

Some "active" vasodilation is also possible. Lindenfeld et al. (1983) found a 24% decrease in pulmonary vascular resistance of normal dogs during treadmill exercise. They wished to determine whether a vasodilating prostaglandin accounted for the decrease. Although following cyclooxygenase inhibition of prostaglandin synthesis, pulmonary vascular resistance increased slightly both at rest and during exercise, the authors concluded that the normal fall in pulmonary vascular resistance during exercise depended largely on factors other than vasodilator prostaglandin production. While there may be active vasodilation of the lung microcirculation during exercise, vascular recruitment and dilation of already recruited vessels may be largely controlled by passive factors, such as intravascular pressure. This largely passive control of the lung circulation is in contrast to the active vasodilation that takes place during exercise in systemic vascular beds such as skeletal muscle and myocardium.

III. Pulmonary Gas Exchange

A. Normal Untrained Individuals

During exercise, completeness of blood oxygenation within the lung is challenged by two major factors. First is the progressive fall in oxygen content and PO_2 of mixed venous blood entering the lung, reflecting increased oxygen extraction by the exercising muscles. Second is the increased velocity of red cells through the pulmonary microcirculation with increased pulmonary blood flow. This curtails the time available for alveolar-capillary gas exchange. If no adjustments occurred in the lung with even moderate exercise, arterial hypoxemia would surely develop. However, two critical adjustments do take place (Dempsey et al., 1980). The pulmonary capillary blood volume expands up to threefold to its maximum capacity, thereby minimizing the reduction in red cell transit time in the pulmonary capillary (transit time = capillary blood volume/blood flow). In addition, alveolar ventilation (VA) rises out of proportion to the coincident increase in cardiac output (Q) and oxygen uptake. As a consequence, overall VA/Q rises from approximately 1 at rest to 3 in moderate exercise, to as high as 5 or 6 with maximum exercise. Hence a rising alveolar PO_2 is assured. Because of this, arterial PO_2 and oxygen content are maintained through maximum work, at least up to an oxygen uptake of about 3500 ml/min.

However, there are some signs of an imperfect response even at relatively moderate work loads. As the level of the alveolar PO_2 rises, arterial PO_2 stays constant, and consequently the alveolar-arterial PO_2 difference doubles, from 5-10 mmHg at rest to 20 in moderate exercise to 25 at heavy exercise. The source of this imperfect response is attributable in part to a signficant increase in the nonuniformity of the VA/Q distribution of the lung from rest to wwork (Gledhill et al., 1977, 1978; Hammond et al., 1986). This was determined by measuring the VA/Q distribution with the multiple inert gas technique, and then using this distribution along with the measured mixed venous blood gas tensions to calculate the pulmonary end-capillary PO_2. The remaining half of the rising alveolar-arterial PO_2 difference during exercise has not been defined. Speculation attributes this portion to two factors: a normal shunt of mixed venous blood amounting to about 1% of the total cardiac output (Gledhill et al., 1977) and an incomplete diffusion equilibrium in the pulmonary capillary as oxygen uptake exceeds 2500 ml/min (Hammond et al., 1986).

Nonuniform Distribution of VA/Q

We emphasize that this increasing VA/Q nonuniformity during exercise is not to be confused with the more uniform topographical VA/Q distribution among lung regions experienced during moderate upright exercise. Thus, whereas VA/Q ratios as measured with radioactive tracer techniques may be two to three times higher in lung apex than base at rest, during exercise VA/Q becomes nearly identical in dependent and apical regions (Bryan et al., 1964; Harf et al., 1978). This qualitative difference between exercise effects on topographical VA/Q versus the "functional" multiple inert gas VA/Q distribution implies that the source of the increased inhomogeneity resides *within* lung regions. Although inhomogeneities in mechanical properties and in the distribution of ventilation do exist within lung regions (Engle et al., 1973), it is not obvious why exercise should increase this inhomogeneity. End-expiratory lung volume is reduced with increasing exercise intensity (Sharatt et al., 1987). If this reduction were sufficient to cause small airway narrowing or even closure during a sufficient fraction of tidal breathing, then the distribution of inspiratory gas might become nonuniform (Henke et al., 1987). Finally, we reemphasize that although the VA/Q distribution is increased and this change contributes significantly to a widening of the alveolar-arterial PO_2 difference during exercise, even the lowest VA/Q region in exercise exceeds the highest VA/Q region at rest. Therefore it is doubtful that any lung regions are really underventilated during exercise. Consequently, alveolar PO_2 is high everywhere and hypoxemia is avoided, at least in normal untrained individuals.

The increased nonuniformity of V_A:Q_c during exercise may also be attributed to a primary effect on perfusion distribution. At rest, in localized underventilated regions of the lung, the low alveolar PO_2 stimulates adjacent blood vessels to constrict, thereby matching V_A/Q (Grover et al., 1983). However, during exercise, the increase in intra-vascular pressures, and in particular the substantial rise in wedge pressure described above, may act to defeat this local hypoxic vasoconstrictor mechanism (Benumof and Wahrenbrock, 1975). As a consequence, V_A/Q matching is disturbed. On the other hand, the increase in alveolar PO_2 throughout the lung during exercise, as just mentioned, would minimize the utilization of localized hypoxic pulmonary vasoconstriction to match V_A/Q. An alternative explanation stems from the observation that the widening of the perfusion distribution during exercise is consistently related to pulmonary arterial pressure (Wagner et al., 1986). This relationship was found to be independent of inspired PO_2 or exercise rate, providing indirect evidence for a role for increased pulmonary vascular pressure as a cause of V_A/Q mismatching during exercise. Of course, many other interpretations of these purely correlative data are feasible.

B. Trained Athletes

There are limits to this homeostasis in healthy persons. These are frequently exceeded by highly trained athletes who are capable of achieving very high work rates and metabolic demands by virtue of the very large capacities of their cardiovascular and skeletal muscle systems (Dempsey, 1986). Often the result is arterial hypoxemia as shown by the contrasting responses in athletes and nonathletes at maximum exercise (Table 3) (Dempsey et al., 1984; Rowell et al., 1964). This hypoxemia in athletes is attributable to two general causes. First, alveolar PO_2 is not as high in the trained as in the untrained for reasons that are not entirely clear but are certainly related to the much higher ventilation required at the athlete's higher maximum oxygen uptake. For example, if the trained runner at an oxygen uptake of 5 liters/min were to achieve the same high alveolar PO_2 and low PCO_2 as in the untrained individual exercising at an oxygen uptake of only 3 liters/min, he would have to sustain a ventilation in excess of 200 liters/min, whereas the untrained individual would only need to achieve about 120 liters/min ventilation (Dempsey, 1986). Second, the athelete at maximum work develops an excessively wide alveolar-arterial PO_2 difference (Table 3).

Nonuniform Distribution of VA/Q

The causes of this excessive alveolar-arterial PO_2 difference are speculative. Any significant contributions from an intrapulmonary shunt were ruled out by showing that slight elevations of inspired PO_2 during heavy exercise raised alveolar

Table 3 Pulmonary Gas Transport During Short-Term Maximum Exercise: Untrained Versus Trained Young Adults

				Pulmonary Capillary							
	VO_2 liter/min	a-v O_2 Diff., m O_2/100 ml	Blood Flow, liters/min	Blood Volume, ml	Transit time available[b] sec	Transit time required,[c] sec	VE, liters/min	Alveolar PO_2, mmHg	Arterial PO_2, mmHg	Alv–art. PO_2 Diff., mmHg	Arterial PCO_2, mmHg
Untrained	3–4	16–17	19–24	175–210	.53–.55	0.4	110–120	120	90	20–30	25–32
Trained	5–6	18–19	28–33	210	.38–.45	0.6	160–180	100	55–75	35–45	35–40

[a]VO_2, oxygen uptake; a-v O_2 diff., arterial–venous blood oxygen content difference; VE, ventilation per minute.
[b]Transit time available = capillary blood volume/blood flow.
[c]Transit time required = time in pulmonary capillary "required" to bring capillary PO_2 into equilibrium with alveolar PO_2. This was estimated (Dempsey, 1987) from the rate of the diffusion equilibration calculations determined by Wagner (1982). Note that in the highly trained athletes, the time *required* for equilibration is longer than that in the untrained and exceeds the time *available* for equilibration. However, not all highly trained athletes show hypoxemia at maximum work (Dempsey et al., 1984).

PO_2 and arterial PO_2 by equal amounts (Dempsey et al., 1984). A worsening of VA/Q distribution with increasing work loads does occur (Gale et al., 1985) and would be expected to contribute more to the increasing alveolar-arterial PO_2 difference as mixed venous PO_2 falls. So, just as in the untrained, the imperfections in VA/Q distribution and the small anatomical shunt in the face of a falling mixed venous PO_2 cause much of the widening of the alveolar-arterial PO_2 difference.

Diffusion Limitation

We think the additional factor brought out by the high work load in the trained athlete is a significant contribution from the inability of mixed venous blood to equilibrate with alveolar gas by the time the desaturated blood reaches the end of the pulmonary capillary, that is, diffusion limitation. Several characteristics of the response to and requirements of very heavy work are ideal for the precipitation of diffusion disequilibrium. Our reasoning follows:

The primary determinants of alveolar-capillary equilibrium include:

1. The *surface area* available for gas exchange, as determined by the maximal expansion and recruitment of the pulmonary capillary bed together with VA/Q distribution
2. The diffusion *distance* from alveolar gas to red cell
3. The *time* available for equilibrium in the pulmonary capillary, as determined by the increase in pulmonary blood flow relative to the expansion of the pulmonary capillary blood volume
4. The *rate* of equilibrium of mixed venous blood with alveolar gas

The high metabolic demand of the athlete creates a susceptibility toward diffusion limitation by exerting negative effects on at least three and possibly all four of these determinants. The transit time in the pulmonary capillary is greatly shortened because blood flow continues to increase after pulmonary capillary blood volume (Vc) has reached its maximum morphologic capacity (Fig. 7). Also, the rate of equilibration is slowed; that is, the time required to reach equilibration of mixed venous blood with alveolar PO_2 is prolonged because of the relatively low alveolar PO_2 and driving pressure for diffusion. These factors would create the dilemma of a shorter time *available* in the pulmonary capillary for equilibration, under circumstances where a longer time is *required* for equilibration. Thus, for the trained runner at maximum oxygen uptake (Table 3; Fig. 7) with an alveolar PO_2 of 100 mmHg and a mixed venous blood PO_2 approximating 20 mmHg, the estimated mean transit time available (0.45 sec) is significantly shorter than the estimated average time required (0.60 sec) for completeness of equilibration of mixed venous blood with alveolar gas by the end of the pulmonary capillary (Wagner, 1982). Since there must be significant variation around this mean transit time, diffusion disequilibrium probably exists in a

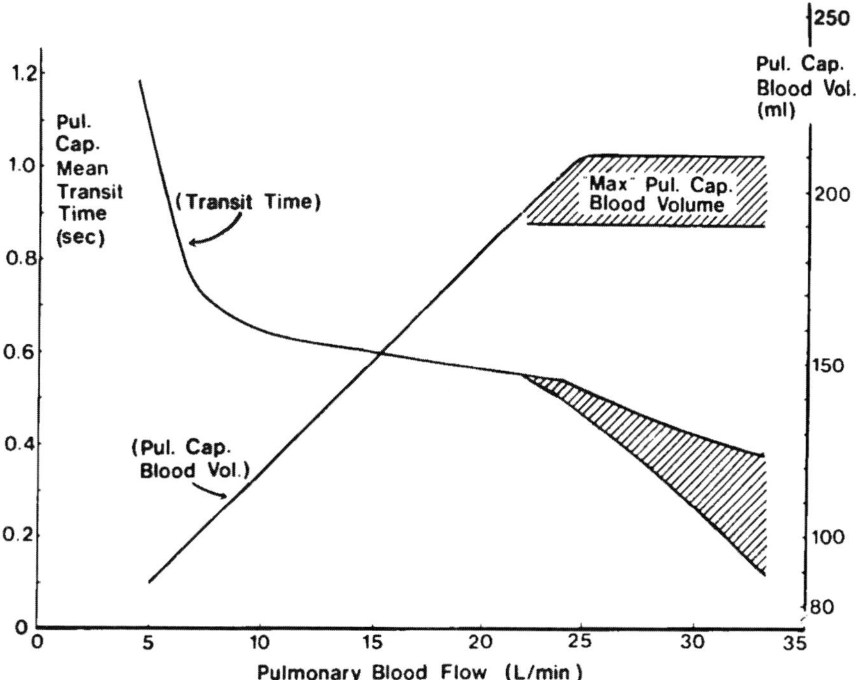

Figure 7 Relationship of increasing pulmonary blood flow (Qc) with increasing exercise load to the expansion of the pulmonary capillary blood volume (Vc), and the effect of this relationship on average red cell transit time through the lung (mean transit time = Vc/Qc). We propose that Vc achieves maximum morphological expansion at about 2.5 times the resting value. Thereafter, as exercise and Qc increase further, transit time will fall precipitously (shaded area). (Reproduced from Dempsey, 1986.)

significant fraction of the pulmonary end capillary blood leaving the trained runner's lung.

We reemphasize that not all athletes capable of achieving very high metabolic rates and blood flows experience inadequate alveolar hyperventilation *or* excessive alveolar-arterial PO_2 differences *or* arterial hypoxemia. We would predict from recent evidence, which is still in a limited population of athletes, that the incidence of moderate hypoxemia (reduction in arterial PO_2 of 10-20 mmHg below rest) occurs in about three-fourths of young adults with maximum oxygen uptakes of 4000 ml/min [> 65 ml/(kg/min)] and that even more severe hypoxemia (arterial PO_2 20-40 mmHg below rest) may occur in over half of this highly fit population. There are probably many reasons for differences among individuals, and one may well be the maximum pulmonary capillary blood volume.

Older fit athletes capable of high maximum oxygen uptake but with normal aging effects on the pulmonary vasculature (see above) and on airway closure may have a fairly high incidence of arterial hypoxemia during heavy exercise.

Interestingly, arterial hypoxemia seems to occur quite consistently in thoroughbred horses running at or near their maximum capacity, which may approximate 125 ml/(kg-min). Exercise-induced pulmonary hypertension in the horse is marked, and alveolar hypoventilation with frank CO_2 retention is common during heavy exercise (Bayly et al., 1983; Dempsey, 1986).

Extravascular Lung Water

The final potential cause of the widened alveolar-arterial PO_2 difference might be found in an increase in extravascular lung water at high work loads, but , to date, findings are inconclusive. Lung lymph flow increased in exercising sheep as much as three- to fourfold with comparable increases in cardiac output (Coates et al., 1984), and this was attributed to an expanding surface area for gas exchange. However, the capacity for lymphatic drainage from the lung is high, so lung water might not actually accumulate in significant amounts. Indeed, dogs showed no change in wet weight/dry weight ratios of the lung following "heavy" exercise (Marshall et al., 1975). However, Younes et al. (1987) have recently shown that the dog lung perfused in situ does accumulate weight as flow is increased to four times the resting level and pulmonary arterial pressure increases to more than 25-30 mmHg even though left atrial pressure is maintained at control levels.

In humans during very heavy exercise, pulmonary arterial pressure can exceed 40 mmHg, and wedge (pulmonary venous) pressure can exceed 30 mmHg (see above), so the potential for excessive leakage into the interstitial fluid space from the plasma does exist. However, indications of extravascular lung water accumulation in the human are indirect and inconsistent. For example, immediately following heavy exercise, residual and closing lung volumes may increase and a relative tachypnea occur (Maron et al., 1979; Younes and Kivinen, 1984), suggesting small airway closure presumably secondary to fluid accumulation in the lung. Unfortunately, these effects are not seen consistently. Sufficiently sensitive techniques for the in vivo measurements of extravascular lung water are sorely needed here.

When lung water does accumulate, it appears first in interstitial fluid "cuffs" around larger extraalveolar vessels and airways. This would probably not affect the alveolar-capillary diffusion distance because the intraalveolar septal diameter apparently does not change in these initial stages (Staub et al., 1967). VA/Q distribution might be affected if cuffing causes increased resistance to blood or air flow in these bronchioles or arterioles, but there is some doubt if vascular or bronchiolar resistance is actually affected by cuffing in these regions (Michel et al., 1987). If the accumulation of extravascular lung water proceeds to the stage of alveolar flooding, then of course the stability of the alveolus would be lost and clearly gas exchange would be severely impaired. However, it is unlikely, with a few rare exceptions (McKechnie et al., 1979) that this extreme would ever be reached in the healthy lung during even extreme exercise.

Exercise Limitations

Do findings of arterial hypoxemia and suspected diffusion disequilibrium in trained athletes implicate the pulmonary circulation as a potential limiting factor to gas transport and hence to exercise performance at sea level? Probably not in the untrained healthy individual who is only capable of working sufficiently hard to achieve a pulmonary blood flow of 20-25 liters/min. This individual can continue to expand his pulmonary capillary blood volume up to the limit of his maximum oxygen uptake, and so alveolar-capillary equilibrium is assured. The problem comes in the trained athletes who fail to undergo adaptation at the level of the lung. As a consequence, the maximum dimensions of the pulmonary capillary bed no longer match the capacity of the cardiovascular and skeletal muscle systems for oxygen. Hence, these individuals might literally have worked themselves to the position where the finite dimensions of the pulmonary capillary bed become a major limiting factor to alveolar-capillary diffusion equilibrium and hence to maximum oxygen transport and exercise performance (Dempsey, 1986). Maximum oxygen uptake seems to be quite sensitive to the level of the arterial oxygen saturation, so that in the range of about 80-92%, maximum oxygen uptake is reduced about 1% for each 1% decrease in arterial oxygen saturation.

IV. Summary

At rest in the supine posture, the topographical distribution of lung perfusion is relatively uniform, the majority of the vascular channels are open, and vascular resistance is low. The increase in blood flow associated with exercise is achieved predominantly by increasing both pulmonary arterial and wedge pressures as well as the driving pressure across the lung, the pressure difference from pulmonary artery to wedge (left atrium). The already low pulmonary vascular resistance decreases only slightly, probably due to the recruitment of parallel capillary channels by the elevation of intravascular pressures.

When the resting subject assumes the upright posture, pulmonary arterial pressure remains constant while wedge pressure and cardiac output fall. The topographical distribution of lung perfusion is no longer uniform, and the increase in calculated pulmonary vascular resistance probably reflects underperfusion of the apical regions of the lung. With the onset of even mild exercise in this upright posture, there is a parallel rise in both pulmonary arterial and wedge pressures, with no increase in driving pressure across the lung. Nevertheless, pulmonary blood flow increases, indicating an abrupt fall in pulmonary vascular resistance approaching the low levels that were present supine. This probably reflects opening of vascular channels in the apical regions as the topographical perfusion of the lung becomes much more uniform. The rise in wedge pressure thus appears to be of major importance in this vascular recruitment, whereas previously the increase in pulmonary arterial pressure had been thought to be the dominant factor.

Subsequently, as the intensity of the upright exercise is increased, the greater blood flow through the lung is achieved largely by an increase in the driving pressure across the lung. The now low vascular resistance again decreases slightly as it follows virtually the same pattern observed during supine exercise.

In spite of these hemodynamic adjustments of the pulmonary circulation during exercise, the efficiency of pulmonary gas exchange is reduced, as evidenced by a widening of the alveolar-arterial PO_2 difference. Contributing factors include less perfect matching of ventilation to perfusion (VA/Q) within local regions of the lung. This tends to lower arterial PO_2 particularly as mixed venous blood PO_2 falls with exercise. However, a significant part of the arterial hypoxemia may be avoided if alveolar PO_2 is raised sufficiently by the hyperventilation of exercise. The increased dispersion of VA/Q may result from greater nonuniformity in the distribution of inspired air during heavy exercise. Interstitial edema may also develop, but this is probably rare.

Inefficiency of pulmonary gas exchange during exercise also results from a failure to achieve equilibrium of PO_2 between alveolar gas and pulmonary end-capillary blood. Because mixed venous blood PO_2 falls to very low levels during heavy exercise, more time is required to reoxygenate this blood. However, with high blood flow during exercise, less time is available – that is, the red cell transit time is shortened. Capillary recruitment (by higher intravascular pressures) tends to reduce red cell velocity through the capillaries and also increases the total surface area for diffusion. Nevertheless, a diffusion limitation probably does develop and may actually act as a significant handicap to the trained athlete who is capable of increasing his work load and pulmonary blood flow beyond the point where the maximum expansion of his pulmonary capillary blood volume has been reached.

References

Bake, B., Wood, L., Murphy, B., Macklem, P. T., and Milic-Emili, J. (1974). Effect of inspiratory flow rate on regional distribution of inspired gas. *J. Appl. Physiol.* *37*:8-17.

Bayly, W. M., Grant, B. D., Breeze, R. G., and Kramer, J. W. (1983). The effects of maximal exercise on acid-base balance and arterial blood gas tensions in thoroughbred horses. In *Equine Exercise Physiology*. Edited by D. H. Snow, S. G. Persson, and R. J. Rose. Granta Editions, Cambridge, pp. 400-404.

Benumof, J. L., and Wahrenbrock, E. A. (1975). Blunted hypoxic pulmonary vasoconstriction by increased lung vascular pressures. *J. Appl. Physiol. 38*: 846-850.

Bevegard, S. (1963). The effects of cardioacceleration by methylscopolamine nitrate on the circulation at rest and during exercise in supine position, with special reference to the stroke volume. *Acta Physiol. Scand. 57*:61-80.

Bevegard, S., Holmgren, A., and Jonsson, B. (1960). The effect of body position on the circulation at rest and during exercise, with special reference to the influence on the stroke volume. *Acta Physiol. Scand. 49*:279-298.

Bevegard, S., Holmgren, A., and Jonsson, B. (1963). Circulatory studies in well trained athletes at rest and during heavy exercise, with special reference to stroke volume and the influence of body position. *Acta Physiol. Scand. 57*:26-50.

Bryan, A. C., Bentivaglio, L. B., Beerel, F., MacLeish, H., Zidulka, A., and Bates, D. V., (1964). Factors affecting regional distribution of ventilation and perfusion in the lung. *J. Appl. Physiol. 19*:395-402.

Coates, G. H., O'Bradovich, H., Jerreries, A. L., and Gray, G. W. (1984). Effects of exercise on lung lymph flow in sheep and goats during normoxia and hypoxia. *J. Clin. Invest. 74*:133-141.

Dempsey, J. A. (1986). Is the lung built for exercise? *Med. Sci. Sports Exercise 18*:143-155.

Dempsey, J. A. (1987). Some exercise-induced imperfections in pulmonary gas exchange. *Canad. J. Sport Sci. 12*: Suppl I, 66-71.

Dempsey, J. A., Vidruk, E. H., and Masterbrook, S. M. (1980). Pulmonary control systems in exercise. *Fed. Proc. 39*:1498-1505.

Dempsey, J. A., Hanson, P., and Henderson, K. (1984). Exercise-induced alveolar hypoxemia in healthy human subjects at sea level. *J. Physiol. (Lond.) 355*:161-175.

Dempsey, J. A., Vidruk, E. H., and Mitchell, G. S. (1985). Pulmonary control systems: update. *Fed. Proc. 44*:2260-2270.

Dexter, L., Whittenberger, J. L., Haynes, F. W., Goodale, W. T., Gorlin, R., and Sawyer, C. G. (1951). Effect of exercise on circulatory dynamics of normal individuals. *J. Appl. Physiol. 3*:439-453.

Ekelund, L. G. (1967). Circulatory and respiratory adaptation during prolonged exercise of moderate intensity in the sitting position. *Acta Physiol. Scand. 69*:327-340.

Engel, L., Wood, L. D., Utz, G., and Macklem, T. P. (1973). Gas mixing during inspiration. *J. Appl. Physiol.* *35*:18-24.

Gale, G. E., Torre-Bueno, J. R., Moon, R. E., Saltzman, H. A., and Wagner, P. D. (1985). Ventilation-perfusion inequality in normal humans during exercise at sea level and simulated altitude. *J. Appl. Physiol.* *58*:978-988.

Gledhill, N., Froese, A. B., and Dempsey, J. A. (1977). Ventilation to perfusion distribution during exercise in health. In *Muscular Exercise and the Lung.* Edited by J. A. Dempsey and C. E. Reed. University of Wisconsin Press, Madison. pp. 325-342.

Gledhill, N., Froese, A. B., Buick, F. J., and Bryan, A. C. (1978). VA/Q inhomogeneity and $AaDO_2$ in man during exercise: effect of SF_6 breathing. *J. Appl. Physiol.* *45*:512-515.

Granath, A., and Strandell, T. (1964). Relationships between cardiac output, stroke volume, and intracardiac pressures at rest and during exercise in supine position and some antropometric data in healthy old men. *Acta Med. Scand.* *176*:447-466.

Granath, A., Jonsson, B., and Strandell, T. (1964). Circulation in healthy old men, studied by right heart catheterization at rest and during exercise in supine and sitting position. *Acta Med. Scand.* *176*:425-446.

Grimby, G., Saltin, B., and Helmsen, L. W. (1971). Pulmonary flow-volume and pressure-volume relationships during submaximal and maximal exercise in young well-trained men. *Bull. Physiol. - Pathol. Resp.* *7*:157-168.

Grover, R. F., Wagner, W. W., Jr., McMurtry, I. F., nd Reeves, J. T. (1983). Pulmonary circulation. In *Handbook of Physiology.* Sect. 2, *The Cardiovascular System.* Vol. III, *Peripheral Circulation and Organ Blood Flow.* Edited by J. T. Shepherd and F. M. Abboud. American Physiological Society, Bethesda, pp. 103-136.

Groves, B. M., Reeves, J. T., Sutton, J. R., Wagner, P. D., Cymerman, A., Malconian, M. K., Rock, P. B., Young, P. M., and Houston, C. S. (1987). Operation Everest II: elevated high altitude pulmonary resistance unresponsive to oxygen. *J. Appl. Physiol.* *63*:521-530.

Gurtner, H. P., Walser, P., and Fassler, B. (1975). Normal values for pulmonary hemodynamics at rest and during exercise in man. *Prog. Resp. Res.* *9*:295-315.

Hammond, M. D., Gale, G. E., Kapiton, K. S., Reis, A., and Wagner, P. D. (1986). Pulmonary gas exchange in humans during exercise at sea level. *J. Appl. Physiol.* *60*:1590-1598.

Harf, A., Pratt, T., and Hughes, J. M. B. (1978). Regional distribution of VA/Q in man at rest and with exercise measured with krypton-81m. *J. Appl. Physiol.* *44*:115-123.

Harris, P., Segel, N., and Bishop, J. M. (1968). The relation between pressure and flow in the pulmonary circulation in normal subjects and in patients with chronic bronchitis and mitral stenosis. *Cardiovasc. Res.* *27*:73-81.

Henke, K. G., Sharratt, M., Pegelow, D., and Dempsey, J. A. (1987). Regulation of end-expiratory lung volume during exercise. *J. Appl. Physiol.* (in press).

Holmgren, A., Jonsson, B., and Sjostrand, T. (1960). Circulatory data in normal subjects at rest and during exercise in recumbent position, with special reference to the stroke volume at different working intensities. *Acta Physiol. Scand. 49*:343-363.

Lindenfeld, J., Reeves, J. T., and Horwitz, L. D. (1983). Low exercise pulmonary resistance is not dependent on vasodilator prostaglandins. *J. Appl. Physiol. 55*:559-561.

McKechnie, J. K., Leary, W. P., Noakes, T. D., Kallmeyer, J. C., MacSearraigh, E. T., and Olivier, L. R. (1979). Acute pulmonary edema in two athletes during a 90 km running race. *S. Afr. Med. J. 56*:261-265.

Maron, M. B., Hamilton, L. H., and Maksud, M. G. (1979). Alterations in pulmonary function consequent to competitive marathon running. *Med. Sci. Sports 2*:244-249.

Marshall, B. E., Soma, L. R., and Neufeld, G. R. (1975). Lung water volume at rest and exercise in dogs. *J. Appl. Physiol. 39*:7-8.

Michel, R. P., Zocchi, L., Rossi, A., Cardinal, G. A., Ploy-Sand, Y., Paulsen, R. S., Milic-Emili, J., and Staub, N. C. (1987). Does interstitial lung edema compress airways and arteries? A morphometric study. *J. Appl. Physiol. 62*:108-115.

Permutt, S. B., Bromberger-Barnea, B., and Bane, H. N. (1963). Alveolar pressure, pulmonary venous pressure, and the vascular waterfall. In *Normal and Abnormal Pulmonary Circulation*. Edited by R. F. Grover. S. Karger, New York, pp. 47-68.

Reeves, J. T., and Groves, B. M. (1984). Approach to the patient with pulmonary hypertension. In *Pulmonary Hypertension*. Edited by E. K. Weir and J. T. Reeves. Futura, Mt. Kisco, NY pp. 1-44.

Reeves, J. T., Grover, R. F., Blount, S. G., Jr., and Filley, G. F. (1961). Cardiac output response to standing and treadmill walking. *J. Appl. Physiol. 16*: 283-288.

Reeves, J. T., Groves, B. M., Sutton, J. R., Wagner, P. D., Cymerman, A., Malkonian, M. K., Rock, P. B., Young, P. M., and Houston, C. S. (1987). Operation Everest II: preservation of cardiac function at extreme altitude. *J. Appl. Physiol. 63*:531-539.

Rowell, L. B., Taylor, H. L., Wang, Y., and Carlson, W. B. (1964). Saturation of arterial blood with oxygen during maximal exercise. *J. Appl. Physiol. 19*: 284-286.

Sharatt, M., Henke, K. G., Aaron, E. A., Pegelow, D., and Dempsey, J. A. (1987). Exercise-induced changes in functional residual capacity. *Resp. Physiol. 70*:313-326.

Staub, N. C., Nagano, H., and Pearce, M. L. (1967). Pulmonary edema in dogs, especially the sequence of fluid accumulation in lungs. *J. Appl. Physiol.* *22*:227-240.

Varnauskas, E. (1955). Studies in hypertensive cardiovascular disease. *Scand. J. Clin. Labl. Invest. Suppl.* *17*:1-117.

Wagner, P. D. (1982). Influence of mixed venous PO_2 on diffusion of O_2 across the pulmonary blood: gas barrier. *Clin. Physiol.* *2*:105-115.

Wagner, P. D., Gale, G. E., Moon, R. E., Tane-Buena, J., Stolpe, B. W., Saltzman, H. A., "Pulmonary gas exchange in Himons at sea-level and simulated altitude." *J. Appl. Physiol.* *61*:260-270, 1986.

Wagner, W. W., Jr., Latham, L. P., and Capen, R. L. (1979). Capillary recruitment during airway hypoxia: role of pulmonary arterial pressure. *J. Appl. Physiol.* *47*:383-387.

West, J. B. (1979). *Respiratory Physiology.* Williams and Wilkins, Baltimore, MD.

Widimski, J., Berglund, E., and Malberg, R. (1963). Effect of repeated exercise on the lesser circulation. *J. Appl. Physiol.* *18*:983-986.

Younes, M. and Kivinen, G. (1984). Respiratory mechanics and breathing pattern during and following maximal exercise. *J. Appl. Physiol.* *57*:1773-1782.

Younes, M., Bshouty, Z., and Ali, J. (1987). Longitudinal distribution of pulmonary vascular resistance with very high pulmonary blood flow. *J. Appl. Physiol.* *62*:344-358.

5

Circulation in the Pregnant and Nonpregnant State

LORNA GRINDLAY MOORE

University of Colorado and University of Colorado Health Sciences Center
Denver, Colorado

I. Introduction

The maternal circulation undergoes profound changes during pregnancy. The pulmonary circulation, like the systemic vascular bed, must accommodate an increased blood volume and cardiac output and undergoes alterations in pulmonary vascular control similar to those observed in the systemic circulation. Despite the profound nature of the circulatory changes imposed on the lung by pregnancy, comparatively little study has been devoted to understanding their occurrence or detailing their mechanisms.

This chapter first reviews the evidence available concerning the effects of pregnancy on the pulmonary circulation. Where applicable to understanding alterations in the pulmonary circulation, information is also drawn from studies of the systemic circulation. Hormones likely to play important roles in the circulatory and vascular effects of pregnancy are then considered. The last section deals with hypertensive disorders in pregnancy and the pulmonary circulation. In particular, the association reported between pregnancy and primary pulmonary hypertension is reviewed.

II. Effects of Pregnancy on the Pulmonary Circulation

Striking maternal circulatory changes occur during pregnancy, surpassed in life perhaps only by those taking place simultaneously in the fetal circulation. A new vascular bed, the uteroplacental circuit, develops. Flow to the uterus changes from the nonpregnant pattern in which the bilateral uterine arteries, emanating from the internal iliac arteries, supply the uterus, to the pregnant pattern in which the uterine arteries are joined by the ovarian arteries for supplying the uterine circulation. An anastomosis develops on either side of the uterus between the main branch of the uterine artery and the tubal branch of the ovarian artery, a vessel that originates from the thoracic aorta below the renal arteries. The resultant arterial manifold on either side of the uterus is the source of an abundant network of small arteries that ramify in a plane parallel to the surface, penetrate the uterine wall, and extend toward the endometrium to terminate in the intervillous space. This new vascular circuit accommodates an extraordinary increase in total uterine blood flow. In the sheep, total uterine flow at term reaches approximately 2 liters/min, which amounts to a more than 70-fold increase over values measured in the nonpregnant state (Meschia, 1983).

While the increase in uterine blood flow clearly takes place outside the pulmonary circulation, the pulmonary circulation is subject to many of the factors involved in accomplishing the observed increase in uterine flow. These factors are the expansion of total blood volume, the increase in total cardiac output, and the reduction in vascular resistance.

Maternal blood volume increases from approximately 3500 to 5000 ml, or by 40%, with pregnancy. The increase in blood volume is detectable as early as the 10th week of gestation and reaches a peak by approximately the 30th week (Longo, 1983). The blood volume increase is due to a 50% expansion in plasma volume, which is greater than the 25% increase in red blood cell volume, resulting in a mild anemia during pregnancy. The increase in plasma volume is thought to be due to the combined actions of estradiol and progesterone on increasing renin production via stimulation of aldosterone secretion and, in turn, renal sodium and water retention (Longo, 1983) (Fig. 1). Erythropoietic actions of progesterone, prolactin, and chorionic somatomammotrophin lead to the increase in red blood cell volume (Longo, 1983). It is not known why the increase in red blood cell volume fails to match the expansion in plasma volume over the prolonged time course of pregnancy.

The increase in blood volume accompanies an increasing cardiac output. The rise in cardiac output begins early in pregnancy and plateaus (Lees et al., 1967) or declines during the third trimester toward values present in the nonpregnant female (Ueland et al., 1964). A pronounced late pregnancy fall occurs in the supine position due to obstruction of venous return by the gravid uterus

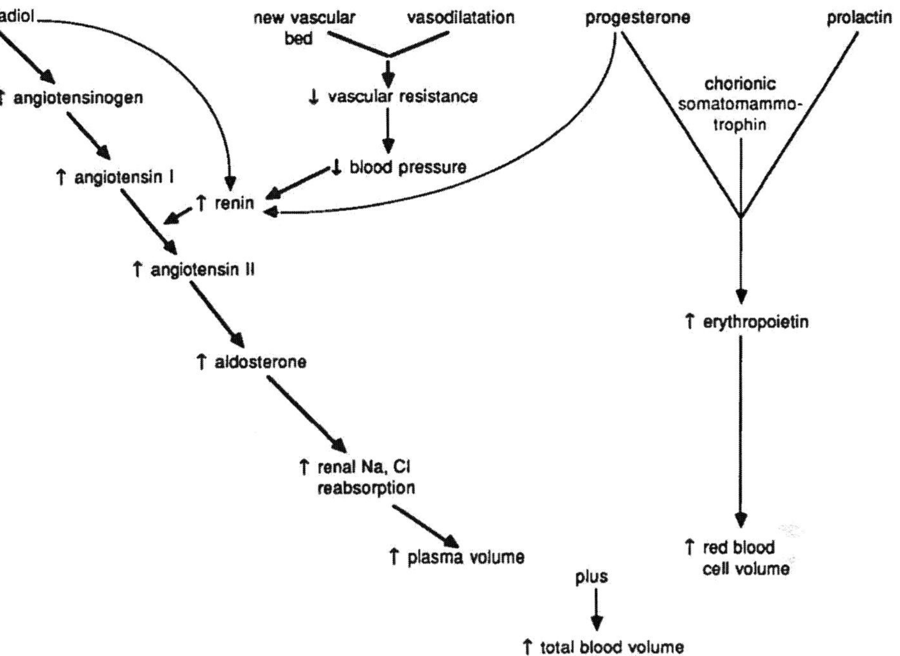

Figure 1 Factors influencing expansion of plasma volume and red blood cell volume during pregnancy.

(Ueland et al., 1964). The late pregnancy decline in cardiac output has not been described in nonhuman species and may result from the constraints of an upright posture. Increases in heart rate (Clapp, 1985) and stroke volume contribute to the rise in cardiac output.

The early onset of the increase in cardiac output suggests hormonal involvement. Estrogen and progesterone, administered separately or in combination, increase cardiac output via stroke volume in the guinea pig (Hart et al., 1985). Progressive left ventricular enlargement occurs in pregnancy, with no apparent changes in contractility or filling pressure (Bader et al., 1955; Katz et al., 1978). The left ventricular size and cardiac output increase were reproduced by chronic estrogen and/or progesterone administration and occurred prior to changes in uterine flow in the guinea pig, suggesting that the sex steroids are involved in a preparatory process by which cardiac output increases before the elevation occurs in uterine blood flow (Hart et al., 1985).

Despite the increase in cardiac output and therefore in pulmonary blood flow, pulmonary arterial and systemic arterial blood pressures fall during pregnancy. Pulmonary arterial pressures average 3-5 mmHg lower in pregnant than in nonpregnant women (Table 1). Systemic arterial pressure also declines, beginning early in gestation and tending to return toward nonpregnant levels near term. From the limited number of observations of pulmonary arterial pressure, a similar time course appears evident (Table 1). The fall in pulmonary and systemic arterial pressures in the face of an increased cardiac output implies a fall in vascular resistance. The gradual restoration of vascular resistance may be responsible for the increasing blood pressure and/or the declining cardiac output near term.

The decrease in pulmonary and systemic vascular resistance in pregnancy may be attributable to three factors: the creation of the new uteroplacental circuit, increased diameters of existing vessels, and decreased contractility to vasoconstrictor stimuli.

The new uteroplacental circuit of pregnancy has been likened to an arteriovenous fistula (Burwell, 1938). The low-resistance uteroplacental bed participates in the reduction of peripheral vascular resistance and manifests itself as a widened pulse pressure with decreased diastolic and mean pressure values. However, the creation of an arteriovenous fistula does not appear able to fully account for the decreased vascular resistance of pregnancy for several reasons. First, the presence of the uteroplacental circuit would be expected to decrease systemic but not necessarily pulmonary vascular resistance. Second, the greatest fall in systemic pressure and vascular resistance occurs before the greatest increase in uterine flow (Hart et al., 1985). Therefore, although quite likely a contributor, the concept of an arteriovenous fistula does not appear sufficient to account for the reduction in systemic and pulmonary vascular resistance in pregnancy.

Certain vessels, namely the uterine and ovarian arteries (Griendling et al., 1985) as well as other vessels (Danforth et al., 1964) increase in diameter and internal radius during pregnancy. The increased diameters of existing vessels would act to expand the vascular bed in pregnancy in much the same way as the new uteroplacental circuit. In the sheep uterine artery, the increased diameter is due to vascular smooth muscle hypertrophy without a change in wall thickness (Griendling et al., 1985). No data are available, to our knowledge, as to whether enlargement of the main pulmonary artery or its branches occurs in pregnancy.

Decreased contractility to vasoconstrictor stimuli may participate in decreasing vascular resistance by maintaining vessels normally in a more fully dilated state. In the systemic circulation, decreased pressor responsiveness to angiotensin II has long been observed in pregnancy (Abdul Karim and Assali, 1961; Chesley et al., 1965). It is unclear, however, whether the decrease in pressor response is due to a true reduction in vasoreactivity or to a decrease in blood flow. Supporting a decrease in vasoreactivity are observations of reduced pressor response to angiotensin II under constant flow conditions (McLaughlin et al.,

Table 1 Pulmonary and systemic Hemodynamics in Normal, Supine Pregnant Women[a]

Condition and Week of gestation	Ppa, mmHg	PVR mmHg/ (liter-min)	CO liters/ min	Psa, mmHg	SVR mmHg/ (liter-min)
Werko, 1954					
Nonpregnant	13	1.99	6.54	89	13.6
Pregnant, wk 16	10 ± 1	1.40 ± 0.15	7.81 ± 0.64	90 ± 5	12.0 ± 0.8
Pregnant, wk 36	10 ± 1	1.52 ± 0.10	6.45 ± 0.44	90 ± 5	14.6 ± 1.3
Bader et al., 1955					
Pregnant, wk 20	10 ± 1	1.56 ± 0.13	6.53 ± 0.21	84 ± 5	12.4 ± 0.8
Pregnant, wk 26	11 ± 1	1.59 ± 0.56	6.96 ± 1.19	83 ± 3	12.4 ± 0.5
Pregnant, wk 29	12 ± 1	1.89 ± 0.19	6.59 ± 1.08	88 ± 3	13.9 ± 1.2
Pregnant, wk 32	11 ± 1	1.93 ± 0.60	5.75 ± 0.72	87 ± 5	14.9 ± 1.6
Pregnant, wk 38	11 ± 1	2.01 ± 0.19	5.53 ± 0.72	90 ± 3	15.9 ± 0.7
Weir et al., 1976					
Nonpregnant	16 ± 1				
Pregnant, wk 18	11 ± 1				
Secher et al., 1982					
Pregnant, wk 11	12 ± 1	2.31	5.18 ± 0.40	85 ± 2	16.4

[a]Ppa, pulmonary arterial pressure, PVR, total pulmonary vascular resistance, CO, cardiac output, Psa, systemic arterial pressure, SVR, total systemic vascular resistance.

1985; Humpheys and Joels, 1981a,b; Dogterom and DeJong, 1974; Fuchs et al., 1982). Under the normal flow conditions of pregnancy, a reduced systemic vascular resistance response and a decreased pressor response to angiotensin II have been observed in sheep (McLaughlin et al., 1985; Naden et al., 1984). However, the pregnant ewes also evidenced a greater fall in cardiac output during angiotensin II infusion (Naden et al., 1984), making it unclear whether the decreased systemic vascular reactivity was due to decreased pressor responsiveness or to decreased flow. We found that decreased systemic vascular resistance responsiveness to angiotensin II was accompanied by a reduced pressor response but similar cardiac output response in pregnant guinea pigs, indicating that pregnancy decreased systemic vascular reactivity to angiotensin II (Harrison and Moore, 1988). Decreased pressor responsiveness to angiotensin II fails to develop in pregnancies complicated by preeclampsia (Gant et al., 1973), suggesting that alterations in vascular or pressor responsiveness in pregnancy may be important.

Pregnancy also appears to reduce vasoreactivity in the pulmonary circulation. Initial observations (Weir et al., 1976) in women undergoing second trimester therapeutic abortion showed a smaller than expected pulmonary pressor response after intramuscular injection of 15-methyl-prostaglandin F_{2a}. Experimental animal studies afford an opportunity to compare pulmonary pressor responses in the same animals while pregnant and postpartum as well as to examine a broader variety of agonists. In anesthetized second or third trimester dogs, the pulmonary arterial and pulmonary arterial-wedge pressor responses to hypoxia were decreased in comparison to values obtained in the same animals postpartum (Fig. 2). Pulmonary vascular resistance was consistently lower in the pregnant animals (Moore and Reeves, 1980). The effect of pregnancy on pulmonary pressor responsiveness did not appear to be selective for hypoxia, since pregnancy also reduced the pulmonary arterial and pulmonary arterial-wedge pressor responses to prostaglandin F_{2a} and norepineprhine (Fig. 2) and decreased the pulmonary vascular resistance response to prostaglandin F_{2a} infusion (Moore and Reeves, 1980). The effect of pregnancy on blunting the pressor response to norepinephrine was similar in the pulmonary and systemic circulations; in each case the pregnant animals evidenced about one-third the peak pressure rise observed in the nonpregnant animals (Moore and Reeves, 1980).

To examine the effect of pregnancy on pulmonary vascular reactivity in a setting where alterations in pressure would not be confounded by changes in flow, Fuchs et al. (1982) examined the pulmonary pressor response in lungs isolated from pregnant and nonpregnant rats. Compared to nonpregnant controls, hypoxic and angiotensin II pressor responses were blunted in lungs perfused with blood from pregnant donors (Fig. 3). In order to separate effects of pregnancy on the lung itself from effects of circulating factors, the pressor responses were compared in lungs from pregnant and nonpregnant animals perfused with blood from nonpregnant and pregnant rats, respectively. The blunting of

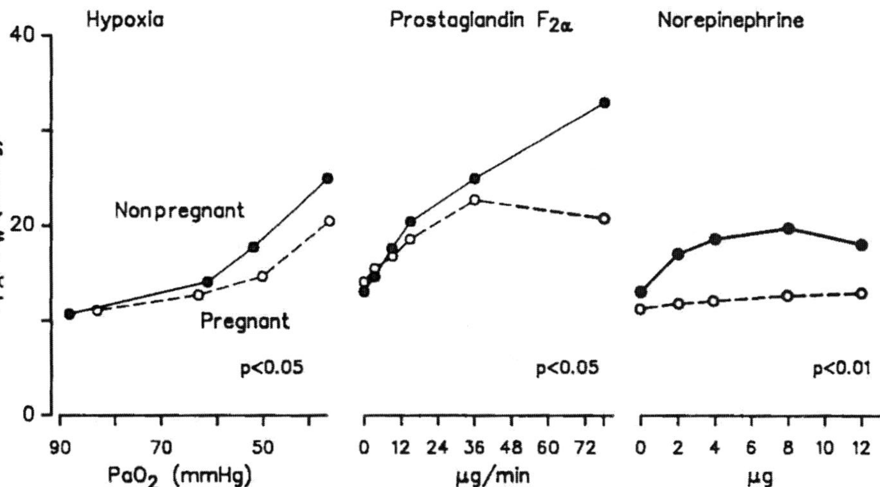

Figure 2 The pressure gradient across the lung (mean pulmonary artery-wedge pressure (ppa - Pw) was decreased during hypoxia, prostaglandin F_{2a} infusion, and norepinephrine injection in eight pregnant dogs compared to the same animals postpartum. (Adapted from Moore and Reeves, 1980).

the hypoxic pressor response appeared to be primarily an effect of some blood-borne substance, whereas the effect of the reduced angiotensin II pressor response with pregnancy appeared to be due to changes with pregnancy in both the lungs and the blood (Fig. 3). The lung- and blood-specific attributes of pregnancy appeared to work synergistically, since the greatest blunting to both hypoxia and angiotensin II was observed when lungs from pregnant rats were perfused with blood from pregnant donors. Studies in the in situ perfused cat lung also demonstrated reduced reactivity to acute hypoxia, angiotensin II, serotonin, histamine, norepinephrine, and epinephrine (Cutaia et al., 1987). The decrease in reactivity (measured as the magnitude of the contractile response) was accompanied by reduced sensitivity (measured as the ED_{50}) only in the case of angiotensin II, whereas sensitivity to the other agonists was similar in the pregnant and nonpregnant groups (Cutaia et al., 1987).

The cause of the reduced systemic and pulmonary vasoreactivity in pregnancy is unclear. In studies concerned with the systemic circulation, interest has been directed toward determining whether the reduced vasoreactivity is generalized for all agonists or specific to stimulation by angiotensin II. A reduced pressor response to angiotensin II has been more consistently observed in pregnancy (Chesley et al., 1965; Lumbers, 1970), but other agonists have also been shown to elicit less pressor responsiveness in the pregnant state (Paller, 1984).

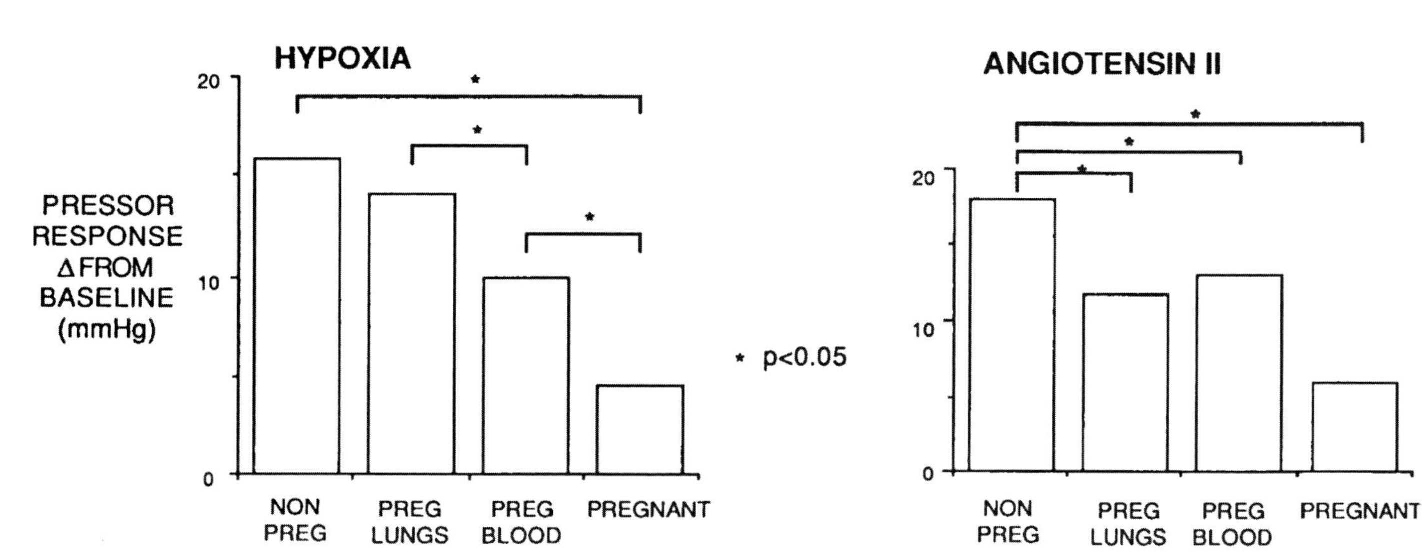

Figure 3 The pressor responses (baseline to peak mean pulmonary arterial pressures) in isolated, perfused rat lungs were reduced to hypoxia and angiotensin II from pregnant compared to nonpregnant animals. Lungs from pregnant donors or blood perfused from pregnant donors had intermediate pressor responses. (Adapted from Fuchs et al., 1982).

In other studies, however, the reduced systemic vascular resistance responsiveness to angiotensin II was not apparent in response to phenylephrine (McLaughlin and Westney, 1985; Harrison and Moore, 1988), perhaps because phenylephrine produced less rise in systemic vascular resistance than angiotensin II, making it difficult to detect differences between the pregnant and nonpregnant animals.

If reduced vasoreactivity is specific to angiotensin II, the possibility exists that alterations in angiotensin II levels or metabolism may be involved. Angiotensin II levels are increased in normal pregnancy (Table 2). Elevation of circulating angiotensin II levels in nonpregnant animals reduced the pressor response to angiotensin II infusion, and reduction of angiotensin II levels in pregnant sheep by administration of converting enzyme inhibitor potentiated pressor responsiveness to angiotensin II in pregnant sheep (Siddiqi et al., 1983). However, the hypothesis that the blunted pressor response is due to increased angiotensin II levels is weakened by the observations that plasma volume expansion does not affect the angiotensin II pressor response despite significant reductions in plasma renin activity and angiotensin II levels (Matsuura et al., 1981). Others have suggested that downregulation of angiotensin II receptor numbers by elevated angiotensin II levels may be involved in reducing pressor responsiveness (Brown and Venuto, 1986). In pregnant rabbits, angiotensin converting enzyme inhibitor normalized receptor numbers and elevated pressor responsiveness (Mah et al., 1985). However, in rats, converting enzyme inhibitor failed to alter angiotensin receptor numbers or angiotensin II pressor responsiveness (Paller, 1984). Metabolic clearance of angiotensin II in pregnant sheep has also been investigated in order to determine whether an increased clearance rate might be responsible for reducing pressor responsiveness to angiotensin II infusion. However, metabolic clearance values attained during angiotensin II infusion were similar in pregnant and nonpregnant sheep (Naden et al., 1985). Thus, despite numerous investigations, clear evidence is lacking in support of reduced pressor responsiveness to angiotensin II being due exclusively to alterations in angiotensin II levels, receptor numbers, or metabolism.

Support for a generalized reduction in vasoreactivity with pregnancy comes from whole animal studies as well as from studies performed in constant flow perfused organs and isolated vessels. Nonspecific blunting of pressor responsiveness to angiotensin II, norepinephrine, and arginine vasopressin was observed in pregnant compared to nonpregnant rats (Paller, 1984). A generalized reduction in the pulmonary pressor responsiveness to hypoxia, prostaglandin $F_{2\alpha}$, norepinephrine, angiotensin II, serotonin, histamine, and epinephrine has been seen in the whole animal and isolated perfused lung preparations (Moore and Reeves, 1980; Fuchs et al., 1982; Cutaia et al., 1987). Data obtained in perfused hind-limb or tail preparations demonstrated reduced pressor response to angiotensin II and to sympathetic stimulation but decreased as well as un-

Table 2 Hormone changes of pregnancy

Hormone	Nonpregnant	Pregnant	Time of Peak
Aldosterone	0.05 ng/ml	0.6 ng/ml[a]	wk 36
Angiotensin II	25 pg/ml	100 pg/ml	wk 25-36
Chorionic ACTH	0	?	?
Cortisol	0.09 mg/ml	0.32 mg/ml	term
Eicosanoids:			
prostaglandin E_2	55 ng/24 hr[b]	280 ng/24 hr	term
prostaglandin F_{2a}	400 ng/24 hr	2200 ng/24 hr	term
prostaglandin 6-keto-F_{1a}	1.5 pg/ml	5 pg/ml	term
Estradiol	0.2 ng/ml	20 ng/ml	term
Estriol	0	30 mg/24 hr[b]	term
Estrone	0.1 ng/ml	7.5 ng/ml	term
Human chorionic gonadotrophin (hCG)	0	60 IU/ml	wk 10

Human chorionic thyrotropin (hCT)	0	?	?
Luteinizing hormone releasing hormone (LHRH-like)	0	?	?
Placental lactogen (hPL)	0	7.5 ng/ml	wk 32
Plasma renin substrate (PRS)	1594 ng/ml	6480 ng/ml	wk 20
Progesterone	4 ng/ml	27 ng/ml	term
Prolactin	35 ng/ml	368 ng/ml	term
Testosterone	0.38 ng/ml	1.45 ng/ml	term
Thyrotropin hormone releasing hormone (TRH-like)	0	?	?

[a]Units of measurement are per milliliter plasma unless noted otherwise.
[b]Urinary excretion per 24 hr.
Source: Casey et al. (1985), Jarnfelt-Samsioe et al. (1985), Pederson et al. (1982), Poindexter et al. (1977), Tagatz and Gurpide (1973), Wilson et al. (1980), Symords (1983), Wintour et al. (1978).

changed pressor responsiveness to alpha-adrenergic agonists (Humprheys and Joels 1981a, b; Dogterom and DeJong, 1974; McLaughlin et al., 1983, 1985). In isolated vessels, pregnancy decreased the contractile response to barium chloride in the rat aorta (Hart, 1982) and portal vein (Hart, 1984), to calcium chloride and potassium chloride in rat small mesenteric arteries (McLaughlin and Keve, 1986), and to alpha-adrenergic agonists in rabbit cranial arteries (Hardebo and Edvinsson, 1977). However, in isolated uterine artery preparations involving removal of the endothelium, unchanged or increased contractile responsiveness has been reported (Moisey and Tulenko, 1983; Annibale et al., 1987).

The presence of the endothelium may be important in modifying contractile responsiveness in pregnancy. Bell observed that acetylcholine, which ordinarily does not provoke vasodilation in the guinea pig uterine artery, became a vasodilator during pregnancy (Bell, 1974). Like the application of exogenous acetylcholine, activation of cholinergic nerves produced vasodilation only during pregnancy (Griess et al., 1967). Perhaps the decreased contractility evidenced in vessels from pregnant compared to nonpregnant animals is due to increased production of endothelium-derived relaxing factor (EDRF).

Several investigators have proposed that the reduction in vasoreactivity observed in pregnancy is due to increased vasodilator prostaglandin production (Everett et al., 1978; Paller, 1984; Venuto et al., 1984). An increase in pressor responsiveness to angiotensin II after indomethacin treatment in pregnant women has been interpreted as support for vasodilator mediation of the blunted pressor response (Everett et al., 1978). However, nonpregnant women were not studied; since angiotensin II is known to induce vasodilator prostaglandin synthesis (McGiff et al., 1970), it is unknown whether the increased pressor responsiveness was unique to or exaggerated in pregnancy. Paller found that meclofenamate restored the systemic pressor response to angiotensin II and to other agonists (Paller, 1984). However, these results could not be confirmed by others using chronically catheterized, unstressed animal preparations (Conrad and Colpoys, 1986; Harrison and Moore, 1988). Meclofenamate failed to restore the pulmonary pressor response to hypoxia, prostaglandin $F_{2\alpha}$, or norepinephrine in pregnant dogs (Moore and Reeves, 1980)

In summary, the lung participates in the circulatory changes of pregnancy by accommodating the increased cardiac output and blood volume and by participating in the decreased vasoreactivity characteristic of the systemic circulation. The decreased vasoreactivity appears to be nonselective, insofar as the pulmonary pressor and vascular responses to hypoxia, as well as to several pharmacological agonists, were reduced by pregnancy in several species including humans, rats, dogs, and cats. The mechanisms responsible for the reduction in vasoreactivity in pregnancy remain unknown. Support for increased prostaglandins, acting as circulating or local vasodilators, is called into question by the inability of prostaglandin synthesis inhibitors to restore vasoreactivity in unstressed pregnant animals to levels observed in the nonpregnant state. The similarity in vascular effects of pregnancy in the pulmonary and systemic circulations suggests the involvement of basic factors underlying vascular control. The functional consequences of alterations in vasoreactivity for maternal and fetal well-being remains poorly understood. Teleologically, the reduced vasoreactivity would appear to be a means for ensuring low vascular resistance and maximal blood flow to the uteroplacental circuit. However, it is puzzling why the reduced reactivity is bodywide, involving both the systemic and pulmonary circulations.

III. Hormonal Influences on the Pulmonary Circulation

A broad range of hormones influence the pulmonary circulation. Interest will be restricted here to those hormones likely to be involved in the pulmonary circulatory changes of pregnancy. Despite the ever-broadening array of biologic actions attributed to these hormones, remarkably little attention has been paid to their influences on the pulmonary circulation. Support for hormonal influences stems from associations between characteristics of the pulmonary circulation and the hormonally altered conditions of pregnancy and of gender as well as from attributes of the lung itself.

Pregnancy is a condition involving some of the most remarkable hormone changes of mammalian physiology (Table 2). By term, the pregnant woman produces a total of several grams of hormones per day. Some of these changes are especially marked in the human female in comparison to other species. For example, the human female produces greater quantities of estrogens than most other mammals due to the greater capacity of the human fetal adrenal to provide the substrate dehydroisoandrosterone sulfate (Casey et al., 1985). Most of these hormones remain at significant levels throughout gestation, and many peak near term (Table 2), a time course that indicates their availability for participating in the observed circulatory and vascular changes. Information on the circulatory and vascular effects of some of these hormones, namely the sex steroids and eicosanoids, will be reviewed below. The circulatory and vascular effects of many of the hormones – including the mineralocorticosteroids, glucocorticosteroids, and protein hormones – have not been well characterized.

Gender differences in pulmonary vascular characteristics suggest hormonal involvement in the pulmonary circulation. The occurrence of high altitude pulmonary edema and chronic mountain sickness has long been known to be more common in men than in women (Arias-Stella, 1971; Penaloza et al., 1971). Increased right ventricular hypertrophy and earlier demise from congestive cardiac failure has also been observed in adult male compared to adult female rats (Smith et al., 1974). Because hypoxic pulmonary vasoconstriction occurs in these conditions, it is possible that gender or gender-related factors influence the pulmonary vascular response to hypoxia. Greater right ventricular hypertrophy after high altitude exposure has been described for males of several species (Burton et al., 1968; McMurtry et al., 1973) and seen in conjunction with increased pulmonary artery pressures in rats (Rabinovitch et al., 1981; Peake et al., 1981). Studies in isolated sheep lungs demonstrate greater vasoconstrictor response to acute hypoxia in adult males than in adult females (Fig. 4) (Wetzel and Sylvester, 1983). That the female hormones may be involved was suggested by finding that postpubertal female sheep lungs had less vasomotor response to hypoxia than postpubertal males or males that had been castrated soon after birth, whereas prepubertal male and female sheep lungs were not different (Wetzel and Sylvester, 1983). Thus, the presence of female hormones was implicated rather than some other attribute of gender in the pulmonary vascular reactivity differences observed (Wetzel and Sylvester, 1983). Rat studies, on the other hand, point to the possible involvement of male hormones, since gender differences were absent in juvenile rats and appeared in adults as a result of the worsening of right ventricular hypertrophy in males (Smith et al., 1974). That testosterone might be involved was suggested by the observation that testosterone increased right ventricular hypertrophy in chronic high-altitude-exposed castrated male rats whereas female hormones (estrogen and progesterone) had no effect (Moore et al., 1980).

The third line of evidence for hormonal influence on the lung comes from attributes of the lung itself. Because the entire cardiac output passes through the lung, the pulmonary circulation is strategically positioned to influence the composition of circulating factors affecting the systemic as well as the pulmonary circulation. The lung, with a vascular and endothelial surface area unrivaled by any other organ, has the capacity to produce, process, and amplify the release of numerous vasoactive substances (Ryan et al., 1985). Furthermore, there is a clear selectivity in the specific processing of hormones; for example, prostaglandins of the E and F series are metabolized, whereas the A series prostaglandins and prostacyclin pass through the lung (Bedwani and Marley, 1978). Thus, the lung can be both an endocrine organ and a metabolic site, determining whether a vasoactive hormone is "local" (i.e., effectively removed by the lung) or "circulating" (i.e., passing through the lung unchanged) (Ben-Harari and Youdim, 1983).

Pregnancy- and gender-related hormones may also affect or be affected by the lung. For example, specific hormone receptors for estrogen and androgen have been found in the lung (Morishige and Uetake, 1978). Nuclear uptake of estrogen, androgen, and progestin has been demonstrated in smooth muscle cells of the heart and major arteries (McGill and Sheridan, 1981; Horwitz and Horwitz, 1982). Not only do sex steroid receptors exist in cardiovascular pulmonary tissues, but pulmonary absorption and metabolism of estradiol, testosterone, and

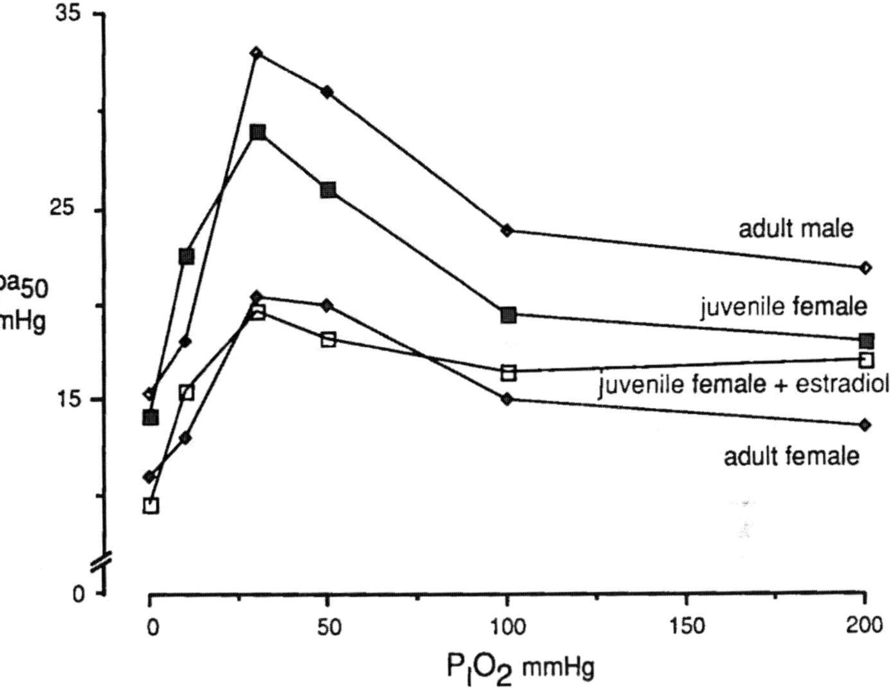

Figure 4 The stimulus-response relationship quantitated by the pulmonary arterial pressure at a flow of 50 ml/kg per minute (Ppa_{50}) evidence reduced peak pressor response in adult females compared to adult males or juvenile females. Juvenile females after 3-5 days of estradiol treatment had reduced peak pressor responses. (Adapted from Wetzel and Sylvester 1983; Wetzel et al., 1984).

progesterone have been demonstrated (Hartiala et al., 1979a, b; Milewich et al., 1980). In vitro metabolism by human lung of both the C_{21} steroids (pregnenolone and progesterone) and the C_{19} steroids (androstenedione, dehydroisoandrosterone, and testosterone) is supportive of the idea that the lung is a steroid-metabolizing organ (Milewich et al., 1980, 1983). Metabolism of 5-hydroxytryptamine, known to be influenced by endogenous steroid levels in target tissues such as the uterus and the ovaries, is also influenced by exogenous or endogenous hormones in the lung (Bakhle and Ben-Harari, 1979). Finally, the lung as an organ of gas exchange may affect hormone production indirectly via alterations in O_2 availability. Hypoxia has been associated with a reduction in serum testosterone levels at high altitude (Pugh, 1962; Vander et al., 1978) and with chronic lung disease (Semple et al., 1980). Aromatization of estrone and estradiol from androstenedione and testosterone in placental microsomes and in cultured choriocarcinoma cells has been shown to be markedly dependent on variations in oxygen concentration within the physiologic range (20-120 mmHg) (Aw et al., 1985).

A. Sex Steroids: Estrogens, Progestins, and Androgens

During pregnancy, the placenta surpasses ovarian and adrenal sites to become the major source of sex steroid production. Extraglandular conversion of androstenedione and testosterone to estrone is an additonal source that, while trivial in pregnancy, accounts for a sizable fraction of estrogen production per day in nonpregnant females and males (Siiteri and MacDonald, 1973). The pathways for steroidogenesis reveal the considerable opportunities that exist for interconversion and hence complexity for the interpretation of steroid effects (Fig. 5).

In the premenopausal female, the ovaries produce nearly all the estrogens and progestins. Daily production rates vary from the follicular to the luteal menstrual cycle phases for estradiol (up to 0.94 mg/day and 0.27 mg/day) and estrone (up to 0.66 mg/day and 0.24 mg/day) (Tagatz and Gurpide, 1973). In the female, the ovaries produce up to half the total androstenedione (3.2 mg/day), which together with the adrenals is responsible for all the testosterone production (26 mg/day) (Tagatz and Gurpide, 1973). After menopause, extraglandular androstenedione becomes the major source of estrone but the adrenals plus extraglandular androstenedione continue to supply testosterone. In males, the testes and adrenals produce significant androstenedione (2.5 mg/day) and testosterone (7.0 mg/day) but little estrogen. Rather, peripheral conversion of plasma androstenedione and testosterone accounts for virtually all the estrone (60 μg/day) and estradiol (40 μg/day) produced in men (Siiteri and MacDonald, 1973).

Vascular effects of sex steroids have been best characterized for estradiol, but even there the understanding is far from complete. Acute estrogen treatment results in vasodilation in uterine tissues and other reproductive tissues (Rosenfeld and Jackson, 1984). While their direct vasodilatory actions appear confined to reproductive tissues, estrogens modify vascular reactivity in the pulmonary circulation and in the systemic circulation in many of the same ways as does pregnancy. The systemic pressor and resistance responses to angiotensin II were blunted in estrogen-pretreated animals (Naden and Rosenfeld, 1985a; Rosenfeld and Jackson, 1984; Tamai et al., 1984). Estradiol-treated dogs exhibited a blunted hypoxic pressor response and a trend toward reduced pressor response to prostaglandin $F_{2\alpha}$ infusion (Moore and Reeves, 1980). In sheep, pretreatment with estradiol reduced pulmonary arterial pressure in in situ perfused lungs from juvenile females (Fig. 4) (Wetzel et al., 1984). The level of hypoxic responsiveness achieved after estradiol treatment was similar to that of postpubertal female sheep, suggesting that the presence of estradiol in females was responsible for the

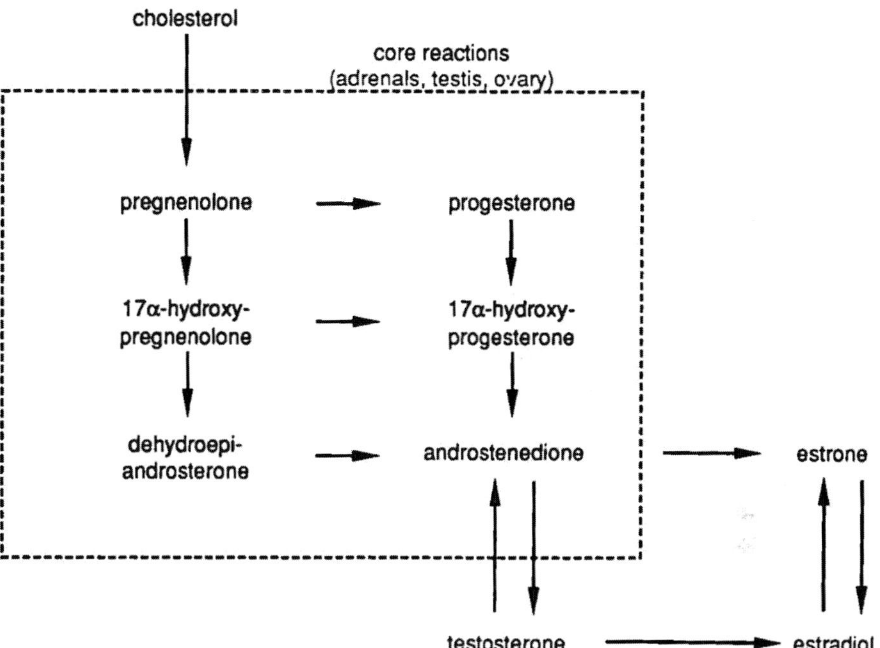

Figure 5 Pathways involved in the synthesis of sex steroids. The delta-5 steroids (left-hand column) are oxidized (right-hand column) and subsequently undergo side-chain cleavage to form dehydroepiandrosterone and androstenedione. Estrogen synthetase ("aromatase") catalyzes the androstenedione to estrone and the testosterone to estradiol reactions. 17-Hydroxysteroid dehydrogenase catalyzes the androstenedione-testosterone and estrone-estradiol reactions. The presence of estrogen synthetase and 17-hydroxysteroid dehydrogenase in tissues other than the adrenals, testes, and ovaries indicates that peripheral conversion of these hormones is possible.

lesser responsiveness observed in adult female compared to adult male sheep (Fig. 4) (Wetzel et al., 1984). However, hypoxic and angiotensin II pressor responses were not significantly blunted in lungs or blood obtained from rats treated for 2 weeks with estradiol (Fuchs et al., 1982). Perhaps species differences, duration of treatment, dosage, or compound employed are factors influencing estrogen's effects on vasoreactivity.

In contrast to the vasodilatory effects of estrogen in the uterine circulation and the reduction in vascular reactivity seen in the systemic and pulmonary beds, estradiol treatment enhanced the vasoconstrictor response to epinephrine, norepinephrine, arginine vasopressin, and oxytocin in terminal mesenteric arteries (Altura and Altura, 1977). Female rats also exhibited greater sensitivity to catecholamines than male rats, whereas arterial constriction induced by dopamine, serotonin, or angiotensin was not influenced by sex or estrogen pretreatment (Altura and Altura, 1977). Estrogen administration increased the alpha-adrenergic receptor binding affinity by approximately the same magnitude as the increase in vasoconstrictor responsiveness observed with estradiol treatment (Colucci et al., 1982). Estrogen receptors exist in vascular smooth muscle, and estrogen administration raises the transmembrane potential (Harder and Coulson, 1979). Perhaps conformational changes in the smooth muscle membrane are responsible for the increased alpha-receptor affinity observed with estrogen treatment.

The mechanisms by which estrogen alters vasoreactivity are unclear. Estrogen's uterine vasodilatory action appears to be a direct, receptor-mediated event leading to new protein synthesis insofar as the administration of cycloheximide, a protein synthesis inhibitor, and of the antiestrogens tamoxifen or nafoxidine prevented the increased uterine blood flow response to estrogen administration (Killam et al., 1973; Majid and Senior, 1982). Whether effects of estrogen on vascular reactivity are directly receptor mediated is unclear. Estrogen receptors exist in vascular smooth muscle, albeit at lower concentrations but with the same physicochemical properties as estrogen receptors in uterine smooth muscle (Harder and Coulson, 1979). Exposure of vascular smooth muscle cells to estrogen caused membrane hyperpolarization and increased the amplitude of action potentials, indicating that estrogen is capable of directly modifying the electrical activity and hence perhaps the contractile properties of vascular smooth muscle.

Estrogens have long been recognized as capable of stimulating prostaglandin synthesis by way of increasing phospholipid synthesis and turnover (Dey et al., 1982) or prostaglandin cyclooxygenase and prostacyclin synthesase activities (Chang et al., 1980). Because the uterus is a rich source of the vasodilator prostacyclin (Gerber et al., 1981) as well as vasoactive E and F series prostaglandins (Clark et al., 1982), a role for prostaglandins in mediating estrogen's vasodilator effects has been suggested. However, cyclooxygenase blockade with indomethacin attenuates but does not completely block estrogen-induced uterine hyperemia (Ryan et al., 1974; Phaily and Senior, 1978) and administration of meclofenamate, another cyclooxygenase inhibitor, had no effect on the increase in uterine blood flow (Mueller et al., 1978). Estrogen also does not appear to act via alterations in lipoxygenase products, since administration of the leukotriene receptor antagonist FPL 55712 failed to prevent estrogen-induced vasodilation (Parisi et al., 1984). Estradiol has also been reported to increase thromboxane release from cultured endothelial cells (Witter and DiBlasi, 1984).

In the sheep lung, the estradiol-induced attentuation of the hypoxic pressor response appeared to be due in part to increased vasodilator prostaglandin production (Gordon et al., 1986). Whereas indomethacin had no effect on hypoxic vasoconstriction in control isolated sheep lungs, indomethacin increased the pulmonary artery pressure in constant flow perfused lungs from animals pretreated with estradiol for 3-5 days. However, the pulmonary artery pressures during hypoxia remained lower than control values, suggesting that vasodilator prostaglandins were only partially responsible for estradiol's attentuating effect. A surprising finding was that indomethacin treatment decreased pulmonary arterial pressures during hyperoxia, suggesting that estradiol treatment may also increase vasoconstrictor prostaglandin production under some conditions (Gordon et al., 1986).

Other vasodilators have been examined as possible mediators of estrogen's systemic vasodilator effect, including histamine, bradykinin, vasoactive peptides, and catecholamines. Pretreatment of rats with H_1 and H_2 histamine receptor blockers failed to prevent estrogen-induced uterine hyperemia (Clark et al., 1977). Vasoactive intestinal peptide, a powerful uterine vasodilator in nonpregnant animals, appears not to have any local uterine vasodilatory effect in pregnancy (Clark et al., 1982). The structural similarity between catecholamines and some estrogens (e.g., the catechol estrogens) has led to consideration of the possibility that estrogen acts by opposing endogenous vasoconstrictors. However, estradiol treatment does not block the uterine vasoconstrictor response to norepinephrine or phenylephrine (Naden and Rosenfeld, 1985b). Uterine vasodilation in nonpregnant animals also does not occur after alpha-adrenergic blockade (Naden and Rosenfeld, 1985b; Clark et al., 1978). The vasodilatory effect of estradiol was not prevented by alpha blockade in sheep (Naden and Rosenfeld, 1985b), although attenuation of the response to estradiol was seen in rats (Clark et al., 1978). Thus, existing data do not clearly identify an endogenous mediator by which estrogen exerts its vasodilatory actions on the uterine circulation.

The marked increase in progesterone levels during pregnancy (Table 2) and the relationship between the effects of progesterone and estrogen have led to consideration of their combined and separate effects on vasoreactivity. In some early reports, progesterone but not estrogen-reduced pressor responsiveness to angiotensin II (Hettiaratchi and Pickford, 1967). Since direct, progesterone receptor-mediated events normally require estrogen to induce the formation of progesterone receptors (Baulieu, 1983), estrogen in settings where progesterone is likely to be present may act by way of induction of progesterone receptors. Actions attributed to estrogen may therefore constitute effects of progesterone on vascular control. Alternatively, progesterone may influence the actions of estrogen by depleting the availability of estrogen receptors (Hsueh et al., 1975) or by acting as an antiestrogen to oppose estrogen's effect. Consistent with an antagonistic effect for progesterone, administration of progesterone suppresses the estrogen-induced increase in uterine blood flow (Resnick et al., 1977). Progesterone enhances prostaglandin E_2 inactivation in the lung in vivo, suggesting that progesterone may also influence vascular tone by modifying levels of circulating prostaglandins (Bedwani and Marley, 1978). The effects of progesterone on prostaglandin production may operate by modulating the phospholipase A_2-stimulating effect of estrogen (Naylor and Poyser, 1975).

Progesterone has also been shown to reduce vasoreactivity to angiotensin II to the in situ perfused hind limb. Pregnant women quickly regain pressor responsiveness to angiotensin II after delivery of the placenta (Worley et al., 1979). Progesterone treatment delays the return of pressor responsiveness in postpartum women (Worley et al., 1979). Infusion of the progesterone metabolite, 5α-dihydroprogesterone but not progesterone reduces pressor responsiveness in preeclamptic women toward values observed in normal pregnancy, suggesting that progesterone metabolites may be important modulators of vascular control (Worley et al., 1979).

Androgen's effects on vascular reactivity have not been studied as extensively as those of the other sex steroids. The intact male rat exhibits a greater systemic pressor response to norepinephrine than the female rat (Baker et al., 1978). That increased contractile response is also seen in the isolated aortas from male compared to female rats and that testosterone pretreatment increases the contractile response suggest that androgens increase vasoreactivity (Ramwell, et al., 1983). Whereas gender differences in pulmonary vascular reactivity have been described in some species (Wetzel and Sylvester, 1983; Vanhoutte, 1987), direct investigation of the influence of androgens has not, to our knowledge, been investigated.

The importance of the vascular endothelium in modifying vascular smooth muscle contractile activity has opened a new area of investigation for studies of vascular control. An intact endothelium appears required for dilations evoked by numerous neurohumoral substances, including acetylcholine, histamine, bradykinin, and substance P. It is currently thought that these substances cause release of endothelium-derived relaxing factor(s) (EDRF), which, in turn, hyperpolarizes the cell membrane, stimulates guanylate cyclase, and increases cyclic GMP production to inhibit the contractile process (Vanhoutte, 1987). Bell recognized that a dilator response, absent in the nonpregnant uterine artery, developed progressively with pregnancy in parallel with rising estrogen levels (Bell, 1974). Cholinergic vasodilator nerves extend along the arteries entering the uterus in the guinea pig (as well as in humans, dogs, and pigs) whereas the adrenergic vasoconstrictor nerves do not. Like the application of exogenous acetylcholine, cholinergic activation produces vasodilation only during pregnancy or after estrogen priming (Bell, 1974; Griess et al., 1967). Sensitization of a vasodilatory response to acetylcholine in the uterine artery was prevented when protein synthesis was prevented over the period of estrogen administration (Bell and Coffey, 1982). While vasodilatory effects of acetylcholine may operate independently of the endothelium, the possibility that the endothelium is involved is strengthened by the observation that estrogen receptors are present in endothelial cell cultures (Colburn and Buonassisi, 1978) and by several recent reports that estrogen treatment enhances endothelial-dependent relaxation to acetylcholine (Gisclard and Vanhoute, 1985; Miller et al., 1987; Williams et al., 1987). An increased sensitivity to endothelium-dependent vasodilatory effects of acetylcholine appears to occur in uterine arteries from pregnant women (Nelson, 1987). Thus, limited observations suggest the intriguing possibility that estrogen may modify vascular reactivity via influences on the production of endothelium-derived substances.

B. Eicosanoids

Prostaglandins exert important influences during pregnancy from the time of conception through the expulsion of fetus and placenta. Eicosanoids are also recognized as having a profound influence on the control of the perinatal pulmonary circulation (Stenmark et al., 1988). The broad topic of the roles played by eicosanoids in the control of the fetal neonatal adult pulmonary circulations has been reviewed elsewhere and will not be addressed here (Voelkel and Chang, 1987; Kadowitz et al., 1982; Weir and Grover, 1978). Rather, studies pertaining to the narrower topic concerning the role of eicosanoids in mediating the pulmonary and systemic vasoreactivity changes of pregnancy will be discussed.

Several groups have postulated that increased vasodilator prostaglandins mediate the decreased pressor responsiveness of pregnancy. Everett and coworkers (1978) found that indomethacin, a prostaglandin synthesis inhibitor, increased pressor response to angiotensin II infusion in pregnant women. However, the effect of indomethacin was not studied in nonpregnant women. Because angiotensin II has been shown to induce vasodilator prostaglandin synthesis (McGiff et al., 1970). The changes in pressor responsiveness after indomethacin need to be compared in pregnant and nonpregnant subjects. Paller (1984) investigated the effects of meclofenamate, another prostaglandin synthesis inhibitor, in pregnant and nonpregnant rats. He found that meclofenamate increased the pressor response to angiotensin II, norepinephrine, and vasopressin in pregnant rats to levels that were not different from the pressor responses seen in nonpregnant animals (Paller, 1984). Data from Venuto and coworkers (1984) also support the involvement of vasodilator prostaglandins in reducing the pressor response to norepinephrine and angiotensin II in rabbit pregnancy. However, it is unclear whether meclofenamate fully restored pressor responsiveness, as blood pressure values still appeared lower in the meclofenamate-treated animals than in the nonpregnant group (Venuto et al., 1984). In contrast, Conrad and Colpoys (1986) found that the blunted pressor responsiveness to angiotensin II or norepinephrine in pregnant rats was unaffected by indomethacin or meclofenamate, two structurally different cyclooxygenase inhibitors. We also previously reported that meclofenamate failed to restore the pulmonary pressor or vascular resistance response to hypoxia, prostaglandin $F_{2\alpha}$, or norepinephrine in pregnant dogs (Moore and Reeves, 1980). More recently, we examined the effect of meclofenamate on vasoreactivity in pregnant guinea pigs (Harrison and Moore, 1988). Our results indicated that meclofenamate, a prostaglandin synthesis inhibitor, did not raise systemic vascular resistance or restore the systemic vascular response to angiotensin II or the contractile response to phenylephrine or norepinephrine in pregnant animals to levels observed in the nonpregnant state. Perhaps the similarity between our results (Harrison and Moore, 1988) and those of Conrad and Colpoys (1986) was related to the use of chronically catheterized, conscious, unstressed animals whereas the animals used by Paller (1984) had undergone catheterization one hour before study. Prostaglandin production is known to be enhanced by anesthesia and conditions of stress (Walker et al., 1982), perhaps especially in pregnant animals (Conrad and Colpoys, 1986).

Thus the evidence available does not support prostaglandins as the mediators of pregnancy-induced reductions in vasoreactivity seen in the systemic as well as the pulmonary circulations. However, they may be involved in the regulation of vascular reactivity and maintenance of blood flow in the uterine, placental, and fetal circulations.

IV. Hypertensive Disorders in Pregnancy and the Pulmonary Circulation

The maternal vascular changes of normal pregnancy operate in a fashion that confers protection against hypertensive stimuli. Paradoxically, pregnancy has also been associated with the onset of primary pulmonary hypertension, a rare but nearly always fatal condition, as well as with the onset of systemic hypertension, the major maternal complication of pregnancy.

Primary pulmonary hypertension is principally a disease of young females (Walcott et al., 1970). Approximately 300-1000 cases of unexplained severe pulmonary hypertension occur per year in the United States (Voelkel, 1987). If half of these cases occur among women of reproductive age, the approximate incidence of young (age 18-44 years) females is 0.5-1.5 cases per 100,000. The disproportionate number of females with the disorder has also been observed when pulmonary hypertension has been involked by ingestion of the appetite depressant drug aminorex (Gurtner, 1978). Not only is the disorder more common among females, but its occurrence is centered in the reproductive years

(Fuster et al., 1984) and has been associated with two conditions involving elevation of female hormones – pregnancy and the use of oral contraceptives (McCaffrey and Dunn, 1964; Gurtner, 1978; Kleiger et al., 1976).

An association between oral contraceptive use and primary pulmonary hypertension was seen in a small number of patients in an early study (Kleiger et al., 1976). Worsening of pulmonary vascular disease shortly after beginning oral contraceptives has also been reported in three patients with congenital septal defects and elevated pulmonary artery pressures (Oakley and Somerville, 1968). However, the associations between oral contraceptives and primary pulmonary hypertension in a large, more recent series was no different than that found in the general population (Fuster et al., 1984).

Several persons have hypothesized that pregnancy may trigger or accelerate the progression of primary pulmonary hypertension (McCaffrey and Dunn, 1964; Gurtner, 1978). If so, the incidence of the disease in association with pregnancy ought to exceed the pregnancy rate in the general population. In 1985, 62.4 births occurred per 1000 women aged 15-44, for a pregnancy rate (ignoring abortions) of approximately 6% (U. S. Bureau of the Census, 1986). Wagenvoort and Wagenvoort (1970) reported eight cases in association with pregnancy in a series of 156, or an incidence of 5%, which is no greater than the pregnancy rate in the general population. However, 51 medical centers were involved and uniform diagnostic criteria may not have been used. More recent studies have reported a higher than expected proportion of cases in association with pregnancy. Fuster et al. (1984) found 14 cases, or 17%, of primary pulmonary hypertension in association with pregnancy among 82 postpubertal patients. However, if the number of patients 20-45 years of age (rather than all postpubertal women) is used in the denominator, 14/55, or 25%, of the cases occurred in conjunction with pregnancy (Fuster et al., 1984). Similarly, Dawkins et al. (1986) found that among 73 patients evaluated for heart-lung transplant, 6, or 8%, of the cases occurred in association with pregnancy. Thus, the more recently compiled data from single centers indicate that the occurrence of primary pulmonary hypertension in relation to pregnancy is greater than the pregnancy rate in the general population.

In the cases where primary pulmonary hypertension occurs in association with pregnancy, the onset of the disease is typically not during but soon after pregnancy itself. In a survey of 23 pregnancies, McCaffrey and Dunn (1964) found that only three of the cases began while the woman was pregnant and that the greatest concentration of cases within a few years of pregnancy was 1-3 years postpartum. The onset of symptoms in five out of six previously asymptomatic patients reported by Dawkins et al. (1986) also occurred postpartum.

The combination of primary pulmonary hypertension and pregnancy is often but not always fatal. In the McCaffrey and Dunn (1964) report, approximately half the women experienced an improvement or no change in symptoms whereas the remainder of the women deteriorated and 9 of the 23 died. The majority (6/9) of the maternal deaths occurred when the woman was in labor or immediately postpartum (McCaffrey and Dunn, 1964). Most authors attribute maternal demise to the eventual collapse of the already compromised maternal circulation by the additional circulatory burdens of pregnancy (McCaffrey and Dunn, 1964; Jewett, 1979; Fuster et al., 1984). However, the time course of the circulatory changes in pregnancy and the timing of death call this interpretation into question. The peak cardiac output is attained by midgestation, with values declining in at least the supine posture by term (Ueland et al., 1964). Labor itself causes a considerable increase in cardiac output and is accompanied by substantial fluid shifts. However, it appeared not so much to be labor itself but the completion of labor that was associated with death (McCaffrey and Dunn, 1964) or the onset of symptoms (Dawkins et al., 1986). In one instance, labor had not even been present, since death had occurred after delivery of the fetus and placenta during cesarean section (McCaffrey and Dunn, 1964). The gradual rise in blood pressure and vascular resistance with advancing gestation may suggest that progressive loss of a protective vasodilator during pregnancy. In such a scenario, it is possible that pregnancy permitted an impaired survival and death ensued when the limited protection afforded by pregnancy was no longer present. If so, perhaps the cessation of pregnancy, more than its presence, is the immediate threat to survival for the primary pulmonary hypertensive patient.

Another way to examine the influence of pregnancy on hypertensive disorders of the pulmonary circulation is to ask whether pregnancy worsens pulmonary hypertension due to other causes. A case report of a woman with pulmonary hypertension due to Eisenmenger's syndrome revealed that the woman experienced an uncomplicated pregnancy until developing preeclampsia at 38 weeks (Jewett, 1979). Following spontaneous delivery of a healthy but low-birth-weight infant, she continued to have systemic hypertension and proteinuria but felt so well that she wanted to go home. Death occurred on the sixth postpartum day after a rapid and irreversible decline in arterial oxygen tensions due to pulmonary vascular intimal obliteration evident upon autopsy (Jewett, 1979). While the occurrence of systemic hypertension is unusual, the timing of the death following parturition resembles that observed in the primary pulmonary hypertension fatalities.

We undertook studies in pregnant cattle as a possible animal model for the effects of pregnancy in the setting of pulmonary hypertension. Some cattle at high altitude are known to be genetically susceptible to pulmonary hypertension and right heart failure (high mountain or brisket disease) (Grover et al., 1963; Will et al., 1962). Anecdotal reports suggested that susceptible cattle survived pregnancy at high altitude but died postpartum, leading us to ask whether pregnancy decreased pulmonary vasoreactivity and protected the animals from pulmonary hypertension. We studied susceptible and resistant cows during progressive hypoxia while pregnant and again 2-4 months postpartum (Moore et al., 1979). We found that neither the resistant nor the susceptible cows experienced a fall in pulmonary arterial pressures with pregnancy. Contrary to our hypothesis, the susceptible cattle had higher pulmonary arterial pressures and pulmonary vascular resistance values when examined in their third trimester than when 2-4 months postpartum. While no maternal deaths occurred in our series, study results suggested that cows may have died postpartum because of augmented pulmonary hypertension during pregnancy. Whether these results can be generalized to humans is uncertain, however, because the normal (resistant) cows did not show the decrease in pulmonary arterial pressure or the reduction in pulmonary vascular reactivity to hypoxia observed in other species (Moore and Reeves, 1980; Fuchs et al., 1982; Cutaia et al., 1987). Perhaps cattle, known to have high pulmonary arterial pressures and vascular reactivity, behave unusually in pregnancy in comparison to other species.

The association between primary pulmonary hypertension and pregnancy or, more specifically, the immediate puerperium suggests the involvement of circulating factors of placental and/or fetal origin. The estrogens and progestins are attractive candidates since they are present in comparatively large amounts during pregnancy as well as in the oral contraceptives marketed earlier when associations with pulmonary vascular disorders were observed (Oakley and Somerville, 1968; Kleiger et al., 1976). However, the etiology by which estrogens and progestins might influence hypertensive disorders of the pulmonary circulation is far from clear.

The pathophysiology of primary pulmonary hypertension indicates intimal cell proliferation and luminal obstruction without marked medial muscular hypertrophy (Voelkel, 1988). While the evidence is limited, reports in the literature suggest the intriguing possibility that pregnancy and/or the sex steroids may be capable of inducing morphological alterations in the vascular wall via several mechanisms.

One route is by invoking changes in collagen and elastin synthesis that could, in turn, alter vascular stiffness or distensibility. Estradiol treatment decreased collagen and increased elastin in the rat aorta, with the net result of decreasing the collagen/elastin ratio (Fischer and Swain, 1977). Estrogen treatment has also been observed to have an inhibitory effect on the increase in collagen and elastin synthesis observed with renal hypertension (Wolinsky, 1972). These estrogen-induced changes in collagen and elastin would be expected to be protective against hypertensive states. However, as reviewed earlier, the hormonal changes of pregnancy involve more than alterations in estrogen levels. The other sex steroids also appear to affect collagen and elastin synthesis. Testosterone treatment increased collagen and decreased elastin in the rat aorta whereas progestin treatment slightly increased collagen and elastin (Fischer and Swain, 1977). In the setting of pregnancy, a decrease in the collagen fraction and no change in elastin occurred in the uterine but not the carotid arteries (Griendling et al., 1985). A decrease in collagen would be expected to increase vessel compliance, but a decrease in vessel stiffness was observed, suggesting that the composition or organization of collagen and elastin fibers may have been altered (Griendling et al., 1985). Sex steroids are also suspected as modulating diabetes-induced increases in collagen cross-linking and stiffness (Williamson et al., 1986).

Smooth muscle hypertrophy and hyperplasia of the vessel wall are a possible second means by which sex hormones might alter vascular morphology. Estrogen influences growth in several settings, including preparation of the endometrium for implantation, accelerating the maturation of the fetal lung (Khosla et al., 1981) and being able to convert cultured cells to release prolactin or growth hormone (Boockfor et all, 1986). In guinea pigs, the widening of uterine arteries with pregnancy or estrogen treatment appears to operate at least somewhat independently of vascular smooth muscle, since wider diameters were observed in pregnant or estrogen-treated animals after incubation in papaverine, a vascular smooth muscle relaxant (Moll and Gotz, 1985). In pregnancy, smooth muscle hypertrophy occurs in the uterine artery, which enables a characteristic increase in internal radius without a change in wall thickness and an increase in the capacity for stress development (Griending et al., 1985). The smooth muscle hypertrophy observed in the uterine artery did not occur in the carotid arteries (Griendling et al., 1985). Intimal hyperplasia has been described at various sites including pulmonary arteries, coronary vessels, mesenteric arteries, and veins in association with pregnancy, the early postpartum, and oral contraceptive use (Irey and Norris, 1973). Intimal thickening appeared to be a proliferative response rather than a consequence of thrombosis or embolization (Irey and Norris, 1973). Pregnancy and oral contraceptive use have also been reported to produce endothelial proliferation and degeneration of elastic membranes and of the media (Altura and Altura, 1977).

A third route may be via influences of sex steroids on capillary permeability that may in turn lead to vascular injury and a proliferative response. Dependent as well as nondependent edema is common in pregnancy and is also a frequent complaint of women during the menstrual cycle. Increased capillary permeability has been reported in pregnancy in some studies (Hunyor et al., 1983; Weissberg et al., 1983). Progesterone has been described as influencing vascular permeability by exerting a protective effect in carrageenin-induced paw edema (Nakagawa et al., 1981). Other hormones may be involved in permeability changes in pregnancy and the menstrual cycle, but their effects have not been well characterized.

V. Summary and Conclusions

Four main points have been addressed in this chapter.

First, the pulmonary circulation undergoes enormous changes with pregnancy. Despite an expansion of blood volume and increase in cardiac output, pulmonary arterial pressure and therefore total pulmonary resistance fall. The changes experienced by the pulmonary circulation are, by and large, similar to those of the systemic circulation, suggesting that pregnancy affects bodywide factors underlying vascular control.

Second, both the pulmonary and systemic circulations undergo alterations in vasoreactivity with pregnancy. The reduction in vasoreactivity is likely to be important in maintaining the low vascular resistance of the pregnant state and, in turn, the conditions conducive for high flow to the uteroplacental vascular bed.

Third, while the precise cause of the blunted vasoreactivity of pregnancy is unknown, influences of hormones in general and the sex steroids in particular are almost certainly involved. The strategic position of the lung as the recipient of the entire cardiac output and the ability of the lung to metabolize sex steroids suggest hormonal involvement. The leading candidate and the most extensively studied of the sex steroids in relation to vascular control is estradiol. Estradiol has been shown to reduce the pulmonary pressor response to hypoxia in some studies and to diminish systemic pressor responsiveness to several agonists. Further studies are warranted to uncover the mechanisms by which estrogen exerts its effects. Other hormones may be involved in regulating vasoreactivity in pregnancy. Despite earlier studies implicating prostaglandins, current evidence does not favor the hypothesis that prostaglandin modulation of vasoreactivity differs in the pregnant and nonpregnant states.

Fourth, the intriguing association between pregnancy, normally a vasodilated state, and primary pulmonary hypertension may offer clues to the etiology of this enigmatic and nearly always fatal condition. From the evidence currently available, it is not possible to determine whether the association with the onset of primary pulmonary hypertension and/or demise is due to the presence or the cessation of pregnancy. Discriminating between these two possibilities would be useful for the search for mechanisms responsible for primary pulmonary hypertension.

It is hoped that this review will prompt additional investigations into the effects of pregnancy and its associated hormones on the pulmonary circulation. Perhaps pregnancy may prove to be an experiment of nature able to provide new insight into factors responsible for the normal and abnormal functioning of the lung circulation.

References

Abdul-Karim, R., and Assali, N. S. (1961). Pressor response to angiotensin in pregnant and nonpregnant women. *Am. J. Obstet. Gynecol. 82*:256-251.

Altura, B. M., and Altura, B. T. (1977). Influence of sex hormones, oral contraceptives and pregnancy on vascular muscle and its reactivity. In *Factors Influencing Vascular Reactivity.* Edited by O. J. Carrier and S. Shibata, Igaku-Shoin, Tokyo, pp. 221-254.

Annibale, D. J., Rosenfeld, C. R., and Kamm, K. E. (1987). Contractile responses of systemic and uterine (Ut) arterial smooth muscle from pregnant (P) and late postpartum (LPP) sheep. *Fed. Proc. 46*:652.

Arias-Stella, J. (1971). Chronic mountain sickness: pathology and definitiion. In *High Altitude Physiology: Cardiac and Respiratory Aspects.* Churchill Livingstone, Edinburgh, pp. 31-40.

Aw, T. Y., Jone, D. P., O'Shannessy, D. J., Priest, J. H., and Priest, R. E. (1985). Oxygen dependence of oestrogen production by human placental microsomes and cultured choriocarcinoma cells. *J. Steroid Biochem. 22* (6): 753-758.

Bader, R. A., Bader, M. E., Rose, D. J., and Braunwald, E. (1955). Hemodynamics at rest and during exercise in normal pregnancy as studied by cardiac catheterization. *Clin. Invest. 34*:1524-1536.

Baker, P. J., Ramey, E. R., and Ramwell, P. W. (1978). Androgen mediated sex differences of cardiovascular responses in rats. *Am. J. Physiol. 235*(2): H242-H246.

Bakhle, Y. S., and Ben-Harari, R. R. (1979). Effects of oestrous cycle and exogenous ovarian steroids on 5-hydroxytryptamine metabolism in rat lung. *J. Physiol. 291*:11-18.

Barrow, S. E., Blair, I. A., Waddell, K. A., Shepherd, G. L., Lewis, P. J. and Dollery, C. T. (1983). Prostacyclin in late pregnancy: analysis of 6-oxo-prostaglandin $F_{1\alpha}$ in maternal plasma. In *Prostacyclin in Pregnancy.* Edited by P. J. Lewis. Raven Press, New York, pp. 79-85.

Baulieu, E. E. (1983). The progesterone receptor. In *Progestogens in Therapy.* Edited by G. Benagrano et al. Raven Press, New York, pp. 27-38.

Bedwani, J. R., and Marley, P. B. (1978). Enhanced inactivation of prostaglandin E2 by the rabbit lung during pregnancy or progesterone treatment. *Br. J. Pharmacol. 53*:547-554.

Bell, C. (1974). Control of uterine blood flow in pregnancy. *Med. Biol. 52*:219-228.

Bell, C., and Coffey, C. (1982). Factors influencing oestrogen-induced sensitization to acetylcholine of guinea-pig uterine artery. *J. Reprod. Fert. 66*:133-137.

Ben-Harari, R. R., and Youdim, B. H. (1983). The lung as an endocrine organ. *J. Br. Pharmacol. 32*(2):189-197.

Boockfor, F. R., Hoeffler, J. P., and Frawley, L. S. (1986). Estradiol induces a shift in cultured cells that release prolactin or growth hormone. *Am. J. Physiol. 250 (Endocinol. Metab. 13)*:E103-E105.

Brown, G. P., and Venuto, R. C. (1986). Angiotensin II receptor alterations during pregnancy in rabbits. *Am. J. Physiol. 251* (*Endocrinol. Metab. 14*): E58-E64.

Burton, R. R., Besch, E. L., and Smith, A. H. (1968). Effect of chronic hypoxia on the pulmonary arterial blood pressure of the chicken. *Am. J. Physiol. 214*:1438-1442.

Burwell, C. S. (1938). The placenta as a modified arteriovenous fistula considered in relation to the circulatory adjustments of pregnancy. *Am. J. Med. Sci. 195*:1.

Casey, M. L., Macdonald, P. C., and Simpson, E. R. (1985). Endocrinological changes of pregnancy. In *Williams, Testbook of Endocrinology*, 17th ed. Edited by J. D. Wilson and D. W. Foster. W. B. Saunders, Philadelphia, PA.

Chang, W. C., Nakao, J., Orimo, H., and Murota, S. (1980). Stimulation of prostaglandin cyclooxygenase and prostacyclin synthetaste activities by estradiol in rat aortic smooth muscle cells. *Biochim. Biophys. Acta 620*: 472-482.

Chesley, L. C., Talledo, E., Bohler, C. S., and Zuspan, F. P. (1965). Vascular reactivity to angiotensin II and norepinephrine in pregnant and nonpregnant women. *Am. J. Obstet. Gynecol. 91*:837-842.

Clapp, J. F., III (1985). Maternal heart rate in pregnancy. *Am. J. Obstet. Gynecol. 152*:659-60.

Clark, K. E., Farley, D. B., Van Orden, D. E. and Brody, M. J. (1977). Estrogen-induced uterine hyperemia and edema persist during histamine receptor blockade. *Proc. Soc. Exp. Biol. Med. 156*:411-416.

Clark, K. E., Baker, H. A., Bhatnagar, R., Van Orden, D. E., and Brody, M. J. (1978). Prevention of estrogen-induced uterine hyperemia by alpha-adrenergic receptor-blocking agents. *Endocrinology 102*:903-909.

Clark, K. E., Austin, J. E., and Stys, S. J. (1982). Effect of vasoactive intestinal polypeptide on uterine blood flow in pregnant ewes. *Am. J. Obstet. Gynecol. 144*:497-503.

Colburn, P., and Buonassisi, V. (1978). Estrogen-binding sites in endothelial cell cultures. *Science 201*:817-8.

Colucci, W. S., Gimbrone, M. A., Jr., McLaughlin, M. K., Halpern, W., and Alexander, R. W. (1982). Increased vascular catecholamine sensitivity and alpha-adrenergic receptor affinity in female and estrogen-treated male rats. *Circ. Res. 50*:805-811.

Conrad, K. P., and Colpoys, M. C. (1986). Evidence against the hypothesis that prostaglandins are the vasodepressor agents of pregnancy. *J. Clin. Invest. 77*:236-245.

Cutaia, M., Friedrich, P., Grimson, R., and Procelli, R. J. (1987). Pregnancy and gender related changes in pulmonary vascular reactivity in the isolated perfused cat lung, in situ. *Exp. Lung Res. 13*:343-357.

Danforth, D. N., Manalo-Estrella, P., and Buckingham, J. C. (1964). The effect of pregnancy and of Enovid on the rabbit vasculature. *Am. J. Obstet. Gynecol. 88*:952-959.

Dawkins, K. D., Burke, C. M., Billingham, M. E., and Jamieson, S. W. (1986). Primary pulmonary hypertension and pregnancy. *Chest 89*:383-388.

Dey, S. K., Hoversland, R. C., and Johnson, D. C. (1982). Phospholipase A_2 activity in the rat uterus: modulation by steroid hormones. *Prostaglandins 23*:619-624.

Dogterom, J., and DeJong, W. (1974). Diminished pressor response to noradrenaline of the perfused tail artery of pregnant rats. *Eur. J. Pharmacol. 25*: 267-269.

Everett, R. B., Worley, R. J., MacDonald, P. C., and Gant, N. F. (1978). Effect of prostaglandin synthetase inhibitors on pressor response to angiotensin II in human pregnancy. *J. Clin. Endocrinol. Metab. 46*:1007-1010.

Fischer, G. M., and Swain, M. L. (1977). Effect of sex hormones on blood pressure and vascular connective tissue in castrated and noncastrated male rats. *Am. J. Physiol. 232* (6):H617-H621.

Fuchs, K. I., Moore, L. G., and Rounds, S. (1982). Pulmonary vascular reactivity is blunted in pregnant rats. *J. Appl. Physiol.: Resp. Environ. Exercise Physiol. 53* (3):703-707.

Fuster, V., Steele, P. M., Edwards, W. D., Gersh, B. J., McGoon, M. D., and Frye, R. L. (1984). Primary pulmonary hypertension: natural history and the importance of thrombosis. *Circulation 70* (4):580-587.

Gant, N. F., Daley, G. L., Chand, S., Whalley, P. J., and MacDonald, P. C. (1973). A study of angiotensin II pressor response throughout primigravid pregnancy. *J. Clin. Invest. 52*:2682-2689.

Gerber, J. G., Payne, N. A., Murphy, R. C., and Nies, A. S. (1981). Prostacyclin produced by the pregnant uterus in the dog may act as a circulating vasodepressor substance. *J. Clin. Invest. 67*:632-636.

Gisclard, V., and Vanhoutte, P. M. (1985). Estrogens and endothelium-dependent responses in the femoral artery of the rabbit (abstr). *Physiologist 28*:324.

Gordon, J. B., Wetzel, R. C., McGeady, M. L., Adkinson, N. F., Jr., and Sylvester, J. T. (1986). Effects of indomethacin on estradiol-induced attenuation of hypoxic vasoconstriction in lamb lungs. *J. Appl. Physiol. 61* (6): 2116-2121.

Griendling, K. K., Fuller, E. O., and Cox, R. H. (1985). Pregnancy-induced changes in sheep uterine and carotid arteries. *Am. J. Physiol. 248 (Heart Circ. Physiol. 17)* :H658-H665.

Griess, F. C., Jr., Gobble, F. L., Jr., Anderson, S. G., and McGuirt, W. F. (1967). Effect of acetylcholine on the uterine vascular bed. *Am. J. Obstet. Gynecol. 99*:1073-1077.

Grover, R. F., Reeves, J. T., Will, D. H., and Blount, S. G. (1963). Pulmonary vasoconstriction in steers at high altitude. *J. Appl. Physiol. 18*:567-574.

Gurtner, H. P. (1978). Pulmonary hypertension "plexogenic pulmonary arteriopathy" and the appetite depressant drug aminorex: post or propter? *Bull. Eur. Physiopathol. Resp. 15*:897-923.

Hardebo, J. E., and Edvinsson, L. (1977). Reduced sensitivity to alpha- and beta-adrenergic receptor agonists of intra- and extracranial vessels during pregnancy. Relevance to migraine. *Acta Neurol. Scand. Suppl. 64*:204-205.

Harder, D. R., and Coulson, P. B. (1979). Estrogen receptors and effects of estrogen on membrane electrical properties of coronary vascular smooth muscle. *J. Cell Physiol. 100*:375-382.

Harrison, G. L., and Moore, L. G. (1988). Blunted vasoreactivity in pregnant guinea pigs is not restored by meclofenamate. *Am. J. Obstet. Gynecol.* (in press).

Hart, J. L. (1982). Barium responsiveness of the rat aorta and femoral artery during pregnancy. *Life Sci. 30*:163-169.

Hart, J. L. (1984). Effects of pregnancy on spontaneous contraction and barium responsiveness of the rat portal vein. *Biol. Res. Pregnancy 5*: (2):78-83.

Hart, M. V., Hosenpud, J. D., Hohimer, A. R., and Morton, M. J. (1985). Hemodynamics during pregnancy and sex steroid administration in guinea pigs. *Am. J. Physiol. 249*:R179-R185.

Hartiala, J., Uotila, P., and Nienstedt, W. (1976). Metabolism of testosterone in isolated perfused rat lungs. *J. Steroid Biochem. 7*:527-533.

Hartiala, J., Uotila, P., and Nienstedt, W. (1979a). Metabolism of estradiol in isolated perfused rat lungs. *J. Steroid Biochem. 13*:571-572.

Hartiala, J., Uotila, P., and Nienstedt, W. (1979b). Metabolism of progesterone in the isolated perfused rat lungs. *J. Steroid Biochem. 11*:1539-1541.

Hettiaratchi, E. S., and Pickford, M. (1967). The effect of oestrogen and progesterone on the pressor action of angiotensin in the rat. *Physiology 196*:447-451.

Horwitz, K. B., and Horwitz, L. D. (1982). Canine vascular tissues are targets for androgens, estrogens, progestins, and glucocorticoids. *J. Clin. Invest. 69*:750-758.

Hsueh, A. J., Peck, E. J., and Clark, J. H. (1975). Progesterone antagonism of estrogen receptor and estrogen-induced uterine growth. *Nature 254*:337.

Humpheys, P. W., and Joels, N. (1981a). The response of the hind-limb vascular bed of the rabbit to sympathetic stimulation and its modification by pregnancy. *J. Physiol. 330*:475-488.

Humpheys, P. W., and Joels, N. (1981b). Reflex response of the rabbit hind-limb muscle vascular bed to baroreceptor stimulation and its modification by pregnancy. *J. Physiol. 330*:461-473.

Hunyor, S. N., McEniery, P. T., Roberts, K. A., Bellamy, G. R., Roffe, D. J., Gallery, E. D. M., Gyory, A. Z., and Boyce, E. S. (1982). Capillary permeability in normal and hypertensive human pregnancy. *Clin. Exp. Pharmacol. Physiol. 10*:345-350.

Irey, N. S., and Norris, H. J. (1973). Intimal vascular lesions associated with female reproductive steroids. *Arch. Pathol. 96*:227.

Jarnfelt-Samsioe, A., Bremme, K., and Eneroth, P. (1985). Steroid hormones in emetic and non-emetic pregnancy. *Eur. J. Obstet. Gynecol. Reprod. Biol. 21*:87-99.

Jewett, J. F. (1979) Pulmonary hypertension and pre-eclampis. *New Engl. J. Med. 301* (19):1063-1064.

Kadowitz, P. J., Lippton, H. L., McNamara, D. B., Spannhake, E. W., and Hyman, A. L. (1982). Action and metabolism of prostaglandins in the pulmonary circulation. *Adv. Prostaglandins, Thromboxase, Leukotrine Res. 10*:333-356.

Katz, R., Karliner, J. S., and Resnik, R. (1978). Effects of a natural volume overload state (pregnancy) on left ventricular performance in normal human subjects. *Circulation 58*:434-441.

Khosla, S. S., Walker Smith, G. J., Parks, P. A., and Rooney, S. A. (1981). Effects of estrogen on fetal rabbit lung maturation: morphological and biochemical studies. *Pediatr. Res.* 15:1274-1281.

Killam, A. P., Rosenfeld, C. R., Battaglia, F. C., Makowski, E. L. and Meschia, G. (1973). Effect of estrogens on the uterine blood flow of oophorectomized ewes. *Am. J. Obstet. Gynecol. 115*:1045-1052.

Kleiger, R. E., Boxer, M., Ingham, R. E., and Harrison, D. C. (1976). Pulmonary hypertension in patients using oral contraceptives. *Chest 69*:144-147.

Lees, M. M., Taylor, S. H., Kerr, D. B., and Scott, D. B. (1967). A study of cardiac output at rest throughout pregnancy. *J. Obstet. Gynaecol. Br. Commonwealth 74*:319-328.

Longo, L. D. (1983). Maternal blood volume and cardiac output during pregnancy: a hypothesis of endocrinologic control. *Am. J. Physiol. 245* (*Reg. Integrative Comp. Physiol. 14*):R720-R729.

Lumbers, E. R. (1970). Peripheral vascular reactivity to angiotensin and noradrenaline in pregnant and non-pregnant women. *Aust. J. Exp. Biol. Med. Sci. 48*:493-500.

McCaffrey, R. M., and Dunn, L. J. (1964). Primary pulmonary hypertension in pregnancy. *Obstet. Gynecol. Surv. 19*:567-591.

McGiff, J. C., Crowshaw, K., Terragno, N. A., and Lonigro, A. J. (1970). Release of a prostaglandin-like substance into renal venous blood in response to angiotensin II. *Circ. Res. 26-27* (suppl. 1):I-121-I-130.

McGill, H. C., Jr., and Sheridan, P. J. (1981). Nuclear uptake of sex steroid hormones in the cardiovascular system of the baboon. *Circ. Res. 48*:238-244.

McLaughlin, M. K., and Keve, T. M. (1986). Pregnancy-induced changes in resistance blood vessels. *Am. J. Obstet. Gynecol. 155*:1296-1299.

McLaughlin, M. K., and Westney, D. J. (1985). An examination of vascular reactivity during pregnancy in the chronic ewe model. *Am. J. Obstet. Gynecol. 151*:479-483.

McLaughlin, M. K., Quinn, P. M., and Farnham, J. S. (1983). Differential sensitivity to angiotensin II in pregnant rabbits. *Am. J. Obstet. Gynecol. 146*:633-638.

McLaughlin, M. K., Quinn, P. M., and Farnham, J. S. (1985). Vascular reactivity in the hind limb of the pregnant ewe. *Am. J. Obstet. Gynecol. 152*:593-598.

McMurtry, I. F., Frith, C. H., and Will, D. H. (1973). Cardiopulmonary responses of male and female swine to simulated high altitude. *J. Appl. Physiol. 35*: 459-462.

Mah, M., Brown, G., Min, I., Barone, P., and Venuto, R. (1985). Captopril acutely alters the pressor response to infused angiotensin II in pregnant rabbits. *Clin. Res. 33*:364A (abstr.)

Majid, E., and Senior, J. (1982). Anti-oestrogen modification of uterine respones to oestrogen in the rat. *J. Reprod. Fert. 66*:79-85.

Matsuura, S., Naden, R. P., Grant, N. F., Jr., and Rosenfeld, C. R. (1981). Effect of volume expansion on pressor response to angiotensin II in pregnant ewes. *Am. J. Physiol. 240 (Heart Circ. Physiol. 9)*:H908-H913.

Meschia, G. (1983). Circulation to female reproductive organs. In *Handbook of Physiology*. Sect. 2, *The Cardiovascular System.* Vol. III. Edited by J. T. Shepherd and F. M. Abboud. Am. Physiological Soc., Bethesda, MD, pp. 241-269.

Milewich, L., Smith, S. L., and MacDonald, P. C. (1980). Nonrespiratory functions of the human lung: in vitro metabolism of tritium-labeled progesterone and pregnenolone. *J. Clin. Endocrinol. Metab. 50*:507-515.

Milewich, L., Hendricks, T. S., and Johnson, A. R. (1983). Metabolism of dehydroisoandrosterone and androstenedione in human pulmonary endothelial cells in culture. *J. Clin. Endocrinol. Metab. 56*:930-935.

Miller, V. M., Aarhus, L. L., and Vanhoutte, P. M. (1987). Estrogen modulates endothelium-dependent responses to oxydoxin in ovarian arteries of rabbits. *Fed. Proc. 46*:828.

Moisey, D. M., and Tulenko, T. (1983). Increased sensitivity to angiotensin in uterine arteries from pregnant rabbits. *Am. J. Physiol. 244* (*Heart Circ. Physiol. 13*):H335-H340.

Moll, W., and Gotz, R. (1985). Pressure-diameter curves of mesometrial arteries of guinea pigs demonstrate a nonmuscular, oestrogen-inducible mechanism of lumen regulation. *Pfluegers Arch. 404*:332-336.

Moore, L. G., and Reeves, J. T. (1980) Pregnancy blunts pulmonary vascular reactivity in dogs. *Am. J. Physiol.* Vol. *293 (Heart Circ. Physiol. 8)*:H297-H301.

Moore, L. G., Reeves, J. T., Will, D. H., and Grover, R. F. (1979). Pregnancy-induced pulmonary hypertension in cows susceptible to high mountain disease. *Am. J. Physiol.* Vol. *46 (Resp. Environ. Exercise Physiol.* (1) 184-188.

Moore, L. G., McMurtry, I. F., and Reeves, J. T. (1980) Effects of sex hormones on cardiovascular and hematologic response to chronic hypoxia in rats. *Proc. Soc. Exp. Biol. Med. 158*:658-662.

Morishige, W. K., and Uetake, C. (1978). Receptors for androgen and estrogen in the rat lung. *Endocrinology 102*:1827-1833.

Mueller, D., Stoehr, B., Jr., Phernetton, T., and Rankin, J. H. (1978). The effects of indomethacin and meclofenamate on estrogen induced vasodilation in the rabbit uterus. *Proc. Soc. Exp. Biol. Med. 159*:25-29.

Naden, R. P., and Rosenfeld, C. R. (1985a). Systemic and uterine responsiveness to angiotensin II and norepinephrine in estrogen-treated nonpregnant sheep. *Am. J. Obstet. Gynecol. 153*:417-425.

Naden, R. P., and Rosenfeld, C. R. (1985b). Role of apha-receptors in estrogen-induced vasodilation in nonpregnant sheep. *Am. J. Physiol. 248 (Heart Circ. Physiol. 17)*:H339-H344.

Naden, R. P., Gant, N. F., Jr., and Rosenfeld, C. R. (1984). The pressor response to angiotensin II: the roles of peripheral and cardiac responses in pregnant and nonpregnant sheep. *Am. J. Obstet. Gynecol. 148*:450-457.

Naden, R. P., Coultrup, S., Arant, B. S., and Rosenfeld, C. R. (1985) Metabolic clearance of angiotensin II in pregnant and nonpregnant sheep. *Am. J. Physiol. 249 (Endocrinol Metab. 23)*:E49-E55.

Nakagawa, H., Min, K. R., and Tsurufuji, S. (1981). Anti-inflammatory action of progesterone and its possible mode of action in rats. *Biochem. Pharmacol. 30*:639-644.

Naylor, B., and Poyser, N. L. (1975). Effects of oestradiol and progesterone on the in vitro production of prostaglandin F_{2a} by the guinea-pig uterus. *Brit. J. Pharmacol. 55*:229-232.

Nelson, S. H. (1987) Pregnancy-induced endothelium-dependent increase in sensitivity to acetylcholine (ACh) in human uterine arteries. *Fed. Proc. 46*: 502.

Oakley, C., and Somerville, J. (1968). Oral contraceptives and progressive pulmonary vascular disease. *Lancet* April 27:890-893.

Paller, M. S. (1984). Mechanism of decreased pressor responsiveness to ANG, NE, and vasopressin in pregnant rats. *Am. J. Physiol.* Vol. *16 (Heart Circ. Physiol.)*:H100-H108.

Parisi, V. M., Rankin, J. H. G., Phernetton, T. M., and Makowski, E. L. (1984). The effect of a leukotriene receptor antagonist, FPL 55712, on estrogen-induced uterine hyperemia in the nonpregnant rabbit. *Am. J. Obstet. Gynecol. 148*:365-369.

Peake, M. D., Harabin, A. L., Brennan, N. J., and Sylvester, J. T. (1981). Steady-state vascular responses to graded hypoxia in isolated lungs of five species. *J. Appl. Physiol.* Vol. *51 (Resp. Environ. Exercise Physiol.)*:1214-1219. 1219.

Pederson, E. B., Cristensen, N. J., Christensen, P., Johannesen, Kornerup, H. J., Kristensen, S., Lauritsen, J. G., Leyssac, P. P., Rasmussen, A. B., an Wohlert, M. (1982). Prostaglandins, catecholamines, renin and aldosterone during hypertensive and normotensive pregnancy. *Clin. Exp. Hyper. – Theory Practice, A4* (9,10):1453-1467.

Penaloza, D., Sime, F., and Ruiz, L. (1971). Cor pulmonale in chronic mountain sickness: present concept of Monge's disease. In *High Altitude Physiology: Cardiac and Respiratory Aspects.* Churchill Livingstone, Edinburgh, pp. 41-60.

Phaily, S., and Senior, J. (1978). Modification of oestrogen-indurec uterine hyperaemia by drugs in the ovariectomized rat. *J. Reprod. Fert. 53*:91-97.

Poindexter, A. N., Buttram, V. C., Besch, P. K., and Lash, B. (1977). Circulating prolactin levels I: normal females. *Int. J. Fertil. 22*:1-5.

Pugh, L. G. C. E. (1962). Physiological and medical aspects of the Himalayan scientific mountaineering expedition. *Birt. Med. J. II*:621-627.

Rabinovitch, M., Gamble, W. J., Miettinen, O. S., and Reid, L. (1981). Age and sex influence on pulmonary hypertension of chronic hypoxia and on recovery. *Am. J. Physiol. 240 (Heart Circ. Physiol. 9)*:H62-H72.

Ramwell, P., Karanian, J., Maggi, F., Myers, A., Penhos, J., Watkins, W., and Ramey, E. (1983). Gonadal steroid regulation of vascular arachidonate metabolites. In *Advances in Prostaglandin, Thromboxane, and Leukotriene Research.* Vol. 12. Edited by B. Samuelson, R. Paolett, and P. Ramwell. Raven Press, New York, pp. 229-234.

Resnk, R., Brink, G. W., and Plummer, M. H. (1977). The effect of progesterone on estrogen-induced uterine blood flow. *Am. J. Obstet. Gynecol. 128*: 251-256.

Rosenfeld, C. R., and Jackson, G. M. (1984). Estrogen-induced refractoriness to the pressor effects of infused angiotensin II. *Am. J. Obstet. Gynecol. 148*: 429-435.

Ryan, K. E., Farley, D. B., Van Orden, D. E., Farley, D., Edvinsson, L., Sjoberg, N. O., Van Orden, L. S., III, and Brody, M. J. (1974). Role of prostaglandins in estrogen-induced uterine hyperemia. *Prostaglandins 5*:257-268.

Ryan, U. S., Ryan, J. W., and Crutchley, D. J. (1985). The pulmonary endothelial surface. *Fed. Proc. 44*:2603-2609.

Secher, N. J., Thayssen, P., Arnsbo, P., and Olsen, J. (1982) Effect of prostaglandin E_2 and F_{2a} on the systemic and pulmonary circulation in pregnant anesthetized women. *Acta Obstet. Gynecol. Scand. 61*:213-218.

Semple, P. D., Beastall, G. H., Watson, W. S., and Hume, R. (1980). Serum testosterone depression associated with hypoxia in respiratory failure. *Clin. Sci. 58*:105-106.

Sheridan, P. J., and McGill, H. C., Jr. (1984). The nuclear uptake and retention of a synthetic progestin in the cardiovascular system of the baboon. *Endocronology 114*:2015-2019.

Siddiqi, T. A., Austin, J. E., Holroyd, J. C., and Clark, K. E. (1983) Modulation of angiotensin II pressor responsiveness by circulating levels of angiotensin II in pregnant sheep. *Am. J. Obstet. Gynecol. 145*:458-464.

Siiteri, P. K., and MacDonald, P. C. (1973). Role of extraglandular extrogen in human endocrinology. In *Handbook of Physiology*. Sect. 7, *Endocrinology*. Vol. II. Am. Physiol. Soc., Bethesda, MD, pp. 615-629.

Smith, P., Moosavi, H., Winson, M., and Heath, D. (1974). The influence of age and sex on the response of the right ventricle, pulmonary vasculature and carotid bodies to hypoxia in rats. *J. Pathol. 112*:11-17.

Stenmark, K. R., Abman, S. H., and Accurso, F. J. (1988). Etiologic mechanisms in persistent pulmonary hypertension of the newborn. In *Pulmonary Vascular Physiology and Pathophysiology*. Edited by E. K. Weir and J. T. Reeves. Marcel Dekker, New York, pp. 355-402.

Symonds, E. M. (1983). Renin-angiotensin system in normal and hypertensive pregnancy. In *Prostacyclin in Pregnancy*. Edited by P. J. Lewis. United Kingdom, pp. 91-98.

Tagatz, G. E., and Gurpide, E. (1973). Hormone secretion by the normal human ovary. In Handbook of Physiology. Sect. 7, *Endocrinology*. Vol. II. Am. Physiol. Soc., Bethesda, MD, pp. 603-613.

Tamai, T., Matsuura, S., Tatsumi, N., Nunotani, T., and Sagawa, N. (1984) Role of sex steroid horomes in relative refractoriness to angiotensin II during pregnancy. *Am. J. Obstet. Gynecol. 149*:177-183.

Ueland, K., Novy, M. J., Peterson, E. N., and Metcalfe, J. (1964). Maternal cardiovascular dynamics. *Am. J. Obstet. Gynecol. 104*:856-864.

U. S. Bureau of the Census (1985). *Statistical Abstract of the United States: 1986*. Washington, D. C.

Vander, A. V., Moore, L. G., Brewer, G. L., Menon, J., and England, B. (1978). Effects of high altitude on plasma concentrations of testosterone and pituitary gonadotrophins. *J. Aero-Space Med. 49* February:356-357.

Vanhoutte, P. M. (1987). Endothelium and the control of vascular tissue. *NIPS 2*:18-22.

Venuto, R., Minn, I., Barone, P., Donker, A. B., and Cunningham, E. (1984). Blood pressure control in pregnant rabbits: norepinephrine and prostaglandin interactions. *Am. J. Physiol. 247* (*Reg. Integrative Comp. Physiol. 16*):R786-R791.

Voelkel, N. F. (1988). Etiologic mechanisms of primary pulmonary hypertension. In *Pulmonary Physiology and Pathophysiology*. Edited by E. K. Weir and J. T. Reeves. Marcel Dekker, New York, Chap. 15.

Voelkel, N. F., and Chang, S. W. (1987). Eicosanoids and pulmonary injury. In *Eicosanoids in Cardiovascular and Renal Systems*. Edited by P. Halushka. MTP Press, Boston. (in press).

Wagenvoort, C. A., and Wagenvoort, (1970). Primary pulmonary hypertension. A pathologic study of the lung vessels in 156 clinically diagnosed cases. *Circulation 42*:1163-1184.

Walcott, G., Burchell, H. B., and Brown, A. L. (1970). Primary pulmonary hypertension. *JAMA 4A*:70-79.

Walker, B. R., Voelkel, N. F., and Reeves, J. T. (1982). Pulmonary pressor response after prostaglandin synthesis inhibition in conscious dogs. *J. Appl. Physiol. 52*:705-709.

Weir, E. K., and Grover, R. F. (1978). The role of endogenous prostaglandins in the pulmonary circulation. *Anesthesiology 48*:201-212.

Weir, E. K., Greer, B. E., Smith, S. C., Silvers, G. W., Droegemueller, W., Reeves, J. T., and Grover, R. F. (1976). Bronchoconstriction and pulmonary hypertension during abortion induced by 15-methyl-prostaglandin $F_{2\alpha}$. *Am. J. Med. 60*:556-562.

Werko, L. (1954). Pregnancy and heart disease. *Acta Obstet. Gynecol. Scand. 33*:162-210.

Weissberg, P. L., Weaver, J., Woods, L. L., West, M. J., and Beevers, D. G. (1983). Pregnancy induced hypertension: evidence for increased cell membrane permeability to sodium. *Brit. Med. J. 287*:709-711.

Wetzel, R. C., and Sylvester, J. T. (1983). Gender differences in hypoxic vascular response of isolated sheep lungs. *J. Appl. Physiol.:Resp. Exercise Physiol. 55* (1):100-104.

Wetzel, R. C., Zacur, H. A., and Sylvester, J. T. (1984). Effect of puberty and estradiol on hypoxic vasomoter response in isolated sheep lungs. *J. Appl. Physiol. : Resp. Environ. Exercise Physiol. 56* (50):1199-1203.

Will, D. H., Alexander, A. F., Reeves, J. T., and Grover, R. F. (1962). High altitude-induced pulmonary hypertension in normal cattle. *Circ. Res. 10*:172-177.

Williams, S. P., Shackelford, P. D., Iams, S. G., and Mustafa, S. J. (1987). Endothelium dependent responses to acetylcholine in estrogen treated spontaneously hypertensive rats. *Fed. Proc. 46*:828.

Williamson, J. R., Rowold, E., Chang, K., Marvel, J., Tomlinson, M., Sherman, W. R., Ackerman, K. E., Berger, R. A., and Kilo, C. (1986). Sex steroid dependency of diabetes-induced changes in polyol metabolism, vascular permeability, and collagen cross-linking. *Diabetes 35*:20-27.

Wilson, M., Morganti, A. A., Zervoudakis, I., Letcher, R. L., Romney, B. M., Von Oeyon, P., Papera, S., Sealey, J. E., and Laragh, J. H. (1980). Blood pressure, the renin-aldosterone system and sex steroids throughout normal pregnancy. *JAMA 68*:97-104.

Wintour, E. M., Coghlan, J. P., Oddie, C. J., Scoggins, B. A., and Walters, W. A. (1978). A sequential study of adrenocorticosteroid level in human pregnancy. *Clin. Exp. Pharmacol. Physiol., Aust. 5*:399-403.

Witter, F. R., and DiBlasi, M. C. (1984). Effect of steroid hormones on arachidonic acid metabolites of endothelial cells. *J. Obstet. Gynecol. 63*:747-751.

Wolinsky, E. H. (1972). Effects of estrogen and progestogen treatment on the response of the aorta of male rats to hypertension. *Circ. Res. 30*:341-349.

Worley, R. J., Gant, N. F., Everett, R. B., and MacDonald, P. C. (1979). Vascular responsiveness to pressor agents during human pregnancy. *J. Reprod. Med. 23*:115-128.

6

Hypobaric Effects on the Pulmonary Circulation and High Altitude Pulmonary Edema

PETER D. WAGNER

University of California, San Diego
La Jolla, California

I. Introduction

No treatise on the pulmonary circulation would be complete without some consideration of the effects of hypoxia on pulmonary pressure-flow relationships, and in almost every chapter of this volume the role of hypoxia is in some way important to the subject at hand. This chapter is, in fact, completely devoted to the effects of hypobaria (i.e., hypoxia) on the pulmonary circulation. This will produce some overlap with many of the other chapters of this volume, but it is hoped that this is neither substantial nor contradictory. It does, however, become important to define what will be covered herein and what will not be addressed.

As the fundamental source within this book for the effects of hypoxia on the pulmonary circulation, there will be some initial basic description of how hypoxia affects pulmonary vascular pressures and flow, with both acute and chronic exposure to a low PO_2. The focus will be on human data, with reference to animal work only as necessary to support hypotheses or mechanisms of effect. Little will be said about structural changes consequent to prolonged hypoxia. Not only does Dr. Reid have a chapter in this volume, but there are a number of descriptions of these changes in considerable detail (Arias-Stella and

Saldana, 1963; Hislop and Reid, 1976; Sobin et al., 1983) available to the interested reader. Nothing will be said about molecular mechanisms for the way in which hypoxia exerts its pressor effect. These are covered in Chapter 8.

Next will follow a contrast between effects of acute and chronic hypoxia on the pulmonary circulation, with some attempts to provide, where known, a rational explanation for the observed differences based on a combination of logic and the literature.

Subsequent to this will be a discussion of the consequences of altered pulmonary pressure-flow relationships on key physiological functions of the lung, especially gas exchange and its determinants, and transcapillary fluid exchange in the lung.

In each of these sections, exercise will be examined along with resting conditions, for two reasons. Very few people ascend to altitude unless they intend to undertake exercise of some sort. Also, exercise is a stress to the pulmonary circulation that amplifies phenomena barely observable at rest.

All of this will lead naturally into a discussion of high altitude pulmonary edema (HAPE) and its pathophysiological basis, as yet incompletely understood.

II. Effects of Hypoxia on the Pulmonary Circulation

A. Acute Hypoxia

Von Euler and Liljestrand (1946) described the pulmonary vascular pressor response to acute hypoxia in the cat and are generally credited with the "discovery" of hypoxic pulmonary vasoconstriction (HPV). However, as pointed out by Fishman (1985) in the *Handbook of Physiology*, Beyne (1942) published the same basic observation 4 years earlier. Whether this pressor response is merely the residual remains of an essential mechanism to reduce total pulmonary blood flow in fetal life or a designed mechanism to counterbalance the effect of local reduction in ventilation throughout life (thus reducing ventilation-perfusion inequality and consequently enhancing gas exchange) is both conjectural and unimportant to the current topic. However, total lung hypoxia, whether reached via nomobaric reduction in inspired O_2 concentration or hypobarically reduced PIO_2 at constant O_2 concentration, clearly causes the hypoxic pulmonary pressor response to be activated. Such global HPV is seen by no investigator as conveying any significant advantage to the individual so exposed. At best, there will be no negative functional consequence (of alveolar hypoxia) for the pulmonary circulation, but prolonged and/or severe hypoxia will, because of HPV, render an individual susceptible to right ventricular failure (from pulmonary hypertension, i.e., increased afterload) and/or a peculiar form of pulmonary edema known as HAPE (high altitude pulmonary edema).

Well-controlled, isolated lung experiments have clearly shown that pulmonary artery pressure at constant, controlled flow rises in response to alveolar hypoxia (Barer et al., 1970) without change in outflow (pulmonary venous) pressure. There is unquestionably an active increase in pulmonary vascular resistance in response to hypoxia. This point is stressed because acute exposure to high altitude in humans considerably raises cardiac output (and hence pulmonary blood flow), both at rest and during exercise, at any given $\dot{V}O_2$ (Alexander et al., 1967; Haab et al., 1967; Korner and Edwards, 1960). Increased pulmonary blood flow per se will be associated with increased pulmonary arterial pressure, even though there is concomitant vascular recruitment and distension (Glazier et al., 1969) that to some extent offsets this pulmonary hypertensive response. In other words, the increase in pulmonary artery pressure seen on altitude exposure is produced by an integrated response involving three interacting phenomena: active pulmonary vasoconstriction due to alveolar hypoxia, increased pulmonary blood flow probably due to hypoxia-induced adrenergic stimulation (Folkow et al., 1965), and offsetting mechanical reduction in vascular resistance due to recruitment and distention.

In intact humans, we see, of course, only the integrated end result of all of these factors. Figure 1 illustrates the mean pulmonary artery pressures and flows in normal, young subjects at rest and during exercise when acutely exposed to moderate altitudes, with sea-level values for comparison (Wagner et al., 1986a). The altitudes, achieved hypobarically in a decompression chamber, were characterized by barometric pressures of 523 torr (10,000 ft equivalent altitude) and 429 torr (15,000 ft equivalent altitude), and mean arterial PO_2 values are shown in the figure for each altitude. Data were obtained from direct pressure measurements by means of a pulmonary arterial catheter, and pulmonary blood flow was measured by mass conservation of tracer inert gases (Fick principle) using directly sampled systemic and pulmonary arterial blood and mixed expired gas. For each altitude, panel A shows pulmonary arterial pressure against work load; panel B, pulmonary blood flow against work load; and panel C, paired mean pulmonary arterial pressure and flow values for the points shown in panels A and B. Panel D shows flow plotted against the driving pressure (mean pulmonary artery-wedge). Because the original data appear elsewhere (Wagner et al., 1986a), standard error bars are omitted for clarity. Panel A shows how pulmonary arterial pressure at a given work load clearly increases with altitude, but panel B suggests that a part of this may be associated with the correspondingly higher cardiac output at a given work load. Panel C demonstrates that the pulmonary arterial pressures and flows increase with altitude in order to produce a single relationship across the three altitudes. However, this should not be taken as evidence that there is no change in pulmonary vascular tone, because the remaining variable, left atrial pressure, must be incorporated into the analysis. When that is done (panel D) (using wedge pressure as the only feasible approximation to left atrial pressure in such studies), it becomes evident that pulmonary vascular resistance at any cardiac output is higher as altitude is increased. It is interesting that the effects are more marked at the highest exercise levels (i.e.,

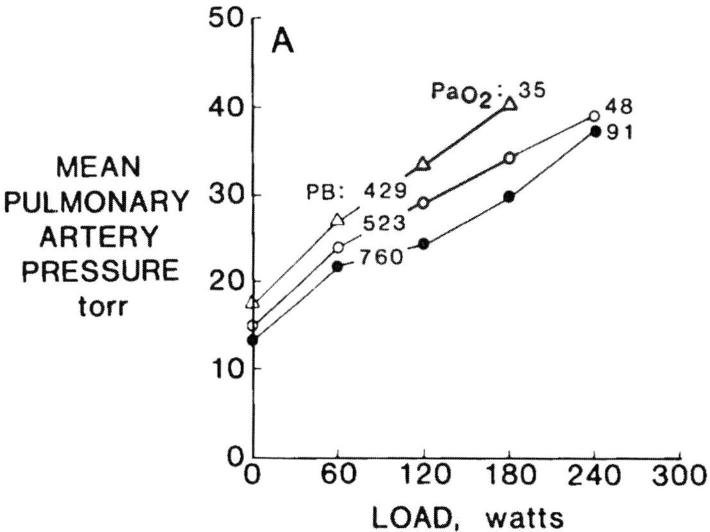

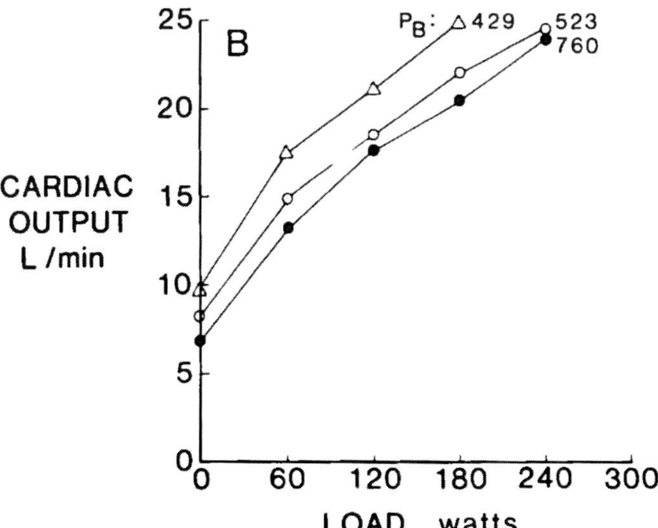

Figure 1 Pulmonary hemodynamics in acute hypobaric hypoxia. Data are from normal subjects studied at rest and several levels of exercise at barometic pressures of 760, 523, and 429 torr. (A,B) Relationship between mean pulmonary artery pressure and work load, and between cardiac output and work load;

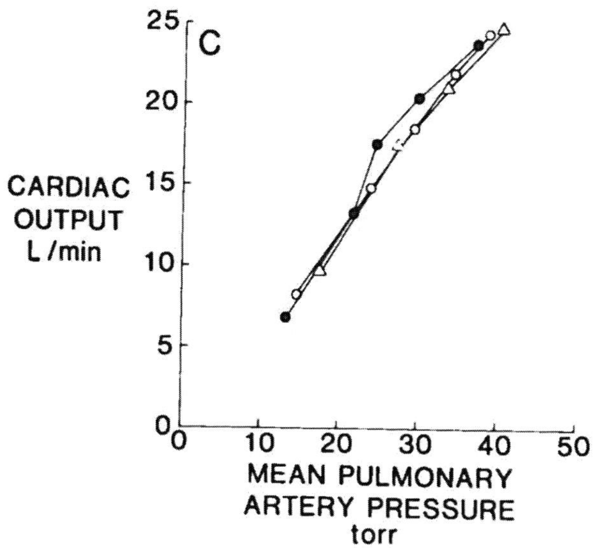

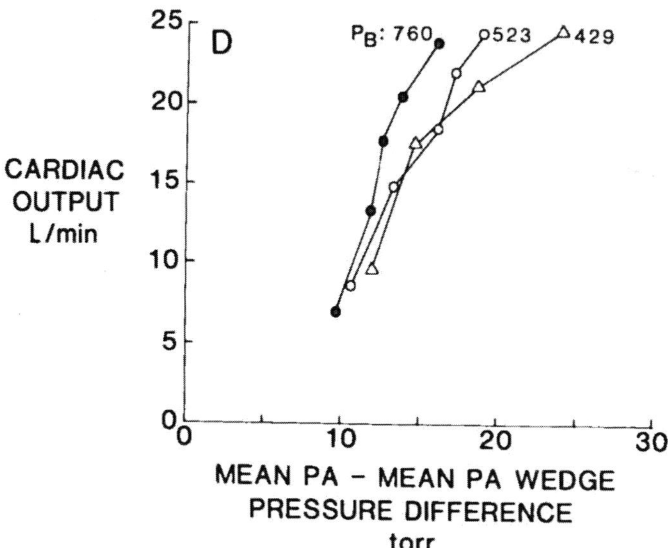

(C,D) pressure-flow relationships. Notice in D that in moderate and heavy exercise, hypobaric hypoxia clearly increases pulmonary vascular resistance. At rest and light levels of exercise, the effect of hypoxia is more subtle.

highest cardiac output values), presumably reflecting the compliance characteristics of the pulmonary circulation.

The effects of hypoxia are substantial (panel D), and it is seen that at cardiac output of 24-25 liters/min at near maximum $\dot{V}O_2$, pulmonary vascular resistance is about 0.7 torr/(liter-min) at sea level and rises to about 1.0 torr/(liter-min) at $P_B = 429$ torr, a 40% increase.

Figure 1 was constructed from the data of eight subjects (Wagner et al., 1986a), averaging results at work loads of 0, 60, 120, 180, and 240 watts. Each subject achieved his own maximum work load at each altitude, and there was some variation among subjects in that load. However, at each subject's maximum load (at each altitude), each was studied breathing ambient air and then again breathing 100% O_2. Figure 2 shows the pressure-flow points comparing air and 100% O_2 against a reproduction of Figure 1D. It shows that all points breathing 100% O_2 revert to positions on, or very close to, the initial sea-level relationship. In other words, relieving the hypoxia while maintaining both exercise and hypobaria completely reverses the vasoconstriction of altitude.

In summary, *acute* hypobaric exposures increasingly cause vasoconstriction due to hypoxia. This is brought out best by exercise but is apparent even at rest. However, such vasoconstriction is not the only reason for elevated pulmonary arterial pressures at altitude: A portion of the increase comes about as a result of an increased cardiac output. A further factor implicit in Figure 1 is that pulmonary artery-wedge pressure, while lying between 3 and 5 torr at rest at both sea level and altitude, appears to rise considerably during heavy exercise. Groves et al. (1987) also found this, and levels of about 20 torr mean are seen during near maximum exercise at sea level with slight reductions [to about 16 torr (Wagner et al., 1986a)] at $P_B = 429$ torr.

B. Cnronic Hypoxia

One-day exposures such as described above are necessarily limited to about 15,000 ft ($P_B = 429$ torr) for reasons of safety. Furthermore, some of the longer term adaptations to altitude cannot develop within a day. However, upon chronic exposure, much higher altitudes are attainable (Riley and Houston, 1951; West et al., 1962; Houston et al., 1987), and both the longer duration and greater severity of hypoxia result in a very different pressure-flow situation in the lungs. Large increases in hemoglobin concentration and hematocrit, together with structural changes (hypertrophy) of both the pulmonary arterial smooth muscle and the right ventricle, develop with severe, prolonged exposure to hypoxia.

Few comprehensive data on pulmonary hemodynamics under such conditions exist, for obvious practical reasons. To collect such data requires multiple pulmonary artery catheterizations, clearly impossible in the field. Conversely.

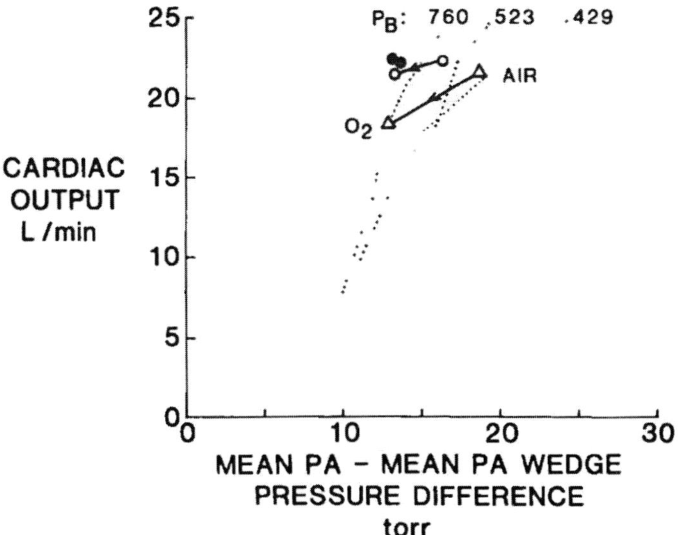

Figure 2 Reversibility of hypoxic vasoconstriction with oxygen breathing in acute hypobaric exposures. Dotted lines are reproduced from Figure 1D, while solid lines show points obtained during heavy exercise breathing ambient air and 100% oxygen at the three barometric pressures. These data, from the same subjects as in Figure 1, show that pressure-flow relationships on oxygen are essentially superimposed on the sea-level line and therefore indicate complete reversibility of the increased pulmonary vascular resistance at altitude.

while long-term field expeditions to great altitude are commonplace, corresponding long-term chamber "ascents" are few and far between, and few of those resort to the repeated degree of invasive catheter placement necessary to collect the necessary data.

In fact, the recently completed simulated ascent of Mt. Everest known as Operation Everest II (OE II) (Houston et al., 1987) is about the only source of such data, and thus for a comparison with the above results obtained during a one-day travel to 15,000 ft, the hemodynamic data from OE II are now presented in an analogous manner.

Figure 3A shows mean pulmonary artery pressure, and Figure 3B, cardiac output at each work load at three altitudes from OE II. Note that despite arterial PO_2 values similar to those at P_B = 429 torr in Figure 1 (acute hypoxia), mean pulmonary artery pressure at altitude in OE II is much higher. Panel B also reveals that cardiac output at a given work load actually *falls* after acclimatization (compare acute hypoxia where cardiac output is increased). The diminished response of cardiac output to exercise in prolonged hypoxia is well-described

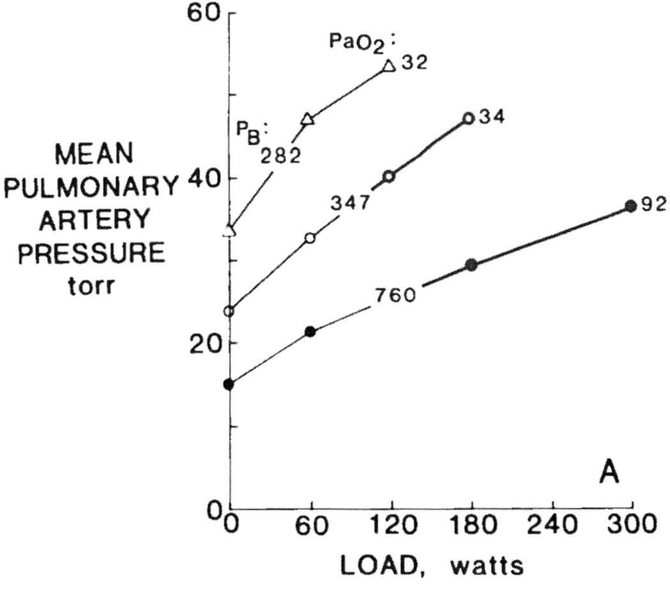

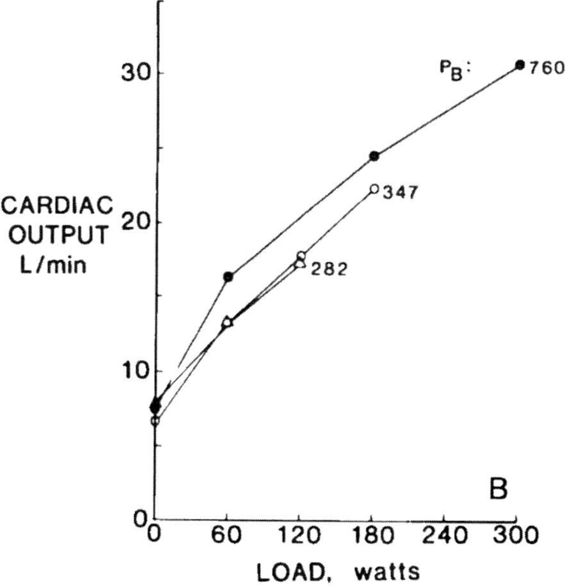

Figure 3 Pulmonary hemodynamics in chronic hypobaric hypoxia. The plots are identical in nature to those of Figure 1 and illustrate the major differences between acute and chronic hypoxia. It is evident from panels A and B that not only is pulmonary artery pressure higher than in acute hypoxia, but cardiac output is conversely lower. This results in major differences (panels C and D) in the

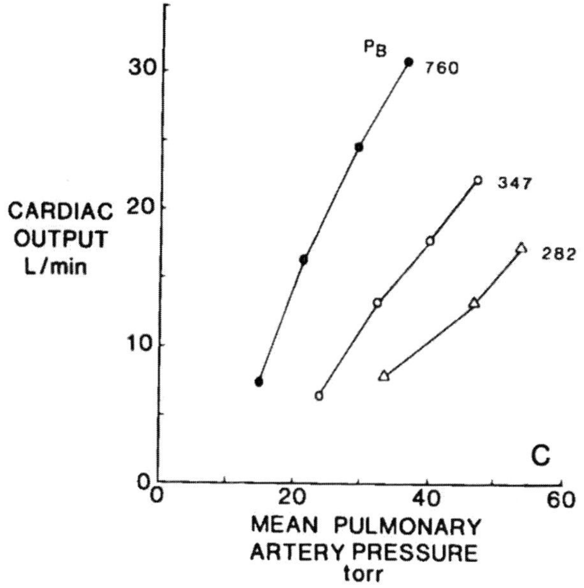

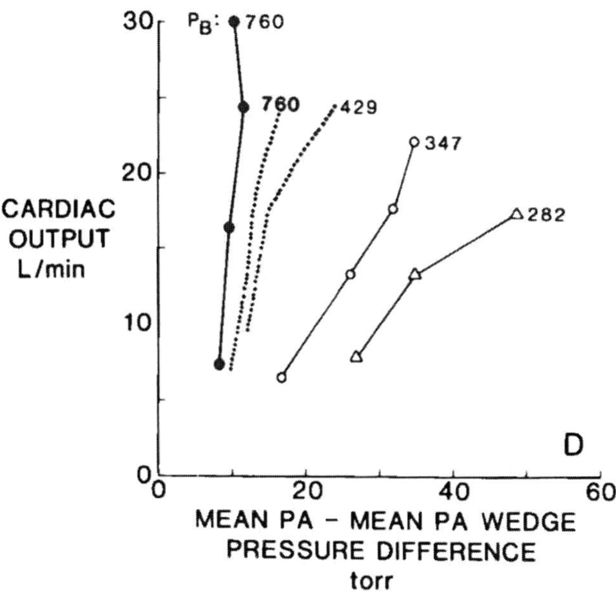

pressure-flow relationships. In panel D, the dotted lines reproduce data from Figure 1D at the indicated barometric pressures for comparison. Pulmonary vascular resistance is greatly increased in chronic hypoxia compared to acute hypoxia.

(Pugh, 1964) but poorly understood (West, 1962), and it is certainly beyond the scope of this chapter to discuss these effects on cardiac output. As a result of these differences, the plots of cardiac output against mean pulmonary artery pressure (panel C) and against driving pressure difference (panel D, solid lines) are grossly different from what is observed in acute hypoxia, even at a similar arterial PO_2 (low to mid-30s as shown). For contrast, the acute hypoxic data of Figure 1 are superimposed on those of OE II in Figure 3, using dotted lines.

Of considerable interest is the response to acute administration of 100% O_2. Just as in the acute hypoxic study described above, the subjects were asked to repeat the heaviest work load (attained on ambient air) while breathing 100% O_2. Including a few minutes of resting O_2 breathing, total duration of inhaling 100% O_2 was 15-20 min. Figure 4 shows (in a manner analogous to Figure 2) the pulmonary hemodynamic consequences of such O_2 breathing during exercise at the three altitudes. In marked contrast to the changes seen in identical manuuvers in acute hypoxia, the reductions in pressures and flows during breathing of O_2 demonstrated no reduction of pulmonary vascular tone: the air breathing and O_2 breathing pressure-flow relationships coincided at each altitude as shown in Figure 4.

Thus, hyperoxia for 15-20 min in this setting is ineffectual in reducing the effect of hypoxia. Whether evidence of diminished tone would have occurred after perhaps an hour of O_2 breathing is a matter of speculation. A reasonable conclusion is that the more severe pulmonary hypertension seen in prolonged hypoxia results more from structural changes in the pulmonary arteries (medial hypertrophy and adventitial thickening) as described in animal studies after prolonged hypoxic exposures (Arias-Stella and Saldana, 1963; Hislop and Reid, 1976; Sobin et al., 1983). An additional but probably lesser contributing factor is the higher hemoglobin concentration at altitude, acting to increase pressure because of increased blood viscosity. In the acute altitude study, hematocrit did not change with altitude (as was expected). In OE II, however, mean hematocrit at sea level was 42%; at 347 torr P_B, it was 51%; and at 282 torr P_B, 54%. These increases are modest due both to the limited duration of hypoxia (35 days to 282 torr) and (especially) to the amount of blood systematically taken from the subjects for multiple investigations.

Yet another factor of interest in interpreting the pulmonary pressure-flow relationships at altitude is blood volume, particularly central blood volume. Neither of the two studies described directly addressed this question, since no measurements were made of central blood volume. Examination of pulmonary artery mean wedge pressures, however, revealed no differences (at the same arterial PO_2) between the acute and chronic experiments, and this indirectly suggests that central blood volume was probably not much different between the two studies.

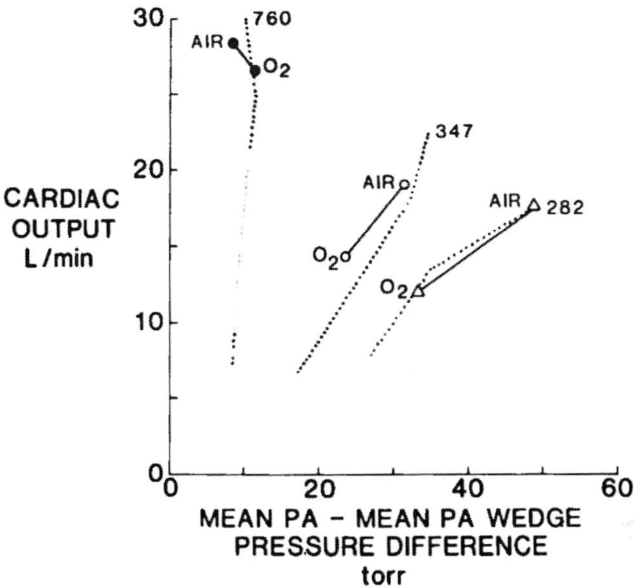

Figure 4 Effects of oxygen breathing on pressure-flow relationships during chronic hypobaric hypoxia. The dotted lines reproduce the data of Figure 3D, while the solid lines show the air and 100% oxygen breathing pressure-flow points at the same heavy levels of exercise at the three indicated barometric pressures. In marked contrast to Figure 2, breathing of oxygen (for 20 min) produces no significant reduction in pulmonary vascular resistance.

It was also possible to calculate an effective lumped parameter (overall) pulmonary diffusing capacity for O_2 during hypoxia (Hammond and Hempleman, 1987; Wagner et al., 1986a, 1987). At the same barometric pressure of 429 torr in the acute and chronic studies, this parameter was remarkably similar, as shown in Figure 5, both at rest and during exercise. To the extent that pulmonary capillary volume partly determines diffusing capacity (Roughton and Forster, 1957), this result is further, if also indirect, evidence against substantial blood volume differences between the acute and chronic situations.

In summary, the pulmonary hemodynamic consequences of prolonged hypoxia in humans are clearly different from those of acute hypoxia at essentially similar values of arterial PO_2. The differences are well brought out by exercise and characterized by modest, rapidly reversible vasoconstriction in acute exposures. Chronic exposure, on the other hand, produces a markedly exaggerated pulmonary hypertension that does not show acute reversibility with O_2 breathing. These differences are logically assumed to be mostly the result of

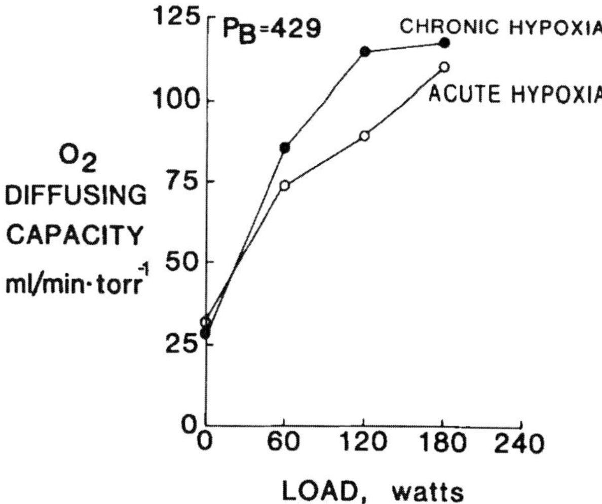

Figure 5 Calculated oxygen-diffusing capacity as a function of work load in acute and chronic hypoxia. Data are from Wagner et al. (1986) (acute hypoxia) and from Wagner et al. (1987) (chronic hypoxia). Diffusing capacity in acute and chronic hypoxia are remarkably similar. The slightly higher values in chronic hypoxia are probably explained by the increased hemoglobin concentration rather than by differences in the true diffusing capacity of the lung.

the structural changes in the pulmonary arteries occurring after prolonged hypoxic exposures.

III. Effects of Altitude-Induced Hemodynamic Changes on Pulmonary Function

A. General Considerations

It is relatively easy to measure gas-exchange variables at rest (and during exercise) together with the hemodynamic changes in experiments such as those described above. It is another matter to decide the extent to which the hemodynamic changes are responsible for those of gas exchange on ascent to altitude, but this will now be attempted.

The two most important processes that can interfere with pulmonary gas exchange at altitude are diffusion limitation of O_2 uptake (Lilienthal et al., 1946; West et al., 1962) and ventilation-perfusion mismatching (Gale et al., 1985; Wagner et al., 1986a). Each of these phenomena in turn can be affected by alterations in the distribution of ventilation on the one hand and blood flow on the other. Thus, for blood flow, not only could perfusion maldistribution develop, along the lines of Hultgren's theories (Hultgren, 1978), but the high pulmonary arterial pressures may produce increased transcapillary fluid movement sufficient to cause edema and affect gas exchange. In fact, high altitude pulmonary edema is a well-recognized complication of ascent to high altitude [although its mechanism remains obscure (Houston, 1960; Hultgren, 1978)]. A third way in which the pulmonary circulation could interfere with gas exchange at altitude is by a short red cell transit time, especially on exercise, leading to diffusion limitation of O_2 uptake.

Four levels of questions may then be posed in approaching the issue of how the pulmonary circulation affects pulmonary gas exchange at altitude.

1. Is there evidence of altered gas exchange other than the obvious changes in arterial PO_2 and PCO_2 from hypoxia and hyperventilation?
2. If so, is it abnormal $\dot{V}A/\dot{Q}$ relationships or diffusion limitation that develop?
3. (a) If $\dot{V}A/\dot{Q}$ mismatching develops, is it based on changes on the gas side or on the blood side of the blood-gas barrier?
   (b) If diffusion limitation occurs, is there evidence for an altered (reduced) diffusing capacity, or is it simply due to the combination of hypoxia and a low red cell transit time?
4. If abnormalities in $\dot{V}A/\dot{Q}$ matching or diffusing capacity occur, what is their pathophysiologic basis?

These questions are now addressed within the framework of the normal asymptomatic subject (i.e., without clinical evidence of high altitude pulmonary edema). Only situations short of frank, clinical high altitude pulmonary edema will be analyzed; pulmonary edema will be dealt with separately later – it is clearly associated with more hypoxemia still.

B. Altered Gas Exchange at Altitude

Few resting measurements useful in defining abnormal gas exchange have been made at altitude, but those available show, on the basis of conventional alveolar-arterial PO_2 difference (A-a DO_2), little or no inefficiency. In particular, the A-a DO_2 is less at altitude than at sea level (due to the shape of the oxyhemoglobin dissociation curve, as is well known), and is between 0 and 5 torr when arterial PO_2 is in the 30-40 torr range (Wagner et al., 1986a).

On exercise, however, there is considerable evidence of abnormal O_2 exchange. The A-a DO_2, which also widens with sea-level exercise (Wasserman and Whipp, 1975; Dempsey et al., 1984; Hammond et al., 1986a) widens considerably on exercise at altutide. This was shown dramatically on the Silver Hut expedition more than 25 years ago (West et al., 1962) by observations that, while ear-oximeter saturation fell substantially, alveolar PO_2 rose with increasing exercise loads. Other similar long-standing observations (Kreuzer et al., 1964; Reeves et al., 1969) confirm that this is characteristic of normal subjects at altitude who have no clinical evidence of high altitude pulmonary edema. More recently, a number of chamber and field studies have demonstrated similar responses in experiments aimed at understanding the physiological basis of the high altitude exercise A-a DO_2 (Torre-Bueno et al., 1985; Wagner et al., 1986a; Bebout et al., 1988), and Figure 6 illustrates the results from OE II (Wagner et al., 1988).

C. Physiological Explanations of the Widened Exercise Alveolar-Arterial PO_2 Difference

An increased A-a DO_2 during hypoxic exercise can, as stated, be due to diffusion limitation or ventilation-perfusion inequality, and additional techniques (beyond measurement of the A-a DO_2 itself) must be used to distinguish between these two general classes of mechanisms. Certainly, as suggested long ago by Lilienthal et al. (1946) and more recently by West and Wagner (1980), it is logically more likely that large A-a DO_2 values on exercise at altitude are caused by diffusion limitation than by $\dot{V}A/\dot{Q}$ mismatch, on the basis of the steepness of the O_2 dissociation curve, but moderate $\dot{V}A/\dot{Q}$ inequality could still be an important component and should be excluded by direct measurement rather than by logic.

The most direct currently available tool for separating the roles of $\dot{V}A/\dot{Q}$ inequality and diffusion limitation in this regard is the multiple inert gas elimination technique (Wagner et al., 1974b; Evans and Wagner, 1977). The power to do so rests in quantitatively comparing inert gas exchange to O_2 exchange. Because inert gases are invulnerable to alveolar-capillary diffusion limitation but are affected by $\dot{V}A/\dot{Q}$ inequality, while O_2 is vulnerable to both mechanisms of hypoxemia, any excess hypoxemia not predicted from simultaneous inert gas measurements is reflective of diffusion limitation (Wagner and West, 1980; Torre-Bueno et al., 1985).

When used in altitude chamber studies (the method is too invasive to use in the field), the inert gas method reveals that both $\dot{V}A/\dot{Q}$ mismatch and diffusion limitation are present and that both together explain the high A-a DO_2 on exercise. Figure 6 shows the relative roles of the two phenomena as measured in OE II (Wagner et al., 1987). Each panel shows the A-a DO_2 as a function of $\dot{V}O_2$ (or exercise level) and illustrates both the total (i.e., measured) A-a DO_2 and that portion predicted on the basis of $\dot{V}A/\dot{Q}$ mismatching alone ("predicted" lines of Fig. 6). It is evident that increasing either the altitude or the exercise level increases that component of the A-a DO_2 due to diffusion limitation (i.e., increases the distance between the measured and predicted curves). However, the predicted curves also demonstrate a systematic, if small, increase with exercise at any altitude (see Fig. 6), indicating worsening $\dot{V}A/\dot{Q}$ relationships on exercise.

In summary, diffusion limitation is the larger factor but $\dot{V}A/\dot{Q}$ inequality is also present and not insignificant.

D. Physiological Explanation of Diffusion Limitation

Classical physiological arguments (Forster, 1957; Piiper and Scheid, 1981) predict that diffusion limitation should become greater with altitude (due to the steep O_2 hemoglobin dissociation curve) and also with exercise due to the reduced transit time found because blood flow increases to a greater degree than capillary blood volume (Johnson et al., 1960).

What needs to be addressed, however, is whether these expected physiological sequelae of hypoxic exercise are sufficient to account for observations such as those of Figure 6, or whether there are also true changes in O_2 diffusing capacity of the lung (DLO_2).

It is possible to compute the DLO_2 that must be present to account for the difference between measured and predicted A-a DO_2 values (Hammond and Hempleman, 1987). In normal lungs, it is not important to such computations how diffusing capacity is assumed to be distributed among the various gas exchange units present (Hammond and Hempleman, 1987), and so the simplest assumption that DLO_2 is distributed uniformly with respect to blood flow is followed (the actual distribution of diffusing capacity cannot be measured). Both in acute (Wagner et al., 1986a) and prolonged (Wagner et al., 1987) hypobaric exposures, such estimates of DLO_2 yield values that are not only very high [> 100 ml/(min-torr)] but, if anything, increase with increasing altitude. Moreover, they are in precisely the range estimated morphometrically by Gehr et al. (1978) for normal human lungs.

Consequently, we suggest that the diffusion limitation seen in Figure 6 simply represents exhaustion of the ability to reach diffusional equilibrium due to rapid red cell transit in combination with the steep O_2 dissociation curve. The high values of DLO_2 found so consistently (Wagner et al., 1986a, 1987) by the method of Hammond and Hempleman (1987) do not suggest that diffusing capacity is significantly impaired by altered ventilation or perfusion distribution or by subclinical pulmonary edema, if the latter is indeed present as suggested (Wagner et al., 1986a) under these conditions.

In summary, it appears that the significant degrees of O_2 diffusion limitation seen during hypoxic exercise are likely the result of a short pulmonary circulation time and not a pathologically abnormal O_2 diffusing capacity.

E. Physiological Explanation of Ventilation-Perfusion Mismatching

Just as with diffusion limitation, it appears that the pulmonary circulation is to blame for the development of $\dot{V}A/\dot{Q}$ mismatch at altitude. There is actually no

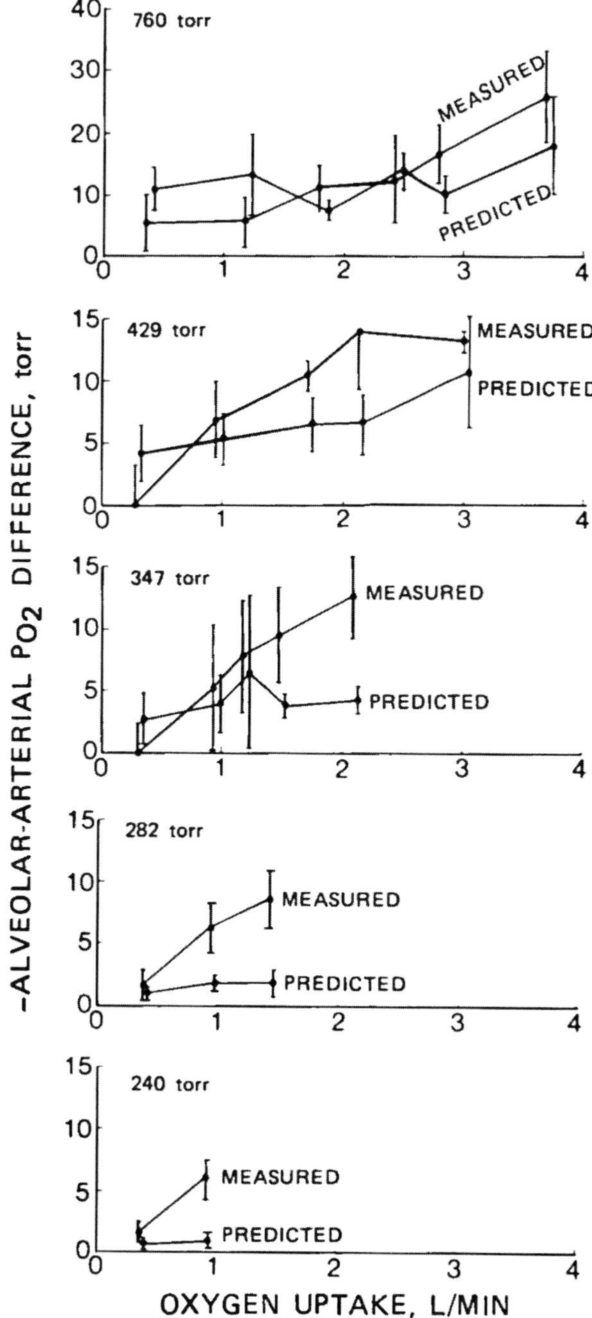
760 torr
MEASURED
PREDICTED
429 torr
MEASURED
PREDICTED
347 torr
MEASURED
PREDICTED
282 torr
MEASURED
PREDICTED
240 torr
MEASURED
PREDICTED
-ALVEOLAR-ARTERIAL P_{O_2} DIFFERENCE, torr
OXYGEN UPTAKE, L/MIN

evidence in the absence of signs of pulmonary edema that events on the gas side of the blood-gas barrier are primarily responsible for the increased VA/Q inequality of altitude, although, to be fair, more work needs to be done in this area. Thus, in OE II, considerable $\dot{V}A/\dot{Q}$ mismatch was found, while at the same time expiratory flow rates were not altered from resting values (Wagner et al., 1986b). This was especially true of the midexpiratory flow rate, which is generally regarded as a sensitive indicator of airway obstruction. Others have found changes in the single-breath N_2 test consistent with interstitial edema (Gray et al., 1975), but no simultaneous spirometric measurement of air flow rates were made, making these results difficult to compare to the above data. Clearly, at some point, edema may lead to at least small airways obstruction when peribronchial cuffing becomes extensive. However, in OE II, the important observation was the simultaneous development of $\dot{V}A/\dot{Q}$ inequality and absence of evidence of airways obstruction.

On the other hand, there is considerable circumstantial evidence that the pulmonary circulation is directly involved in the abnormal $\dot{V}A/\dot{Q}$ relationships of hypoxic exercise. The clearest data came from acute hypoxic studies (Wagner et al., 1986a); those from OE II (Wagner et al., 1987) are more difficult to assess because of the associated structural changes in the pulmonary arterial musculature discussed above.

The evidence is as follows. In acute hypoxia (Wagner et al., 1986a), a single relationship is observed between mean pulmonary arterial pressure and the amount of $\dot{V}A/\dot{Q}$ inequality (Fig. 7) irrespective of altitude, FIO_2, or exercise level. Moreover, the $\dot{V}A/\dot{Q}$ deterioration can be immediately reversed by breathing 100% O_2 (Wagner et al., 1986a), while in prolonged hypoxia (such as in OE II, where it was pointed out that hypoxic vasoconstriction is not reduced by 20 min of 100% O_2 breathing) there is also no reduction in $\dot{V}A/\dot{Q}$ mismatch with O_2 (Wagner et al., 1987). Furthermore, the amount by which $\dot{V}A/\dot{Q}$ inequality increases on exercise is greater in hypoxia than in normoxia (Hammond et al., 1986b). This happens with no substantial difference in minute ventilation levels comparing hypoxia and normoxia [the exercise load is necessarily lower in

---

Figure 6 Alvolar-arterial PO_2 differences in chronic hypoxia (Wagner et al., 1988) as a function of oxygen uptake. Data are shown for five altitudes, and at each the line labeled "measured" indicates the total, or actual, alveolar-arterial PO_2 difference. The line labeled "predicted" represents the alveolar-arterial difference due to $\dot{V}A/\dot{Q}$ inequality and shunt when present. The difference between measured and predicted relationships is accounted for by alveolar-end capillary diffusion limitation of oxygen. Diffusion limitation becomes a larger and larger factor with increasing altitude and increasing exercise. At extreme altitude, the slightest exercise produces diffusion limitation.

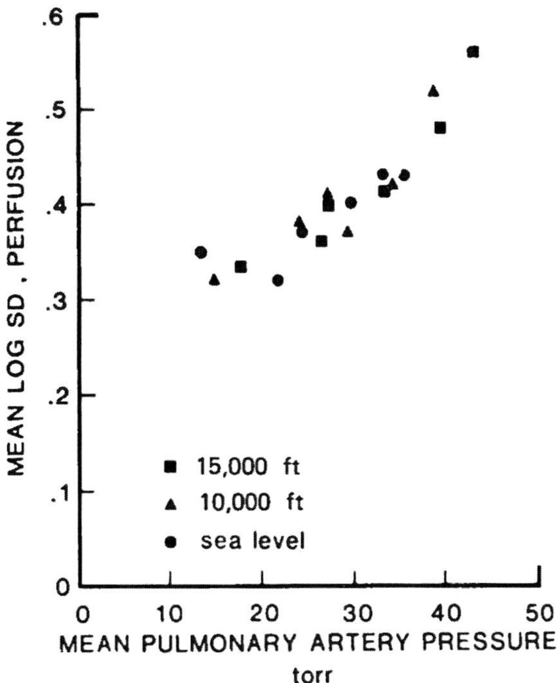

Figure 7 Relationship between the amount of ventilation-perfusion mismatch expressed as the second moment of the perfusion distribution on a logarithmic scale and mean pulmonary artery pressure in acute hypoxia (Wagner et al., 1986a). Each point represents the average data from eight subjects at the indicated altitudes (barometric pressures of 760, 523, and 429 torr), and multiple points at each altitude refer to values at rest and several levels of exercise. A single strong relationship is observed encompassing all altitudes and excercise levels, associating $\dot{V}A/\dot{Q}$ inequality with pulmonary artery hypertension.

hypoxia, but ventilation is about the same (Wagner et al., 1986a)].

In summary, it appears that the genesis of the increase in $\dot{V}A/\dot{Q}$ inequality seen on ascent to altitude lies in the pulmonary circulation rather than in some defect in ventilation.

F. Pathophysiological Basis of VA/Q Inequality

While there is no evidence that the reasons for O_2 diffusion limitation are anything other than that the diffusional transport capabilities of the normal lung are exceeded due to rapid red cell transit, it is hard to account for the $\dot{V}A/\dot{Q}$ mismatch on other than pathological grounds, although direct proof remains to be gathered.

Only two pathophysiological mechanisms for the way in which the pulmonary circulation impairs $\dot{V}A/\dot{Q}$ relationships come to mind. One is nonuniform hypoxic vasoconstriction, which by definition could be responsible for uneven perfusion and hence $\dot{V}A/\dot{Q}$ mismatch. This would fit with the theory advanced by Hultgren to account for high altitude pulmonary edema (Hultgren, 1978). Acute hypoxic studies (Gale et al., 1985; Hammond et al., 1986b; Wagner et al., 1986a) are not incompatible with this explanation, since the nature of the $\dot{V}A/\dot{Q}$ inequality is just a slight increase in dispersion about the mean. However, in OE II we frequently observed either shunt or areas of very low ventilation-perfusion ratio, especially at times of rapid ascent (Wagner et al., 1987). To the extent that all the altitude-induced $\dot{V}A/\dot{Q}$ changes reported from our several studies are based on the same pathophysiological process, only varying in magnitude according to the severity of the responsible causative factor, it becomes difficult to explain shunt and very low $\dot{V}A/\dot{Q}$ regions on the basis of nonuniform blood flow alone.

Thus, one is left with considerable suggestive evidence implicating interstitial, and on occasion scattered alveolar, edema as the most likely pathophysiological basis for the pulmonary functional changes with altitude.

That $\dot{V}A/\dot{Q}$ mismatch appears to be related to mean pulmonary arterial pressure (Fig. 6) is complementary to Hultgren's evidence (1978) that pulmonary wedge pressures are normal in high altitude edema. However, because it is so difficult to directly measure small degrees of increased lung water content under any circumstances, let alone those of high altitude chamber studies, we must still await direct measurement of the degrees of edema and of $\dot{V}A/\dot{Q}$ mismatch at the same time before firmer conclusions can be reached.

In summary, current evidence strongly suggests, but only circumstantially, that ascent to altitude leads to $\dot{V}A/\dot{Q}$ mismatching due to small degrees of pulmonary interstitial edema. When ascent is rapid and altitude extreme, these mild changes in $\dot{V}A/\dot{Q}$ relationships progress to shunting and eventually to clinical evidence of high altitude edema. This continuum of responses seems intimately related to the degree of pulmonary hypertension that develops, which leads to a discussion of high altitude pulmonary edema.

IV. High Altitude Pulmonary Edema

This subject has already been extensively described and discussed in this series by Hultgren (1978). Lamentably, there is little further insight into the mechanism (or mechanisms) by which HAPE is produced. Consequently, the present chapter is not meant to be the vehicle for an extensive reexamination of this complex issue, and only a general overview will be given. There seems to be little problem with diagnosis and even less with treatment (evacuation to low altitude and the breathing of O_2 are, of course, specific). Therefore, the important question is, why does HAPE occur?

Any hypothesis must account for the common observations summarized in Table 1.

The combination of case reports and prospective research upon which Table 1 is based strongly suggests the following:

1. The problem is *not* left ventricular failure (Fred et al., 1962; Hultgren et al., 1964; Penaloza and Sime, 1969; Roy et al., 1969).
2. The problem is *not* diagnostic confusion with infection (Arias-Stella and Kruger, 1963; Nayak et al., 1964).
3. It is very difficult to sort out the primary etiological factor(s) from those that may supervene later to worsen the lesion in a vicious cycle.
4. HAPE *need not* be accompanied by neurologic signs of acute mountain sickness, suggesting that it is not primarily a neurogenic edema.
5. All data point to a key role for the degree of pulmonary hypertension: Prior HAPE victims have a greater hypoxic pressor response (Fasules et al., 1985); pulmonary artery pressure is generally marked in HAPE (Hultgren, 1978); incidence is higher in juveniles who, at least in South America, have a higher pulmonary arterial pressure than adults (Penaloza and Gamboa, 1987); incidence and severity appear more marked in those rare cases of unilateral absence of a pulmonary artery (Hackett et al., 1980); there is a clear-cut association with rapidity of ascent and exercise, both of which are known to be associated with even more or more rapidly developing pulmonary hypertension (than slow ascent at rest).
6. There are intriguing, possibly genetic factors, as shown in cattle (Weir et al., 1974) and suggested by the relationship of HAPE to postrecovery hypoxic pressure response in humans (Fasules et al., 1985).
7. The degree to which hormonal factors are of primary influence is uncertain, but the gender distribution with respect to age (Hultgren, 1961; Sophocles, 1986; and Table 1) and supporting animal work (Wetzel and Sylvester, 1983; Wetzel et al., 1984) suggest that estrogens are protective.
8. Whether capillary permeability is primarily increased in hypoxia and contributes to edema is difficult to ascertain.
9. The role of physical factors as a primary cause (i.e., shear stress from high blood flow and also high pressure) as opposed to playing a secondary role after the problem is initated is also unclear.

Table 1 Epidemiological, Clinical, and Physiological Accompaniments of HAPE

Epidemiology

1. Most frequently seen in children or adolescents of either sex.
2. Virtually confined to males in adulthood.
3. Probability increased by rapidity of ascent and by exercise.
4. Prior HAPE victims appear to have greater hypoxic pressor response than normal.
5. Risk is higher with increasing altitude.

Clinical markers

1. Edema is characteristically patchy.
2. There is a continuum of severity from rales without CXR changes to full-blown radiological edema.
3. Arterial desaturation is marked, as is hyperpnea.
4. Pulmonary hypertension is marked with EKG evidence of right ventricular strain.
5. Usually accompanied by signs of acute mountain sickness (headache, tachycardia, nausea, fatigue) and cough.
6. In severe cases there may be hemoptysis and coma.
7. Occurs without preexisting cardiopulmonary disease or respiratory infections.

Physiological features

1. Pulmonary hypertension is marked; pulmonary artery wedge pressure is normal.
2. Whether edema is from high pressure alone or increased permeability as well is not clear.
3. Lung lavage material shows inflammatory cells and increased protein concentration.
4. Edema is more likely and more severe in unilateral absence of pulmonary artery.
5. Whatever the initiating cause, endothelial damage from high pressures and/or velocity of flow may worsen the problem.
6. Role of hormonal factors and formed elements in either primary or secondary damage is unclear.
7. Role of body fluid balance is unclear.

10. The role of clotting factors, inflammatory mediators, and formed elements of the blood as primary factors is also unclear; these may have important secondary effects subsequent to vascular change.

The situation is evidently very complex and will be difficult to unravel because the incidence of HAPE is low (< 1% in adults), is unpredictable among the general public, and develops in the field. Recent lung lavage measurements on Mount McKinley (Schoene et al., 1986a, b) are an exciting addition to the usual approaches to studying HAPE and clearly show increased protein and inflammatory cells. However, whether this reflects a primary component of HAPE or a secondary inflammatory response cannot be deduced from the data.

As one surveys the literature, the likely scenario for the development of HAPE is as follows: There is increased transcapillary fluid movement due to high pulmonary arterial pressure, possibly involving nonuniform, hypoxic vasoconstriction as postulated by Hultgren (1978). The high pulmonary arterial pressures and flows may also damage the pulmonary vascular endothelium for physical reasons, perhaps setting in motion a host of mechanisms related to inflammation and coagulation that worsen lung damage in a viciously cyclic manner, thus presenting a picture of edema with an inflammatory component by the time clinical examination and evaluation such as lung lavage is performed. The physiologic consequences of edema (i.e., reduced arterial saturation) further compound the problem by increasing vascular tone. The entire development of this complex is enhanced by genetic and hormonal factors that influence susceptibility and explain why HAPE is seen more in certain age groups. However, this overall interpretation should be regarded as a set of working hypotheses and not yet be taken as fact.

Acknowledgments

This work was supported by NIH grant HL 17731. I wish to thank Tania Davisson for the preparation of this chapter.

References

Alexander, J. K., Hartley, L. H., Modelski, M., and Grover, R. F. (1967). Reduction of stroke volume during exercise in man following ascent to 3,100 m altitude. *J. Appl. Physiol. 23* (6):849-858.

Arias-Stella, J., Kruger, H. (1963). Pathology of high altitude pulmonary edema. *Arch. Pathol. 76*:147-157.

Arias-Stella, J., and Saldana, M. (1963). The terminal portion of the pulmonary arterial tree in people native to high altitudes. *Circulation 28*:915-925.

Barer, G. R., Howard, P., and Shaw, J. W. (1970). Stimulus-response curves for the pulmonary vascular bed to hypoxia and hypercapnia. *J. Physiol. (Lond.) 211*:139-155.

Bebout, D. E., Story, D., Roca, J., Gonzalez, A., Haab, P., Hogan, M., Ueno, S., and Wagner, P. D. (1988). Effects of altitude acclimatization of the alveolar-arterial PO_2 difference in man. *The FASEB Journal* 2(6):8272.

Beyne, J. (1942). Influence de l'anoxemie sur la grande circulation et sur la circulation pulmonaire. *C. R. Soc. Biol. Paris 136*:399-400.

Dempsey, J. A., Handson, P. G., and Henderson, K. S. (1984). Exercise-induced arterial hypoxaemia in healthy human subjects at sea level. *J. Physiol. (Lond.) 355*:161-175.

Euler, U. S. von, and Liljestrand, G. (1946). Observations on the pulmonary arterial blood pressure in the cat. *Acta Physiol. Scand. 12*:301-320.

Evans, J. W., and Wagner, P. D. (1977). Limits on VA/Q distributions from analysis of experimental inert gas elimination. *J. Appl. Physiol. 42*:889-898.

Fasules, J. W., Wiggins, J. W., and Wolfe, R. R. (1985). Increased lung vasoreactivity in children from Leadville, Colorado, after recovery from high-altitude pulmonary edema. *Circulation 72*: (5):957-962.

Fishman, A. P. (1985). Pulmonary circulation. In *Handbook of Physiology*. Sect. 3, *The Respiratory System*. Vol. I. Edited by A. P. Fishman, A. B. Fisher, and S. R. Geiger. American Physiological Society, Bethesda, MD.

Folkow, B., Heymans, C., and Neil, E. (1965). Integrated aspects of cardiovascular regulation. In *Handbook of Physiology*. Sect. 2, *Circulation*. Vol. III. Edited by W. F. Hamilton and P. Dow. American Physiological Society, Bethesda, MD.

Forster, R. E. (1957). Exchange of gases between alveolar air and pulmonary capillary blood: pulmonary diffusing capacity. *Physiol. Rev. 37*:391-452.

Fred, H., Schmidt, A., Bates, T., and Hecht, H. (1962). Acute pulmonary edema of altitude. Clinical and physiologic observations. *Circulation 25*:929-937.

Gale, G. E. Torre-Bueno, J., Moon, R. E., Saltzman, H. A., and Wagner, P. D. (1985). Ventilation-perfusion inequality in normal humans during exercise at sea level and simulated altitude. *J. Appl. Physiol. 58* (3):978-988.

Gehr, P., Bachofen, M., and Weibel, E. R. (1978). The normal human lung: ultrastructure and morphometric estimation of diffusion capacity. *Resp. Physiol. 32*:121-140.

Glazier, J. B., Hughes, J. M. B., Maloney, J. E., and West, J. B. (1969). Measurements of capillary dimensions and blood volume in rapidly frozen lungs. *J. Appl. Physiol. 26* (1):65-76.

Gray, G. W., McFadden, D. M., Houston, C. S., and Bryan, A. C. (1975). Changes in the single-breath nitrogen washout curve on exposure to 17,600 ft. *J. Appl. Physiol. 39* (4):652-656.

Groves, B. M., Reeves, J. T., Sutton, J. R., Wagner, P. D., Cymerman, A., Malconian, M. K., Rock, P. B., Young, P. M., and Houston, C. S. (1987). Operation Everest II: high altitude pulmonary resistance unresponsive to oxygen. *J. Appl. Physiol. 63*(2):521-530.

Haab, P. E., Held, D. R., and Farhi, L. E. (1967). Readjustments of ventilation/perfusion relationships in the lung at altitude. In *Exercise at Altitude.* Edited by R. Margaria. Excerpta Medica Foundation, Amsterdam, pp. 108-111.

Hackett, P. H., Creagh, C. E., Grover, R. F., Honigman, B., Houston, C. S., Reeves, J. T., Sophocles, A. M., and Van Hardenbroek, M. (1980). High-altitude pulmonary edema in persons without the right pulmonary artery. *New Engl. J. Med. 302* (19): 1070-1073.

Hammond, M. D., and Hempleman, S. C. (1987). Oxygen diffusing capacity estimates derived from measured VA/Q distributions in man. *Resp. Physiol. 69*:129-147.

Hammond, M. D., Gale, G. E., Kapitan, K. S., Ries, A. and Wagner, P. D. (1986a). Pulmonary gas exchange in humans during exercise at sea level. *J. Appl. Physiol. 60* (5):1590-1598.

Hammond, M. D., Gale, G. E., Kapitan, K. S., Ries, A., and Wagner, P. D. (1986b). Pulmonary gas exchange in humans during normobaric hypoxic exercise. *J. Appl. Physiol. 61* (5):1749-1757.

Hislop, A., and Reid, L. (1976). New findings in pulmonary arteries of rats with hypoxia-induced pulmonary hypertension. *Brit. J. Exp. Pathol. 57*: 542-554.

Houston, C. (1960). Acute pulmonary edema of high altitude. *New Engl. J. Med. 263*:478-480.

Houston, C. S., Sutton, J. R., Cymerman, A., and Reeves, J. T. (1987). Operation Everest II: man at extreme altitude. *J. Appl. Physiol. 63*(2):877-882.

Hultgren, H. N. (1961). High altitude pulmonary edema. *Medicine 40*:289-313.

Hultgren, H. N. (1978). High altitude pulmonary edema. In *Lung Water and Solute Exchange.* Vol. 7. Edited by N. C. Staub. Marcel Dekker, New York, Chap. 15:437-469.

Hultgren, H., Lopez, C., Lundberg, E., and Miller, H. (1964). Physiologic studies of pulmonary edema at high altitude. *Circulation 29*:393-408.

Johnson, R. L., Jr., Spicer, W. S., Bishop, J. M., and Forster, R. E. (1960). Pulmonary capillary blood volume, flow and diffusing capacity during exercise. *J. Appl. Physiol. 15*:893-902.

Korner, P. I., and Edwards, A. W. (1960). The immediate effects of acute hypoxia on the heart rate, arterial pressure, cardiac output, and ventilation in the unanesthesized rabbit. *Quart. J. Exp. Physiol. 45*:113-122.

Kreuzer, F., Tenney, S. M., Mithoeffer, J. C., and Remmers, J. (1964). Alveolar-arterial oxygen gradient in Andean natives at high altitude. *J. Appl. Physiol. 19* (1):13-16.

Lilienthal, J. L., Jr., Riley, R. L., Proemmel, D. D., and Franke, R. E. H. (1946). An experimental analysis in man of the oxygen pressure gradient from alveolar air to arterial blood during rest and exercise at sea level and at altitude. *Am. J. Physiol. 147*:199-216.

Nayak, N., Roy, S., and Narrayanan, D. (1964). Pathologic features of altitude sickness. *Am. J. Pathol. 45*:381-391.

Penaloza, D., and Gamboa, R. (1987). Hipertension pulmonar. In *Cardiologia Pediatrica.* Salvat, Madrid.

Penaloza, D., and Sime, F. (1969). Circulatory dynamics during high altitude pulmonary edema. *Am. J. Cardiol. 23*:369-378.

Piiper, J., and Scheid, P. (1981). Model for capillary-alveolar equilibration with special reference to 0_2 uptake in hypoxia. *Resp. Physiol. 46*:193-208.

Pugh, L. G. C. E. (1964). Cardiac output in muscular exercise at 5,800 m (19,000 ft). *J. Appl. Physiol. 19* (3):441-447.

Reeves, J. T., Halpin, J., Cohn, J. E., and Daoud, F. (1969). Increased alveolar-arterial oxygen difference during simulated high-altitude exposure. *J. Appl. Physiol. 27* (5):658-661.

Riley, R. L., and Houston, C. S. (1951). Composition of alveolar air and volume of pulmonary ventilation during long exposure to high altitude. *J. Appl. Physiol. 3*:526-534.

Roughton, F. J. W., and Forster, R. E. (1957). Relative importance of diffusion and chemical reaction rates in determining rate of exchange of gases in the human lung, with special reference to true diffusing capacity of pulmonary membrane and volume of blood in the lung capillaries. *J. Appl. Physiol. 11* (2):290-302.

Roy, S., Guleria, J. S., Khanna, P. K., Manchanda, S. C., Pande, J. N., and Subba, P. S. (1969). Hemodynamic studies in high altitude pulmonary edema. *Brit. Heart J. 31*:52-58.

Schoene, R. B., Hackett, P. H., Henderson, W. R., Sage, E. H., Chow, M., Roach, R. C., Mills, W. J., Jr., and Martin, T. R. (1986a). High-altitude pulmonary edema. Characteristics of lung lavage fluid. *JAMA 256*:63-69.

Schoene, R. B., Swenson, E. R., Pizzo, C., Maunder, R. J., Roach, R. C., Hackett, P. H., Mills, W. J., Jr., and Martin, T. R. (1986b). High altitude pulmonary edema: comparison with other forms of lung injury. *Am. Rev. Resp. Dis. 133* (4):A269.

Sobin, S. S., Tremer, H. M., Hardy, J. D., and Chiodi, H. P. (1983). Changes in arteriole in acute and chronic hypoxic pulmonary hypertension and recovery in rat. *J. Appl. Physiol. 55*:1445-1455.

Sophocles, A. M., Jr. (1986). High-altitude pulmonary edema in Vail, Colorado, 1975-1982. *West J. Med. 144*:569-573.

Torre-Bueno, J., Wagner, P. D., Saltzman, H. A., Gale, G. E., and Moon, R. E. (1985). Diffusion limitation in normal humans during exercise at sea level and simulated altitude. *J. Appl. Physiol. 58* (3):989-995.

Wagner, P. D., and West, J. B. (1980). Ventilation-perfusion relationships. In *Pulmonary Gas Exchange*. Vol. 1. Edited by J. B. West. Academic Press, Orlando, FL, Chap. 7, pp. 219-262.

Wagner, P. D., Laravuso, R. B., Uhl, R. R., and West, J. (1974a). Continuous distributions of ventilation-perfusion ratios in normal subjects breathing air and 100% O_2. *J. Clin. Invest. 54*:54-68.

Wagner, P. D., Naumann, P. F., and Laravuso, R. B. (1974b). Simultaneous measurement of eight foreign gases in blood by gas chromatography. *J. Appl. Physiol. 36*:600-605.

Wagner, P. D., Gale, G. E., Moon, R. E., Torre-Bueno, J., Stolp, B. W., and Saltzman, H. A. (1986a). Pulmonary gas exchange in humans exercising at sea level and simulated altitude. *J. Appl. Physiol. 60* (1):260-270.

Wagner, P. D., Sutton, J. R., Malconian, M. K., Cymerman, A., Groves, B. M., and Reeves, J. T. (1986b). Lung volumes and flow rates in man during a simulated ascent of Mt. Everest. *Am. Rev. Resp. Dis. 133* (4):A76.

Wagner, P. D., Sutton, J. R., Reeves, J. T., Cymerman, A., Groves, B. M., and Malconian, M. K. (1988). Pulmonary gas exchange throughout a simulated ascent of Mt. Everest: Operation Everest II. *J. Appl. Physiol. (1988) 63* (6):2348-2359.

Wasserman, K., and Whipp, B. J. (1975). Exercise physiology in health and disease. *Am. Rev. Resp. Dis. 112*:219-249.

Weir, E. K., Tucker, A., Reeves, J. T., Will, D. H., and Grover, R. F. (1974). The genetic factor influencing pulmonary hypertension in cattle at high altitude. *Cardiovasc. Res. 8*:745-749.

West, J. B. (1962). Gas exchange at altitude. In *Oxygen Transport to Human Tissues*. Edited by J. A. Leoppky and M. L. Riedesel. North-Holland, Amsterdam, pp. 205-212.

West, J. B., and Wagner, P. D. (1980). Predicted gas exchange on the summit of Mt. Everest. *Resp. Physiol. 42*:1-16.

West, J. B., Lahiri, S., Gill, M. B., Milledge, J. S., Pugh, L. G., and Ward, M. P. (1962). Arterial oxygen saturation during exercise at high altitude. *J. Appl. Physiol. 17*:617-621.

Wetzel, R. C., and Sylvester, J. T. (1983). Gender differences in hypoxic vascular response of isolated sheep lungs. *J. Appl. Physiol. 55*:100-104.

Wetzel, R. C., Zacur, H. A., and Sylvester, J. T. (1984). Effect of puberty and estradiol on hypoxic vasomotor response in isolated sheep lungs. *J. Appl. Physiol. 56*:1199-1203.

7

Pulmonary Circulation in Diving and Hyperbaric Environment

CLAES E. G. LUNDGREN and LEON E. FARHI

State University of New York at Buffalo
School of Medicine
Buffalo, New York

I. Introduction

The hyperbaric or high pressure environment is encountered in diving, caisson work, and activities in hyperbaric chambers.* While the depth record for air-breathing animals presumably is held by the humpback whale, which is known to reach depths of more than 1000 m, the most severe pressure exposures endured by humans, to the equivalent of 686 m (2250 ft), have occurred in experiments in hyperbaric chambers (Bennett et al, 1982). Routine diving to serve the offshore oil and gas industry can currently be performed down to about 500 m.

There are several factors that may conceivably influence the pulmonary circulation during diving and hyperbaric exposures:

Pressure per se
Gas density

*The relationships between some commonly used depth and pressure units are given in Table 1.

Table 1 Pressure Conversion Factors[a]

	Standard Abbreviation	Pa N/m^2	ATA	bar	torr, mmHg	psi	msw	fsw
Pascal, or newton per square meter	Pa, N/m^2	1	9.869×10^{-6}	1×10^{-5}	7.501×10^{-3}	1.450×10^{-4}	9.940×10^{-5}	3.261×10^{-4}
Atmospheres absolute	ATA	1.013×10^{5}	1	1.013	760	14.7	10.07	33.05
Bar	bar	1×10^{5}	9.869×10^{-1}	1	7.501×10^{2}	14.5	9.939	32.61
Torr (1 mmHg at 0°C)	torr, mmHg	1.333×10^{2}	1.316×10^{-3}	1.333×10^{-3}	1	1.934×10^{-2}	1.324×10^{-2}	4.347×10^{-2}
Pounds per square inch	psi	6.895×10^{3}	6.805×10^{-2}	6.895×10^{-2}	51.715	1	6.848×10^{-1}	2.247
Meters sea water	msw	1.006×10^{4}	9.927×10^{-2}	1.006×10^{-1}	75.5	1.460	1	3.281
Feet sea water	fsw	3.067×10^{3}	3.026×10^{-2}	3.067×10^{-2}	23.0	4.445×10^{-1}	3.048×10^{-1}	1

[a]To arrive at desired unit (top), multiply given unit (left) by conversion factor.

Source: Adapted with permission from pressure conversion tables in *Undersea Biomedical Research* (1974, 1987).

Hydrostatic pressure distribution

Pharmacologic effects of inhaled gases

While pathophysiological in nature, important effects on the pulmonary circulation may arise in conjunction with excessive exposures to pressure and pressure changes. Such influences include

Excessive chest compression (squeeze)

Gas embolism due to pulmonary barotrauma or decompression sickness

Toxic effects of oxygen

II. Pressure per se

Some components of the circulatory system are known to be susceptible to direct pressure effects. Slowing of the beating frequency of the heart at high pressures has frequently been observed in humans (e.g., Heller et al., 1897; Shilling et al., 1936; Hamilton, 1967; Raymond et al., 1968; Flynn et al., 1972; Fagraeus, 1974; Kerem and Salzano, 1974). Judging from animal experiments, one etiologic component in such bradycardia is a direct pressure effect on the heart. When pharmacological effects of gases at high pressures were avoided by using liquid-breathing mice, compression still caused bradycardia (Lundgren and Örnhagen, 1976). A reduction in heart rate to 48% of the 1 atm value was noted at 169 atm. The same occurred in the autonomically blocked animal. This phenomenon, called hyperbaric bradycardia, has also been demonstrated as a reduction in beating frequency of the excised sinus nodes of several species (Örnhagen and Hogan, 1977) and is considered a direct pressure effect on the pacemaker cells, action by decreasing the rate of diastolic depolarization. In the intact air-breathing organism, there is an additional element of negative chronotropic effect from high oxygen pressures (Schilling et al., 1936; Tauton et al., 1970; Fagraeus, 1974). However, there is no evidence that this hyperbaric bradycardia is coupled with changes in cardiac output and thus in pulmonary blood flow. Likewise, there are no studies that can illuminate the question of whether direct pressure effects are exerted on the tone and resistance of pulmonary vessels or any other vascular beds.

III. Gas Density

As the environmental pressure increases, so does the density of the respired gases. There are few studies on the effect of gas density on pulmonary circulation. However, dogs that were exposed to a roughly 50-fold range of gas densities displayed a distinct drop in alveolar-arterial oxygen pressure difference

$P(A\text{-}a)O_2$ when ventilated with the densest gas mixture (Martin et al., 1972). A helium-oxygen mixture at 1 ATA was used as one density extreme, and a sulfur hexafluoride-oxygen mixture at 4 ATA as the other. The $P(A\text{-}a)O_2$ was significantly reduced by the denser gas mixture in each of the nine animals studied; in five of these, the $P(A\text{-}a)O_2$ decreased by 10 mmHg or more. The authors suggested that this phenomenon reflected an increased efficiency in pulmonary gas exchange due to decreased variation of $\dot{V}A/\dot{Q}$ within the lungs. They considered the possibility that the density of the inhaled medium might have modified the distribution of perfusion. This possibility was, however, dismissed on the grounds that although 16 times denser than air, the SF_6 mixture at 4 ATA would still have a density of only about 2% that of water (or blood).

On the basis of circumstantial evidence, the authors suggested a mechanism for dense gas to increase the ventilation of lung regions with low $\dot{V}A/\dot{Q}$. These would be regions with low compliance and low flow resistance, which would receive relatively more ventilation because the higher gas density would require increased ventilatory pressure swings. Another proposed mechanism was that the high density gas improves convective mixing in the airways, thereby eliminating preexisting stratified inhomogeneities of gas tension.

IV. Hydrostatic Pressure Distribution

A. Diving with Breathing Gear

The diving environment exposes the body to hydrostratic pressure inequalities that may have profound effects on both circulatory and respiratory function. As will be noted in the following, there may be considerable interaction between these two functions during immersion and diving. Primarily, water exerts its effects due to its high density, which means that, for instance, in the erect body posture the legs are influenced by a water pressure that may exceed the pressure acting at the level of the head by 150 cmH_2O. This situation, known as the immersion effect, pertains not only to the head-out swimmer, but also to a diver (Fig. 1). In the upright posture, the intrathoracic pressure, largely determined by the breathing gas pressure, will be considerably lower than the pressure in dependent regions of the body. By contrast, when the diver assumes a head-down posture the intrathoracic gas pressure will be relatively high.

Redistribution of Blood Volume

The most commonly encountered and studied situation is that of the erect diver (equivalent to head-out immersion), in which blood is redistributed from dependent regions into the chest (Fig. 2). This is partly because the normal gravity-induced blood pooling in the legs of a nonimmersed person is counteracted by the external water column and partly because of the effects of negative pressure

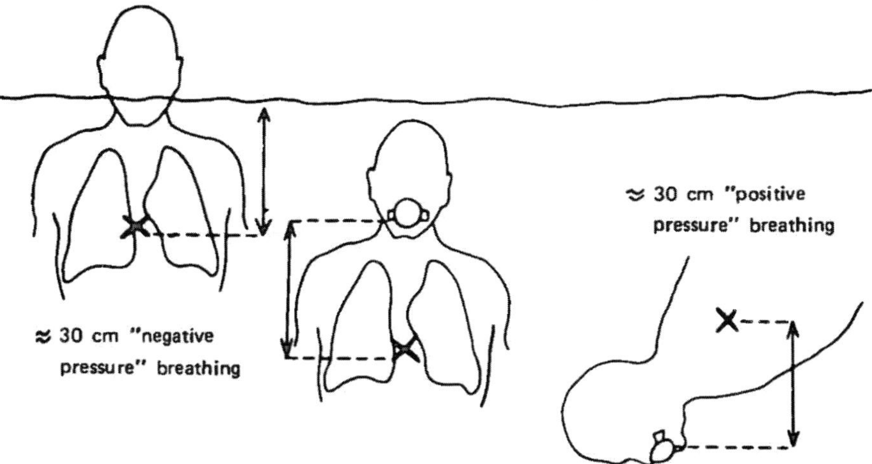

Figure 1 Pressure difference between breathing gas at mouth/nose and center of pressure of the chest (marked X) may induce negative- or positive-pressure breathing (static lung loads) depending on body posture and type of breathing gear. (Reproduced with permission from Lundgren, 1984.).

in the chest during immersion. About 700 ml of blood is redistributed into the thorax in the transition from the nonimmersed sitting posture to head-out immersion in thermoneutral (35°C) water (Arborelius et al., 1972a). A question arises as to how this volume of blood is accommodated. The distensibility of the blood-containing structures within the chest deserves attention. The compliance of the intrathoracic vascular bed may be calculated on the basis of the changes in intrathoracic blood volumes and the concomitant change in right atrial pressure in two subjects in the study of Arborelius et al. (1972a). Such calculations yield values of effective compliance (see below) of 0.78 and 0.42 ml/mmHg per kilogram body weight. This may be compared with values determined in eight subjects by Echt et al. (1974), who made transfusions and withdrawals of blood in combination with norepinephrine infusion and/or lower body positive pressure. Using the term "effective compliance" to recognize that the measurements may have been influenced by arterial hemodynamics and venous tone (in addition to elastic properties of the vascular bed), the authors arrived at values between 0.9 and 1.2 ml/mmHg per kilogram body weight.

As for the distribution within the chest of the blood it receives during immersion, there is evidence that the heart accommodates a fairly large fraction. Based on radiographic measurements, it has been determined that the heart increases in size by about 180 ml (Lange et al., 1974) to 250 ml (Risch et al.,

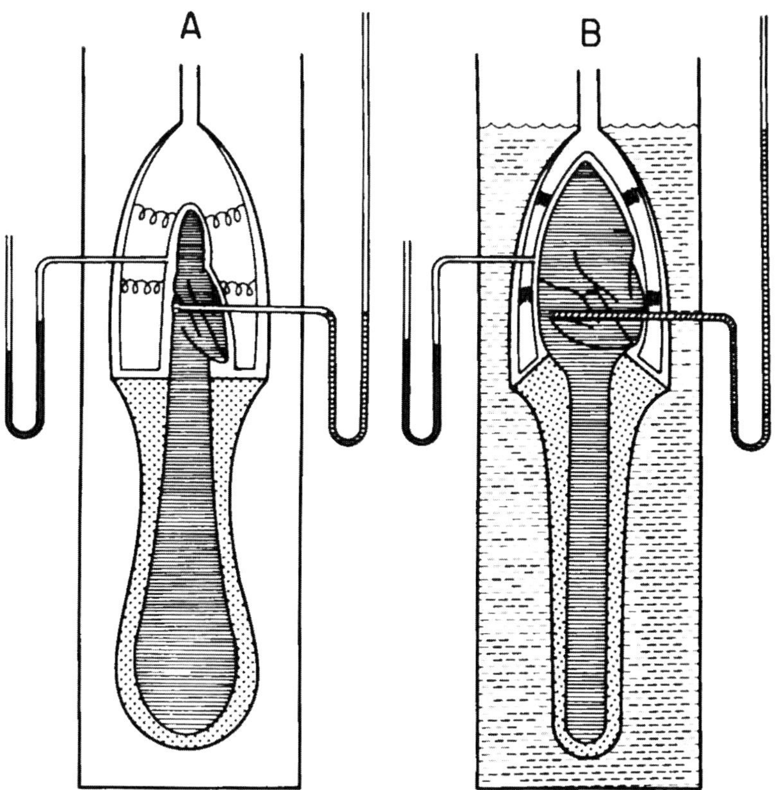

Figure 2 Schematic illustration of the effect of immersion with the head above water on the distribution of blood between dependent regions of the body and the thorax. The springs represent the elastic element of the lung tissue. Dotted areas: incompressible but resilient tissues. Hatched areas: blood. The left manometer (black fluid column) indicates the pleural pressure; the right manometer (hatched fluid column) indicates the right atrial pressure. The difference between right atrial pressure and pleural pressure reflects atrial transmural pressure gradient. (A) Erect body position in the nonimmersed situation; blood pooled in the vascular bed below the heart. Atrial pressure is almost zero, and pleural pressure is negative. Right atrial transmural pressure gradient is small. Apical regions of lungs poorly perfused. (B) Erect body position during immersion with the head above water; redistribution of blood toward the heart and intrathoracic vascular bed, distending these structures. Atrial pressure is raised, and pleural pressure almost zero. Right atrial transmural pressure gradient is increased. Apical regions of lungs are well perfused. (Reproduced with permission of *Aviation, Space, and Environmental Medicine*, from Arborelius et al., 1972a.)

1978a). Given that the total redistribution of blood amounts to about 700 ml, these authors concluded that the major proportion of this blood must be accommodated by the pulmonary vascular bed. However, this suggestion has not been tested by comprehensive measurements, although changes in the amount of blood contained in the capillary segment of the pulmonary circulation have been recorded. According to Löllgen et al., (1980), the average pulmonary capillary volume in six subjects, which was 73.7 ml before immersion, increased to 124.8 ml during head-out immersion in water at 35°C. This modest increase of 51 ml is in good agreement with observations of immersed subjects by Guyatt et al. (1965), and it accounts for only about 7% of the total 700 ml. However, other measurements indicate that the increase in pulmonary capillary blood volume may be considerably larger. From the figures of Farhi and Linnarsson (1977) on so-called equivalent tissue volume during immersion and nonimmersion, the difference in capillary blood volume can be calculated as 200 ml.

Changes in total lung capacity (TLC) have also given some clues to the distribution of the intrathoracic blood volume during immersion. The combined effects of hydrostatic chest compression and blood redistribution accounted for an average TLC reduction of 0.43 liter in the subjects of Dahlbäck and coworkers (1978). They determined that only 0.13 liter of this reduction was due to the intrathoracic blood pooling. For this reason, Dahlback (1978) concluded that the blood moving into the chest as a result of neck-deep immersion serves both to expand the thorax and to reduce lung volume through competition for air space. Furthermore, Dahlbäck et al. (1978) determined that the average reduction in vital capacity (VC) of 0.28 liter (equivalent to 5.3%) in their subjects was entirely due to the blood redistribution. This contrasts with earlier studies that ascribed only 33% (Agostoni et al., 1966) or 60% (Hong et al., 1969) of the VC reduction to this mechanism. In this context it is noteworthy that the intrathoracic redistribution of blood due to immersion and its effects on pulmonary circulation have typically been studied in subjects immersed in thermoneutral water (35°C). However, the change in VC as an indicator of this blood redistribution is profoundly influenced by water temperature. Thus, while the vital capacity was reduced by about 5.5% during head-out immersion in water at 35°C, this reduction disappeared in water at 40°C and increased to about 12% in water at 20°C (Kurss et al., 1981). Using arterial tourniquets on arms and legs, the authors ascertained that the VC changes at 35 and 20°C were indeed due to blood redistribution. To what extent the pulmonary vascular bed shared in accommodating these fluctuations in intrathoracic blood pooling has, however, not yet been systematically studied.

Ventilation-Perfusion Effects

The intrathoracic blood pooling caused by immersion in water of thermoneutral temperature enhances diastolic filling and preload (Arborelius et al., 1972a;

Risch et al., 1978a, b) and increases stroke volume and cardiac output. The latter increases have been measured at between about 30% (Arborelius et al., 1972a; Löllgen et al., 1980) and 60% (Farhi and Linnarsson, 1977), the difference being due to various degrees of orthostatic load in the nonimmersed control situations. The enhanced pulmonary blood flow and changes in mechanical loads on the lung predictably cause changes in ventilation-perfusion distribution.

This translocation of blood is accommodated partly by the heart, which increases its stroke volume by 35% in response to an increased preload, with peak right atrial filling pressures of up to 30 mmHg. The resulting rise in cardiac output (about 32%) must increase pulmonary blood flow by an equal amount.

The pulmonary blood flow distribution during immersion has been subject to studies with various techniques. Using ^{133}Xe-radiospirometry, Arborelius et al. (1972b) recorded the distribution of ventilation and blood flow in two large apical and two large basal lung regions in erect subjects before and after immersion to the neck. This maneuver resulted in a redistribution of circulation and also, to a lesser degree, ventilation toward the apical regions. The net result, discussed in more detail later in this chapter, was a generally more even ventilation-perfusion distribution. Injecting tagged albumin particles and using scintigraphy, Risch et al. (1978a) demonstrated a 35% increase. This increase was due primarily to enhanced perfusion in apical regions in the lung area defined by the 15% isocount line on the lung scintigrams during immersion.

It has been suggested that the improved apical blood flow was due to several factors including increased total pulmonary blood flow and pressure. Arborelius et al. (1972a) recorded an average increase in pulmonary arterial mean pressure of 17 mmHg, which would appear adequate to fill lung vessels up to the very apices of the lungs. In addition, those authors pointed out that air-trapping in dependent lung regions, which may be induced by immersion (cf. Dahlbäck and Lundgren, 1972; Dahlbäck, 1975), would cause local hypoxia. This local hypoxia could also cause redistribution of blood flow toward better ventilated, in this case apical, parts of the lungs (Arborelius, 1969).

The possibility that the immersion-induced changes in ventilation-perfusion matching may influence gas exchange should be considered. A significant drop (by 10 mmHg) in PaO_2 in subjects exposed to head-out immersion was recorded by Cohen et al. (1971). This drop in five subjects out of seven appeared to be due to a true venous admixture, because oxygen breathing did not diminish the alveolar-arterial oxygen gradient. In two remaining subjects the $P(A\text{-}a)O_2$ was changed by oxygen inhalation and was ascribed to more uneven ventilation-perfusion distribution during immersion. In the 11 subjects of Arborelius et al. (1972b) there was no significant change in PaO_2 during immersion. The discrepancy between these two studies may be explained on the basis of the studies of Prefuat and co-workers, who showed that the $P(A\text{-}a)O_2$ as well as the diffusing capacity may respond differently to immersion (to the neck) depending on the subject's breathing pattern, which in turn appeared to be influenced by the subject's age and body build (Prefaut et al., 1978). They recognized three groups among their subjects with regard to the relationship between closing volume (CV) and FRC level: (1) younger and lighter individuals who breathed outside the CV, (2) individuals who were intermediate in age and/or body weight and who breathed partly within their CV envelopes, and (3) a group of older and/or heavier subjects whose breaths were taken within the CV envelope. These breathing patterns, which are illustrated in Figure 3, were linked to different effects of immersion on $P(A\text{-}a)O_2$ and diffusing capacity ($DL_{CO}/\dot{V}$). The relationships between these measures of lung function and breathing patterns are shown in Figures 4 and 5, which are reproduced from Prefaut et al. (1978). The subjects would largely be distributed along the horizontal axes of those figures, with the younger and/or lighter subjects toward the left and the older and/or heavier toward the right.

The airway closure during water immersion to the neck depends primarily on the intrathoracic blood pooling induced by immersion (Dahlbäck, 1975). Similarly, the increase in CV resulting from immersion was only half as large if tourniquets were applied to all four limbs of subjects immediately prior to immersion (Bondi et al., 1976). This coupling between pulmonary gas content and circulation was attributed by Dahlbäck (1975) to the increased pulmonary arterial pressure, which had been observed by Arborelius et al. (1972a) in immersed subjects. The suggested mechanism is the erectile effect on the lungs due to vascular engorgement, which was first shown by von Basch (1887). This erectile effect would increase the amount of air held by the lungs at the time when airway closure is caused by immersion (Dahlbäck, 1975). There may also be another mechanism stiffening the lungs secondary to the hemodynamic changes. A gradual, linear decrease in dynamic compliance in eight air-breathing subjects reaching 13.2% after 30 min of head-out immersion was observed by Baer et al. (1987). One mechanism suggested to cause this phenomenon, in addition to a possible gradual increase in the intravascular fluid compartment, was an expansion of the interstitial fluid volume.

As for mechanisms enhancing airway closure, it may be hypothesized that the vascular engorgement due to immersion may also contribute to airway narrowing. Expansion of the intrathoracic blood volume due to other causes, such as plasma expansion, has been implicated in airway closure (Collins et al., 1973). Closure of small airways in dependent regions of the lung in patients with hepatic cirrhosis has also been ascribed to dilatation of blood vessels (Ruff et al., 1971). An additional factor is the increased amount of blood in the pulmonary vascular bed, which boosts lung weight and in turn will tend to increase pleural pressure around the dependent parts of the lungs, thus further narrowing the airways.

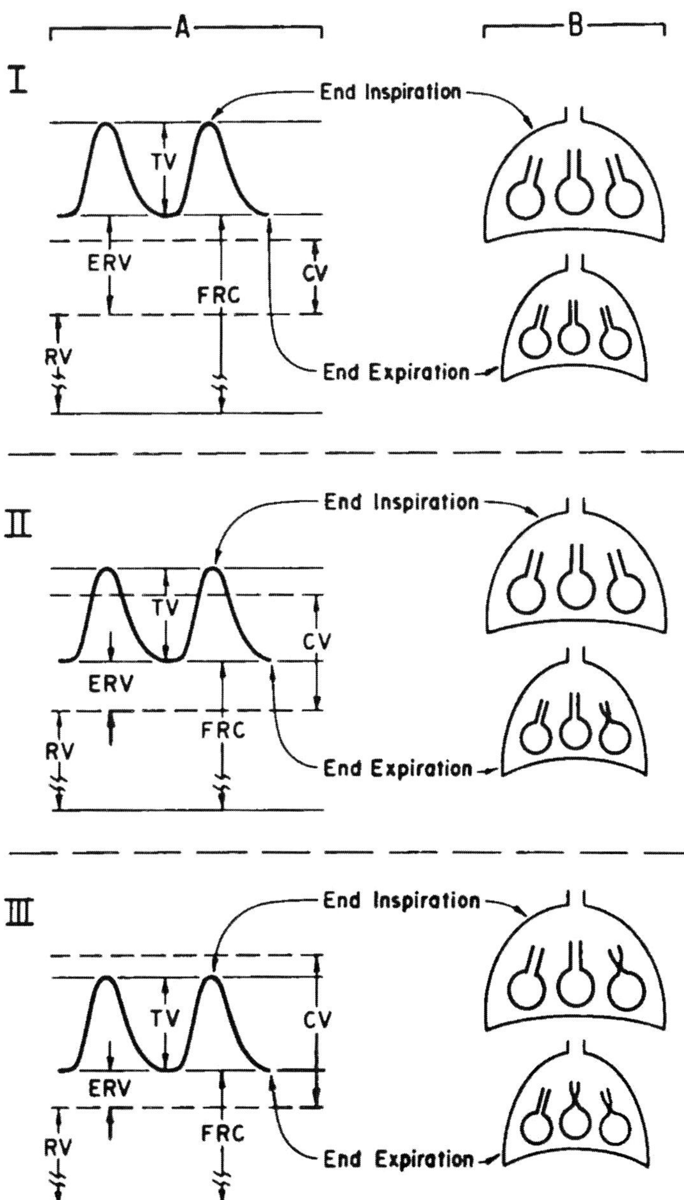
A
B
I
End Inspiration
TV
ERV
CV
FRC
RV
End Expiration
II
End Inspiration
TV
CV
ERV
FRC
RV
End Expiration
III
End Inspiration
TV
CV
ERV
FRC
RV
End Expiration

Figure 3

With regard to ventilation-perfusion matching, Prefaut et al. (1978) theorized that those subjects who breathed within their CV had shunting and loss of functional diffusing area in closed lung regions with a consequent increase in $P(A\text{-}a)O_2$. By contrast, in subjects breathing above their CV, the improved apical perfusion should, in theory, allow an increased diffusing capacity to dominate the oxygen exchange situation (Prefaut et al., 1978).

The mechanisms underlying the changes in $P(A\text{-}a)O_2$ and DL_{CO} were further explored in another study by Prefaut et al. (1979). They recorded the distribution of pulmonary blood flow and ventilation in seven subjects standing in air and during immersion to the neck. In four subjects the CV exceeded expiratory reserve volume (ERV) during immersion and the normal perfusion distribution became inverted so that the regions at the apices of the lungs received a greater blood supply than those at the bases. A change in the same direction, although not a complete inversion of the flow distribution, had been observed earlier by Arborelius et al. (1972a), who discussed several possible mechanisms for the change in perfusion distribution during immersion to the neck. Among these mechanisms were, in addition to the increase in pulmonary arterial pressure mentioned earlier, changes in lung mechanics and especially a reduction in pulmonary recoil and increase in pleural pressure at the bases of the lungs mostly due to the elevated diaphragm. This would lead to increased pressure on the outside surface of extraalveolar blood vessels, a reduction in their caliber, and an increased vascular resistance. Similar flow distribution changes have been observed when the lung volume is reduced in the nonimmersed situ-

---

Figure 3 Schematic illustration of three types of respiratory pattern during immersion, as described by Prefaut et al. (1978). Relationship between breathing range (ERV + TV) and closing volume (CV): effects on patency of airways during breathing cycle. Panels (A) represent hypothetical spirograms and show relative positions of end inspiration, and expiration (i.e., tidal volume or TV), upper limit of functional residual capacity (FRC), expiratory reserve volume (ERV), residual volume, (RV), and closing volume (CV). Panels (B) represent lungs and lung units with open or closed airways at end inspiration or end expiration. Panels IA and B refer to a young healthy, nonimmersed person whose entire breathing cycle is outside the CV envelope; panels IIA and B represent a situation of immersion that reduces ERV and increases CV so that breathing occurs partially within the CV envelope: some airways close toward end of expiration. Panels IIIA and B show a situation in, for instance, an older and/or overweight person in whom immersion causes substantial enlargement of the CV so that breathing occurs wholly within the CV envelope and the airways of some lung units remain closed even at end inspiration. From Lundgren and Norfleet, 1987. Respiratory Function in Hyperbaric Environments. *Main in Stressful Environments: Diving, Hyper- and Hypobaric Physiology*. Edited by K. Shiraki, and M. K. Yousef. By Courtesy of Charles C. Thomas, Publisher, Springfield, Illinois.

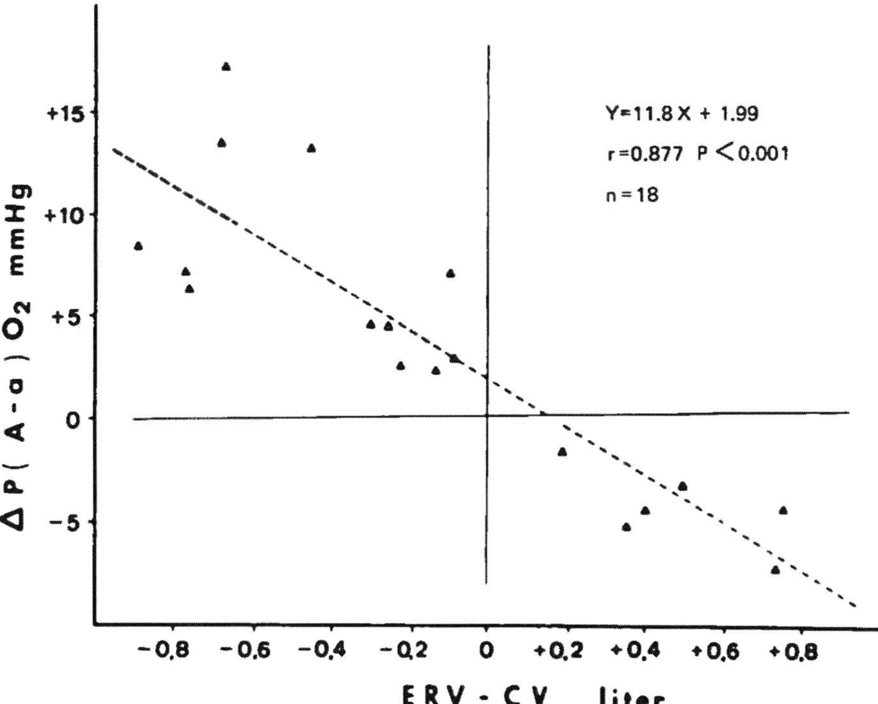

Figure 4 Relationship between $P(A\text{-}a)O_2$ in water minus $P(A\text{-}a)O_2$ in air and expiratory reserve volume (ERV) minus closing volume (CV) in water. (Reproduced with permission from Prefaut et al., 1978.)

ation (Hughes et al., 1967). This explanation was also supported by Prefaut et al. (1979(, as was the role of increased pulmonary arterial pressure. However, they pointed out that it could not explain the actual reversal of flow distribution (diminution of flow in basal regions) that they observed.

The increased lung weight and reduced elastic recoil that were mentioned earlier as contributing to airway closure could also, in theory, lead to increased vascular resistance. On the other hand, the vascular engorgement would tend to decrease flow resistance. It is not clear which of these conflicting influences dominates during immersion, and complexity is added to the picture by the tendency for hypoxia and local vasoconstriction in the lung regions where air trapping occurs as described earlier. This is another mechanism that would tend to redistribute blood flow from dependent lung regions toward the apices during erect immersion, as pointed out by Arborelius et al. (1972a).

The circulatory adjustments to immersion that occur rapidly (in 3-5 sec) will be manifest in about 6 sec in terms of a steady-state increase in heart size

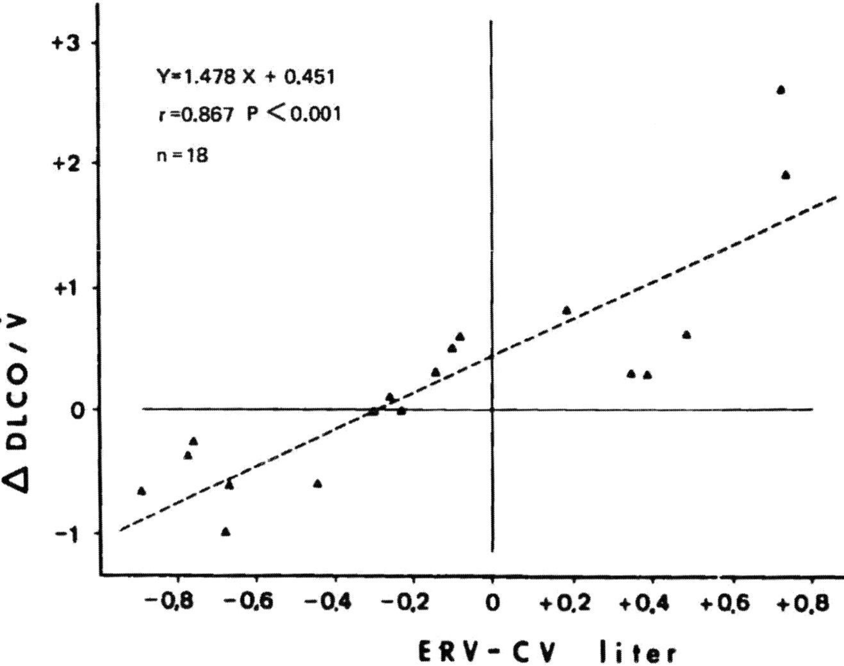

Figure 5 Relationship between DL_{CO}/V in water minus DL_{CO}/V in air and expiratory reserve volume (ERV) minus closing volume (CV) in water. (Reproduced with permission from Prefaut et al., 1978.)

and venous pressure according to Risch et al. (1978b). The same authors pointed out that, in addition to the normal cardiac output, several hundred milliliters of the total 700 ml (Arborelius et al., 1972a) translocated during the immersion would be forced through the right ventricle in the aforementioned short period of time. The rapidity of this adjustment as well as the fast shift of central blood volume in connection with orthostasis and exposure to high gravitational forces was seen as support for the idea that peripheral capacitance vessels and the pulmonary circulation form a functional unit as the low pressure system (Risch et al., 1978b). An overview of the effects of immersion on the chest organs and their functions is offered in Figure 6.

B. Snorkel Breathing and Breath-Hold Diving

Special cases of the immersion effect are presented by snorkel breathing and deep breath-hold diving. In theory, both these activities may expose the circulatory structures in the chest to very large transmural pressure gradients.

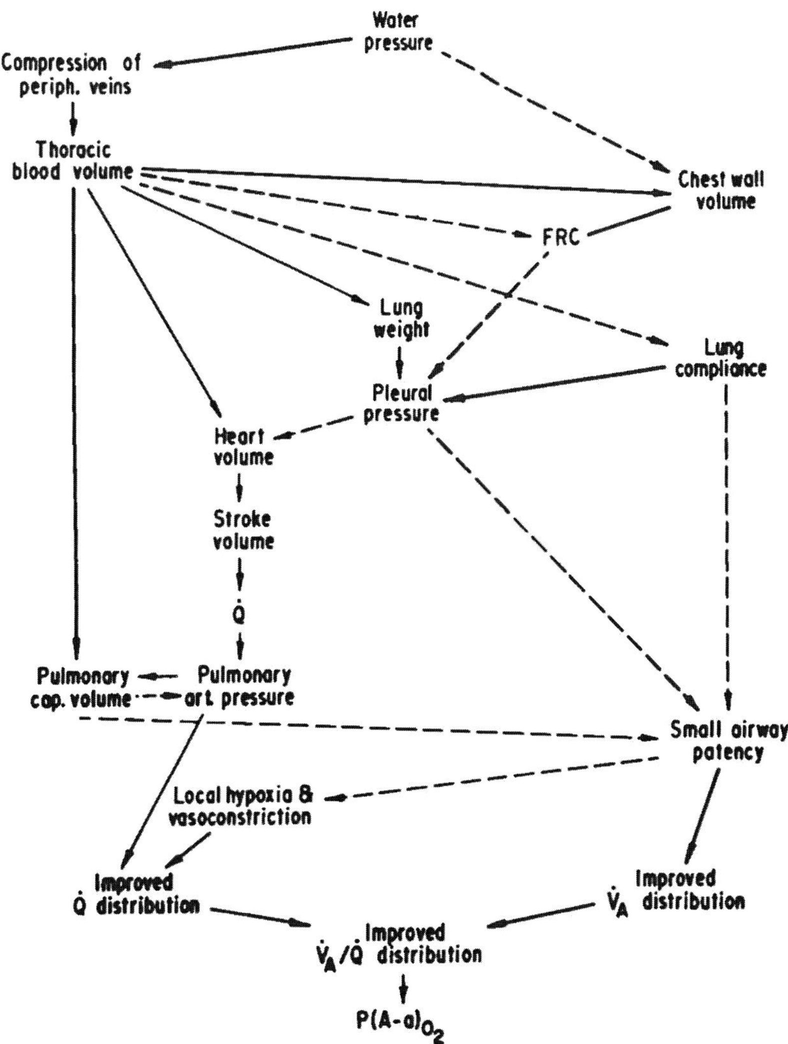

Figure 6 Interaction of cardiopulmonary variables during immersion. The figure shows the effects of immersion to the neck in water at thermoneutral temperature (35°C) compared the nonimmersed situation in a person assuming the erect posture. Positive relationships are indicated by continuous arrows, negative relationships by dashed arrows. Factors on the left describe circulatory variables.

A snorkel or breathing tube allows the alveolar space to communicate with the atmospheric air above the water surface, thus establishing an air pressure of 1 ATA (disregarding small fluctuations due to respiration) in the alveolar gas (Fig. 7), while the external pressure on the rest of the body is 1 ATA plus the pressure exerted by the external water column. By definition, the transmural pressure gradient of a blood-containing structure in the chest will be determined by the difference between the hydrostatic pressure of the blood on the inside and the pressure on its outside surface. The outside pressure would be 1.0 ATA in the case of, for instance, alveolar wall capillaries, and it would be the pleural pressure in the case of the heart and larger vessels; the intraluminal pressure is determined by the physiologic blood pressure plus atmospheric pressure plus that fraction of the ambient water pressure that is transmitted to the blood.

However, very little is known in quantitative terms about the effects of snorkel breathing on the function of the central circulation, including the pulmonary circulation. On the other hand, from the clinical point of view, there are a few observations of relatively alarming effects of snorkel breathing during deep submersion as well as during head-out immersion. Early in this century, R. Stigler (1911), studying the force of the inspiratory muscles, unsuccessfully attempted to breathe, for a few seconds, through a long tube while his chest was about 2 m under the surface. In the process he suffered "delirium cordis" (atrial fibrillation) and acute heart dilatation. This serious mishap may have been due to two different mechanisms acting in unison. The possibility that an intolerably high preload on the heart may be generated in deep snorkel breathing is suggested by the fact that signs of marked engorgement have been noted even in subjects undergoing immersion only to the neck. Thus, the mean right atrial transmural pressure increase was 13 mmHg in response to the intrathoracic redistribution of 700 ml of blood in the subjects of Arborelius et al. (1972a). Individual right atrial pressure peaks reached about 30 mmHg in one subject, and several showed the exaggerated so-called X and Y descents creating the W pattern (Fig. 8) described as typical for constrictive pericarditis with right heart engorgement (quoted from Arborelius et al., 1972a). Extrasystoles were also recorded.

It seems likely that during deep snorkel breathing larger volumes than the 700 ml found in head-out immersion may be forced into the chest, thus creating an even larger preload. That larger volumes of blood may be redistributed by severe hydrostatic pressure differences on the body is suggested by observations in breath-hold divers as will be explained in the following.

The effect of immersion on the left heart should, as pointed out by Lanari et al. (1960), be to increase the afterload as the pressure of the external water column acts on the systemic circulation. These investigators recorded increases in arterial pressure (both systolic and diastolic) that actually somewhat exceeded the water pressure in subjects who were breathing through a hose to the surface

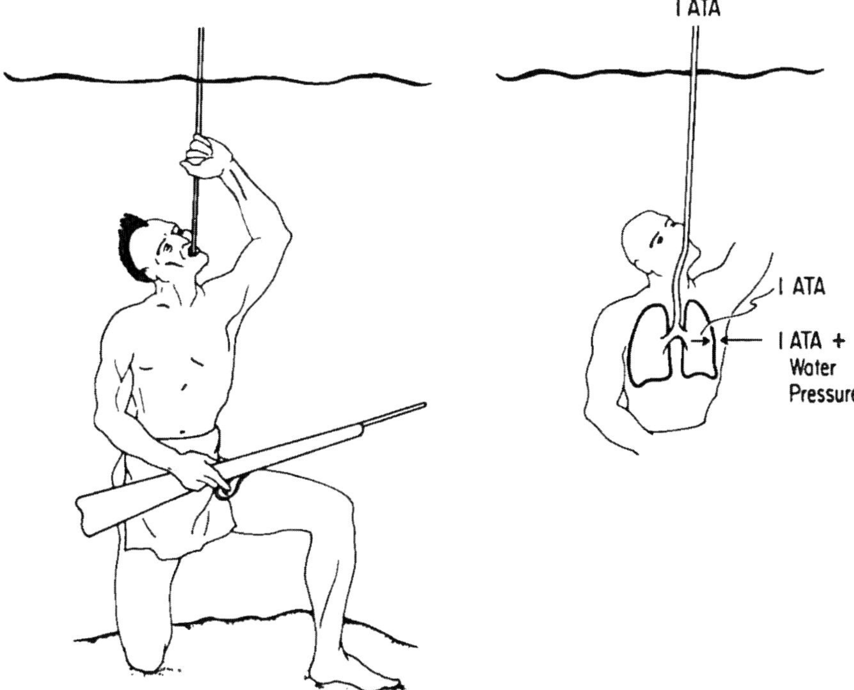

Figure 7 The legendary hero escaping his pursuers by hiding on the bottom of a stream and breathing through a straw. Note several problems: There is risk of dangerous chest squeeze at excessive depth (see text); straw has very high breathing resistance; it is difficult to keep powder dry.

while lying recumbent at a depth of about 100 cmH_2O (equivalent to about 75 mmHg). Extrasystoles were also noted, and Lanari et al. (1960) called attention to the risk of pulmonary edema and rupture of bronchial arteries (the only systemic vessels that are not supported by the external water column) if the immersion were to be too long lasting or deep. The possibility that the increased afterload caused his own heart dilatation during his submergence to 2 m of depth was actually discussed by Stigler (1911).

Using the conventional old type of rigid diving helmet and flexible suit makes a diver vulnerable to a mishap that could greatly exaggerate the type of injuries a long snorkel can cause. Rupture of the air hose high above the diver (assuming a faulty one-wave valve in the helmet) can suddenly reduce the air pressure in the lungs and suit to equal the pressure at the level of the hose rupture. A similar mechanism may be evoked by a rapid fall under water if the air

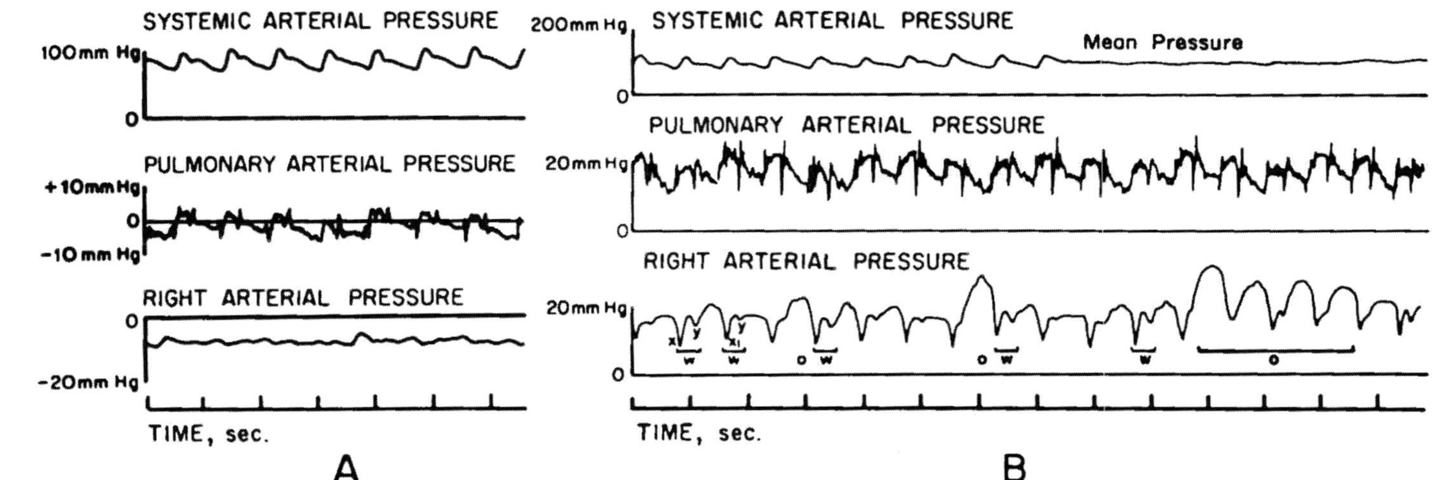

Figure 8 (A) Pressure recordings from subject sitting in air. (B) Pressure recordings from same subject sitting for 10 min immersed to the neck in water of thermoneutral temperature (35°C). Notice the W-formed complexes (marked W) in which the depressions x and y are prominent and similar to those seen in constrictive pericarditis with right heart congestion. Notice also the higher pressures (up to about 30 mmHg) in some cycles (marked O) in which right heart engorgement was more pronounced. (Reproduced with permission from Arborelius et al., 1972a).

supply does not keep up with the external pressure increase. The relatively higher water pressure will force the diver's tissues to fill void space in the helmet; cause pulmonary vessel distention, rupture, and bleeding; and crush the chest ("chest squeeze").

The capacitance function of the blood-containing organs in the chest apparently plays an important physiological role for human adaptation to deep breath-hold diving. The theoretical depth limit for breath-hold diving was at one time thought to be set by the relationship between an individual's total lung capacity (TLC) and residual volume (RV). Assuming that a dive would start after inspiration to TLC and proceed until the pressure at depth had compressed the chest and lungs down to RV, the permissible final pressure would be given by Boyle's law (disregarding, for simplicity, the presence of water vapor).

$$\text{TLC} \times P_{bar} = \text{RV} \times P_f$$

where TLC and RV are defined above, P_{bar} = barometric pressure at sea level, and P_f = total pressure at maximum depth.

With reasonable numbers inserted:

$$6.5 \text{ liters} \times 1.0 \text{ ATA} = 1.5 \text{ liters} \times P_f$$

$$P_f = \frac{6.5 \text{ liters} \times 1.0 \text{ ATA}}{1.5 \text{ liters}} = 4.33 \text{ ATA}$$

That is to say, at a total pressure of 4.33 ATA, equivalent to 110 ft of depth, the chest and lungs would appear to have reached their minimum volume. It is understandable that concerns about possible damage, were the compression to be carried any further, would arise. Certainly, the depth record of 105 m (346 ft) Missiroli and Rizzato, 1984) with its associated 11.5-fold compression of intrathoracic gas, was not anticipated although the underlying physiological mechanism had been identified earlier.

The possibility that movement of blood into the thorax could enhance the depth tolerance in breath-hold diving was first considered by Rahn (1965) and more fully developed by Craig (1968) and Schaefer et al. (1968). To achieve full pressure equilibration in the lungs while descending to the record depth of 105 m, J. Mayol, with a TLC of about 7.2 liters and an RV of about 1.9 liters (Schaefer et al., 1968) would, in theory, have had to rely on an intrathoracic blood volume increase of about 1.3 liters. Because this assumes that there was no net gas transfer from the alveolar space to the blood, the latter figure is probably too low. Indirect proof of the importance of redistribution of blood into the thorax was provided by Craig (1968) in experiments in which esophageal pressure was recorded in subjects who expired to RV and then descended (feet first) to a depth of as much as 4.75 m. No change in esophageal pressure was recorded. This was taken to indicate that blood had provided the necessary bulk to allow complete pressure equilibration between the gas in the lung and ambient water despite, at RV, a very unyielding chest wall. The calculated extra volume needed for this purpose was 600 ml.

Schaefer et al. (1968) used measurements of electrical impedance of the thorax to attempt to deduce the volume of blood shifted into the chest of a subject who performed breath-hold dives to 90 and 130 ft. The changes in impedance in these dives were said to correspond to blood volume increases in the chest of 1047 and 850 ml, respectively. The pressure differences between the chest cavity and the rest of the body are qualitatively the same as in head-out immersion, but deep breath-hold dives have the potential of making these differences even more pronounced, as indicated by the larger blood volumes apparently being relocated. The distribution of the blood between the various blood-containing structures within the chest in such dives has not been studied and would, of course, depend on the relative compliance of these structures as these larger volumes move into the chest. To the extent that the filling pressures increase in these structures and they reach their limits of physiological expansion, several different failure modes can be envisioned. Heart dilatation, arrhythmias, and bleeding in the lungs have already been discussed in conjunction with snorkel breathing. A likely complication of severe pulmonary engorgement is pulmonary edema.

Given the very deep dives performed by the individuals competing for the breath-hold diving depth records, there is a remarkable scarcity of reports of injuries. One case suggesting thoracic squeeze as a result of breath-hold diving has been described by Strauss and Wright (1971). It concerns a 28-yr-old man who was performing breath-hold dives to 80 feet seawater (fsw). He was found "floating" unconscious at 40 fsw. When brought to the surface, he was apneic and frothy bright red blood was coming from the mouth. Within 10 min of the accident he had intermittent clonic seizures and hemoptysis; given supportive therapy, he gradually regained consciousness but developed shock and died of cardiac arrest 3 hr after the accident. The autopsy showed diffuse bilateral vascular injury with intravascular congestion, interstitial edema, diffuse disruption of small vessels, and intraalveolar hemorrhage.

As pointed out earlier (Hickey and Lundgren, 1984), the modest diving depth of 80 fsw would not be conducive of thoracic squeeze unless the dive was initiated after a less than full predive inspiration. Furthermore, the possibility of the lung injuries being caused by frank drowning can probably not be excluded (Hickey and Lundgren, 1984). Another somewhat similar case involved repeated breath-hold dives to 100 ft (Khan, 1979). The diver was found unconscious at 50 ft and brought to the surface within 3-4 min. Frothy hemoptysis was noted; positive-pressure breathing with 100% oxygen immediately started; on auscultatation, highly resonant scattered notes were heard over the chest, and the patient repeatedly coughed up small amounts of clotted blood; about 2 hr after the accident, hypotension refractive to plasma transfusion and plasma expanders developed and the patient died. On autopsy the lungs were dark red and hemorrhagic. Cut sections showed consolidation with purplish parenchyma exuding large amounts of blood-stained fluid.

V. Decompression

The pulmonary circulation plays important roles in diving-induced embolism. Gas emboli, as well as secondary emboli from blood constituents, are important etiologic factors in decompression sickness. The emboli may arrive from the tissues to the lungs and become trapped in the microcirculation, or they may slip through and enter the arterial side. Moreover, gas emboli may originate in the lung in connection with pulmonary barotrauma during ascent.

A. Decompression Sickness

It has long been known that decompression sickness may cause venous gas embolization. The primary condition for the appearance of free gas in the circulation in diving is that the inert gas component of the breathing gases is dissolved in the blood and tissues and accumulates in proportion to the respired inert gas partial pressure, which typically increases with depth. If the subsequent ascent is carried out too rapidly, the excess gas will be released in free form in the tissues and blood. Established decompression routines prescribe a controlled rate of ascent (decompression), which assumes that the inert gas, while still in solution, is eliminated by the blood into the lungs. Freedom from symptoms of decompression sickness has traditionally been considered proof of the adequacy of a particular compression routine.

The symptoms connected with inadequate (too rapid) decompression are quite varied and include, but are not limited to, neurological dysfunction and pain in various locations and most often in relation to the large joints (bends). Of particular interest to the current discussion are the symptoms known as the chokes. The chokes often begin as a mild substernal distress developing into pain that is initially noticeable only on deep inspiration but that forces the victim to gradually breathe less and less deeply. Attempts at deeper inspirations will provoke severe paroxysmal coughing. Dyspnea and respiratory distress and cyanosis ensue, and the condition is commonly considered life-threatening if not treated by recompression. The etiology of the chokes is usually ascribed to venous gas emboli lodging in the lungs. As a secondary effect, one can expect impairment of the pulmonary circulation.

Such involvement was evident in experiments performed by Bove et al. (1974) in which chloralose-anesthetized air-breathing dogs were exposed to severe decompression stress, which produced decompression sickness (40 min at 220 fsw equivalent with rapid decompression). The decompression sickness manifested by signs of spinal cord dysfunction. Typically, the animals showed significant pulmonary artery or right ventricular systolic pressure elevations as well as pulmonary arterial diastolic pressure increases. Cerebrospinal fluid pressure also increased, and tachycardia developed. Following the circulatory changes, signs of spinal cord dysfunction would appear. The circulatory involvement would proceed with a doubling of pulmonary vascular resistance (compared to control), and as signs of decompression sickness developed, arterial oxygen pressure fell significantly. Moreover, an ultrasound Doppler probe in the aorta indicated passage of bubbles through the lungs. In parallel with these developments, cinevenography of the epidural vertebral venous system by various routes revealed positive stasis, venous congestion, and areas of regional obstruction due to bubble emboli. This venous stasis was considered to contribute importantly to the mechanism of decompression-induced spinal cord injury.

It has been suggested that the rise in central venous pressure in dogs subjected to decompression stress may contribute to the stasis in the thoracic epidural veins (Bove et al., 1974). This would occur by retrograde transmission of the central venous pressure increase through patent azygos and intravertebral veins. However, on the basis of extensive additional experimentation in dogs, Hallenbeck (1976) has emphasized that this retrograde action of the pulmonary hypertension and central venous congestion were not absolutely essential for the development of spinal cord involvement. This is in agreement with the well-known fact that, in humans, spinal cord decompression sickness may occur without overt pulmonary symptoms. Moveover, as pointed out by Hallenbeck (1976), "chokes" is a relatively common symptom in decompression sickness provoked by decompression to altitude, while spinal cord involvement is not, and the reverse is true in diving-induced decompression sickness. It is also noteworthy that considerable gas embolism to the lung may occur without overt symptoms of any kind. Indeed, operationally well-established and clinically safe decompression routines have been shown to allow relatively profuse venous gas embolism in divers. This was first demonstrated when the ultrasound Doppler probe was put to use for bubble detection (Spencer, 1976).

The cardiopulmonary effects of symptom-free venous gas emboli (VGE) produced in sheep by simulated (dry) dives to 6.03 ATA were studied quantitatively by Neuman et al. (1980). The 15 dives lasting 15 or 17.5 min invariably produced VGE detectable by an ultrasound Doppler technique. The cardiac output ($\dot{Q}$) fell on the average 20% while the pulmonary vascular resistance (PVR) rose 60% compared to a control group that was not exposed to high pressure. The rise in PVR reaching its maximum 60-100 min after the hyperbaric exposures was considerably above what could be predicted from the fall in $\dot{Q}$. The possible action of the so-called smooth muscle acting factor that may be released in the lungs in decompression sickness (Cryssanthou et al., 1970) was considered an explanation for the PVR increase.

No indications of right or left ventricular failure were recorded, and scans for ventilation/perfusion ($\dot{V}A/\dot{Q}$) distribution using ^{133}Xe revealed no changes. The authors suggested that the lack of change in overall $\dot{V}A/\dot{Q}$ distribution despite a significant obstruction of the pulmonary vasculature was due to the venous gas emboli being so small that they would lodge in the most distal branches of the pulmonary vasculature. It is also noteworthy that there were no significant changes in blood gases.

The lungs thus serve as an important filter for the gas emboli and other embolic material secondary to the gas liberation. Such material has its origin in the ability of gas bubbles to activate intravascular coagulation and the liberation of fat emboli as discussed in an overview by Leitch and Hallenbeck (1984).

Gas trapped in the capillaries of the lungs is eliminated by diffusion into the alveolar space. Indeed, it has been suggested that subclinical gas embolization to the lung may enhance nitrogen elimination during decompression. This unorthodox notion was based on the observation that human subjects exposed to identical air dives (40 min at 100 fsw) would eliminate nitrogen at different rates during oxygen-helium breathing at decompression stages at different depths (Kindwall et al., 1975). Thus, the washout was faster at both 10 and 50 fsw than at 100 fsw. The tentative explanation for this was that the lesser depths would be more conducive to (silent) bubble formation, adding to the nitrogen-transporting capacity of the blood, since a gas bubble carries 100 times more nitrogen than the same volume of blood saturated with N_2. The idea of inert gas elimination being enhanced by embolization to the lung is, however, contradicted by the observations of Hlastala et al. (1979), who caused embolization in dogs by inert gas (N_2 He, or SF_6) infusion and recorded nitrogen clearance of the blood during oxygen breathing. Normally 4% of the nitrogen was retained in the blood during lung passage. With embolization, the nitrogen retention almost doubled.

Given that the lungs seem to be able to receive relatively large amounts of venous gas emboli without serious harm, the question arises as to what the risks are that gas may penetrate the pulmonary vascular bed to form arterial emboli. Injecting calibrated air bubbles with mean diameters ranging from 14 to 300 μm into the venous system of anesthetized dogs, Butler and Hills (1979) determined that normally the lungs are a superb filter and retain any bubble whose diamater is more than 22 μm. However, bubbles reached the arterial side, as evidenced by ultrasound Doppler probe, when the lungs were severely overloaded with gas (20 ml) or when vasodilatation was induced by administration of aminophylline before the bubble injection

In a later study, the same authors (Butler and Hills, 1985) determined that, for dogs, the trapping of venous bubbles was complete when the rate of air infusion was kept below the threshold value of 0.30 ml/kg. The initial bubble diameter was about 0.5 mm. As for the size of bubbles generated in actual decompression a range of 19-700 μm has been recorded in dogs subjected to decompression stress (Hills and Butler, 1981). This was considered to be a size range that would be filtered out by the lungs unless the organ had been insulted.

Considering that it required either pharmacological vasodilatation or a large dose of air to cause arterial embolism in Butler's and Hill's dogs, it is noteworthy that arterial emboli have been recorded in humans in conjunction with symptom-free deompressions (Brubakk et al., 1981). However, there is also the possibility of bubbles passing through an atrioseptal defect. About 30% of a healthy population have been estimated to have such a defect (Lynch et al., 1984); passage would be facilitated by the pressure changes induced by straining or an increased pulmonary vascular resistance in the case of massive embolization to the lung vessels.

B. Barotrauma

Pulmonary barotrauma may result when, during ascent from a dive, the expanding air in the lung is not allowed to escape and therefore overstretches the lung tissue to the point of rupture. The gas in the lungs in its entirety may be withheld if the diver holds his breath during ascent. This happens sometimes in the aftermath of having run out of air in the breathing apparatus. (The proper technique consists in letting excess air bubbles out past the loosely closed lips during the ascent.) A more insidious mechanism consists in air trapping in a part of the lung due to a variety of localized lung pathology as reviewed by Hallenbeck and Andersen (1982). On ascent the trapped gas will expand and, without the diver knowing it, overdistend the lung to the point of rupture. Another condition predisposing to pulmonary barotrauma has been suggested by Colebatch et al. (1976). They recorded significantly lower static lung compliance in six young divers who had suffered pulmonary barotrauma than in matched controls and suggested that in the former unevenly distributed lung elastance may predispose low-elastance lung areas to overstretching and rupture.

If lung rupture occurs, the escaping air can take two different routes (Fig. 9). The most serious consequences stem from the air entering the pulmonary circulation and causing arterial embolism. Cerebral symptoms with sudden unconsciousness and death are not uncommon, although rapid treatment in a recompression chamber can often completely resolve severe cases. In many instances the air escaping from the alveolar space accumulates in the mediastinum, sometimes making its way up under the skin on the neck, where it can be felt as creptitations. It is not clear what factors determine that, on occasion, rather

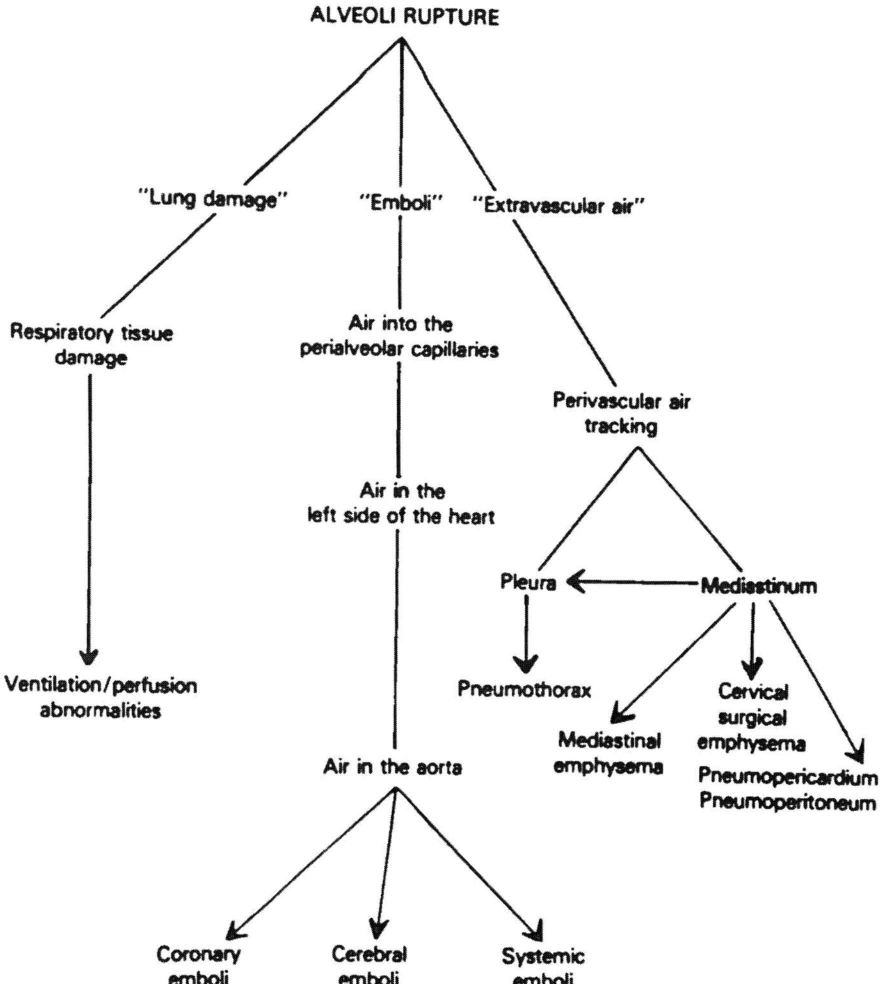

Figure 9 Pulmonary barotrauma of ascent; sequence in the center reflects direct involvement of pulmonary circulation. (Reproduced with permission from Edmonds et al., 1984.)

large mediastinal emphysemas may develop in the absence of apparent vascular involvement, whereas at other times arterial embolism is the striking feature. In a review of 140 cases of pulmonary barotrauma on record at the British Insititute of Naval Medicine, Leitch and Green (1986a) noted 23 uncomplicated cases and 117 cases with clinically manifest cerebral arterial gas embolism of which 58 had respiratory manifestations. The total incidence of arterial gas embolism on record at the institute was 1 per 34,000 dives between 1965 and 1977 and 1 per 19,800 dives between 1978 and 1986 (Leitch and Green, 1986b). It is noteworthy that subclinical cerebral embolism is suggested by the observation that 3.5% of a group of submarine escape trainees (in whom the condition is more common than in divers) showed abnormal focal EEG changes; some of these were recorded after apparently uneventful ascents (Ingvar et al., 1973).

VI. Hyperoxia

A. Oxygen Toxicty

Oxygen toxicity is an important issue in hyperbaric exposures and diving. The increase in oxygen partial pressure in the gas in the lungs may be due to increased total pressure or to a change in the oxygen fraction of the inhaled gas. The extreme example of the latter occurs in clinical hyperbaric oxygen treatment in which the patient may be administered oxygen at pressures up to 2.8 ATA (*U. S. Navy Diving Manual*, 1978). In diving, the desirability of keeping the PI_{O2} at levels that are low enough to be safe may be at conflict with concerns about decompression sickness since it is advantageous to keep the oxygen fraction in the breathing gas mixture as high as possible, thereby reducing the exposure to the diluent inert gas and easing the decompression precautions that must be observed in order to avoid decompression sickness.

The two organs most prone to clinically significant oxygen intoxication in diving and hyperbaric operations are the lung and the brain. Given sufficient exposure time the lung may be damaged at relatively modest oxygen pressures. As noted in an extensive review by Clark (1982), there is a substantial amount of data on humans indicating that, with regard to lung function, a PI_{O2} of 0.5 ATA (equivalent to breathing air at about 2.4 ATA) is a safe upper limit for multiday exposures in man.

At PI_{O2} levels between 0.75 and 2.0 ATA, lung involvement becomes gradually more apparent, with a reduction in vital capacity of 4% appearing after exposure times ranging from 24 hr at the lower oxygen concentration to 5 hr at the higher (Clark and Lambertsen, 1971). As shown in Figure 10, an array of intensifying symptoms of pulmonary irritation culminating in dyspnea accompanied exposures that were pursued until about 10% of the VC had been (temporarily) lost. A causal correlation between oxygen-induced changes in the pulmonary circulation and signs and symptoms of pulmonary dysfunction has not been established in healthy experimental subjects, although changes in the lung circulation apparently occur early in hyperoxia. Reductions in pulmonary capillary blood volume (Vc) and carbon monoxide diffusing capacity (DL_{CO}), were noted by Puy et al. (1968) in six subjects who inhaled 99.8% oxygen at 2

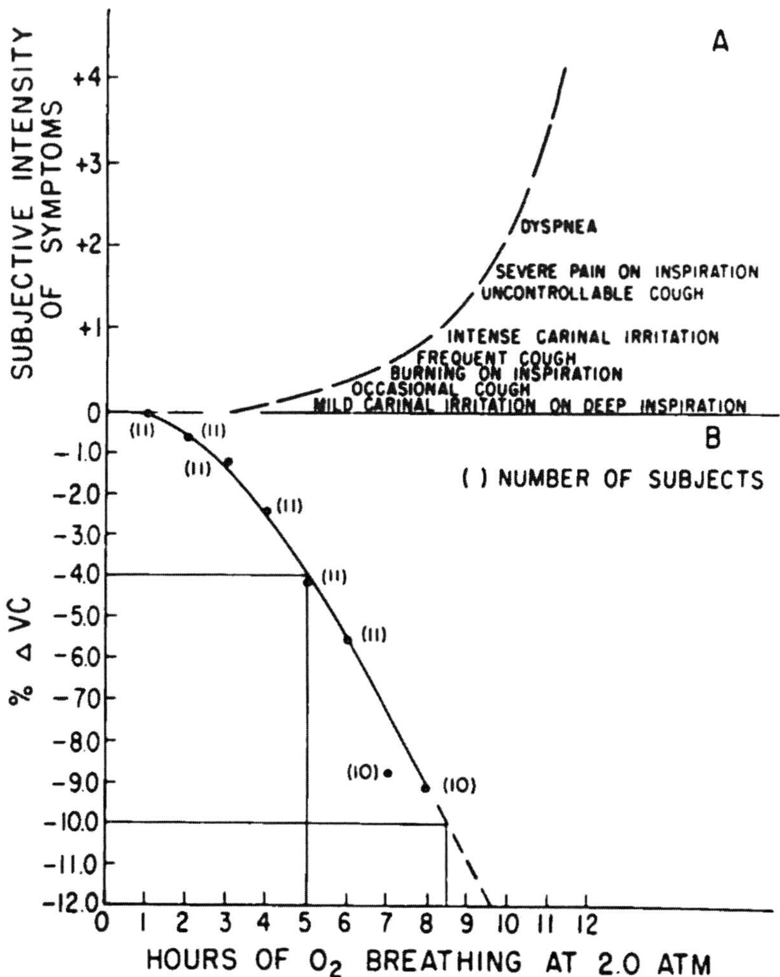

Figure 10 Average rate of decrease in vital capacity and increasing severity of symptoms during continuous oxygen breathing at 2.0 ATA in 10 to 11 men. Hypothetical curve showing rate of development of symptoms during oxygen breathing at 2.0 ATA was obtained from combined subjective observations. Durations of oxygen breathing that caused average vital capacity decrements of 4% and 10% are shown. (Reproduced with permission from Clark, 1982.)

ATA for between 6 and 11 hr. The drop in DL_{CO} measured within 5 hr after the oxygen exposure was 9% on the average; a repeat measurement 11 hr post-exposure showed a 16% reduction. The corresponding figures for Vc were reductions of 22 and 30%, respectively. Among various explanations for the reduction in Vc, the authors proposed either a generalized pulmonary vasoconstriction or direct injury of the pulmonary capillary vessels or a combination of these factors. It was suggested that the DL_{CO} depression was the result of the reduced pulmonary capillary blood volume (Puy et al., 1968). In support of these notions, the authors pointed to the local destructive damage associated with decreased pulmonary capillary blood volume demonstrated during oxygen poisoning in the rat (Kistler et al., 1967). However, there are apparently species differences, since no change in capillary volume could be detected in monkeys exposed to oxygen at a pressure of 750 mmHg (Kapanci et al., 1969). Of particular interest are the recordings of circulatory blood gas variables in animals subjected to lethal exposures of oxygen at 1 ATA. Again, remarkable species differences have been noted. Thus, six sheep that died from hyperoxia after an average of 80 hr exposure still showed no changes in arterial and mixed venous gas tension after 40 hr, and subsequently Pa_{O2} decreased gradually but remained above 200 mmHg at death (Matalon et al., 1982). A major sign of respiratory inadequacy was the steep rise in Pa_{CO2} occurring simultaneously and reaching an average of about 100 mmHg in the final hours. Remarkably, right atrial and pulmonary arterial pressures remained normal throughout the exposures. Autopsy offered the classic macroscopic picture of lethal pulmonary oxygen damage, the lungs appearing consolidated and hemorrhagic and with copious amounts of clear fluid in the airways.

In contrast to the hypoventilation connected with hypercapnea and uncompensated respiratory acidosis in the sheep reported by Matalon et al.(1982) are the observations by Harabin and Farhi (1987) in 10 rabbits also exposed to oxygen at 1 ATA. The mean survival time was about 60 hr, during which the Pa_{CO2} rose only moderately, and the Pa_{O2} was maintained until within 4.9 hr of death, after which it fell precipitously to hypoxic levels. This fall coincided with a marked increase in the shunt fraction (Fig. 11). However, some animals died with unchanged pulmonary oxygen exchange. Among the possibilities for terminal fatal mechanisms, the authors felt that an overall cardiac insufficiency could not be excluded, and they pointed out that the terminal stages of oxygen toxicity in dogs are dynamic and rapidly changing but that cardiovascular changes precede gas exchange effects as shown by Harabin et al. (1984). In the latter study, it was also shown that the capacity of the pulmonary endothelial cells to metabolize angiotensin I was reduced before changes in hemodynamics, permeability, or gas exchange occurred (Harabin et al., 1984). It was noted that the metabolic disturbances were consistent with the magnitude of endothelial cell damage that has been particularly well described in studies on monkeys (Kapanci et al., 1969) and rats (Kistler et al., 1967). However, on the basis of review of the literature, Harabin et al. (1984) also stressed the species differences in pulmonary response to hyperoxia.

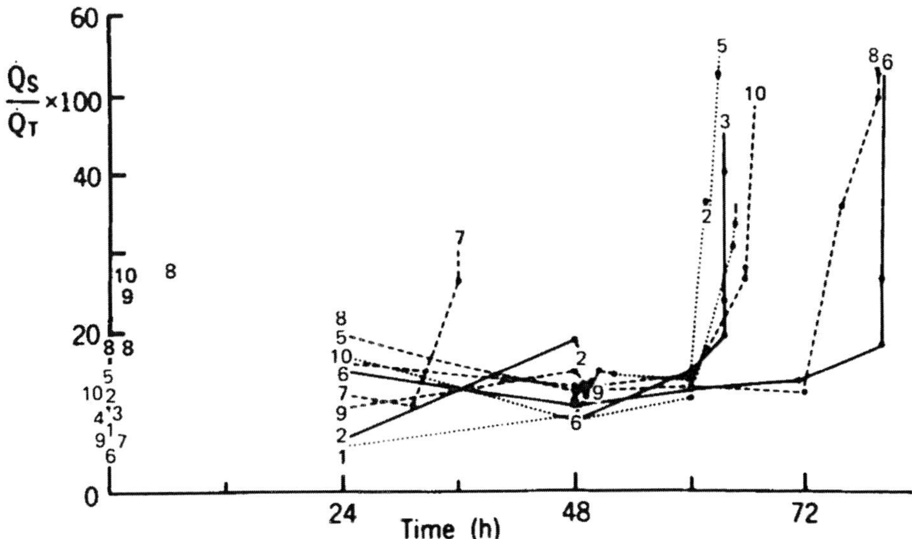

Figure 11 Time course of the percent shunt fraction in 10 conscious rabbits breathing O_2 at normobaric pressure. Note that shunt fraction was well maintained until terminal stage. (Reproduced with permission from Harabin and Farhi, 1987.)

In a review of the alterations in mammalian blood-gas barrier to abnormal oxygen exposure, Matalon and Nickerson (1986) mention that normobaric hyperoxia damages all components of the blood-gas barrier and that permeability changes are important in several species. Quoting observations in the rabbit, they emphasize that increases in endothelial and epithelial permeability occur before overt clinical symptoms and accumulation of inflammatory cells in the lung parenchyma. In addition to oxygen damage to the alveolar epithelium and interstitial space, they consider progressive endothelial damage to be a factor causing an interstitial and alveolar permeability type of edema that ultimately leads to the rabbit's death in arterial hypoxemia (Matalon and Nickerson, 1986). Indeed, ultrastructural studies of oxygen poisoning in the rat lung by Kistler et al. (1967) have shown endothelial damage to be the primary lesion. Increased alveolar permeability to solutes reflects such damage. It is interesting that Holm et al. (1985) demonstrated that protein levels in bronchoalveolar lavage that had increased in rabbits exposed for 64 hr to oxygen at 1 ATA (indicating albumin leakage) were normal after 200 hr of recovery in air. This coincided with the disappearance of pulmonary edema.

The information on the reversibility of oxygen-induced permeability changes in the lung has been reviewed by Matalon and Nickerson (1986). The figures given in the literature are variable both because of species differences and because of differences in the extent of damage before recovery was attempted. Another problem is that in addition to capillary endothelial damage, other factors are involved in the occurrence of increased permeability of the alveolar membrane due to hyperoxia. In addition, there may be marked, and as yet unexplained, differences between individual animals. This is exemplified by the observation by Holm et al. (1985). Rabbits exposed to oxygen at 1 ATA for 64 hr had a mean Pa_{O2} of 80 mmHg 1 hr after return to room air. A further reduction of the Pa_{O2} to 40-60 mmHg occurred during the ensuing 12-48 hr in air, while there was no change in the alveolar permeability to solute compared to the value recorded after 64 hr in oxygen. While 35% of the rabbits died, the 65% that survived had normal blood gases and alveolar permeability after 8 days of air breathing.

The earlier mentioned moderate decreases in DL_{CO} and Vc recorded at the end of 6-11 hr of oxygen exposure at 2 ATA in humans were largely unchanged in repeat measurements after 10-15 hr of recovery in a normal air atmosphere (Puy et al., 1968). Further followup of these measurements was not reported.

There must, for obvious reasons, be considerable uncertainty about the detailed structural and functional impairment of the pulmonary circulation in normal humans exposed to clinically significant hyperoxia. However, morphological observations similar to those reported in many animal studies were made by Nash et al. (1967), who described postmortem findings in 70 patients subjected to artificial ventilation with mechanical ventilators and varying levels of hyperoxia. The control group consisted of patients who had not been ventilated artificially. The authors showed that there was a positive and statistically significant correlation between certain pulmonary changes and higher doses of oxygen. The changes were described as the lungs appearing heavy, "beefy," and edematous; microscopically two phases were recognized that merged and were not distinct. Some changes that suggested pulmonary vascular involvement paralleled some of those observed in animals as mentioned above. In an early exudative phase the microscopic picture showed congestion, alveolar edema, intraalveolar hemorrhage, fibrin exudate, and hyaline membranes; a later proliferative phase also was marked by alveolar edema in addition to various cellular changes.

While inhalation of 100% O_2 is part of hyperbaric oxygen therapy, it is the exception in diving and is used mostly in closed-circuit breathing gear for certain military applications. The largest amount of diving is still carried out with compressed air, and in deep saturation diving a very large fraction of the respired gas mix must consist of inert gases (typically helium, sometimes with an admixture of nitrogen).

To retain an oxygen pressure of, for instance, 0.4 ATA, a dive to 300 msw (30.78 ATA) will require 98.7% inert gas in the breathing mixture. Because, as mentioned earlier, it is desirable to keep the oxygen pressure as high as can safely be done, the question arises as to whether the diluent gases will modify the toxic limits determined for pure oxygen and, for this presentation in particular, the limits with regard to the primary site of the oxygen damage, that is, the pulmonary capillary endoethelium.

Little information is available that speaks to the susceptibility of the pulmonary circulation to oxygen damage and possible modifying effects of inert gas. However, Norman et al. (1971) recorded a distinctly slower progress of lung changes both macroscopically and histologically (including congestion, atelectasis, and hepatiziation) in rats and mice breathing oxygen at 2 ATA in combination with 1 ATA of nitrogen than when the breathing gas was oxygen at 2 ATA alone. Mortality was drastically different: 2 mice out of 30 in the former group versus 20 out of 30 in the latter after 15 hr of exposure but equal (30/30) after 24 hr. The reason for the protective effect was not clear, although the authors forward some argument as to why the ability of nitrogen to counteract absorption atelectases may have played a role.

A protective effect by nitrogen against oxygen lung damage was also noted by Powell and Fust (1981) who compared mice exposed to oxygen at 1.75 bars and oxygen at 1.75 bars plus nitrogen at 1.75 bars until death from pulmonary oxygen damage. Their findings are summarized in Figure 12. Death was clearly delayed, and both changes in lung morphology and increases in lung to body weight ratio developed more slowly in animals who breathed the oxygen-nitrogen combination. No explanation was offered for the protective effect of nitrogen.

In contrast with these observations is the lack of protection provided by nitrogen against respiratory distress and death in mice exposed to nitrogen at 13.8 ATA in combination with oxygen at either 1.0 or 1.5 ATA compared to oxygen alone at the latter pressures (Rokitka and Rahn, 1977). As reviewed, it is possible that when no protective effects or even deleterious effects on oxygen tolerance have been recorded in the presence of even higher gas pressure (e.g., Thompson et al., 1970), this has been due to carbon dioxide retention in the animals, which in turn may enhance oxygen toxicity. The possibility that exposure of the lungs to increased carbon dioxide tensions may enhance the toxic potency of oxygen should be considered because carbon dioxide retention is a distinct possibility in diving. High inert gas densities, hyperoxia, and inert gas narcosis are conducive to hypoventilation and carbon dioxide retention (Lanphier and Camporesi, 1982). Furthermore, exercising divers as a group have been shown to have a higher tendency to retain carbon dioxide during oxygen breathing (1 ATA) than nondivers; this has been attributed partly to a reduced central responsiveness to CO_2 (Kerem et al., 1980). Faulty breathing gear may also cause hypercapnia in a diver by increasing the carbon dioxide level in the inspired gas.

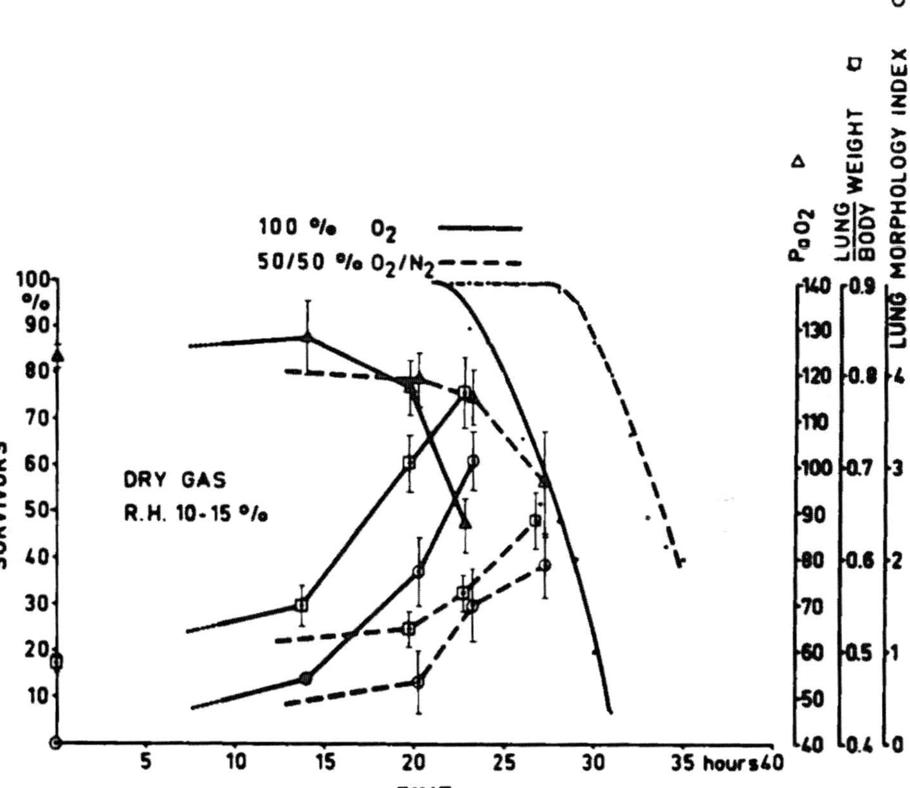

Figure 12 Percent survival (●), arterial oxygen tension (▲), lung/body weight ratio (□ x 100), and lung morphology index (○) as a function of time for mice in oxygen (1.75 bars, continuous lines) and an oxygen-nitrogen mixture (1.75/1.75 bars, dashed lines). Lung morphology index: 0 = normal, 1 = minimal congestion, 2 = small areas of atelectasis, 3 = predominant collapse in one or both lungs, 4 = complete collapse in both lungs, "hepatization." Mean values ± SEM; n = 15 in each series. (Reproduced by permission from Powell and Fust, 1981.)

Early studies of carbon dioxide effects on oxygen-induced lung damage were performed by Olsson (1947). Rabbits exposed to oxygen (80-90%) with an admixture of 3-3.5% CO_2 survived half as long (1.5-3 days) as animals not exposed to carbon dioxide (a 3-3.5% carbon dioxide admixture with air was well tolerated). The carbon dioxide effect appeared to be due to the more rapid development of pulmonary damage. With regard to involvement of the pulmonary circulation, both groups showed marked capillary hyperemia, edema, and, in the carbon dioxide group, hemorrhages.

An extensive, relatively recent study of the effects of hypercapnia on oxygen tolerance in rats has been published by Clark (1981). Acute exposure at 1.0 ATA to oxygen with an admixture of carbon dioxide at 60 mmHg gave a mortality of 93%, while it was 70% in 100% oxygen (exposure terminated after 14 days). Lung weights, however, were not different, and carbon dioxide caused no marked difference in survival at oxygen pressures of 1.5 and 2.0 ATA. However, adaptation to an environment of 60 mmHg PI_{CO2}/130 mmHg PI_{O2} with a balance of N_2 for 5 days had no effect on the tolerance to oxygen at 1.0 ATA in rats but markedly reduced their tolerance to the earlier described oxygen-carbon dioxide combination at 1.0 and 1.5 ATA. The author (Clark, 1981) stated that mechanisms behind the reduced tolerance to oxygen in the acute oxygen-carbon dioxide exposures of nonadapted rats was unknown. However, he pointed out that the greatly reduced tolerance in the carbon dioxide-adapted rats may depend on their being more vulnerable due to detrimental pulmonary effects of hypercapnia that is progressive with time. Specifically, he referred to the fact that prolonged exposure to PI_{CO2} levels of between 20 and 200 mmHg is able to cause hyaline membranes and perivascular and alveolar edema in rats and guinea pigs as demonstrated by Niemoeller and Schaefer (1962).

It is known that various physiological factors may modify the pulmotoxic effects of oxygen. Thus, suppression of both the sympatho-adrenomedullary and hypophyseal-andrenocortical activities provide some protection, as does experimental hypothyroidism. For an overview of these interactions as well as other endocrine, metabolic, and nutritional factors, the review of Clark (1982) is useful.

B. Absorption Atelectasis

The toxic effects of oxygen in the lungs discussed so far can be ascribed primarily to such reactive oxygen radicals as the superoxide anion radical, the hydroxyl radical (H_2O_2), and singlet O_2 (Freemand and Crapo, 1982). However, there is another mechanism that, during oxygen breathing, has been shown to cause considerably more dramatic reductions in VC in humans than classic oxygen intoxication. Thus, Balldin and co-workers (1971) recorded an average reduction in VC of 22.4% in 13 healthy subjects breathing oxygen for only 2 hr during head-out immersion. Noting that immersion (during air breathing) by itself caused a 7.8% VC reduction, they ascribed the larger effect during oxygen breathing to atelectasis formation. The various mechanisms by which airway closure may be promoted during immersion have been discussed earlier in this chapter. It is conceivable that oxygen could get into lung regions that are closed off most of the time during immersion. All it would take is for the subject to take occasional deep breaths so as to open up the blocked lung compartment and remove the nitrogen by dilution. Alternatively, nitrogen may be washed out of a closed compartment by the local circulation. In either case, the formation of absorption atelectasis would be enhanced.

This is not to say that the entire loss of VC must be due to actual loss of lung volume by atelectasis. Restriction of respiratory excursions needed to deliver a VC for measurement may in part have been due to the pain that coincided with atelectasis. The importance of keeping the lungs inflated has been demonstrated in experiments with positive-pressure breathing at 1.5 kPa (11.3 mmHg) in combination with oxygen breathing and head-out immersion for 1 hr (Dahlback and Balldin, 1983). This induced a 70% increase in the expiratory reserve volume. While the control experiments (without positive-pressure breathing) caused an average drop of VC of 42%, there was no loss in three subjects and a halving of the VC reduction in two subjects when positive pressure was used. The authors recognized that there probably were two aspects to the pressure effects, namely, the aforementioned distention of the lungs as well as a reduction of intrathoracic blood pooling.

The importance of these mechanisms for practical diving was borne out by VC measurements in four divers who breathed oxygen for 30 min using two versions of closed-circuit breathing apparatus while assuming a prone swimming position underwater (Dahlback and Balldin, 1985). One apparatus had the rebreathing bag placed on the back of the diver, exposing him to a negative static lung load of -2 kPa (-15 mmHg); and in the other the bag was worn on the chest, inducing a static load of +1-2 kPa (7.5-15 mmHg). Three of the divers showed substantial reductions in VC of between 0.8 and 1.9 liters when exposed to the negative static load as compared to the positive. The fourth diver had small reductions in VC with both types of gear, and it was suggested that this may have been an individual with little tendency for airway closure at the level of negative static load imposed [cf. discussion of the work by Prefaut et al. (1978 and 1979) earlier in this chapter]. In addition, as in the earlier studies of oxygen effects during head-out immersion, the negative static load induced burning sensations in the chest and coughing attacks.

C. Fetal Pulmonary Circulation

Hyperoxia has been used in the study of the mechanisms responsible for transition from fetal to adult pulmonary circulation at birth (e.g., Assali et al., 1968; Heymann et al., 1969; Accurso et al., 1986; Morin et al., 1986a, b, 1987b). The rationale for this experimental approach is the desire to distinguish between possible effects of the mechanical events in the lung and chest as the first breaths of air are taken, on the one hand, and the changes in lung PO_2 that those breaths bring about, on the other.

Early observation of increased pulmonary blood flow in animal fetuses in response to oxygen inhalation by the pregnant mother animal have been reviewed by Assali et al. (1968). These authors used hyperbaric oxygen at 3 ATA on pregnant ewes near term, which raised the fetal pulmonary blood flow by nearly threefold in conjunction with an increase in fetal pulmonary artery blood PO_2 from 16 mmHg (ewe breathing air) to 47 mmHg. While the fall in blood flow through the ductus arteriosus was from 126 ml/min per kilogram (control) to 41 ml/min per kilogram, the pulmonary arterial pressure fell by an average of 5 mmHg, indicating that the primary reason for the increased pulmonary blood flow was a dilatation of the pulmonary vasculature and consequent drop in flow resistance.

While the study just mentioned was performed in acutely prepared anesthetized animals and with the fetuses marsupialized, Morin et al. (1987a) used fully recovered animals with the instrumented fetus in utero. They studied the dependence of the fetal pulmonary vascular response on oxygen in relation to gestational age. Hyperbaric oxygen inhalation by the ewes at 3 ATA increased the fetal PaO_2 from an average of 25 mmHg (control) to 55 mmHg in 11 near-term fetuses (132-146 days gestation); this was coupled with an increase in the proportion of right ventricular output distributed to the lungs from 8% to 59%. In five very immature fetuses (94-101 days gestation), the fetal PaO_2 increased from an average of 27 mmHg to 174 mmHg when the ewes inhaled hyperbaric oxygen. Yet there was no change in the lungs' share of the right ventricular output (8% vs. 9%). It was concluded that the pulmonary circulation of the fetal sheep does not respond to an increased oxygen tension before 101 days gestation. However, once it is fully developed the oxygen response alone can induce the entire increase in pulmonary blood flow that normally occurs following the onset of breathing at birth. As an important practical consideration, the authors pointed to the possibility that an nonphysiological enhancement of the pulmonary blood flow may occur at the expense of placental blood flow in the fetus should a pregnant woman engage in diving (Morin et al., 1987a).

The mediating mechanism between an increased fetal oxygen tensionand the enhancement of pulmonary blood flow has not been conclusively identified. Experimental evidence reviewed by Heymann et al. (1969) has shown that bradykinin is capable of constricting the ductus arteriosus as well as dilating the pulmonary vascular bed in the fetal lamb. For this reason, these authors studied the bradykinin production of the fetal lamb in association with hyperoxygenation. They concluded that increased production of bradykinin is associated with the pulmonary vasodilatation occurring with the onset of respiration and that the bradykinin production is oxygen dependent and not initiated by mechanical lung expansion. However, they cautioned that their findings did not exclude an independent direct vasodilator effect of oxygen.

Prostaglandins as possible mediators were studied by Morin et al. (1987b). They found that while hyperbaric oxygenation at 3 ATA in pregnant ewes increased fetal PaO_2 from an average of 25 mmHg during normoxia to 56 mmHg during hyperoxia and caused increases in pulmonary blood flow from 33 to 293 ml/min per kilogram, the plasma concentrations of 6-keto-PGE_{II}, the hydrolysis product of PGE_{II}, did not change (208 pg/ml during normoxia versus 235 pg/ml during hyperoxia). Furthermore, blocking prostaglandin synthesis by administration of indomethacin could be done without affecting the pulmonary blood flow response to hyperoxia. The authors therefore ruled out prostaglandin as the mediator.

VII. Concluding Remarks

Physiologists have traditionally devoted much attention to the ventilatory function of the lung when studying the effects of hyperbaric exposures and diving. We hope that this chapter has shown that the function of the pulmonary circulation is equally important; one must wonder at the remarkable adaptability to environmental stress of the lesser circulation on the one hand and its unique vulnerability on the other. To recall but two examples: It is the ability of the blood-containing structures in the chest to accept translocation of large volumes of blood from the periphery that has allowed breath-hold diving humans to descend, without crush injury, to a depth of about 300 ft which is far beyond the limit set by chest wall compressibility. In contrast, damage to blood vessels of the lung by hyperoxia is important in making the lung the most sensitive major organ with regard to the toxic effects of increased oxygen tensions. Finally, the reader whose interests are primarily in the area of pulmonary circulatory function under normal environmental conditions or common diseases may want to take note of the good use that can be made of the hyperbaric and simulated diving environment to understand function. Examples range from the study of the normal transition from fetal to adult pulmonary circulation to the fundamental roles of oxygen radicals in the process of aging, action of ionizing radiation, or leukocyte function, to name but a few examples (cf. Freeman and Crapo, 1982).

Acknowledgment

Supported in part by NHLBI contract HL34323 and by USN Naval Medical R & D Command, Office of Naval Research, contract N0001486C0106.

References

Accurso, F. J., Albert, B., Wilkening, R. B., Peterson, R. G., and Merschia, G. (1986). Time-dependent response of fetal pulmonary blood flow to an increase in fetal oxygen tension. *Resp. Physiol. 63*:43-52.

Agostoni, E., Gurtner, G., Torri, G., and Rahn, H. (1966). Respiratory mechanics during submersion and negative pressure breathing. *J. Appl. Physiol. 21*:251-258.

Arborelius, M., Jr. (1969). Influence of unilateral hypoventilation on distribution of pulmonary blood flow in man. *J. Appl. Physiol. 26*:101-104.

Arborelius, M., Jr., Balldin, U. I., Lilja, B., and Lundgren, C. E. G. (1972a). Hemodynamic changes in man during immersion with the head above water. *Aerosp. Med. 43*:592-598.

Arborelius, M., Jr., Balldin, U. I., Lilja, B., and Lundgren, C. E. G. (1972b). Regional lung function in man during immersion with the head above water. *Aerosp. Med. 43*:701-707.

Assali, N. S., Kirschbaum, T. H., and Dilts, P. V. Jr. (1968). Effects of hyperbaric oxygen on uteroplacental and fetal circulation. *Circ. Res. 22*:573-588.

Baer, R., Dahlbäck, G. O., and Balldin, U. I. (1987). Pulmonary mechanics and atelectasis during immersion in oxygen breathing subjects. *Undersea Biomed. Res. 14*(3):229-240.

Balldin, U. I., Dahlbäck, G. O., and Lundgren, C. E. G. (1971). Changes in vital capacity produced by oxygen breathing during immersion with the head above water. *Aerosp. Med. 42*:384-387.

Basch, S. von (1887). Über eine Funktion des Capillardruckes in den Lungenalveolen. *Weiner Med. Blätter 15*:465-467.

Bennett, P. B., Coggin, R., and McLeod, M. (1982). Effect of compression rate on use of trimix to ameliorate HPNS in man to 686 m (2250 ft). *Undersea Biomed. Res. 9*:335-351.

Bondi, K. R., Murray Young, J., Bennett, R. M., and Bradley, M. E. (1976). Closing volumes in man immersed to the neck in water. *J. Appl. Physiol. 40*:736-740.

Bove, A. A., Hallenbeck, J. M., and Elliott, D. H. (1974). Circulatory responses to venous air embolism and decompression sickness in dogs. *Undersea Biomed. Res. 1*(3):207-220.

Brubakk, A. O., Grip, A., Holand, B., Onarheim, J., and Tønjum, S. (1981). Arterial gas bubbles following ascending excursions during He-O_2 saturation diving. In *Program and Abstracts*, Undersea Medical Society Annual Scientific Meeting, May 25-29, 1981. *Undersea Biomed. Res. 8*(1 Suppl): A6.

Butler, B. D., and Hills, B. A. (1979). The lung as a filter for microbubbles. *J. Appl. Physiol. 47*(3):537-543.

Butler, B. D., and Hills, B. A. (1985). Transpulmonary passage of venous air emboli. *J. Appl. Physiol. 59*:543-547.

Clark, J. M. (1981). Effects of acute and chronic hypercapnia on oxygen tolerance in rats. *J. Appl. Physiol.: Resp. Environ. Exercise Physiol. 50*:1036-1044.

Clark, J. M. (1982). Oxygen toxicity. In *The Physiology and Medicine of Diving*. Edited by P. B. Bennett and D. H. Elliott. Best Publishing, San Pedro, CA, pp. 200-238.

Clark, J. M., and Lambertsen, C. J. (1971). Rate of development of pulmonary 0_2 toxicity in man during 0_2 breathing at 1.0 Ata. *J. Appl. Physiol. 30*: 739-752.

Cohen, R. Bell, W. H., Saltzman, H. A., and Kylstra, J. A. (1971). Alveolar-arterial oxygen pressure difference in man immersed up to the neck in water. *J. Appl. Physiol. 30*:720-723.

Colebatch, H. J. H., Smith, M. M., and Ng, C. K. Y. (1976). Increased elastic recoil as a determinant of pulmonary barotrauma in divers. *Resp. Physiol. 26*:55-64.

Collins, J. V., Cochrane, G. M., Davis, J., Benatar, S. R., and Clark, T. J. H. (1973). Some aspects of pulmonary function after rapid saline infusion in healthy subjects. *Clin. Sci. Mol. Med. 45*:407-410.

Craig, A. B., Jr. (1968). Depth limits of breath hold diving (an example of Fennology. *Resp. Physiol. 5*:14-22.

Cryssanthou, C., Teichner, F., Goldstein, G., Kalberer, J., and Antopol, W. (1970). Studies on dysbarism III. A smooth muscle-acting factor (SMAF) in mouse lungs and its increase in decompression sickness. *Aerosp. Med. 41*(1):43-48.

Dahlbäck, G. O. (1975). Influence of intrathoracic blood pooling on pulmonary air-trapping during immersion. *Undersea Biomed. Res. 2*:133-140.

Dahlbäck, G. O. (1978). Lung mechanics during immersion in water. Thesis, Laboratory of Aviation and Naval Physiology, Institute of Physiology and Biophysics, University of Lund, Lund, Sweden.

Dahlbäck, G. O., and Balldin, U. I. (1983). Positive-pressure oxygen breathing and pulmonary atelectasis during immersion. *Undersea Biomed. Res. 10*: 39-44.

Dahlbäck, G. O., and Balldin, U. I. (1985). Pulmonary atelectasis formation during diving with closed-circuit oxygen breathing apparatus. *Undersea Biomed. Res. 12*:129-137.

Dahlbäck, G. O., and Lundgren, C. E. G. (1972). Pulmonary air-trapping induced by water immersion. *Aerosp. Med. 43*:768-774.

Dahlbäck, G. O., Jönsson, E., and Liner, M. H. (1978). Influence of hydrostatic compression of the chest and intrathoracic blood pooling on static lung mechanics during head-out immersion. *Undersea Biomed. Res. 5*:71-85.

Echt, M., Düweling, J., Gauer, O. H., and Lange, L. (1974). Effective compliance of the total vascular bed and the intrathoracic compartment derived from changes in central venous pressure induced by volume changes in man. *Circ. Res. 34*:61-68.

Edmonds, C., Lewry, C., and Pennefather, J. (1984). Diving and subaquatic medicine. Diving Medical Center Biomedical Marine Services, Seaforth, Australia.

Fagraeus, L. (1974). Cardiorespiratory and metabolic functions during exercise in the hyperbaric environment. *Acta Physiol. Scand. Suppl. 414*:1-40.

Farhi, L. E., and Linnarsson, D. (1977). Cardiopulmonary readjustments during graded immersion in water at 35°C. *Resp. Physiol. 30*:35-50.

Flynn, E. T., Berghage, T. E., and Coil, E. F. (1972). Influence of increased ambient pressure and gas density on cardiac rate in man. U. S. Navy Experimental Diving Unit Report 4-72, NEDU, Washington, DC.

Freeman, B. A., and Crapo, J. D. (1982). Biology of disease: free radicals and tissue injury. *Lab. Invest. 47*:412-426.

Guyatt, A. R., Newman, F., Cinkotai, F. F., Palmer, J. I., and Thomson, M. L. (1965). Pulmonary diffusing capacity in man during immersion in water. *J. Appl. Physiol. 20*(5):878-881.

Hallenbeck, J. M. (1976). Cinematomicrography of dog spinal vessels during cord-damaging decompression sickness. *Neurology (Minneapolis) 26*:190-199.

Hallenbeck, J. M., and Andersen, J. C. (1982). Pathogenesis of the decompression disorders. In *The Physiology and Medicine of Diving*. Edited by P. B. Bennett and D. H. Elliott. Best Publishing, San Pedro, CA.

Hamilton, R. W., Jr. (1967). Physiological responses at rest and in exercise during saturation at 20 atmospheres of He-O_2. In *Proceedings Symp. Underwater Physiology*. Vol. 3. Edited by C. J. Lambertsen. Williams and Wilkins, Baltimore.

Harabin, A. L., and Farhi, L. E. (1987). Blood-gas transport in awake rabbits exposed to normobaric hyperoxia. *Undersea Biomed. Res. 14*:133-147.

Harabin, A. L., Homer, L. D., and Bradley, M. E. (1984). Pulmonary oxygen toxicity in awake dogs: metabolic and physiologic effects. *J. Appl. Physiol. 57*:1480-1488.

Heller, R., Mager, W., and von Schrotter, H. (1897). Uber das physiologische Verhalten des Pulses bei Veranderungen des Luftdruckes. *Z. Klin. Med. 33*:341-384.

Heymann, M. A., Rudolph, A. M., Nies, A. S. and Melmon, K. L. (1969). Bradykinin production associated with oxygenation of the fetal lamb. *Circ. Res. 25*:521-534.

Hickey, D. D., and Lundgren, C. E. G. (1984). Breath hold diving. In *The Physician's Guide to Diving Medicine*. Edited by C. W. Shilling, C. B. Carlston, and R. A. Mathias. Plenum Press, New York, pp. 206-221.

Hills, B. A., and Butler, B. D. (1981). Size distribution of intravascular air emboli produced by decompression. *Undersea Biomed. Res. 8*(3):163-170.

Hlastala, M. P., Robertson, H. T., and Ross, B. K. (1979). Gas exchange abnormalities produced by venous gas emboli. *Resp. Physiol. 36*:1-17.

Holm, B. A., Notter, R. H., Siegle, J., and Matalon, S. (1985). Pulmonary physiological and surfactant changes during injury and recovery from hyperoxia. *J. Appl. Physiol. 59*:1402-1409.

Hong, S. K., Cerretelli, P., Cruz, J. C., and Rahn, H. (1969). Mechanics of respiration during submersion in water. *J. Appl. Physiol. 27*:535-538.

Hughes, J. M. B., Glazier, J. B., Maloney, J. E., and West, J. B. (1967). Effect of interstitial pressure on pulmonary blood flow. *Lancet 1*:192-193.

Ingvar, D. H., Adolfson, J., and Lindemark, C. O. (1973). Cerebral air embolism during training of submarine personnel in free escape: an electroencephalographic study. *Aerosp. Med. 44*:628-635.

Kapanci, Y., Weibel, E. R., Kaplan, H. P., and Robinson, F. R. (1969). Pathogenesis and reversibility of the pulmonary lesions of oxygen toxicity in monkeys. II. Ultrastructural and morphometric studies. *Lab. Invest. 20*: 101-118.

Kerem, D., and Salzano, J. (1974). Effect of high ambient pressure on human apneic bradycardia. *J. Appl. Physiol. 37*:108-111.

Kerem, D. D., Melamed, Y., and Moran, A. (1980). Alveolar PCO_2 during rest and exercise in divers and nondivers breathing 0_2 at 1 ATA. *Undersea Biomed. Res. 7*:17-26.

Khan, M. (1979). Fatal thoracic squeeze. *J. Indian Med. Assoc. 73*:38-39.

Kindwall, E. P., Baz, A., Lightfoot, E. N., Lanphier, E. H., and Seireg, A. (1975). Nitrogen elimination in man during decompression. *Undersea Biomed. Res. 2*:285-297.

Kistler, G. S., Caldwell, P. R. B., and Weibel, E. R. (1967). Development of fine structural damage to alveolar and capillary lining cells in oxygen-poisoned rat lungs. *J. Cell Biol. 32*:605-628.

Kurss, D. I., Lundgren, E. G., and Påsche, A. J. (1981). Effect of water temperature on vital capacity in head out immersion. In *Underwater Physiology VII*. Edited by A. J. Bachrach and M. M. Matzen. *Undersea Med. Soc.*, Bethesda, MD, pp. 297-301.

Lanari, A., Lambertini, A., Zubiaur, F. L., and Bromberger Barnea, B. (1960). Las modificaciones de la presion intratoracica, arterial sistemica, y venosa periferica durante la sumersion. *Medicina (Buenos Aires) 20*:159-163.

Lange, L., Lange, S., Echt, M., and Gauer, O. H. (1974). Heart volume in relation to body posture and immersion in a thermo-neutral bath. A roentgenometric study. *Pflugers Arch. 352*:219-226.

Lanphier, E. H., and Camporesi, E. M. (1982). Respiration and exercise. In *The Physiology and Medicine of Diving*. Edited by P. B. Bennett and D. H. Elliott. Best Publishing, San Pedro, CA, pp. 99-156.

Leitch, D. R., and Green, R. D. (1986a). Pulmonary barotrauma in divers and the treatment of cerebral arterial gas embolism. *Avait. Space Environ. Med. 57*:931-938.

Leitch, D. R., and Green, R. D. (1986b). Recurrent pulmonary barotrauma. *Aviat. Space Environ. Med.* *57*(11):1039-1043.

Leitch, D. R., and Hallenbeck, J. M. (1984). Neurological forms of decompression sickness. In *The Physicians Guide to Diving Medicine*. Edited by C. W. Schilling, C. B. Carlston, and R. A. Mathias, Plenum Press, New York, pp. 316-324.

Löllgen, H., Nieding, G. von, and Horres, R. (1980). Respiratory and hemodynamic adjustment during head-out water immersion. *Int. J. Sports Med.* *1*:25-29.

Lundgren, C. E. G. (1984). Respiratory functions during simulated wet dives. *Undersea Biomed. Res.* *11*:139-147.

Lundgren, C. E. G., and Norfleet, W. T. (1987). Respiratory function in hyperbaric environments. In *Stressful Environments: Diving, Hyper- and Hypobaric Physiology*. Edited by K. Shiraki and M. K. Yousef. Springfield, Illinois, Charles C. Thomas Publishers, pp. 21-40.

Lundgren, C. E. G., and Örnhagen, H. C. (1976). Heart rate and respiratory frequency in hydrostatically compressed, liquid breathing mice. *Undersea Biomed. Res.* *3*:303-320.

Lynch, J. J., Schuchard, G. H., Gross, C. M., and Wann, L. S. (1984). Prevalence of right-to-left atrial shunting in a healthy population: detection by valsalva maneuver contrast echocardiography. *Am. J. Cardiol.* *53*:1478-1480.

Martin, R. R., Zutter, M., and Anthonisen, N. R. (1972). Pulmonary gas exchange in dogs breathing SF_6 at 4 ATA. *J. Appl. Physiol* *33*:86-92.

Matalon, S., and Nickerson, P. (1986). Alterations in mammalian blood-gas barrier exposed to hyperoxia. In *Physiology of Oxygen Radicals*. Edited by A. E. Taylor, S. Matalon, and P. A. Ward. Williams and Wilkins, Baltimore, MD, for American Physiological Socity, pp. 55-69.

Matalon, S., Nesarajah, M. S., and Farhi, L. E. (1982). Pulmonary and circulatory changes in conscious sheep exposed to 100% 0_2 at 1 ATA. *J. Appl. Physiol.: Resp. Environ, Exercise Physiol.* *53*:110-116.

Missiroli, F. M., and Rizzato, B. (1984). Mayol a 105 metri. *Mondo Sommerso* *272*:32-37.

Morin, F. C., Egan, E. A., Ferguson, W., and Lundgren, C. E. G. (1986a). The development of the pulmonary vascular response to oxygen. *Pediatr. Res.* *20*:370A, Abstr. 1260.

Morin, F. C., Egan, E. A., and Lundgren, C. E. G. (1986b). The pulmonary vascular response of the fetal lamb to an increase in oxygen tension is not mediated by prostaglandins. *Pediatr. Res.* *20*:370A, Abstr. no. 1261.

Morin, F. C., Egan, E. A., Ferguson, W., and Lundgren, C. E. G. (1987a). Development of the pulmonary vascular response to oxygen in the sheet fetus. *Undersea Biomed. Res. Suppl.* *14*(2):33, Abstr. no. 62.

Morin, F. C., III, Egan, E. A., and Norfleet, W. T. (1987b). Raising oxygen tension in the fetal lamb increases pulmonary blood flow to newborn levels and this increase is not mediated by prostaglandins. *FASEB 46*: 1118, Abstr. 4675.

Nash, G., Blennerhassett, J. B., and Pontoppidan, H. (1967). Pulmonary lesions associated with oxygen therapy and artificial ventilation. *New Engl. J. Med. 276*:368-374.

Neuman, T. S., Spragg, R. G., Wagner, P. D., and Moser, K. M. (1980). Cardiopulmonary consequences of decompression stress. *Resp. Physiol. 41*:143-153.

Niemoeller, H., and Schaefer, K. E. (1962). Development of hyaline membranes and atelectases in experimental chronic respiratory acidosis. *Proc. Soc. Exp. Biol. Med. 110*:804-808.

Norman, J. N., MacIntyre, J., Ross, R. R., and Smith, G. (1971). Etiological studies of pulmonary oxygen poisoning. *Am. J. Physiol. 220*:492-498.

Olsson, W. T. L. (1947). A study on oxygen toxicity at atmospheric pressure. *Acta Med. Scand. 128*, Suppl. *190*:1-93.

Örnhagen, H. Ch., and Hogan, P. M. (1977). Hydrostatic pressure and mammalian cardiac-pacemaker function. *Undersea Biomed. Res. 4*:347-358.

Powell, M. R., and Fust, H. D. (1981). The influence of inert gas concentration on pulmonary oxygen toxicity. In *Underwater Physiology* VII. *Proceedings of the Seventh Symposium on Underwater Physiology*. Edited by A. J. Bachrach and M. M. Matzen. Undersea Medical Society, Bethesda, MD, pp. 113-120.

Prefaut, Ch., Ramonatxo, M., Boyer, R., and Chardon, G. (1978). Human gas exchange during water immersion. *Resp. Physiol. 34*:307-318.

Prefaut, Ch., Dubois, F., Roussos, Ch., Amaral-Marques, R., Macklem, P. T., and Ruff, F. (1979). Influence of immersion to the neck in water on airway closure and distribution of perfusion in man. *Resp. Physiol. 37*:313-323.

Puy, R. J. M., Hyde, R. W., Fisher, A. B., Clark, J. M., Dickson, J. and Lambertsen, C. J. (1968). Alterations in the pulmonary capillary bed during early O_2 toxicity in man. *J. Appl. Physiol. 24*:537-543.

Rahn, H. (1965). The physiological stresses of the Ama. In *Physiology of Breath-hold Diving and the Ama of Japan.* Edited by H. Rahn and T. Yokoyama. Publication 1341. National Academy of Sciences, National Research Council, Washington, DC, pp. 113-138.

Raymond, L. W., Bell, W. H., II, Bondi, K. R., and Lindberg, C. R. (1968). Body temperature and metabolism in hyperbaric helium atmospheres. *J. Appl. Physiol. 24*:678-684.

Risch, W. D., Koubenec, H. J., Beckmann, U., Lange, S., and Gauer, O. H. (1978a). The effect of graded immersion on heart volume, central venous pressure, pulmonary blood distribution and heart rate in man. *Pflüegers Arch. 374*:115-118.

Risch, W. D., Koubenec, H. J., Gauer, O. H., and Lange, S. (1978b). Time course of cardiac distension with rapid immersion in a thermoneutral bath. *Pfleugers Arch.* *374*:119-120.

Rokitka, M. A., and Rahn, H. (1977). Effects of high 0_2 and N_2-0_2 pressures on the physical performance of deer mice: preliminary studies. *Aviat. Space Environ. Med.* *48*:323-326.

Ruff, F., Hughes, J. M. B., Stanley, N., McCarthy, D., Greene, R., Aronoff, A., Clayton, L., and Milic-Emili, J. (1971). Regional lung function in patients with hepatic cirrhosis. *J. Clin. Invest.* *50*:2403-2413.

Schaefer, K. E., Allison, R. D., Dougherty, J. H., Jr., Carey, C. R., Walker, R., Yost, F., and Parker, D. (1968). Pulmonary and circulatory adjustments determining the limits of depths in breathhold diving. *Science* *162*:1020-1023.

Shilling, C. W., Hawkins, J. A., and Hansen, R. A. (1936). The influence of increased barometric pressure on the pulse rate and arterial blood pressure. *U. S. Naval Med. Bull.* *34*:39-47.

Spencer, M. P. (1976). Decompression limits for compressed air determined by ultrasonically detected blood bubbles. *J. Appl. Physiol.* *40*:229-235.

Stigler, R. (1911). Die Kraft unserer Inspirationsmuskulatur. *Pflügers Arch.* *139*:234-254.

Strauss, M. B., and Wright, P. W. (1971). Thoracic squeeze diving casualty. *Aerosp. Med.* *42*:673-675.

Taunton, J. E., Banister, E. W., Patrick, T. R., Oforsagd, P., and Duncan, W. R. (1970). Physical work capacity in hyperbaric environments and conditions of hyperoxia. *J. Appl. Physiol.* *28*:421-427.

Thompson, R. E., Nielsen, T. W., and Akers, T. K. (1970). Synergistic oxygen-inert gas interactions in laboratory rats in a hyperbaric environment. *Aerosp. Med.* *41*:1388-1392.

Undersea Biomedical Research (1974). Pressure conversion table. *Undersea Biomed Res.* *1*:iv.

Undersea Biomedical Research (1987). Pressure conversion table. *Undersea Biomed. Res.* *14*:185.

U. S. Navy Diving Manual (June 1978). Change 2. Vol. 1. NAVSEA 0994-LP-001-9010. U. S. Navy Department, Washington, DC, pp. 8-23 to 8-25.

8

Mechanisms of Acute Hypoxic and Hyperpoxic Changes in Pulmonary Vascular Reactivity

STEVEN L. ARCHER

University of Minnesota
School of Medicine and
VA Medical Center
Minneapolis, Minnesota

E. KENNETH WEIR

VA Medical Center and
University of Minnesota
School of Medicine
Minneapolis, Minnesota

IVAN F. McMURTRY

University of Colorado
Health Sciences Center
Denver, Colorado

I. Introduction

In the mature animal, the pulmonary vascular bed is a low-resistance circuit that accommodates the entire cardiac output at roughly one-fifth the pressure found in the systemic circulation. The tone of the pulmonary arteries and hence the distribution of pulmonary blood flow is actively regulated. While pulmonary vascular tone can be modulated by the autonomic nervous sytem as well as a plethora of constrictor substances, the primary physiological determinant of vascular resistance in the healthy lung is alveolar oxygen concentration. Pulmonary arteries constrict on exposure to hypoxia (Madden et al., 1985; Peake et al., 1981; Sylvester et al., 1980) (hypoxic pulmonary vasoconstriction) and dilate in response to hyperoxia (Madden et al., 1985; Peake et al., 1981; Sylvester et al., 1980). The opposite response to oxygen tension is usually seen in systemic arteries (Chang and Detar, 1980; Coburn, 1977).

While humans have occasionally been exposed to hypoxia in the course of evolution (e.g., during the course of lung diseases or with residence at altitude), hyperoxia is a relatively recent challenge. Inhalation of oxygen concentrations in the hyperoxic range (between 21 and 100%) causes a small, dose-dependent, reversible pulmonary vasodilation (Tucker et al., 1976). In addition, hyperoxia decreases pulmonary reactivity to several pressor stimuli (Tucker et al., 1976), while hypoxia enhances it (Lonigro and Dawson, 1975).

This chapter will deal with the mechanisms by which acute, normobaric hyperoxia and hypoxia alter pulmonary vascular tone and reactivity. The effects of chronic exposure to hyperoxia and hypoxia are considered in Chapter 16. Hyperbaric effects are discussed in Chapter 7.

II. Hyperoxia

Oxygen is the divalent cation that fuels aerobic metabolism and makes the production of large quantities of high-energy triphosphates possible in all advanced life forms. Joseph Priestly recognized the potential for oxygen to function as both a physiologic and a toxic substance:

> Though pure dephlogestated air might be very useful in medicine, it might not be so proper for us in the usual healthy state of the body; for, as a candle burns so much faster in dephlogestated air, so we might, as may be said, live out too fast and the animal powers be too soon exhausted.*

Since Priestly's time, oxygen has become a widely used therapeutic agent, and as the dose and duration of oxygen supplementation has increased it has become clear that it can cause toxicity and even death in most species (Deneke and Fanburg, 1980; White et al., 1986). Since the lung is the only visceral organ that interfaces directly with the environment, it is not surprising that the effects of hyperoxia are predominantly seen in the lung (Deneke and Fanburg, 1980; Turrens et al., 1982b).

The unique circumstances that occur in the lung as a result of hyperoxic ventilation may reflect differences in the source of oxygen sensed by the pulmonary vasculature (alveolar oxygen) as opposed to the systemic vessels (oxyhemoglobin plus dissolved oxygen). Inhalation of 100% oxygen at sea level results in an alveolar oxygen tension that exceeds 700 mmHg. This is probably the level of oxygen "seen" by the small, precapillary, muscular arteries that regulate pulmonary vascular resistance in response to alveolar oxygen tension (Conhaim and Staub, 1980; Jameson, 1964; Sobol et al., 1963). Staub demonstrated that these small arteries are located within and adjacent to terminal respiratory units, placing them in an anatomically suitable site to permit direct oxygenation from the alveolus (Staub, 1963). Several investigators, using different techniques, have demonstrated rapid transfer of oxygen to these precapillary vessels from the alveolus (Conhaim and Staub, 1980; Jameson, 1964; Sobol et al., 1963).

---

*Quoted in Nunn (1985).

Systemic organs are relatively protected from hyperoxia, in part because they are oxygenated by the blood and in part because of the loss of oxygen that occurs as blood progresses to the small systemic arteries that regulate vascular tone (Duling and Berne, 1970). Hemoglobin is 96-98% saturated during normoxia, and hyperoxia adds primarily a small amount of dissolved oxygen to the systemically available pool. The mixed venous PO_2, which approximates the oxygen level seen in most systemic organs, remains less than 50 mmHg during hyperoxia (Turrens et al., 1982b). Although the oxygen tensions seen by small pulmonary arteries are probably much higher than those found in small systemic arteries at all levels of alveolar oxygen tension, there is also some evidence that the vessels intrinsically differ in their response to oxygen (Harder et al., 1985a) and elevation of transmural pressure (Davis et al., 1981). Lombard et al. (1986) have shown that whereas isolated small pulmonary arteries depolarize in response to hypoxia, systemic arteries hyperpolarize or display a decreased frequency of spontaneous depolarizations at low oxygen tensions.

A. The Biochemistry of Hyperoxia

Prior to reviewing the hemodynamic manifestations of hyperoxia in the lung, it is useful to consider the biochemical changes that precede and may explain the alterations in vascular reactivity. Much of the information on the biology of hyperoxia derives from studies of oxygen toxicity. Gerschmann et al. (1954) noted similarities between the pulmonary effects of hyperoxia and x-irradiation. They postulated a common mechanism of injury, namely, generation of oxygen-based free radicals in the lung. The major reactive oxygen metabolites produced in the lung during hyperoxia are superoxide anion O_2- and hydrogen peroxide (H_2O_2) (Freeman et al., 1982; Turrens et al., 1982a; Crapo and Tierney, 1974). Initially, these oxygen species were considered to be toxic and their role, in all cases, to be one of causing cell damage. The realization that oxygen radicals are produced in the course of numerous physiologic reactions, such as oxidative phosphorylation (Freeman et al., 1982) and arachidonic acid metabolism (Kontos et al., 1985), and that they exist in the healthy lung organelles in measurable levels (Yusa et al., 1984) caused a reconsideration of their role (Archer et al., 1986c).

Bishop et al. (1984) measured the effect of oxygen tension on the production of oxygen radicals in lung homogenates. They used potassium cyanide to inhibit the quadravalent reduction of oxygen by the electron transport chain. The residual utilization of oxygen ("cyanide-resistant respiration") is believed to reflect the generation of partially reduced oxygen species (e.g., O_2-, and H_2O_2). Cyanide-resistant respiration increased linearly with the ambient oxygen tension. Under normoxic conditions, 5% of total respiration was cyanide resistant, while this fraction increased to 20% with hyperoxia. Freeman et al. (1982) demonstrated an increase in cyanide-resistant respiration, from 7 to 17% of total respiration, as the ambient 0_2 was increased from room air to 80%. They also found acute increases in lung thiobarbituric acid levels, which could be blocked by addition of superoxide dismutase or catalase. This implies that acute hyperoxic ventilation can increase lung radical production and cause lipid peroxidation. Removal of oxygen from the system caused radical production to fall to unmeasurable levels in rat lung mitochondria (Turrens et al., 1982b). Elevated levels of oxygen radical production are sustained with prolonged hyperoxia. Freeman et al. (1982) noted that cyanide-resistant respiration was still enhanced after 7 days exposure of the rat to an inspired oxygen concentration (Fi_{02}) of 0.85. The lung responds to this sublethal oxidant stress by increasing levels of key antioxidant enzymes (e.g., glutathione peroxidase, catalase, superoxide dismutase) (Tierney et al., 1977). Rats in whom tolerance to hyperoxia has been induced by sublethal exposure to intermittent or moderate hyperoxia have lung levels of superoxide dismutase and glutathione peroxidase two to five times those of control animals (Frank et al., 1978; Kimball et al., 1976; Rister and Bachner, 1976). Warshaw et al. (1985) have found increased levels of glutathione and antioxidant enzymes in human lung explants cultured in a hyperoxic environment.

Animals that, due to immaturity or species variation, cannot induce production of catalase or superoxide dismutase in response to hyperoxia tend to be intolerant to hyperoxia and have a higher mortality rate than animals that can respond appropriately (Deneke and Fanburg, 1980; Frank et al., 1978). Similarly, protection from the lethal effects of inhaling 100% oxygen can be provided by exposing the animal to a sublethal oxidant stress (e.g., endotoxin or 80% oxygen inhalation) prior to the more severe hyperoxia (Crapo and Tierney, 1974). This protection apparently relies on the ability of the milder stress to "prime" the cell and allow it to reset its antioxidant enzyme "set point" to accommodate a higher level of oxygen radicals while avoiding cell damage.

Where are oxygen radicals being generated in the lung? Turrens et al. (1982b) found that the lung mitochondria and submitochondrial particles from rats and pigs had the ability to generate oxygen radicals in response to hyperoxia.

Yusa et al. (1984) showed that NADH-dependent superoxide generation increased from 0 to 2.21±0.11 nmol/min per milligram of protein in porcine lung cell nuclei during "exposure to 100% oxygen." NADPH-dependent 0_2 generation increased to 0.45±0.09 nmol/min per milligram of protein with 100% oxygen in these microsomes. Nuclear 0_2^- generation also increased in hepatocyte nuclei during hyperoxia in this experiment. Compared to hepatocytes, lung cells are always relatively hyperoxic in vivo. Turrens et al. (1982b) have stated that during normoxia the lung mitochondria exist at a PO_2 of 100-110 mmHg, while exposure to 100% O_2 increases this level to 670 mmHg. Other organs have mitochondrial PO_2 levels of 40-50 mmHg, and thus the lung would be expected to be the primary site of radical generation during exposure to acute or chronic hyperoxia. Although oxygen radicals can result from many reactions (arachidonate metabolism, cytochrome P-450 activity, phagocytosis, metabolism of xenobiotics), the bulk of molecular oxygen used by the cell is employed in the mitochondria in the tightly coupled pathways of oxidative phosphorylation and the electron transport chain. It therefore seems probable, although not certain, that the majority of the H_2O_2 and superoxide anion produced in the lung in response to varying oxygen tensions results from these mitochondrial processes. Freeman and Crapo (1981) found that cyanide-resistant respiration accounted for 18% of total respiration during hyperoxia and that 15 ± 3% of this could be attributed to a mitochondrial source. They found that hyperoxia causes production of H_2O_2, most of which derives from dismutation of O_2^- produced in the mitochondria by autooxidation of components of the electron transport chain (Freeman and Crapo, 1981). Turrens et al. (1982b) identified two sites in the electron transport chain at which oxygen radicals could be generated: (1) NADH dehydrogenase complex and (2) the ubiquinone-cytochrome b region. The mitochondrion is rich in superoxide dismutase (SOD), an enzyme that greatly accelerates the conversion of superoxide anion to H_2O_2, and catalase, which converts H_2O_2 to H_2O (Fig. 1). It makes sense teleologically to put superoxide dismutase in the mitochondria only if there is a reasonable expectation that they will need to dismute superoxide. Indeed, Kimura et al. (1983) found that exposure of neonatal rats to 100% O_2 caused reversible inhibition of oxidative phosphorylation, which occurred in the absence of significant pulmonary edema. This study suggests that the lung mitochondria may be a victim of their own metabolic function during hyperoxia by generating levels of oxygen radical beyond the "buffering" capacity of the available levels of antioxidant enzyme.

Understanding of the hemodynamic effects of oxygen radicals generated endogenously, in response to hyperoxia, has been greatly facilitated by the use of drugs that generate similar partially reduced oxygen metabolites. Examples of such drugs include xanthine/xanthine oxidase (X/XO) (Weir et al., 1985), which generates $O_2^{\cdot}$ (Fig. 2); glucose/glucose oxidase (G/GO), which produces H_2O_2 (Burghuber et al., 1984); and tert-butylhydroperoxide, which itself is similar to H_2O_2 (Reeves et al., 1985; Weir and Will, 1982).

The effects of oxygen radicals on vascular tone have been the subject of considerable controversy in the literature. Depending on dose, route of administration, type of radical administered, and, possibly, vessel type, oxygen radicals can cause vasodilatation (Weir et al., 1985), vascular paresis (Kontos et al., 1983), vasoconstriction (Tate et al., 1984, or a mixed response (Rosenblum, 1983). Tate et al. (1984) found that X/XO caused pulmonary vasoconstriction and pulmonary edema within 30 min of administration. The dose of X/XO used

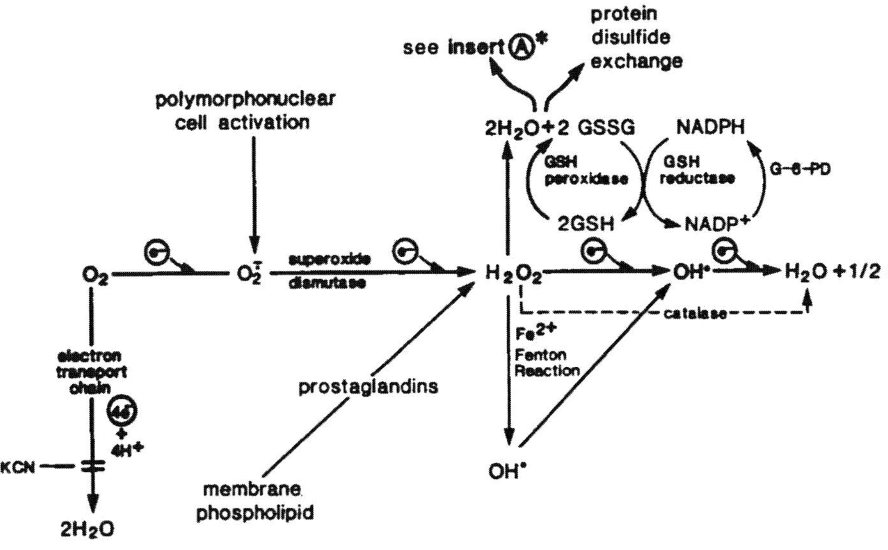

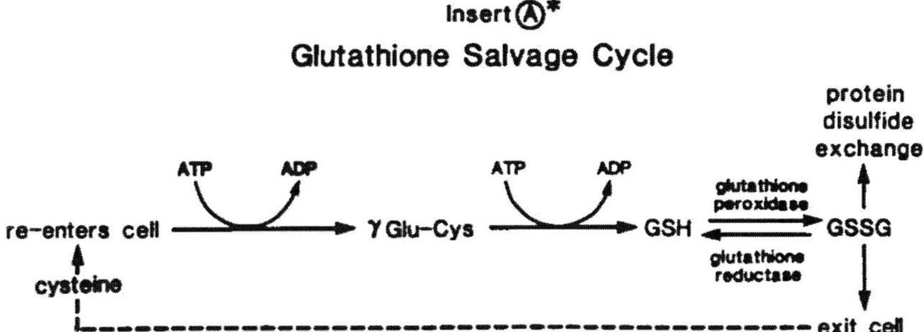

Figure 1 Schematic representation of physiologic sources of partially reduced oxygen species and homeostatic mechanisms that regulate the redox status of the cell. (From Archer et al., 1986c.)

in their study was 20 times greater than was used in the protocol of Weir et al. (1985).

Kontos et al. (1983) and Kontos (1985) reported vasodilatation and irreversible vascular paresis in cerebral vessels exposed to topically applied oxygen radicals. The loss of vascular reactivity was associated with structural damage to the endothelium. These changes could be prevented by prior administration of antioxidants. Rosenblum (1983) found that the effect of oxygen radicals on the

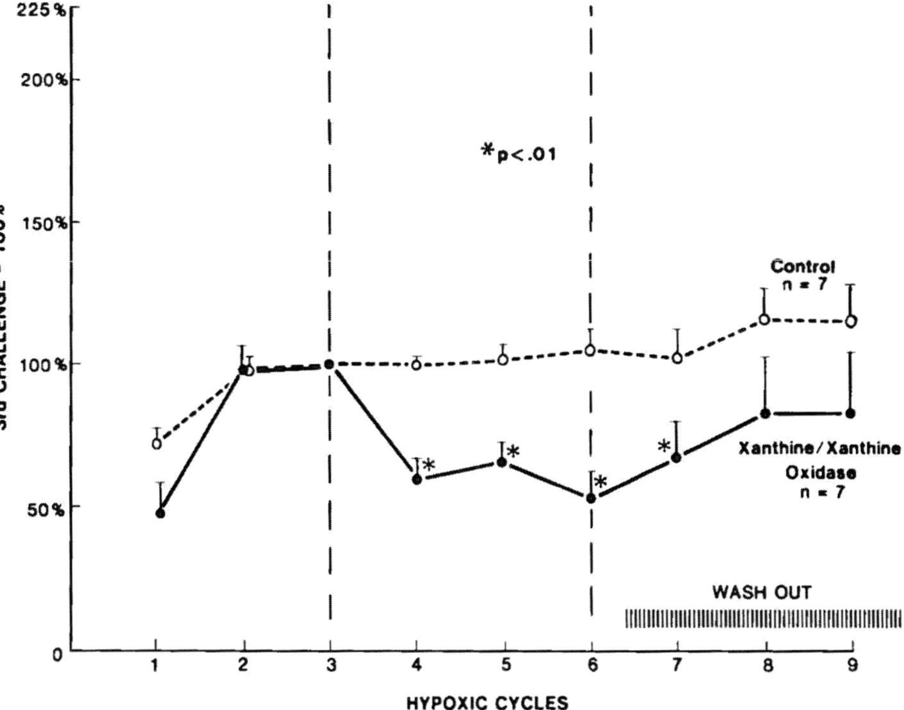

Figure 2 Xanthine/xanthine oxidase reduces the pressor response to hypoxia in isolated perfused rat lungs. The numbers on the horizontal axis represent individual hypoxic challenges. Xanthine/xanthine oxidase was added to the perfusate after the third challenge. The increase in pulmonary arterial pressure (Y axis) caused by the third challenge was defined as 100%. (From Archer et al., 1986c.)

vascular reactivity of mouse pial vessels differed according to the dose administered. Higher doses of acetaldehyde/xanthine oxidase caused initial vasoconstriction followed by reversible vasodilatation, while lower doses resulted in only the vasodilatory phase of the response. Unlike Kontos's model, Rosenblum's system utilized continuous suffusion of the brain surface with fresh solution during the course of the experiment, thereby preventing the accumulation of toxic levels of oxygen metabolites. The effects of the radicals could be blocked by mannitol, catalase, or superoxide dismutase (Rosenblum, 1983). It appears to be the amount of radical administered rather than the means of generation of the radicals that determines the vascular effects. Lamb and Webb (1984) decreased the vascular reactivity of several types of systemic arteries to KCl and norepinephrine using radicals generated by electrical stimulation. As with X/XO-generated radicals, the vasoinhibitory effects of electrically generated radicals could be inhibited by SOD or CAT.

Each of these sources of oxygen radicals will reverse hypoxic pulmonary vasoconstriction and decrease pulmonary vascular reactivity to various pressors. If given in small enough doses, they accomplish these effects without causing overt lung toxicity or an increase in lung wet/dry weight ratio (Reeves et al., 1985; Weir and Will, 1982). Higher doses of these drugs cause pulmonary edema, lipid peroxidation, and pulmonary vasoconstriction (Tate et al., 1984). In certain cases there is evidence that the pulmonary vasoconstriction induced by high doses of an oxidant (e.g., tert-butylhydroperoxide) occurs via a different mechanism than the low-dose vasodilatory effects of the same drug. Farrukh et al. (1985), for example, found that the pulmonary pressor response to tert-butylhydroperoxide was due to thromboxane release, while other studies (Weir and Will, 1982), using low-dose tert-butylhydroperoxide, showed that cyclo-oxygenase blockade did not prevent the inhibition of hypoxic pulmonary vasoconstriction. At high doses, oxidants may cause nonspecific damage that could mask their potentially physiological role in modulating pulmonary vascular tone. It is evident from the preceding discussion that radicals are not only present in the lung but furthermore may, like radical-generating drugs, alter pulmonary vascular tone.

B. The Effects of Hyperoxia on Pulmonary Vascular Reactivity

During normoxic ventilation, the pulmonary vascular bed is maintained in a relatively relaxed state with a mean pulmonary arterial pressure (PAP) of 13 ± 4 mmHg (SD) and pulmonary vascular resistance (PVR) of 1.5 ± 0.6 mmHg/liter-min in healthy young adults (Reeves and Groves, 1984). Hyperoxia can cause a modest but consistent fall in both variables (Tucker et al., 1976). This acute response is not associated with significant alterations of cardiac output or systemic blood pressure. Madden et al. (1985) demonstrated that hyperoxia (tissue bath $PO_2 > 300$ mmHg) decreased vascular tone in isolated small pulmonary arteries (Fig. 3). Micropuncture studies revealed a direct, oxygen tension-dependent effect on the membrane potential of these vessels. Hyperoxia caused an increase in membrane potential and a decrease in the frequency of the action potentials seen at lower oxygen tension (Madden et al., 1985) (Fig. 4).

Historically, oxygen was considered a specific pulmonary vasodilator and was thought only to counteract the constriction induced by hypoxia. Lonigro and Dawson (1975) found, to the contrary, that the pulmonary pressor response to prostaglandin $F_{2\alpha}$ in the cat decreased by mild hyperoxia and enhanced by hypoxia. This vasoinhibitory effect of oxygen did not appear to reflect non-specific vascular toxicity, since the constrictor responses to serotonin and norepinephrine were preserved. Reeves et al. (1972) had previously noted de-

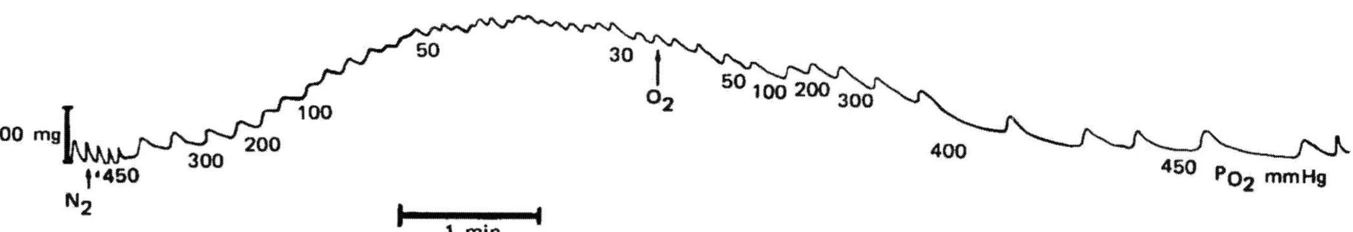

Figure 3 Original chart record depicting O_2-dependent contraction and relaxation from a segment of small (250 μm outer diameter) pulmonary artery. As can be seen, spontaneous rhythmic activity occurs throughout this particular experiment. Active forced development initially occurs at a PO_2 of 250-300 mmHg. Note the increase in duration of the rhythmic components as PO_2 begins to fall. The steepest portion of the curve falls between 150 and 50 mmHg. After sustained periods of low PO_2 (50 to 30 mmHg), one observes a small reduction in active force generation. When PO_2 is elevated, there is a small "rebound" contraction prior to O_2-dependent relaxation. (From Hearder et al., 1985.)

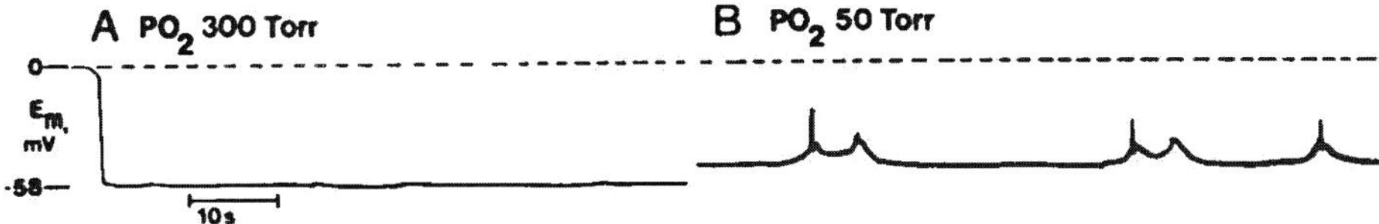

Figure 4 Original chart records of intracellular membrane potential (E_m) measurments from a small (260 μm O.D.) pulmonary artery pressurized to 10 mmHg. (A) Record depicting a stable E_m of -54 mV when the preparation is suffused with solutions containing an 0_2 tension of 300 mmHg. (B) Record depicting membrane depolarization and action potential generation in the same cell (same impalement) 6 min after reduction of $P0_2$ to 50 mmHg. Time and voltage calibrations are the same in both panels. (From Harder et al., 1985.)

creased pulmonary vasoconstriction in response to endotoxin in calves ventilated with 100% oxygen. Tucker and co-workers (1976) likewise found a decrease in sensitivity of the dog pulmonary vasculature to the constrictor effects of prostaglandin F_{2a} during acute hyperoxic ventilation. The reactivity of the vascular bed to 5-hydroxytryptamine was not reduced by hyperoxia in this study.

If inhalation of pure oxygen is contained for several days, pulmonary vascular reactivity is lost to many physiologic (e.g., hypoxia) and pharmacologic (e.g., PGF_{2a}, thromboxane, PGH_2) constrictor stimuli. This phenomenon, which is called vascular paresis, has been demonstrated in rats (Newman et al., 1981), sheep (Newman et al., 1983), and rabbits (Gurtner et al., 1985). Newman et al. (1981) noted a diminished pressor response to acute hypoxia in lungs from rats exposed to 100% oxygen for 48 hr. They observed restoration of reactivity to hypoxia following administration of meclofenamate and postulated that hyperoxia resulted in elaboration of a vasodilatory prostanoid. Subsequently, Newman et al. (1983) showed that hypoxic pulmonary vasoconstriction was impaired in awake sheep by hyperoxia, in a manner that varied directly with the duration of hyperoxia and that could not be attributed to a vasodilatory prostaglandin. Gurtner et al. (1985) found that hyperoxic vascular paresis in the rabbit lung could be inhibited by pretreatment of the animal with antioxidants (butylated hydroxytoluene or vitamin E). They noted that hyperoxia resulted in impaired pulmonary vasoconstriction in response to endogenous thromboxane and speculated that this paresis resulted from oxygen radicals injuring "the normal contractile mechanism of pulmonary vascular smooth muscle." This suggests that while acute hyperoxia causes selective reversible decreases in vascular reactivity, more prolonged inhalation causes a generalized, nonspecific loss of responsiveness.

There are a number of mechanisms by which hyperoxia might cause pulmonary vascular paresis. Reduced pulmonary reactivity might result from indirect effects of oxygen on the lung at a site removed from the vessel, such as release and/or synthesis of a vasodilator substance. Alternatively, hyperoxia might act directly on the vessel through changes in the function of the endothelium or vascular smooth muscle cells. Each possibility will be considered in turn.

Indirect Effects of Hyperoxia

The report of the generation of a vasodilatory prostanoid following hyperoxic ventilation of rats (Newman et al., 1981) would support the indirect hypothesis for the mechanism of vascular paresis. However, most studies of hyperoxic paresis show that the phenomenon persists despite adequate cyclooxygenase blockade (Gurtner et al., 1985). There are no other reports of circulating vasodilators that are induced by hyperoxia.

Direct Effects of Hyperoxia

There is ample evidence of a direct effect of hyperoxia on endothelial cell structure and function in the hyperoxic lung. Vader et al. (1981) demonstrated impaired catabolism of prostaglandins in vivo and in vitro in hyperoxic lungs. Lung endothelial angiotensin converting enzyme (ACE) activity is also depressed by hyperoxia in vitro (Gillis and Catravas, 1982). Toivonen et al. (1981) found that 36 hr of hyperoxic ventilation (FiO^2 0.95) increased the survival of prostaglandin E_2 in isolated perfused rat lungs by 300%. Peptide metabolism (Angiotensin II, bradykinin) was less sensitive to elevated levels of inspired oxygen but was impaired after 48 hr of hyperoxia. The metabolism of both the prostanoids and peptides returned to normal shortly after return to room air. In contrast, Sventek and Zambraski (1985) found that 8 hr of hyperoxia in the dog did not alter the systemic reactivity of prostaglandin E_2 and enhanced the effects of angiotensin I and II on mean systemic arterial pressure. Block et al. (1986) explored the mechanism by which hyperoxia alters the metabolic processing of vasoactive substances by the pulmonary endothelium. They found that hyperoxia altered the membrane fluidity of the endothelial cell but did not alter the cellular ATP content or membrane Na^+/K^+ATPase activity. They postulated that some metabolite of oxygen (e.g., an oxygen radical) might alter the fluidity of the endothelium by inducing peroxidation of key membrane lipids. Membrane fluidity is felt to be important in facilitating the internalization of various pressor substances and their precursors, and interference with this function could impair vascular reactivity. Superoxide anion has also been shown to alter the activity of endothelium-dependent relaxing factor elicited by activation of muscarinic receptors (e.g., by acetylcholine) (Rubanyi and Vanhoutte, 1986). Wolin and co-workers have suggested that oxygen radicals and/or hydrogen peroxide may cause pulmonary vasodilation by increasing vascular cyclic GMP levels (Wolin and Burke, 1987).

C. Summary

Acute hyperoxia decreases pulmonary vascular reactivity to certain constrictor agents. More prolonged exposure causes a generalized loss of vascular responsiveness to hypoxia, thromboxane, and other pressor agents. Evidence from in vitro studies shows that oxygen radicals are produced in the lungs in proportion to oxygen tension. Experiments using low doses of radical-generating enzyme/substrate pairs have shown that exogenous radicals can, like hyperoxia, decrease pulmonary vascular reactivity without causing overt lung toxicity. Antioxidants protect the pulmonary vascular reactivity from the effects of hyperoxia and radical-generating drugs. These findings suggest that endogenously produced oxygen radicals may modulate pulmonary vascular tone and reactivity in response to varying oxygen exposures.

III. Hypoxia

Hypoxic pulmonary vasoconstriction (HPV) is found in species as disparate as amphibians and humans (Shelton, 1970; Motley et al., 1947). Its function has been speculated to be twofold. In the fetus, the pulmonary vascular bed is a high-resistance circuit that carries very low flow. It is maintained in this state by active (and reversible) vasoconstriction. At birth, pulmonary vascular resistance falls rapidly due to a rise in alveolar oxygen tension and, to a lesser extent, the mechanical expansion of the lung (Cassin et al., 1964; Cook et al., 1963). HPV in utero could be useful in reducing perfusion of the fetal lung, whose activity is not crucial to survival. Although it has been argued that hypoxic pulmonary vasoconstriction is merely a fetal reflex that persists into adult life, HPV also serves a useful function in the mature animal. Localized areas of alveolar hypoxia, which occur in pneumonia, atelectasis, or chronic lung disease, result in localized pulmonary vasoconstriction (Zasslow et al., 1982). This diverts blood flow to adequately oxygenated areas of the lung and minimizes hypoxemia. Reversal of HPV in experimental models of pneumonia and atelectasis results in systemic hypoxemia (Colley et al., 1979; Hiser et al., 1975; Goldzimer et al., 1978). Hypoxic ventilation not only causes pulmonary vasoconstriction but also enhances the pressor response to many constrictor substances (Tucker et al., 1976). Hypoxia has also been shown to impair the spontaneous vasodilatation that follows vasoconstriction caused by substances such as angiotensin II, KCl, and bradykinin (Voelkel et al., 1981).

A. Hypoxic Pulmonary Vasoconstriction — Definition and Description

Although hypoxia-related pulmonary hypertension was noted as early as 1904 (Plumier, 1904) and acute hypoxic pulmonary vasoconstriction was described in detail in 1946 by von Euler and Liljestrand (von Euler and Liljestrand, 1946), the underlying mechanism by which alveolar oxygen tension alters pulmonary vascular tone remains obscure. However, certain key experiments have been performed in the intervening 40 years that allow definition, if not explanation, of the essential attributes of this phenomenon. These cardinal features of the pressor response provide criteria that must be satisifed by any putative mediator of hypoxic pulmonary vasconstriction. The criteria will be listed, and then the experimental evidence for their inclusion will be discussed.

1. *Site*: HPV is intrinsic to the lung and occurs in isolated lungs (even those perfused without blood) (McMurtry et al., 1976) and small isolated pulmonary arteries (<300 μm) (Madden et al., 1985)
2. *Threshold*: HPV occurs at fairly high FiO_2 (PaO_2 up to 55 mmHg) (Fig. 3) and may be decreased by severe hypoxia or anoxia (Sylvester et al., 1980). HPV exhibits a rapid onset (1-4 min) and recovery (1-3 min) (Peake et al., 1981).
3. *Requirement for extracellular calcium*: HPV is very sensitive to calcium channel antagonists (e.g., nifedipine, nisoldipine) (Archer et al., 1985) and agonists (e.g. BAY K 9644) (McMurtry, 1985; Tollins et al., 1986), being inhibited by the former and enhanced by the latter (Fig. 5).
4. *Relationship to depolarization of plasma membrane*: Hypoxia decreases the resting membrane potential of isolated small pulmonary arteries with an associated generation of action potentials (Madden et al., 1985) (Fig. 4).

These hallmarks of HPV are of value in sifting through the many agents that cause pulmonary vasoconstriction and may even modify hypoxic pulmonary vasoconstriction but are not involved in the fundamental transduction of alveolar oxygen tension into pulmonary vascular tone.

Hypoxic pulmonary vasoconstriction results from constriction of small, muscular pulmonary arteries (several hundred micrometers in diameter) in response to reduced alveolar oxygen tension. This was initially suggested by von Euler and Liljestrand (1946) and confirmed by Kato and Staub (1966), who used a rapid freeze technique to examine the caliber of various vascular components (arteries, capillaries, veins) during HPV. They found that hypoxia primarily constricted small muscular arteries in the region of the terminal respiratory units. This site was confirmed by analysis of pulmonary arteriograms in the cat (Shirai et al., 1986) and by the demonstration of hypoxic vasoconstriction primarily in 30-200 μm pulmonary arteries in the bullfrog lung (Koyama and Horimoto, 1983). The direct micropuncture studies of Nagasaka et al. (1984) demonstrated a predominant role for the muscular precapillary artery in

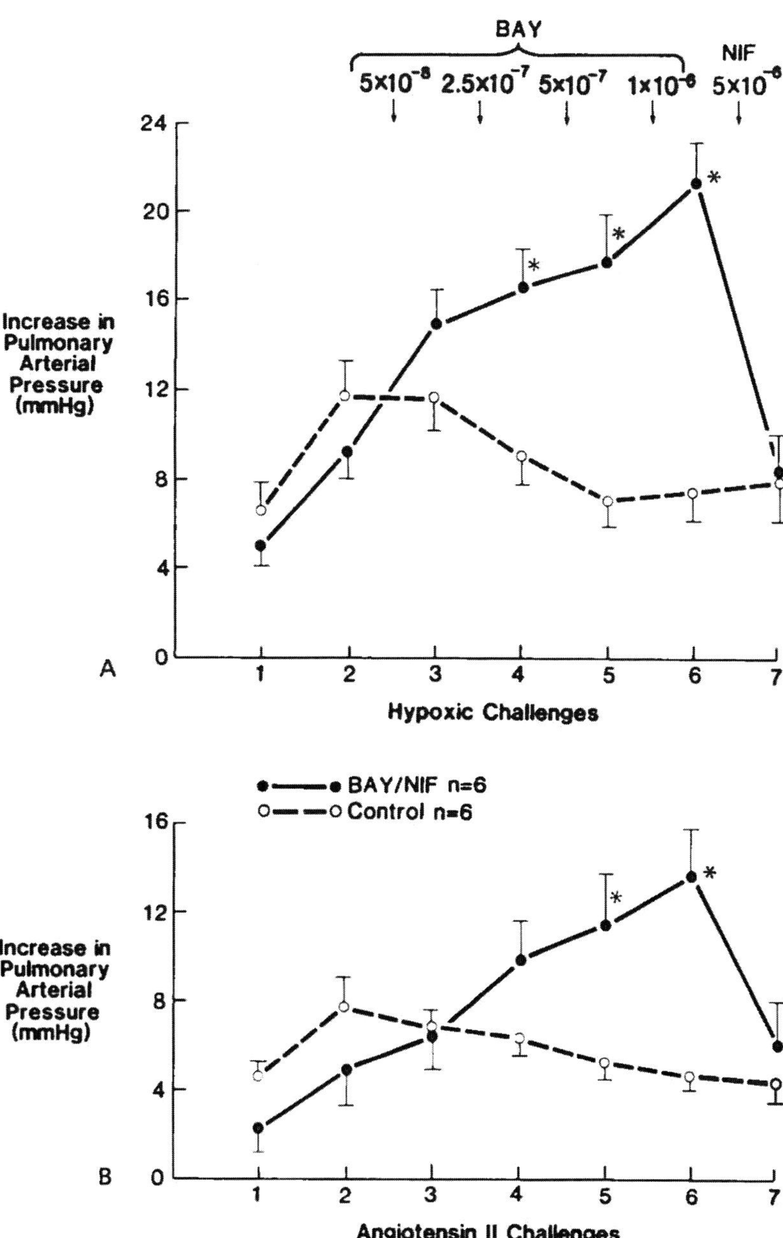

BAY
NIF
5x10⁻⁸ 2.5x10⁻⁷ 5x10⁻⁷ 1x10⁻⁶ 5x10⁻⁶
Increase in Pulmonary Arterial Pressure (mmHg)
0
4
8
12
16
20
24
A
1 2 3 4 5 6 7
Hypoxic Challenges
BAY/NIF n=6
Control n=6
Increase in Pulmonary Arterial Pressure (mmHg)
0
4
8
12
16
B
1 2 3 4 5 6 7
Angiotensin II Challenges

Figure 5

the development of the hypoxic pressor response. They showed a drop in pulmonary arterial pressure from 28.3 ± 2.6 mmHg in the main pulmonary artery to 19.0 ± 3.7 mmHg in the arteriole (<50 μm vessel). The remainder of the pressure drop across the pulmonary circuit (10 mmHg) occurs in the capillaries and veins. The importance of this information is frequently overlooked, as evidenced by the large number of experiments that have attempted to explore HPV using models that studied the reactivity of large pulmonary arteries. These tissues are easily harvested, but conclusions regarding the reactivity of the precapillary arteries probably should not be drawn from the response of these vessels, which do not actively participate in HPV. Madden et al. (1985), for example, found that isolated pulmonary arteries greater than 500 μm in diameter did not constrict in response to hypoxia.

The characteristics of the hypoxic pressor response are somewhat influenced by the volume of lung that is rendered hypoxic. Marshall and Marshall (1980) demonstrated an inverse relationship between the amount of lung made hypoxic and the magnitude of the pressor response. If the area of alveolar hypoxia is localized, the pulmonary vasoconstriction is also restricted to that area. This results in diversion of blood from areas of alveolar hypoxia to better oxygenated alveoli, which optimizes systemic oxygen supply without increasing the pulmonary arterial pressure. This focal response, as might occur with atelectasis, does not fatigue with time. In contrast, ventilation of the entire lung with hypoxic gas causes generalized constriction of the small pulmonary arteries with an attendant decrease in lung blood volume. There is diversion of blood to the lung apices, and the net pulmonary arterial pressure rises. In some species (e.g., the dog), but not all, the hypoxic pressor response to diffuse hypoxia fades with time (Tucker and Reeves, 1975). The adaptive value of such a generalized response is obscure, and this may not be the situation for which HPV was "designed" in the adult. Zasslow et al. (1982) expressed the pressor response to hypoxia as an index relating flow through the segment of lung made hypoxic to the cardiac output. Like the Marshalls, they found that small hypoxic segments caused HPV without increasing pulmonary arterial pressure but noted no diminution of the HPV index with increasing size of the test segment. Instead, as segment size was increased, the manifestation of HPV changed from redistribution of pulmonary blood flow to elevation of pulmonary arterial pressure.

Figure 5 (A) Pressor responses to repeated hypoxic challenges in six control rat lungs (open circles) are compared with responses in six lungs given increasing doses of BAY K 8644 (closed circles). Nifedipine (NIF) was given to BAY rats prior to last challenge. (B) Pressor responses to repeated bolus injections of angiotensin II (0.15 μg) in control (open circles) and BAY (closed circles) rats. Bath concentrations (M) of BAY and nifedipine are shown at top. *$P < 0.05$ for difference between control and BAY-treated lungs. (From Tollins et al., 1986).

Hauge (1969) and subsequently Marshall and Marshall (1983) demonstrated that the most important stimulus for hypoxic pulmonary vasoconstriction is alveolar oxygen tension rather than the mixed venous O_2 saturation of pulmonary arterial blood. They showed that at alveolar oxygen tensions in excess of 60 mmHg, mixed venous O_2 was relatively unimportant, while as alveolar O_2 falls, the mixed venous oxygen concentration could significantly contribute to pulmonary vasoconstriction. Hughes and Rubin (1984) showed, in the open-chest dog, that both mixed venous and alveolar oxygen tension exerted direct effects on vascular tone but that the relative influence of mixed venous oxygen tension was dependent on alveolar oxygen tension, being significant only at low levels of alveolar oxygen tension. Pease et al. (1982) speculated that since mixed venous hypoxemia caused pulmonary vasoconstriction only when alveolar oxygen tension was less than 50 mmHg, intravascular hypoxemia was acting primarily to cause alveolar hypoxia. Although there is some dissent, it appears that mixed venous oxygen tension plays a role in determining pulmonary vascular resistance in certain situations. Thus, in healthy individuals, at physiologic levels of hypoxia, HPV largely reflects alveolar hypoxia, while in patients with severe alveolar hypoxia (e.g., those with chronic obstructive lung disease) mixed venous O_2 saturation may contribute significantly to the pressor response.

The finding that HPV is preserved in pulmonary arteries in vitro was instrumental in allowing assessment of the biochemistry of HPV and the role of the blood and autonomic nervous system in this response. Lloyd (1965) described HPV in isolated dog lungs and the constriction of large isolated pulmonary artery strips in response to hypoxia. Hauge (1969) demonstrated hypoxic pulmonary vasoconstriction in the isolated perfused rat lung. McMurtry et al. (1976) noted inhibition of HPV in rat lungs by verapamil, a calcium channel inhibitor. More recently, Harder and Madden were able to isolate small pulmonary arteries (<300 μm) from cat lung and show reversible constriction in response to hypoxia (Harder et al., 1985). They also found that this constricting response could be blocked by verapamil. These findings suggest that the blood, autonomic nervous system, and lung parenchyma are not essential to HPV. They can, however, play a significant role in modulating pulmonary pressure and reactivity in vivo.

It has long been debated whether there are intrinsic differences between pulmonary and systemic arteries in regard to their reactivity to oxygen tension. Pulmonary arteries respond to alveolar hypoxia with constriction, while most systemic vessels dilate in response to hypoxemia. Lombard et al. (1986) showed that isolated systemic vessels display membrane hyperpolarization and loss of spontaneous action potentials on exposure to hypoxia, while similarly exposed pulmonary arteries display depolarization and increased frequency of action potentials as assessed by direct micropuncture of isolated small arteries. It has also been found that explanted pulmonary arteries placed in the hamster cheek pouch display different responses to increases in transmural pressure at varying oxygen tensions compared to adjacent systemic vessels. However, a pressor response to hypoxia was not found in either vessel type (Davis et al., 1981). Although it appears that there may be intrinsic differences in the response of the systemic and pulmonary arteries to oxygen tension, the basis for the difference is unknown. It is possible that the vessels are conditioned to respond differently to oxygen due to the quite different oxygen tension to which each is normally exposed (see Sec. II) Block et al. (1986) have shown, for example, higher levels of antioxidant enzymes in endothelial cells from pulmonary arteries than those from aortas. If O_2 radicals or cellular redox status are of importance in regulating vascular tone, as discussed in the hyperoxia section, then such differences could result in ambient O_2 radical availability at any given FiO_2 varying between systemic and pulmonary arteries.

Hypoxia not only causes pulmonary vasoconstriction but also enhances the constrictor effects of various pressor substances (e.g., $PGF_{2\alpha}$) (Tucker et al., 1976). Lonigro and Dawson (1975) showed that each of a number of pulmonary pressors had an optimal P_AO_2 for induction of maximal pulmonary vasoconstriction; however, in general, each agonist had its constrictor effects optimized by hypoxia and minimized by hyperoxia. The mechanism for this potentiating effect of hypoxia is uncertain but might be related to partial depolarization of the vascular smooth muscle.

B. Mechanisms of Hypoxic Pulmonary Vasoconstriction

Introduction

The search for the mechanism of HPV has proceeded along two dissimilar lines, with some investigators searching for an indirect action of hypoxia on the lung (e.g., release of a constrictor substance) and others examining direct effects of oxygen on the tone of the small pulmonary artery. The investigation of the mechanism of HPV has been the subject of several recent reviews (Archer et al., 1986c; Voelkel, 1986). The "indirect action hypothesis" states that hypoxia causes the synthesis and/or release of a constrictor substance external to the vascular smooth muscle that is specific for, or localized to, the pulmonary vascular bed. Candidates that have come and gone include histamine, bradykinin, serotonin, angiotensin II, prostaglandins, and products of the autonomic nervous sytem. Each has been able to cause pulmonary vasoconstriction, but none proved essential for HPV (Archer et al., 1986c). These substances can modulate pulmonary vascular tone and may be important in certain disease states but are not essential to the coupling of oxygen and vascular tone. The only endogenous pressor substances currently being studied as potential mediators of HPV are the leukotrienes C_4 and D_4.

The direct action model of hypoxic pulmonary vasoconstriction cites an effect of oxygen on the pulmonary vascular bed without release of an extravascular constrictor substance. There are a number of apparently different theories as to how oxygen might exert a direct effect on vascular tone, but, as will be discussed, these hypotheses (e.g., phosphate potential, redox status) may be more interrelated than is initially apparent (Fig. 6).

Any of the theories that attempt to explain HPV must account for the delivery of cytoplasmic calcium to the contractile apparatus. Whether the proposed signal coupling oxygen tension and pulmonary vascular tone is adenosine triphosphate (ATP) level, phosphate potential (ATP/ADP + Pi), sulfhydryl redox status, oxygen radical flux, or leukotriene production, it must ultimately act by regulating the availability of calcium to the contractile apparatus or altering the sensitivity of the contractile apparatus to a given amount of calcium. For this reason, calcium homeostasis in vascular smooth muscle will be reviewed before discussing the individual theories of pulmonary tone control.

The Role of Calcium in Hypoxic Pulmonary Vasoconstriction

The contractile apparatus of vascular smooth muscle consists of actin and myosin filaments attached to dense bodies (instead of the Z line seen in skeletal muscle). Although the model for cellular excitation-contraction coupling is constantly increasing in complexity as new investigative tools become available (e.g., nuclear magnetic resonance spectroscopy, single-channel voltage clamps, calcium probes), for purposes of this discussion a simplified schematic will be used. Contraction of vascular smooth muscle occurs when calcium binds to calmodulin, resulting in activation of a light chain kinase that phosphorylates myosin light chains, allowing interaction of actin and myosin (Bohr, 1977). This information has been the subject of several recent reviews (Somlyo, 1985; Weiss, 1985). The sarcolemma is relatively impermeable to calcium, and the extracellular concentration of Ca^{2+} is 10,000-fold greater than that in the cytoplasm (Bohr, 1977). Intracellularly, calcium is distributed in compartments or "pools" (e.g., mitochondria, sarcoplasmic reticulum), which, through a dynamic equilibrium with each other and the transsarcolemmal Ca^{2+} flux, control the level of free Ca^{2+} ion in the cytoplasm. The relative importance of intracellular calcium compartments versus transmembrane calcium flux in regulation of vascular tone is an area of ongoing debate.

Calcium Regulation in Vascular Smooth Muscle

In reviewing calcium homeostasis in vascular smooth muscle, Van Breeman et al., (1980) emphasized the multiplicity of calcium pools within the cell and the variety of channels to facilitate entry of this divalent cation across an otherwise impermeable cell membrane. There are voltage-dependent channels that open

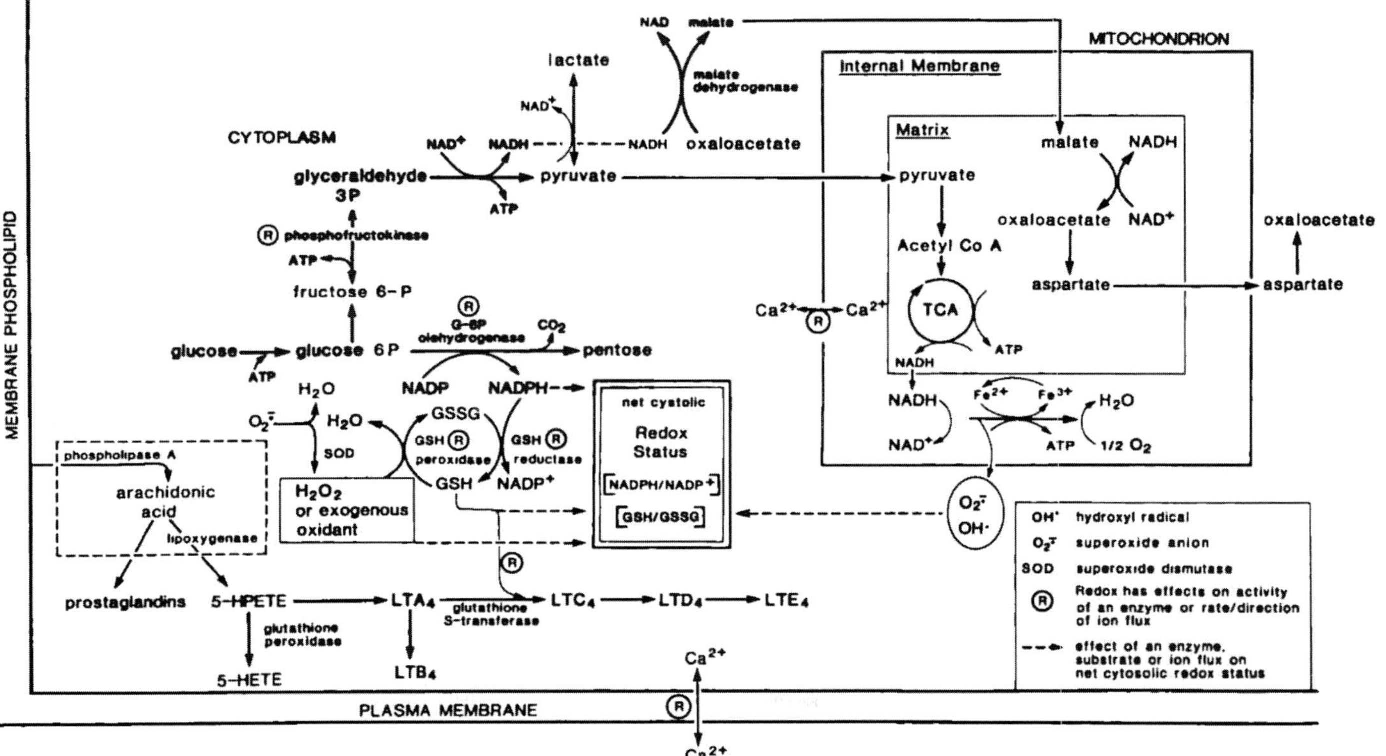

Figure 6 Relationship of cellular metabolism, calcium homeostasis, leukotriene synthesis, and oxygen radical formation to redox status NADPH/NADP, GSH/GSSG. (From Archer et al. 1986c.)

with depolarization of the membrane (presumably those activated by hypoxia or KCl) and receptor-activated channels (such as those activated by various catechols and prostanoids). The calcium flux through these two types of channels is additive, and each channel can be selectively inhibited. Angiotensin II, histamine, and prostaglandin F_{2a} cause vasoconstriction primarily through their effect on the receptor-activated channels and their ability to release a small pool of calcium located superficially within the smooth muscle cell.

In the relaxed state, essentially all calcium is sequestered (probably in the endoplasmic reticulum and mitochondria), leaving the contractile proteins inactive (Van Breeman et al., 1980). Removal of cytosolic calcium following vasoconstriction occurs by an ATP-requiring mechanism that translocates calcium to intra- and extracellular sites by routes independent of calcium inflow channels. The use of relatively specific inhibitors and promoters of calcium flux across the calcium channel has added to the understanding of the effects of oxygen tension on pulmonary vascular tone. The dihydropyridine derivatives include both calcium channel antagonists (e.g., nitrendipine, nifedipine) and agonists (BAY K 8644, CGP 28392). BAY K 8644 and CGP 28392 are agonists for the voltage-dependent calcium channel. BAY K 8644 dramatically enhances hypoxic pulmonary vasoconstriction without increasing normoxic pulmonary arterial pessure (McMurtry, 1985; Tollins et al., 1986) (Fig. 5). Kokubun and Reuter (1984) used patch clamping to show that these lipophilic agonists prolonged the mean "open time" of calcium channels in cardiac cells. In contrast to calcium influx initiated by β-adrenergic agonists, these calcium channel agonists promote calcium uptake without increasing intracellular cAMP (Kokubun and Reuter, 1984). Hess et al. (1984) found that nitrendipine, a calcium channel antagonist, increased the likelihood that the calcium channel would be found "closed," while BAY K 8644 caused the channel to spend more time in a "prolonged open-short closure" mode. The dihydropyridine nifedipine decreases HPV (Archer et al., 1985).

The study of the chemistry of agonist and antagonist dihydropyridines may provide clues to the mechanism by which oxygen tension influences the open/closed status of the channel. The molecular structures of BAY K 8644 and the antagonist dihydropyridines are very similar. How can their opposing hemodynamic effects be understood? Marinov and Saxon (1985) reported that calcium channel antagonists of several types differed from the agonist BAY K 8644 in their redox properties. BAY K 8644 and CGP 28392 acted as electron acceptors, while the calcium channel antagonists functioned as electron donors. Their "in vitro" study assessed the tendency of agonists and antagonists to (1) donate electrons (to the electron acceptors eosin and myoglobin) and, (2) acquire unpaired electrons (generated by flash photolysis). The ranking of calcium channel antagonist predisposition to donate electrons was: felodipine > ryocidil > diltiazem = verapamil. The order of ranking of potency as electron donors was the same as the potency ranking for these drugs with respect to their inhibition of smooth muscle contraction, suggesting that redox and hemodynamic properties of these compounds may be interrelated.

The calcium channel agonist, BAY K 8644, did not donate but rather tended to acquire electrons (act as an oxidant). This study suggests that the differences in the redox properties of the agents account for their opposing effects on the function of the calcium channel and raises the possibility that an oxygen radical (essentially an unpaired, reactive electron source) could, if generated in proximity to the calcium channel, modulate its activity. This concept will be discussed in detail later.

Due to the technical difficulties involved in measuring intracellular calcium levels, evidence that oxygen tension can modulate cytoplasmic calcium levels has been slow to accumulate. Many of the data have been obtained using indirect markers of calcium flux (e.g., static calcium levels, assessment of effects of calcium channel agonists/antagonists). Haack et al. (1974) demonstrated increased intracellular calcium levels in pulmonary vascular smooth muscle from rats and swine following exposure to chronic hypoxia. Oxygen tension-related changes in membrane calcium permeability have also been noted in other types of smooth muscle (Bohr, 1977). Bergofsky and Holtzman (1967) studied the effects of hypoxia on large systemic and pulmonary arteries as well as on pulmonary veins and found that the pulmonary arterial strip was unique in that it lost potassium and gained sodium in a reversible manner in response to hypoxia. This was felt to reflect a hypoxia-induced partial depolarization of smooth muscle cells that would favor pulmonary vasoconstriction. McMurtry et al. (1976) implicated the extracellular calcium pool as being critical in HPV by showing that verapamil, a calcium channel blocker, inhibited HPV in isolated rat lungs.

More direct assessment of the relationship of transmembrane calcium flow was provided by Harder et al. (1985a, b). They showed that the constrictions induced by hypoxia in isolated small pulmonary arteries were associated with a partial depolarization of the cell membrane and the development of action potentials. The decrease in membrane potential and occurrence of action potentials could be inhibited by verapamil, suggesting that the depolarization reflected altered calcium flux, presumably at the level of the calcium channel.

Despite the preceding evidence for the importance of transsarcolemmal calcium flux in HPV, uncertainty remains. Is extracellular calcium merely a "charge carrier" in the action potential? Does extracellular calcium act directly on the contractile apparatus or, perhaps, stimulate the release of intracellular stores?

There is very little information on the role of intracellular calcium pools in regulation of pulmonary vascular tone. Many of the data were derived from studies of other vascular smooth muscle. Somlyo (1985) noted that during brief contractions of isolated smooth muscle, $^{45}Ca^{2+}$ influx was below measurable levels. Bond et al. (1984a, b) found that there is enough releasable intracellular calcium in the guinea pig portal vein to cause vasoconstriction. Somlyo (1985) suggested that in view of the small amount of calcium influx with each action potential and the relatively high calcium requirements for initiation of contraction "it is unlikely that influx of Ca^{2+} makes a major contribution" to the calcium pool required for constriction.

If extracellular calcium were not the sole or major source of calcium for excitation-contraction coupling, where else might the critical Ca^{2+} pool be located? The mitochondria can certainly sequester calcium. However, they appear to function as a sink for calcium within the cell and probably do not regulate vascular smooth muscle cytoplasmic calcium levels under normal conditions. The role of intracellular calcium in regulating vascular tone is considered further in the redox section toward the end of the chapter.

While a final conclusion regarding the relative contribution of intracellular versus extracellular calcium to pulmonary tone cannot yet be made, the potential importance of this controversy is significant both to our understanding of HPV and to the planning of therapeutic intervention for treatment of pulmonary hypertension. Currently, the transmembrane flux of calcium through the voltage-dependent calcium channel is thought to be the most important factor in control of HPV. In the following section each proposed model of HPV should be examined for its ability to control calcium flux within and into the pulmonary vascular smooth muscle cell.

Indirect Mechanisms for Hypoxic Pulmonary Vasoconstriction

Autonomic Nervous System

The autonomic nervous system can modulate the reactivity and basal tone of the pulmonary vasculature (Barer, 1966; Porcelli and Bergofsky, 1973). However, innervation is not essential for HPV (Malik and Kidd, 1973), which is preserved in the denervated, isolated, perfused lung (McMurty et al., 1975).

Mediators

It has been suggested that endogenous vasoconstrictor substances may mediate HPV. Each of the following substances has been investigated as a potential mediator: histamine (Bergofsky, 1979; Haas and Bergofsky, 1972), angiotensin II (Berkov, 1974, McMurtry et al. (1984), 5-hydroxytryptamine (Glazier and Murray, 1971), prostaglandins (Said et al., 1974), and catecholamines (Barer, 1966). HPV persists in the presence of antihistamines (Hales and Kazemi, 1975; Tucker et al., 1976), saralasin (Hales and Kazemi, 1975), lysergic acid diethylamide (LSD) (Barer, 1966; Barer et al., 1978), meclofenamate (Vaage et al., 1975; Weir et al., 1976), and phentolamine (Malik and Kidd, 1973; Lewis et al., 1976). Consequently, it is unlikely that any one of the substances listed is the mediator of HPV.

Leukotrienes and Hypoxic Pulmonary Vasoconstriction

The only intrinsic pulmonary vasconstrictor substances currently under active consideration as possible mediators of hypoxic pulmonary vasoconstriction are the leukotrienes (LTC_4 and LTD_4 in particular) (Ahmed and Oliver, 1983; Morganroth et al. 1985). These lipoxygenase products were historically known as "slow-reacting substance of anaphylaxis." Several observations support the involvement of leukotrienes in HPV. Administration of LTC_4 or LTD_4 increases pulmonary vascular resistance in neonatal piglets and newborn lambs (Leffler et al., 1984; Yokochi et al., 1982). This is not a universal finding. LTD_4 (20 μg/kg) caused no pulmonary vasoconstriction in anesthetized monkeys (Casey et al., 1982) and only weakly constricted isolated human pulmonary arteries (Hanna et al., 1981; Schellenberg and Foster, 1984). The apparent differences probably reflect species variation in bioactivity of the leukotrienes. The mechanism by which leukotrienes cause pulmonary vasoconstriction is uncertain. In the awake adult sheep (Ahmed et al., 1985), leukotriene-induced pulmonary vasoconstriction could be blocked by indomethacin (Ahmed et al., 1985). Kadowitz and Hyman (1984) demonstrated a 50% decrease in LTD_4-induced pulmonary vasoconstriction in anesthetized sheep treated with a thromboxane synthetase inhibitor. The effects of LTD_4 and LTC_4 may be due in part or totally to release of constrictor prostaglandins in some species; however, Fedderson et al. (1983) found no evidence for release of thromboxane B_2 (TXB_2) or 6-keto-$F_{1\alpha}$ in isolated rat lungs treated with LTC_4 or LTE_4. In a recent review, Kulik and Lock (1987) indicated that further work needs to be done to establish how much of the constrictor effect of the leukotrienes is due to prostaglandin release, reasoning that since prostaglandins do not mediate HPV, agents that act through prostaglandin release would not mediate this response either.

Endogenous LTC_4 has been detected in lung lavage fluid from isolated perfused lungs during hypoxia but not following pulmonary vasoconstriction with potassium chloride (Morganroth et al., 1984b). Several studies have shown that hypoxia elevates pulmonary vascular resistance in a manner that can be blocked by inhibitors of leukotriene synthesis or receptor antagonists (Goldberg et al., 1985; Gottlieb et al., 1984; Morganroth et al., 1984a). Unfortunately, many of the leukotriene synthesis inhibitors are nonspecific and also function as antioxidants (Kulik and Lock, 1987). Leukotrienes are synthesized at several sites in the lung including the mast cells. These cells, which have a perivascular distribution, have been shown to degranulate during severe hypoxia (Haas and Bergofsky, 1972). Ahmed and co-workers (Ahmed and Oliver, 1983; Ahmed et al., 1982) have suggested that leukotrienes released from mast cells might be responsible for hypoxic pulmonary vasoconstriction. They showed that disodium cromoglycate DCG [3 mg/kg-min)] blocked HPV in unsedated ewes (Ahmed and Oliver, 1983). Similarly, FPL-527231 [2 mg/kg-min)], a leukotriene receptor antagonist, inhibited the development of HPV and reversed established HPV.

On the other hand, there is evidence that leukotrienes may not be essential for hypoxic pulmonary vasoconstriction. Rengo et al. (1979) found that although DCG (8 mg/kg) blocked HPV in the anesthetized dog, pretreatment with atropine prevented the effect of DCG, suggesting that at high dose the effects of DCG were vagally mediated. In addition, the occurrence of acute HPV and chronic hypoxic pulmonary hypertension in mice lacking mast cells indicates that mast cells per se are not essential for the pressor response in all species (Zhu et al., 1983).

While the preceding evidence refutes the requirement for mast cells in HPV, there are additional data that relate more specifically to the likelihood that leukotrienes mediate this response. Mammel et al. (1986) also failed to demonstrate an effect on hypoxic pulmonary vasoconstriction in anesthetized cats following treatment with the leukotriene synthesis inhibitors diethylcarbamazine (DEC) (10 mg/kg) and LY-83583 (3 mg/kg). Leffler et al. (1984) found at FPL 55712 [100 μg/(kg-min)], DEC (2.5 mg/ml left pulmonary arterial blood flow), and nordihydroguairetic acid (an inhibitor of leukotriene synthesis) (5×10^{-5} Mol) had no effects on normoxic hemodynamics or hypoxic pulmonary vasoconstriction in the neonatal pig. This study is particularly important since the dose of FPL 55712 used was shown to block the effects of exogenous LTC_4 and D_4. Three other groups have recently reported that inhibition of leukotriene synthesis, or receptor blockade, did not reduce HPV in the dog (Schuster and Dennis, 1987; Garrett et al., 1987; Ovetsky et al., 1987). Ovetsky et al. (1987) showed that HPV was maintained while the level of immunoreactive leukotrienes was markedly reduced.

There are features of the constrictor leukotrienes that suggest that they are not ideally suited to mediate HPV. Leffler et al. (1984) demonstrated a pulmonary pressor response to exogenous LTD_4 but found it to be a fairly weak vasoconstrictor (5% as potent as equivalent doses of $PGF_{2\alpha}$). While potency is not an absolute requirement for a mediator substance, it may be a pertinent consideration in this case, for in addition to elevating pulmonary vascular resistance, LTD_4 (100-10,000 ng IV) caused dose-dependent hypotension, depression of cardiac output, bronchospasm and increased capillary permeability (Leffler et al., 1984). These effects are not characteristic of the acute response to hypoxia. Morganroth has pointed out the long time to offset of pulmonary vasoconstriction induced by leukotrienes in comparison to the quick reversal of hypoxic pulmonary vasoconstriction that follows ventilation with normoxic gas (Morganroth et al., 1985; Hultgren et al., 1971).

While leukotrienes do not appear to mediate HPV, they may modulate the magnitude of the response. Synthesis of leukotrienes may be related to HPV through effects of hypoxia on sulfhydryl redox status, which could in turn affect the availability of glutathione (GSH), which is required for the synthesis of these sulfidopeptides. GSH is required for conversion of LTA_4 to LTC_4. In addition, glutathione peroxidase and transferase are involved in their production (Fig. 6) (Kosower et al., 1972). Future experiments should include the use of leukotrienes in human pulmonary arteries, since the problem of species variability makes extrapolation of animal data hazardous. Increased attention should be paid to accurate measurement of leukotriene levels, especially in studies where an "inhibitor" is employed, to ensure that the dose of inhibitor used is effective.

Summary

The list of neurohumoral mediators that have been suspected off linking hypoxia and pulmonary vasoconstriction is long and varied. Each has failed in some way to meet the criteria discussed earlier in this chapter. The fact that an indirect mechanism for HPV has not yet been proved does not exclude the possibility that one exists.

Direct Mechanisms of Hypoxic Pulmonary Vasoconstriction

Oxidative Phosphorylation and Hypoxic Pulmonary Vasoconstriction

The possibility that HPV results from inhibition of oxidative phosphorylation was initially suggested by the knowledge that hypoxia decreased oxidative phosphorylation and the empirical observation that inhibitors or uncouplers of this pathway induced pulmonary vasoconstriction (Lloyd, 1965; McMurtry et al., 1982; Rounds and McMurtry, 1981). Furthermore, this cascade of electron-transferring components contains substances that are sensitive to oxygen tension (e.g., cytochrome C).

Lloyd (1965) shosed that 2,4-dinitrophenol (2,4-DNP), an uncoupler of oxidative phosphorylation, caused normoxic pulmonary vasoconstriction in isolated dog lungs. This pressor response could be reversed by hyperoxic ventilation. Pulmonary vasoconstriction was also noted with administration of potassium cyanide (KCN), which is an inhibitor of oxidative phosphorylation (Lloyd, 1964). Rounds and McMurtry (1981) expanded on Lloyd's observations and studied the hemodynamic effects of four chemically dissimilar inhibitors of oxidative phosphorylation in isolated, perfused rat lungs. Antimycin A, azide, cyanide, and rotenone caused reversible pulmonary vasoconstriction during normoxia. These constrictions, like those induced by hypoxia, could be inhibited by the calcium channel blocker verapamil. The time to onset of constriction for each agent (less than 3 min) was also similar to the delay between initiation of hypoxic ventilation and development of HPV.

Postulating that the hemodynamic effects of these compounds resulted from a property they shared with hypoxia, the ability to inhibit oxidative phosphorylation, Stanbrook and McMurtry (1983) examined the effects of inhibition of glycolysis on hypoxic pulmonary vasoconstriction. They reasoned that since glycolysis (favored by hypoxia) attempts to compensate for the loss of the cell's normal energy source (oxidative phosphorylation), inhibition of this compensatory pathway should increase hypoxic pulmonary vasoconstriction. Administration of inhibitors of glycolysis, iodoacetate and 2-deoxyglucose, enhanced the pressor responses to hypoxia but not angiotensin II. In an hypothesis paper, this group speculated that hypoxic inhibition of oxidative phosphorylation resulted in a "signal" (e.g., decreased cellular ATP levels, altered phosphate potential ATP/ADP + Pi), which in turn altered the membrane potential of the pulmonary vascular smooth muscle cell with subsequent inflow of calcium and vasoconstriction (McMurtry et al., 1981, McMurtry et al., 1982) (Fig. 7). Since vasoconstriction and subsequent relaxation require energy, such a theory implies that the "signal" is generated before ATP levels become critically depleted.

Initially, it appeared that changes in oxidative phosphorylation would be unlikely to serve as the oxygen sensor coupling FiO_2 to vascular tone, since cellular respiration was shown to be independent of oxygen availability to very low oxygen levels (Fisher and Dodia, 1981). Fisher and Dodia (1981) found that ATP levels did not fall, or lung lactate production increase, with alveolar oxygen tensions as low as 7 mmHg. Furthermore, Buescher et al. (1987) used nuclear magnetic resonance (NMR) spectroscopy to demonstrate that lung levels of ATP were not significantly reduced during mild hypoxia in isolated lungs. A decrease in lung ATP levels resulted with severe but not moderate hypoxia. Since moderate hypoxia causes pulmonary vasoconstriction while severe hypoxia or anoxia causes pulmonary vasodilation (Sylvester et al., 1980; Harabin et al., 1981), the relevance of energy changes at the extremes of hypoxia is questionable. A number of attempts have been made to explain how a critical "microenvironment" of very low oxygen tension might exist under conditions of "physiologic" hypoxia. Pittman and Duling (1973) estimated that oxygen gradients in vascular strips could result in a core oxygen tension low enough to limit the function of the respiratory chain, assuming the traditionally held limits of oxidative phosphorylation. Recent work suggests that an anoxic core need not be present to explain the effects of varying oxygen tensions on oxidative phosphorylation. Chang and Detar (1980) found that the dose-dependent depression of contractile response to agonists caused by hypoxia occurred at high levels of oxygen tension in tissue bath and speculated that in these systemic vessels an "anoxic core" did not account for the oxygen-dependent changes in vascular tone. Wilson has shown that while net cellular respiration does not change in tumor cells during moderate hypoxia, the redox status of cytochrome C changes as oxygen tension is varied from 240 μmol downward (Wilson et al. 1979). This was associated with alterations in the ratio of ATP to ADP + Pi. They showed

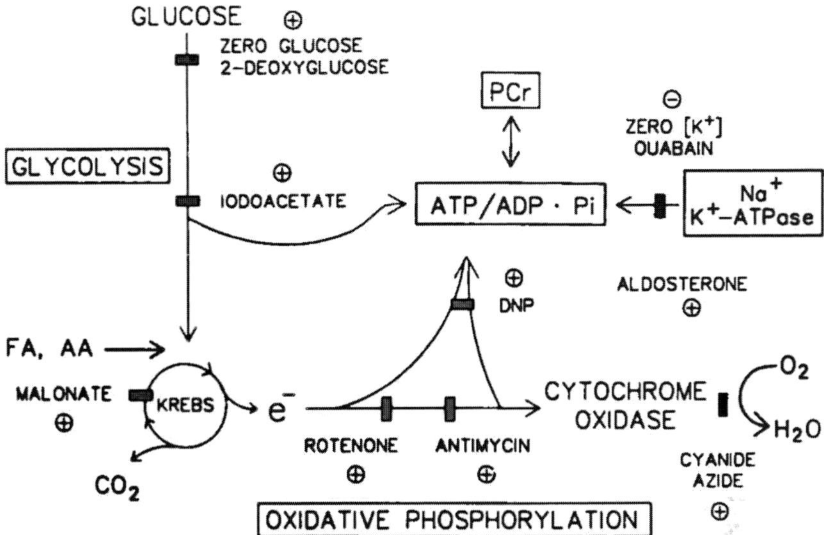

Figure 7 Schematic representation of the oxidative phosphorylation model for control of the pulmonary pressor response to hypoxia (see text for details). (From McMurtry et al. 1982.)

that a threefold change in the ATP to ADP + Pi ratio occurred as tissue oxygen tension varied from 0.5 to 90 mmHg. This change in phosphate potential preceded any decrease in ATP levels. The means by which cytochrome C redox status or phosphate potential could regulate transmembrane calcium flux in pulmonary vascular smooth muscle is unknown. These observations led to the development of a model of coronary artery vasoregulation based on redox regulation of mitochondrial oxidative phosphorylation by oxygen tension (Nuutinen et al., 1982).

Nuutinen et al. (1982) showed that the ratio of ATP to ADP + Pi was decreased in isolated rat hearts after they were challenged with various vasodilatory stimuli (hypoxia, amobarbital, increased work load). They concluded that mitochondrial oxidative phosphorylation served as the link between oxygen tension and coronary blood flow. These findings have not been duplicated in the lung, and there are several considerations that still raise concern regarding the extrapolation of data from the coronary to the pulmonary circulation. First, the primary role of blood flow in the heart is delivery of oxygen and substrate for energy production, while pulmonary flow is not designed to supply the lungs metabolic demands but functions primarily to optimize gas exchange with the alveoli. Second, the cardiac arterial smooth muscle senses the systemic arterial oxygen tension, while the pulmonary arterial smooth muscle at the level involved with vasoregulation senses the alveolar oxygen tension (which is higher). An energy-regulating system based on sensing phosphate potential makes teleologic sense for an organ like the heart. Its applicability to the lung, which is trying to regulate O_2 uptake rather than ATP production, is not clear.

Another caveat regarding this theory was noted by Rounds and McMurtry (1981), who found that the metabolic inhibitors used to cause pulmonary vasoconstriction left the pulmonary vasculature relatively unreactive to hypoxia or angiotensin II. Although this was thought to be a dose effect similar to the reduction in pulmonary pressor reactivity that severe hypoxia can produce (Sylvester et al., 1980), it is a matter for concern that such modest constriction (e.g., < 10 mmHg for azide) should render the vascular bed unreactive. Also, as mentioned by Sylvester et al. (1980), these inhibitors have numerous actions other than their effects on cellular energetics. Iodoacetate is illustrative of this potential source of confusion. At high doses, iodoacetate inhibits glycolysis, while at lower doses the drug may act primarily as a sulfhydryl redox agent (Liang, 1977; Pagliara et al., 1975). Although efforts have been made to control for nonspecific activity through the use of multiple unrelated compounds, it must be remembered that these inhibitors affect cellular functions other than oxidative phosphorylation. The observation by Madden et al. (1985) that oxygen tension-induced constriction of isolated small pulmonary arteries occurred at oxygen tensions as high as 250 mmHg and was maximal at 50 mmHg is difficult to reconcile with this theory, since these oxygen tensions exceed those required for optimal activity of oxidative phosphorylation. However, the possibility remains that the rate of oxidative phosphorylation regulates pulmonary vascular tone. It is possible that oxygen-mediated regulation of cellular energetics has relevance to other proposed mechanisms of HPV (e.g., the redox model, Fig. 6).

Cytochrome P-450 as the Mediator of HPV

Cytochrome P-450 is a hemoprotein that binds oxygen (Longmuir et al., 1973; Rosen and Stier, 1973) reversibly. This oxygen-binding ability, together with the demonstration that cytochrome P-450 is present in the lung (Bend and Hook, 1977), suggests that it could function as a pulmonary oxygen sensor. To fulfill this role, it is necessary that oxygen tension-dependent alterations of cytochrome P-450 activity be able to modulate vascular tone (directly or through some product such as oxygen radicals) and that it respond to variance in O_2 tension over the physiologic range. Duke and Killick (1952) found that carbon monoxide (CO), an inhibitor of cytochrome P-450, caused pulmonary vasodilation and reversed pulmonary vasoconstriction induced by "inert" gases (e.g., nitrogen). Sylvester and McGowan (1978) speculated that any agent that can "saturate" cytochrome P-450 (by binding the heme iron), be it oxygen or CO, would decrease pulmonary vascular tone. They used two inhibitors of cytochrome P-450 (metyrapone and CO) in an isolated pig lung model of HPV and found that both agents decreased HPV; however, both agents also decreased the pressor response to prostaglandin F_{2a} (PGF_{2a}). This suggests the possibility that the cytochrome P-450 inhibitors employed may have been toxic to the pulmonary vasculature and their effects on the hypoxic pressor response nonspecific.

Miller and Hales (1979) performed experiments in anesthetized dogs and found that CO and metyrapone inhibited HPV, but in their study the pressor responses to angiotensin II and PGF_{2a} were preserved. Like most chemical inhibitors, CO and metyrapone are not specific. Carbon monoxide can inhibit other cytochromes, and metyrapone inhibits the synthesis of steroids. Miller and Hales attempted to control for the "other functions" of these drugs by giving hydrocortisone to some of the dogs. The administration of hydrocortisone did not change the effects of either inhibitor on HPV. Their study employed lower doses of CO than have been used in previous studies in an attempt to avoid generalized poisoning of the cytochromes. This lower dose of CO was still effective in blocking hypoxic pulmonary vasoconstriction.

One point supporting the contention that cytochrome P-450 could be involved in the pulmonary pressor response is the observation that in the lung its time to onset of substrate metabolism is roughly the same as the time from onset of hypoxia to HPV (Sylvester and McGowan, 1978). However, while oxygen and carbon monoxide cause similar hemodynamic effects (pulmonary vasodilatation), they exert opposite effects on the hydroxylation reactions that are catalyzed by cytochrome P-450. Therefore, this activity of the enzyme is unlikely to be the means of transducing oxygen tension to vascular tone.

While cytochrome P-450 is an oxygen-dependent heme protein and could therefore represent the "oxygen sensor" linking alveolar 0_2 and vascular tone, there are some problems with this hypothesis. The K_m for oxygen of cytochrome P-450 (in the liver) is near 1 mmHg (Coburn, 1977). If lung cytochrome P-450 had such kinetics, it would remain fully oxidized over the entire range of physiologically tolerable oxygen concentrations. If the redox status of cytochrome P-450 were to serve as a modulator of pulmonary vascular tone it would be necessary that lung cytochrome P-450 have a significantly higher K_m for oxygen. This possibility exists because some cytochromes do have much higher K_m values for oxygen than that measured in the liver (e.g., rabbit brain cytochrome oxidase) (Rosenthal et al., 1976). However, prelminary work by Custer et al. (1985) found that cytochrome P-450 was not detectable in lamb lungs during the "newborn period". These lungs exhibited a normal pressor response to hypoxia that was not diminished by metyrapone. It is also disconcerting that partial reduction of cytochrome P-450 (by hypoxia) produces vasoconstriction while complete reduction (by carbon monoxide) causes vasodilatation. Even if cytochrome P-450 does not function as the only oxygen sensor for the pulmonary vasculature, it may affect vascular tone through its ability to alter the metabolism of mediator substances or the generation of vasoactive substances as a result of its enzymatic activity. A point in favor of the latter possibility is the observation that activation of cytochrome P-450 results in the generation of superoxide anion (White and Coon, 1980). Gonder et al. (1985) showed that mice with genetically inducible cytochrome P-450 enzyme systems (e.g., increased cytochrome P-450 activity occurs on exposure to 100% O_2) had a greater sensitivity to hyperoxia than a similar strain of mouse with genetically noninducible cytochrome P-450 exposed to hyperoxia. The possibility that O_2 radical production by cytochrome P-450 occurs in response to alterations in oxygen tension may provide a link between this heme protein and the redox model of hypoxic pulmonary vasoconstriction, to be discussed subsequently. At this time, no explanation exists that would allow cytochrome P-450 to be the mediator of oxygen-related pulmonary vascular tone. Questions that need to be answered include: (1) What is the K_m for lung cytochrome P-450 humans? (2) Can the reduction/oxidation state of cytochrome P-450 control calcium flux in vascular smooth muscle?

Redox Model of HPV

A redox (reduction-oxidation) reaction is a chemical concept describing the interchange of one or more electrons between two substances. Acceptance of an electron is called reduction; donation of an electron is oxidation. The redox model of hypoxic pulmonary vasoconstriction states that oxygen, or some partially reduced oxygen species, acts directly on key sulfhydryl groups in the pulmonary vasculature, thereby regulating calcium flux into pulmonary vascular smooth muscle cells and thus controlling vascular tone (Archer et al., 1986c). The nature of the link between oxygen tension and sulfydryl redox status is uncertain. Oxygen radicals and hydroperoxides produced during normal oxidative metabolism are likely candidates for the role of an oxygen tension-sensitive vasoactive mediator. Short-lived oxygen metabolites, such as the superoxide anion, react readily with sulfhydryl groups because of an unpaired electron in their outer orbital. The redox theory does not specify whether oxygen-induced changes in sulfhydryl reduction/oxidation status occur in the entire cell, in a subcellular compartment, or solely at the level of the calcium channel. There is also ambiguity as to the specific cell type where redox regulation would occur (e.g., endothelial cells, vascular smooth muscle cells, or both).

The following observations are fundamental to the construction of a redox model of HPV:

1. Superoxide anion and hydrogen peroxide are produced in lung mitochondria in proportion to oxygen tension over the physiological spectrum from hypoxia to hyperoxia (Turrens et al., 1982a, b).
2. Exogenous oxygen radicals are vasoactive in the lung (Weir et al., 1985).

3. Oxygen tension alters lung sulfhydryl redox balance as reflected by the ratio of reduced to oxiolized glutathione (GSH/GSSG) and pyridine nucleotides (see Sec. II) (White et al., 1986; Warshaw et al., 1985; Patterson et al., 1985).
4. Oxygen and oxidant drugs can alter calcium homeostasis in vitro (Orrenius et al., 1983).
5. Drugs that act as oxidants of the sulfhydryl tripeptide glutathione prevent hypoxic pulmonary vasoconstriction (Weir et al, 1982; Archer et al., 1986c).
6. The sulfhydryl redox status of the calcium channel is an important determinant of its structure and function (Schmid et al., 1986).
7. Calcium channel agonists and antagonists often have similar structures but differ in their redox properties (Marinov and Saxon, 2985).

The information regarding the interrelationship of inspired oxygen concentration and oxygen radical production as well as the effect of oxygen in cellular redox status has been discussed in Section II. The preceding list will be discussed beginning with a review of the ability of oxidant drugs to regulate pulmonary vascular reactivity.

Oxidant Vasodilators

Weir and Will (1982) described a new class of pulmonary vasodilators, the oxidants. This heterogeneous group of drugs have in common their ability to enter cells and rapidly oxidize glutathione and presumably other sulfhydryl compounds. Such oxidants as diamide and 2-butanone hydroperoxide reverse HPV in vivo and in vitro.

Diamide is the prototype of sulfhydryl oxidant vasodilators (Kosower and Kosower, 1976). It is a diazene compound that rapidly oxidizes glutathione. In low doses it is quite specific for glutathione, while at higher doses it may alter other sulfhydryl groups. The oxidation of GSH by diamide is reversible due to the homeostatic effects of glutathione reductase (Kosower and Kosower, 1976). While the specificity of diamide for GSH is not absolute, it tends to affect this antioxidant peptide prior to depleting other critical sulfhydryl groups. The effect of diamide on pulmonary vascular reactivity is not the result of random damage to the pulmonary vasculature or vascular paresis (Fig. 8). Diamide (5 mg/kg IV bolus) rapidly obliterates hypoxic pulmonary vasoconstriction without decreasing the pulmonary pressor response to angiotensin II or altering systemic hemodynamics (Weir and Will, 1983). The effect of diamide on HPV can be prevented by augmentation of the animal's supply of expendable sulfhydryl groups with *N*-acetylcysteine or coincubation of diamide with reduced glutathione prior to its administration (Weir, 1984). In addition to its biochemical

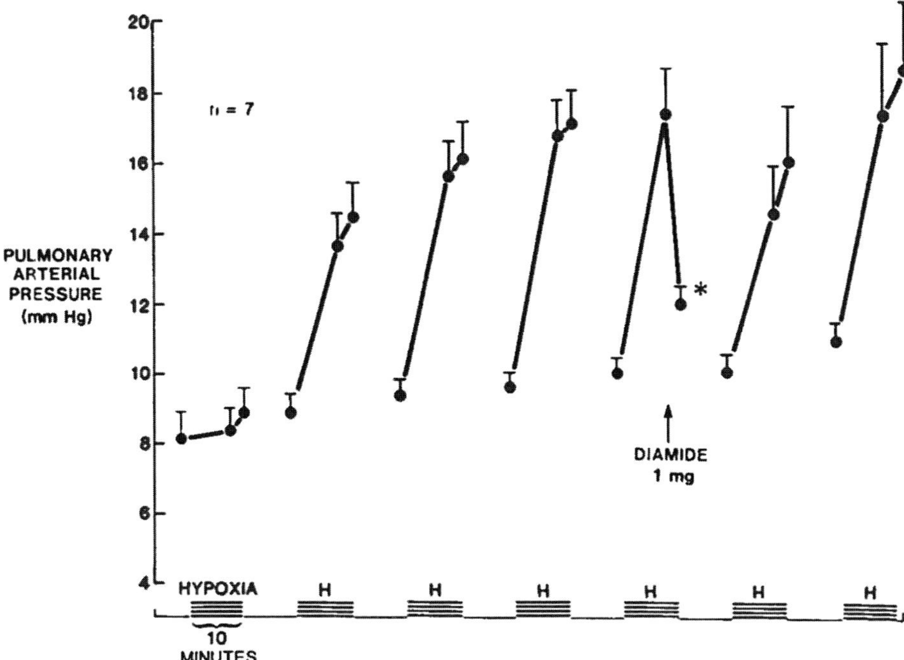

Figure 8 Diamide causes reversible inhibition of hypoxic pulmonary vasoconstriction in the blood-perfused rat lung. (From Weir et al., 1985.)

effects, Kosower (1970) has shown that diamide rapidly and reversibly inhibits contraction of cultured skeletal muscle cells.

Diamide and its congeners (DIP, DIP + 2) are not the only vasoactive sulfhydryl oxidants. Peroxides (e.g., tert-butylhydroperoxide, 2-butanone hydroperoxide) also reduce HPV (Weir and Will, 1982). In addition, enzyme-substrate pairs that generate oxygen radicals or hydroperoxides [e.g., xanthine-xanthine oxidase (X/XO) (Weir et al., 1985) and glucose-glucose oxidase (G/GO) (Burghuber et al., 1984)] reduce hypoxic pulmonary vasoconstriction. They do so in a manner that can be blocked by superoxide dismutase (SOD) and catalase (CAT) (Archer et al., 1986) or allopurinol (Weir et al., 1985).

As discussed in Section II. B, the dose of "oxidant" is a critical determinant of the effect of the drug on the pulmonary pressor response to hypoxia. Low doses of tert-butyl hydroperoxide and X/XO reverse HPV without increasing the wet/dry ratio of the lungs or destroying the reactivity of the pulmonary vasculature to angiotensin II, whereas high doses of each produce pulmonary vasoconstriction and nonspecific lung injury and/or vascular paresis (Gurtner et al., 1985; Farrukh et al., 1985).

Part of the problem in assessing the dose of radicals administered in a given experiment is the evanescent nature of these substances. This makes in vivo measurement of radical levels very difficult. Superoxide, for example, can account for up to 17% of the total electron flow in the electron transport chain, and yet, due to its rapid destruction by SOD, it is rarely measurable outside the cell (Fridovich, 1983). Fridovich (1983) estimates an average cellular concentration of $O_2^{\cdot}$ of 1×10^{-11} M. In the presence of SOD (roughly 1×10^{-6} M in most tissues), superoxide is destroyed 10^6-fold faster than would occur with spontaneous dismutation (Fridovich, 1983).

The vasodilatory effects of exogenous radicals appear similar to that of inhaled oxygen (which itself increases endogenous radical production). This raises the possibility that hypoxic pulmonary vasoconstriction is the response of the vasculature to loss of an endogenous normoxic vasodilator (a peroxide or oxygen radical). This concept may be termed "normoxic vasodilation." It implies that the low resting tone of the pulmonary arteries during normoxia, or even lower tone during hyperoxia, is an active process due to a vasodilator effect of oxygen, which is lost with reduction of oxygen tension.

In order to validate the redox theory of pulmonary vascular control it is necessary to establish a clear link between F_IO_2 and cellular redox state. It is possible that the mediator (e.g., an oxygen radical) would act locally on the calcium channel without producing perturbation in the overall smooth muscle cell redox status. Indeed, pulmonary redox changes would need to be somewhat localized to avoid the many other consequences of widespread alterations in redox status [e.g., inhibition or inactivation of key enzymes or protein synthesis (Kosower and Kosower, 1976)]. Prolonged or intense exposure of the lung to extremes of oxygen tension, as occurs with pathologic processes, would be more likely to produce generalized changes in lung redox status of glutathione and NADPH (White et al., 1986) than would the brief, milder changes in F_IO_2 that occur under physiologic conditions.

Preliminary evidence has shown that red blood cell (RBC) GSH concentration is inversely proportional to F_IO_2 (Archer et al., 1986a). In this study changes in GSH were noted after less than 10 min ventilation at a given F_IO_2 over a range of inspired oxygen concentrations from 10 to 100%. Pulmonary arterial pressure varied directly with RBC GSH in these dogs. It was not determined whether these rapid changes reflected altered synthesis and/or utilization of glutathione or merely the release of glutathione from mixed disulfide reserves during hypoxia.

While the effects of administration and removal of exogenous radicals on pulmonary vascular reactivity have been studied, the effect of scavenging endogenous radicals has not. Part of the difficulty in assessing this area is the poor permeability of cells to exogenous CAT or SOD. Superoxide dismutase, for example, has a half-life of only 6 min when administered intravenously (Fridovitch, 1983), largely due to excretion of this poorly absorbed enzyme. The uptake of SOD by the lung can be increased by administering this enzyme in liposomes (Michelson and Puget, 1980). These lipid microspheres allow the lungs to rapidly remove as much as 21% of a dose of SOD from the circulation. Administration of CAT plus SOD either free or in liposomes blocked the effects of X/XO on hypoxic pulmonary vasoconstriction in the isolated perfused rat lung (Archer et al., 1986b). The liposome-entrapped enzymes enhanced the pulmonary vascular reactivity to hypoxia and angiotensin II. This was not seen with an equal amount of free enzyme or with administration of an equal weight of albumin in liposomes. The alteration of pulmonary vascular reactivity by administration of antioxidant enzymes suggests that endogenous radicals may participate in determining pulmonary vascular tone.

If oxygen radicals are important modulators of pulmonary vascular tone in response to F_IO_2, where are they produced? While radicals can be produced by phagocytosis (Harada et al., 1984) or arachidonic acid metabolism (Kontos et al., 1985), it is more probable that production of radicals involved in coupling oxygen tension and vascular tone are generated via an oxygen-sensitive pathway (e.g., electron transport chain). The evidence that this occurs in the lung mitochondria has been discussed.

The redox hypothesis regarding regulation of pulmonary vascular tone needs further assessment. The need to correlate the level of oxygen radical production (in vivo) in the lung with pulmonary vascular tone is paramount. In addition it is uncertain which redox pool (e.g., GSH or NADPH) might be critical in regulating calcium flux. Does some reactive metabolite of oxygen (e.g., H_2O_2 or $O_2^{\cdot}$) act directly on the voltage-dependent calcium channel? Although further investigation is needed, there are examples of other organ systems where sulfhydryl redox status serves a regulatory function.

In the pancreatic β cell, transmembrane calcium flux (which is coupled to insulin release) is controlled by the redox state of glutathione and/or NADPH (Ammon et al., 1983; Malaisse et al., 1982). In the β cell, secretagogues (glucose, leucine, 2-ketoisocaproate) have been shown to shift the NADPH/NADP and GSH/GSSG ratios to a more reduced state. Inhibition of this shift by diamide or tert-butyl hydroperoxide prevents insulin release (Ammon et al., 1979; Sener et al., 1984), much as it prevents hypoxic pulmonary vasoconstriction in the lung. In the β cell it is thought that redox changes in the sulfhydryl groups of the cell membrane and cytosol result in decreased potassium conductance and depolarization of the plasma membrane (Ammon et al., 1983; Lebrun et al., 1983). The effect of altered potassium conductance has a parallel in the lung. Bergofsky and Holtzmann (1967) showed that hypoxia causes decreased potassium conductance in pulmonary, but not systemic, vessels. Glucose-stimulated insulin release in rats can be blocked by calcium channel blockers (Kanatsuna et al., 1985) in a manner analogous to the inhibition of hypoxic pulmonary vasoconstriction by these agents. Calcium influx in the β cell, whether achieved in a voltage-dependent, redox-influenced manner (e.g., secretagogues) (Anjaneyulu et al., 1982) or by membrane potential-independent (redox-independent) agonists (e.g., glibenclamide), results in insulin release (Ammon et al., 1984; Sener et al., 1984). It is interesting that both insulin release and pulmonary vasoconstriction can occur by voltage-dependent (hypoxic pulmonary vasoconstriction) or receptor operated and voltage-independent (AII, $PGF_{2\alpha}$, etc.) mechanisms. The similarities in regulation of the β cell's release of insulin and the pulmonary pressor response to hypoxia have been discussed in a previous review (Archer et al., 1986c).

As mentioned earlier in this chapter, putative mechanisms for mediation of HPV must explain how increased calcium is delivered to the contractile apparatus or how the sensitivity of the contractile apparatus to available calcium is altered by changes in oxygen tension. What evidence is there that redox status of sulfhydryl groups can alter these events?

Redox Regulation of Calcium Flux in Mitochondria

There is evidence that manipulation of sulfhydryl redox status can alter calcium homeostasis in the mitochondria, in the endoplasmic reticulum, and possibly across the sarcolemma. The calcium within the mitochondria of some cells represents a large reservoir of intracellular calcium, the physiological role of which is poorly understood. In the hepatocytes, it is speculated that mitochondria provide a high-capacity calcium sink that "buffers" the cytoplasmic calcium level, preventing excessive fluctuations of this important variable. It is not known whether mitochondria can release calcium to the contractile apparatus during hypoxia or sequester calcium during normoxia and hyperoxia. Certainly mitochondria isolated from vascular smooth muscle contain more calcium and can more rapidly transport calcium than can mitochondria from other tissues (Vallieres et al., 1975). In rat portal veins, hypoxia causes dilation with an associated decrease in calcium granules within the mitochondria (Ebeigbe, 1980). In addition, calcium is taken up by mitochondria during normoxia, but not hypoxia, in the rabbit aorta (Karki et al., 1982). These findings suggest, but certainly do not prove, that calcium balance in the mitochondria may be linked to vascular tone, at least in some vessels.

While HPV is assumed to be predominantly mediated by flow of extracellular calcium across the plasma membrane, the potential for intracellular pools to be involved in supply of calcium to or its removal from the contractile apparatus cannot be discounted. The smooth muscle of the main pulmonary artery can constrict in an essentially calcium-free medium (Devine et al., 1972) whereas the dog coronary artery displays an absolute requirement for extracellular calcium (Van Breeman et al., 1980).

There is evidence that the redox status (ratio of reduced to oxidized) of the pyridine nucleotide NADPH or glutathione can alter calcium flow across the mitochondrial membrane (Lehninger et al., 1978; Lotscher et al., 1979, 1980). Treatment of rat liver mitochondria with hydroperoxides alters their NADPH/NADP+ ratio and causes release of intramitochondrial calcium (Lotscher et al., 1979, 1980). While the effects of oxygen on mitochondrial calcium have not been similarly studied, oxygen can produce significant changes in NADPH and GSH levels.

How does the redox status of NADPH or GSH control mitochondrial calcium flux? To retain calcium within the mitochondria, magnesium adenine dinucleotide phosphate (MgADP) is required in adequate amounts in association with the inner mitochondrial membrane (Roth and Dikstein, 1982; Harris et al. 1979, Le-Quoc and Le-Quoc, 1982). Reduced glutathione and NADPH promote a tight association between the internal mitochondrial membrane and ATP. The need for both ATP and specific redox parameters in the regulation of calcium homeostasis suggests an interface between the redox and oxidative phosphorylation hypotheses. There appears to be a direct relationship between flux of electrons through the electron transport chain and flow of calcium into the mitochondria. To maintain an adequate supply of GSH, NADPH is required. NADPH is produced by an ATP-requiring transhydrogenation reaction. Depletion of ATP or alteration of mitochondrial redox potential (as represented by GSH/GSSG, NADPH/NADP) can alter calcium homeostasis; whether it does so in vivo and whether such changes are relevant to pulmonary vascular tone is not known.

Redox Regulation of Ca^{2+} in Extramitochondrial Pools

As in the mitochondria, the redox status of glutathione can affect calcium flux in the endoplasmic reticulum (Jewell et al., 1982). Orrenius et al. (1983) manipulated cellular redox status using various oxidant drugs and concluded that thiol (GSH/GSSG) rather than pyridine nucleotide (NADPH/NADP+) redox status was important in altering the size of the extramitochondrial calcium pool. tert-Butyl hydroperoxide was used to increase the cytoplasmic ratio of GSSG/GSH. This effect was enhanced by administration of *N*,*N*-bis (2-chloroethyl)-*N*-nitrosourea (BCNU), an inhibitor of glutathione reductase. The mitochondrial calcium pool was relatively unaffected by these changes despite the alterations in the extramitochondrial pool, raising the possibility that different calcium compartments respond to relatively specific redox signals. The importance of the sarcoplasmic reticulum in pulmonary vascular tone is essentially unexplored.

Redox Regulation of Calcium Flux Through the Voltage-Dependent Channel

There is considerable evidence cited in this chapter that inflow of calcium through the voltage-dependent calcium channel is a prerequisite for hypoxic pulmonary vasoconstriction. There have been very few studies designed to assess the effects of oxygen or oxidant vasodilation on this critical mechanism. However, circumstantial evidence points to the feasibility of redox regulation of this flow. The ability of agonist dihydropyridines to markedly augment HPV in a manner that can be blocked by antagonists has been discussed (Fig. 5). The receptor protein for these drugs has been isolated and its chemical structure determined (Borsotto et al., 1984, 1985; Curtis and Catterall, 1984). This protein is presumed, but not proved, to be the actual calcium channel protein (Schmid et al., 1986). Schmid et al. performed immunochemical analyses of 1,4-dihydropyridine receptors in smooth muscle and found that, as in the heart and skeletal muscle, it was a glycoprotein composed of a large polypeptide connected to a smaller polypeptide by disulfide bridges. Exposure of the BAY K 8644 binding protein to an oxidant environment resulted in disassociation of the complex molecule into its components. This raises the possibility that adding or removing an electron from the calcium channel could induce conformational or electrostatic changes that might "open" or "close" the channel. The fact that chemically similar dihydropyridines may be sorted into "agonists" or "antagonists" of the calcium channel on the basis of their tendency to donate or receive an electron also is consistent with speculation that local redox changes near or in the calcium channel regulate its activity.

Studies of the pancreatic β cell have provided supportive evidence for the ability of sulfhydryl redox status to regulate plasma membrane calcium flux. Ammon et al. (1983) have shown that oxidation of intracellular glutathione by a diazene (related to diamide) inhibits glucose-stimulated $^{45}Ca^{2+}$ uptake in the β cell. The parallels between redox regulation models for the β cell and the pulmonary vascular smooth muscle cell are numerous.

C. Summary

The redox theory can be summarized as follows: Oxygen tension regulates pulmonary vascular tone over the entire spectrum of F_IO_2 by producing a mediator (possibly an oxygen radical or peroxide) in the wall of small pulmonary arteries. Through direct action on the redox status of sulfhydryl groups in the cacium channel proteins, possibly in conjunction with the effects of changes in redox status on the intracellular calcium compartments, this oxygen-derived mediator controls transmembrane calcium flux and hence tone (Archer et al., 1986c). There is evidence for redox-based regulatory mechanisms in other organs, including the pancreas.

IV. Conclusion

This chapter has reviewed the effects of acute hyperoxia and hypoxia on pulmonary vascular tone and reactivity. Research in these two areas has traditionally been focused at one or other extreme of the oxygen spectrum. The data presented in this chapter suggest that hypoxia and hyperoxia are probably just opposite ends of a spectrum in which normoxia is our reference point. A theory that explains pulmonary vasoconstriction in response to hypoxia should be able to account for vasodilation during hyperoxia. The long search for chemical mediation of hypoxic pulmonary vasoconstriction or hyperoxic vascular paresis has provided enormous insight on the modulation of pulmonary hemodynamics but has failed to produce a unifying hypothesis for vasoregulation. While absence of evidence is not evidence of absence, it appears that investigation of direct effects of oxygen on vascular biochemistry, regulation of smooth muscle membrane potential, and control of the voltage-dependent calcium channel is more likely to produce a unifying model of pulmonary vascular tone control over the entire range of oxygen tensions to which we are exposed.

References

Ahmed, T., and Oliver, W., Jr. (1983). Does slow-reacting substance of anaphylaxis mediate hypoxic pulmonary vasoconstriction? *Am. Rev. Resp. Dis. 127*:566-571.

Ahmed, T., Oliver, W., Jr., Frank, B. L., and Robinson, M. J. (1982). Hypoxic pulmonary vasoconstriction in conscious sheep. *Am. Rev. Resp. Dis. 126*: 291-297.

Ahmed, T., Marchette, B., Wanner, A., and Yerger, L. (1985). Direct and indirect effects of leukotriene D_4 on the pulmonary and systemic circulations. *Am. Rev. Resp. Dis. 131*:554-558.

Ammon, H., P. T., Hoppe, Akhtar, M. S., and Niklas, H. (1979). Effect of leucine on the pyridine nucleotide contents of islets and on the insulin released interactions in vitro with methylene blue, thiol oxidants, and *p*-chloromercuribenzoate. *Diabetes 28*:593-599.

Ammon, H. P. T., Hagele, R., Youssif, N., Eujen, R., and El-Amri, N. (1983). A possible role of intracellular and membrane thiols of rat pancreatic islets in calcium uptake and insulin release. *Endocrinology 112*:720-726.

Ammon, H. P. T., Abdel-Hamid, M., Rao, P. G., and Enz, G. (1984). Thiol-dependent and non-thiol-dependent stimulations of insulin release. *Diabetes 33*:251-257.

Anjaneyulu, K., Anjaneyulu, R., Sener, A., and Malaisse, W. J. (1982). The stimulus-secretion coupling of glucose-induced insulin release. Thiol: disulfide balance in pancreatic islets. *Biochimie 64*:29-36.

Archer, S. L., Nelson, D., Eaton, J., and Weir, E. K. (1986a). Changes in glutathione status parallel changes in pulmonary vascular reactivity. *Proc. Int. Union Physiol. Sci. 16*:448.

Archer, S. L., Nelson, D., Kelly, S., Peterson, D., and Weir, E. K. (1986b). Antioxidant enzymes protect hypoxic pulmonary vasoconstriction against oxygen radical-mediated vasodilatation. *Fed. Proc. 45*:2310.

Archer, S. L., Yankovich, R. D., Chesler, E., and Weir, E. K. (1985). Comparative effects of nisoldipine, nifedipine and bepridil on experimental pulmonary hypertension. *J. Pharmacol. Exp. Ther. 233*:12-17.

Archer, S. L., Will, J. A., and Weir, E. K. (1986c). Redox status in the control of pulmonary vascular tone. *Herz 11*:127-141.

Barer, G. R. (1966). Reactivity of the vessels of collapsed and ventilated lungs to drugs and hypoxia. *Cir. Res. 18*:366-378.

Barer, G. R., Emery, C. J., Mohammed, F. H., and Mungall, I. P. F. (1978) H_1 and H_2 histamine actions on lung vessels; their relevance to hypoxic vasoconstriction. *Quart. J. Exp. Physiol. 63*:157-169.

Bend, J., and Hook, G. (1977). Hepatic and extrahepatic mixed-function oxidases. In *Handbook of Physiology*. Section. *Reaction to Environmental Agents*. Edited by D. Lee, H. Falk, S. Murphy, and S. Geiger. American Physiological Society, Washington, D.C.

Bergofsky, E. H. (1979). Active control of the normal pulmonary circulation. In *Pulmonary Vascular Diseases*. Edited by K. M. Moser. Marcel Dekker, New York.

Bergofsky, E. H., and Holtzman, S. (1967). A study of the mechanisms involved in the pulmonary arterial pressor response to hypoxia. *Circ. Res. 20*:506-509.

Berkov, S. (1974). Hypoxic pulmonary vasoconstriction in the rat. *Circ. Res. 35*: 256-261.

Bishop, C. T., Freeman, B. A., and Crapo, J. D. (1984). Free radicals and lung injury. In *Free Radicals in Molecular Biology, Aging, and Disease*. Edited by D. Armstrong, R. S. Sohal, R. G. Cutler, and T. F. Slater. Raven Press, New York.

Block, E. R., Patel, J. M., Angelides, K. J., Sheridan, N. P., and Garg, L. C. (1986). Hyperoxia reduces plasma membrane fluidity: a mechanism for endothelial cell dysfunction. *J. Appl. Physiol. 60*:826-835.

Bohr, D. F. (1977). The pulmonary hypoxic response. *Chest 71*:244-246.

Bond, M., Kitazawa, T., Somlyo, A. P., and Somlyo, A. V. (1984a). Release and recycling of calcium by the sarcoplasmic reticulum in guinea pig portal vein smooth muscle. *J. Physiol. (Lond.) 355*:677-695.

Bond, M., Shuman, H., Somlyo, A. P., and Somlyo, A. V. (1984b). Total cytoplasmic calcium in relaxed and maximally contracted rabbit portal vein smooth muscle. *J. Physiol. (Lond.) 357*:185-201.

Borsotto, M., Barhanin, J., Norman, R. A., and Lazdunski, M. (1984). Purification of the dihydropyridine receptor of the voltage-dependent calcium channel from skeletal muscle transverse tubules. *Biochem. Biophy. Res. Commun. 122*:1357-1366.

Borsotto, M., Barhanin, J., Fosset, M., and Lazdunski, M. (1985). The 1,4-dihydropyridine receptor associated with the skeletal muscle voltage-dependent calcium channel. *J. Biol. Chem. 260*:14255-14263.

Buescher, P., Litt, M., Perse, D., Pillai, R., Eichorn, G., Mitchell, M., Michael, J., and Sylvester, J. T. (1987). Comparison of lung adenosine triphosphate (ATP) measured by enzyme assay high pressure liquid chromatography (HPLC) and 31-P NMR. *Fed. Proc. 46*:520.

Burghuber, O., Mathies, M. M., McMurtry, I. F., Reeves, J. T., and Voelkel, N. F. (1984). Lung edema due to hydrogen peroxide is independent of cyclooxygenase products. *J. Appl. Physiol. 56*:900-905.

Casey, L., Clarke, J., Fletcher, J., and Ramwell, P. (1982). Cardiovascular, respiratory, and hematologic effects of leukotriene D_4 in primates. In *Leukotrienes and Other Lipoxygenase Products*. Edited by B. Samuelsson and R. Paoletti. Raven Press, New York.

Cassin, S., Dawes, G. S., Mott, J. C., Ross, B. B., and Strang, L. B. (1964). The vascular resistance of the foetal and newly ventilated lung of the lamb. *J. Physiol. 171*:61-79.

Chang, A. E., and Detar, R. (1980). Oxygen and vascular smooth muscle contraction revisited. *Am. J. Physiol. 238*:H716-H728.

Coburn, R. F. (177). Oxygen tension sensors in vascular smooth muscle. *Adv. Exp. Med. Biol. 78*:101-115.

Colley, P. S., Cheney, F. W., and Hlastala, M. P. (1979). Ventilation-perfusion and gas exchange effects of sodium nitroprusside in dogs with normal and edematous lungs. *Anesthesiology 50*:489-495.

Conhaim, R. L., and Staub, N. C. (1980). Reflection of spectrophotometric measurement of 0_2 uptake in pulmonary arterioles of cats. *J. Appl. Physiol. 48*:848-856.

Crapo, J. D., and Tierney, D. F. (1974). Superoxide dismutase and pulmonary oxygen toxicity. *Am. J. Physiol. 226*:1401-1407.

Curtis, B. M., and Catterall, W. A. (1984). Purification of the calcium antagonist receptor of the voltage-sensitive calcium channel from skeletal muscle transverse tubules. *Proc. Natl. Acad. Sci. USA 79*:6707-6711.

Custer, J., Zhu, Y., and Hales, C. (1985). Pulmonary alveolar hypoxic vasoconstriction (PAHVC) in lambs is not affected by blockade of cytochrome P450 by metyrapone. *Am. Rev. Resp. Dis. 131*:A399.

Davis, M. J., Gilmore, J. P., and Joyner, W. L. (1981). Responses of pulmonary allograft and cheek pouch arterioles in the hamster to alterations in extravascular pressure in different oxygen environments. *Circ. Res. 49*:133-140.

Deneke, S. M., and Fanburg, B. L. (1980). Normobaric oxygen toxicity of the lung. *New Engl. J. Med. 303*:76-86.

Devine, C. E., Somlyo, A. V., and Somlyo, A. P. (1972). Sarcoplasmic reticulum and excitation-contraction coupling in mammalian smooth muscles. *J. Cell Biol. 52*:690-718.

Duke, H., and Killick, E. M. (1952). Pulmonary vascular responses of isolated perfused cat lungs to anoxia. *J. Physiol. 117*:303-316.

Duling, B. R., and Berne, R. M. (1970). Longitudinal gradients in periarteriolar oxygen tension. *Circ. Res. 27*:669-678.

Ebeigbe, A. B. (1980). Vascular smooth muscle responses to hypoxia and calcium withdrawal: ultrastructural and mechanical observations. *IRCS Med. Sci. 8*:549.

Euler, U. S., and Liljestrand, von G. (1946). Observations on the pulmonary arterial blood pressure in the cat. *Acta Physiol. Scand. 12*:301-320.

Farrukh, I. S., Michael, J. R., Summer, W. R., Adkinson, N. F., Jr., and Gurtner, G. H. (1985). Thromboxane-induced pulmonary vasoconstriction: involvement of calcium. *J. Appl. Physiol. 58*:34-44.

Fedderson, O. C., Mathias, M., Murphy, R. C., Reeves, J. T., and Voelkel, N. F. (1983). Leukotriene E_4 causes pulmonary vasoconstriction, not inhibited by meclofenamate. *Prostaglandins 26*:869-883.

Fisher, A. B., and Dodia, C. (1981). Lung as a model for evaluation of critical intracellular P_{O2} and P_{CO2}. *Am. J. Physiol. 241*:E47-E50.

Frank, L., Bucher, J. R., and Roberts, R. J. (1978). Oxygen toxicity in neonatal and adult animals of various species. *J. Appl. Physiol. 45*:699-704.

Freeman, B. A., and Crapo, J. D. (1981). Hyperoxia increases oxygen radical production in rat lungs and lung mitochondria. *J. Biol. Chem. 256*:10986-10992.

Freeman, B. A., Topolosky, M. K., and Crapo, J. D. (1982). Hyperoxia increases oxygen radical production in rat lung homogenates. *Arch. Biochem. Biophys. 216*:477-484.

Fridovich, I. (1983). Superoxide radical: an endogenous toxicant. *Ann. Rev. Pharmacol. Toxicol. 23*:239-257.

Garrett, R. C., Foster, S., and Thomas, H. M. (1987). Lipoxygenase and cyclo-oxygenase blockade by BW 755C enhances pulmonary hypoxic vasoconstriction. *J. Appl. Physiol. 62*:129-133.

Gerschman, R., Gilbert, D. L., Nye, S. W., Dwyer, P., and Fenn, W. O. (1954). Oxygen poisoning and x-irradiation: a mechanism in common. *Science 119*:623-626.

Gillis, C. N., and Catravas, J. D. (1982). Altered removal of vasoactive substances in the injured lung: detection of lung microvascular injury. *Ann. NY Acad. Sci. 384*:458-474.

Glazier, J. B., and Murray, J. F. (1971). Sites of pulmonary vasomotor reactivity in the dog during alveolar hypoxia and serotonin, and histamine infusion. *J. Clin. Invest. 50*:2550-2580.

Goldberg, R. N., Suguihara, C., Ahmed, T., Deseda de Cudemus, B., Barrios, P., Setzer, E. S., and Bancalari, E. (1985). Influence of an antagonist of slow-reacting substance of anaphylaxis on the cardiovascular manifestations of hypoxia in piglets. *Pediatr. Res. 19*:1201-1205.

Goldzimer, E. K., Konopka, R. G., and Moser, K. M. (1978). Reversal of the perfusion defect in experimental canine lobar pneumococcal pneumonia. *J. Appl. Physiol. 37*:85-91.

Gonder, J. C., Proctor, R. A., and Will, J. A. (1985). Genetic differences in oxygen toxicity are correlated with cytochrome P-450 inducibility. *Proc. Natl. Acad. Sci. USA 82*:6315-6319.

Gottlieb, J., McGeady, M., Adkinson, N. F., Hayes, E., and Sylvester, J. T. (1984). Inhibition of hypoxic pulmonary vasoconstriction in ferret lungs by nordihydroguaiaretic acid (NDGA) (Abstr.). *Am. Rev. Resp. Dis. 129*: A343.

Gurtner, G. H., Michael, J. R., Farrukh, I. S., Sciuto, A. M., and Adkinson, N. F. (1985). Mechanism of hyperoxia-induced pulmonary vascular paralysis: effect of antioxidant pretreatment. *J. Appl. Physiol. 59*:953-958.

Haack, D. W., Abel, J. H., Jr., and Jaenke, R. S. (1974). Effects of hypoxia on the distribution of calcium in arterial smooth muscle cells of rats and swine. *Cell Tiss. Res. 157*:125-140.

Haas, F., and Bergofsky, E. H. (1972). Role of the mast cell in the pulmonary pressor response to hypoxia. *J. Clin. Invest. 51*:3154-3162.

Hales, C. A., and Kazemi, H. (1975). Role of histamine in the hypoxic vascular response of the lungs. *Resp. Physiol. 24*:81-88.

Hanna, C. J., Bach, M. F., Pare, P. D., and Schellenberg, R. R. (1981). Slow-reacting substances (leukotrienes) contract human airway and pulmonary vascular smooth muscle *in vitro*. *Nature 290*:343-344.

Harabin, A. L., Peake, M. D., and Sylvester, J. T. (1981). Effect of severe hypoxia on the pulmonary vascular response to vasoconstrictor agents. *J. Appl. Physiol. 50*:561-565.

Harada, R. N., Vatter, A. E., and Repine, J. E. (1984). Macrophage effector function in pulmonary oxygen toxicity: hyperoxia damages and stimulates alveolar macrophages to make and release chemotaxins for polymorphonuclear leukocytes. *J. Leukocyte Biol. 35*:373-383.

Harder, D. R., Madden, J. A., and Dawson, C. (1985a). A membrane electrical mechanism for hypoxic vasoconstriction of small pulmonary arteries from cat. *Chest 88*:234S-245S.

Harder, D. R., Madden, J. A., and Dawson, C. (1985b). Hypoxic induction of Ca^{2+}-dependent action potentials in small pulmonary arteries of the cat. *J. Appl. Physiol. 59*:1389-1393.

Harris, E. J., Al-Saikhaly, M., and Baum, H. (1979). Stimulation mitochondrial calcium ion efflux by thiol-specific reagents and by thyroxine. *Biochem. J. 182*:455-464.

Hauge, A. (1969. Hypoxia and pulmonary vascular resistance. The relative effects of pulmonary arterial and alveolar PO_2. *Acta Physiol. Scand. 76*: 121-130.

Hess, P., Lansman, J. B., and Tsien, R. W. (1984). Different modes of Ca channel gating behaviour favoured by dihydropyridine Ca agonists and antagonists. *Nature 311*:538-544.

Hiser, W., Penman, R. W., and Reeves, J. T. (1975). Preservation of hypoxic pulmonary pressor response in canine pneumoccal pneumonia. *Am. Rev. Resp. Dis. 112*:817-822.

Hughes, J. D., and Rubin, L. J. (1984). Relation between mixed venous oxygen tension and pulmonary vascular tone during normoxic, hyperoxic and hypoxic ventilation in dogs. *Am. J. Cardiol. 54*:1118-1123.

Hultgren, H. N., Grover, R. F., and Hartley, L. H. (1971). Abnormal circulatory responses to high altitude in subjects with a previous history of high-altitude pulmonary edema. *Circulation 44*:759-770.

Jameson, A. G. (1964). Gaseous diffusion from alveoli into pulmonary arteries. *J. Appl. Physiol. 19*:448-456.

Jewell, S. A., Bellomo, G., Thor, H., and Orrenius, S. (1982). Bleb formation in hepatocytes during drug metabolism is caused by disturbances in thiol and calcium ion homeostasis. *Science 217*:1257-1259.

Kadowitz, P. J., and Hyman, A. L. (1984). Analysis of responses to leukotriene D_4 in the pulmonary vascular bed. *Circ. Res. 55*:707-717.

Kanatsuna, T., Nakano, K., Mori, H., Kano, Y., Nishioka, H., Kajiyama, S., Kitasawa, Y., Yoshida, T., Kondo, M., Nakamura, N., et al. (1985). Effects of nifedipine on insulin secretion and glucose metabolism in rats and in hypertensive type 2 (non-insulin dependent) diabetics. *Arzneimittelforsch. 35*:514-517.

Karki, H., Suzuki, T., Oxaki, H., Urakawa, N., and Ishida, Y. (1982). Dissociation of K^+-induced tension and cellular Ca^{2+} retention in vascular and intestinal smooth muscle in normoxia and hypoxia. *Pfluegers Arch. 394*: 118-123.

Kato, M., and Staub, N. C. (1966). Response of small pulmonary arteries to unilobar hypoxia and hypercapnia. *Circ. Res. 19*:426-440.

Kimball, R. E., Reddy, K., Peirce, T. H., Schwartz, W., Mustafa, M. G., and Cross, C. B. (1976). Oxygen toxicity: augmentation of antioxidant defense mechanisms in rat lung. *Am. J. Physiol. 230*:1425-1430.

Kimura, R. E., Thulin, G. E., Wender, D., and Warshaw, J. B. (1983). Decreased oxidative metabolism in neonatal rat lung exposed to hyperoxia. *J. Appl. Physiol. 55*:1501-1505.

Kokubun, S., and Reuter, H. (1984). Dihydropyridine derivatives prolong the open state of Ca channels in cultured cardiac cells. *Proc. Natl. Acad. Sci. USA 81*:4824-4827.

Kontos, H. A. (1985). Oxygen radicals in cerebral vascular injury. *Circ. Res. 57*: 508-516.

Kontos, H. A., Wei, E. P., Christman, C. W., Levasseur, J. E., Povlishock, J. T., and Ellis, E. F. (1983). Free oxygen radicals in cerebral vascular responses *Physiology 26*:165-181.

Kontos, H. A., Wei, E. P., Ellis, E. F., Jenkins, L. W., Povlishock, J. T., Rowe, G. T., and Hess, M. L. (1985). Appearance of superoxide anion radical in cerebral extracellular space during increased prostaglandin synthesis in cats. *Circ. Res. 57*:142-151.

Kosower, E. M. (1970). A role for glutathione in muscle contraction. *Experientia 26*:760-761.

Kosower, E. M., and Kosower, N. S. (1976). Chemical basis of the perturbation of glutathione-glutathione disulfide status of biological systems by diazenes. In *Glutathione: Metabolism and Function*. Edited by I. M. Arias and W. B. Jacoby. Raven Press, New York.

Kosower, E. M., Correa, W., Kinon, B. J., and Kosower, N. S. (1972). Glutathione VII. Differentiation among substrates by the thiol-oxidizing agent, diamide. *Biochem. Biophys. Acta 264*:39-44.

Koyama, T., and Horimoto, M. (1983). Blood flow reduction in local pulmonary microvessels during acute hypoxic imposed on a small fraction of the lung. *Resp. Physiol. 52*:181-189.

Kulik, T. J., and Lock, J. E. (1987). Leukotrienes and the immature pulmonary circulation. *Am. Rev. Resp. Dis. 136*:220-222.

Lahiri, S. (1981). Chemical modification of carotid body chemoreception by sulfhydryls. *Science 212*:1065-1066.

Lamb, F. S., and Webb, R. C. (1984). Vascular effects of free radicals generated by electrical stimulation. *Am. J. Physiol. 247*:H709-H714.

Lebrun, P., Malaisse, W. J., and Herchuelz, A. (1983). Impairment by amino-oxyacetate of ionic response to nutrients in pancreatic islets. *Am. J. Physiol. 245*:E38-E46.

Leffler, C. W., Mitchell, J. A., and Green, R. S. (1984). Cardiovascular effects of leuikotrienes in neonatal piglets. Role in hypoxic pulmonary vasoconstriction? *Circ. Res. 55*:780-787.

Lehninger, A. L., Vercesi, A., and Bababunmi, E. A. (1978). Regulation of Ca^{2+} release from mitochondria by the oxidation-reduction state of pyridine nucleotides. *Proc. Natl. Acad. Sci. USA 75*:1690-1694.

Le-Quoc, K., and Le-Quoc, K. (1982). Central of mitochondrial inner membrane permeability by sulfhydryl groups. *Arch. Biochem. Biophys. 216*:639-651.

Lewis, A. B., Heyman, M. A., and Rudolph, A. M. (1976). Gestational changes in pulmonary vascular responses in fetal lambs in utero. *Circ. Res. 39*:536-541.

Liang, C. S. (1977). Metabolic control of circulation: effects of iodoacetate and fluoroacetate. *J. Clin. Invest. 60*:61-69.

Lloyd, T. C. (1965). Pulmonary vasoconstriction during histotoxic hypoxia. *J. Appl. Physiol. 20*:488-490.

Lloyd, T. C., Jr. (1964). Effect of alveolar hypoxia on pulmonary vascular resistance. *J. Appl. Physiol. 19*:1086-1094.

Lombard, J. H., Smeda, J., Madden, J. A., and Harder, D. R. (1986). Effect of reduced oxygen availability upon myogenic depolarization and contraction of cat middle cerebral artery. *Circ. Res. 58*:565-569.

Longigro, A. J., and Dawson, C. A. (1975). Vascular responses to prostaglandin $F_{2\alpha}$ in isolated cat lungs. *Circ. Res. 36*:706-712.

Longmuir I., Sun, S., and Soucie, W. (1973). Possible role of cytochrome P-450 as a tissue oxygen carrier. In *Oxidases and Related Redox Systems*. Edited by T. King, H. Mason, and M. Morrison, New York.

Lotscher, H. R , Winterhalter, K. H., Carafli, E., and Richter, C. (1979). Hydroperoxides can modulate the redox state of pyridine nucleotides and the calcium balance in rat liver mitochondria. *Proc. Natl. Acad. Sci. USA 76*: 4340-4344.

Lotscher, H. R., Winterhalter, K. H., Carafoli, E., and Richter, C. (1980). Hydroperoxide-induced loss of pyridine nucleotides and release of calcium from rat liver mitochondria. *J. Biol. Chem. 255*:9325-9330.

McMurtry, I. F. (1984). Angiotensin is not required for hypoxic constriction in salt solution-perfused rat lungs. *J. Appl. Physiol. 56*:375-380.

McMurtry, I. F., Davidson, A. B., Reeves, J. T., and Grover, R. F. (1976). Inhibition of hypoxic pulmonary vasoconstriction by calcium antagonists in isolated rat lungs. *Circ. Res. 38*:99-104.

McMurtry, I. F., Rounds, S., and Stanbrook, H. S. (1981). Studies of the mechanism of hypoxic pulmonary vasoconstriction. *Adv. Shock Res. 8*:21-33.

McMurtry, I. F. (1985). BAY K 8644 potentiates and A23187 inhibits hypoxic vasoconstriction in rat lungs. *Am. J. Physiol. 18*:H741-H746.

McMurtry, I. F., Stanbrook, H. S., and Rounds, S. (1982). The mechanisms of hypoxic pulmonary vasoconstriction: a working hypothesis. In *Oxygen Transport to Human Tissues*. Edited by J. A. Loeppky and M. L. Riedesel. Elsevier North-Holland, New York.

Madden, J. A., Dawson, C. A., and Harder, D. R. (1985). Hypoxia-induced activation in small isolated pulmonary arteries from the cat. *J. Appl. Physiol. 59*:113-118.

Malaisse, W. J., Malaisse-Lagae, F., and Sener, A. (1982). The stimulus-secretion coupling of glucose-induced insulin release: effect of aminooxyacetate upon nutrient-stimulated insulin secretion. *Endocrinology 111*:392-397.

Malik, A. B., and Kidd, B. S. L. (1973). Adrenergic blockade and the pulmonary vascular response to hypoxia. *Resp. Physiol. 19*:96-106.

Mammel, M. C., Edgren, B. E., Gordon, M. J., and Boros, S. J. (1986). Failure of two leukotriene synthesis inhibitors to reverse hypoxic pulmonary vasoconstriction. *Clin. Res. 34*:153A.

Marinov, B. S., and Saxon, M. E. (1985). Dihydropyridine Ca^{2+} agonists and channel blockers interact in the opposite manner with photogenerated unpaired electrons. *FEBS 86*:251-254.

Marshall, C., and Marshall, B. (1983). Site and sensitivity of hypoxic pulmonary vasoconstriction. *J. Appl. Physiol. 55*:711-716.

Michelson, A. M., and Puget, K. (1980). Cell penetration by exogenous superoxide dismutase. *Acta Physiol. Scand. 492*:67-80.

Miller, M. A., and Hales, C. A. (1979). Role of cytochrome P-450 in alveolar hypoxic pulmonary vasoconstriction in dogs. *J. Clin. Invest. 64*:666-673.

Morganroth, M. L., Murphy, R. C., Stenmark, K. R., Reeves, J. T., and Voelkel, N. F. (1985). Possible contribution of leukotrienes to hypoxic pulmonary vasoconstriction. *Prog. Resp. Res. 20*:11-16.

Morganroth, M. L., Reeves, J. T., Murphy, R. C., and Voelkel, N. F. (1984a). Leukotriene synthesis and receptor blockers block hypoxic pulmonary vasoconstriction. *J. Appl. Physiol. 56*:1340-1346.

Morganroth, M. L., Stenmark, K., Zirrolli, J. A., Mathias, M., Reeves, J. T., Murphy, R. C., and Voelkel, N. F. (1984b). Leukotriene C_4 production during hypoxic pulmonary vasoconstriction in isolated rat lungs. *Prostaglandins 28*:867-875.

Motley, H. L., Cournand, A., Werko, L., Himmelstein, A., and Dresdale, D. (1947). The influence of short periods of induced acute anoxia upon pulmonary artery pressures in man. *Am. J. Physiol. 150*:315-320.

Nagasaka, Y., Bhattacharya, J., Nanjo, S., Gropper, M. A., and Staub, N. C. (1984). Micropuncture measurement of lung microvascular pressure profile during hypoxia in cats. *Circ. Res. 54*:90-95.

Newman, J. H., McMurtry, I. F., and Reeves, J. T. (1981). Blunted pulmonary pressor responses to hypoxia in blood perfused, ventilated lungs isolated from oxygen toxic rats: possible role of prostaglandins. *Prostaglandins 22*: 11-20.

Newman, J. H., Loyd, J. E., English, D. K., Ogletree, M. L., Fulkerson, W. J., and Brigham, K. L. (1983). Effects of 100% oxygen on lung vascular function in awake sheep. *J. Appl. Physiol. 54*:1379-1386.

Nunn, J. F. (1985). Oxygen-friend and foe. *J. Roy. Soc. Med. 78*:618-622.

Nuutinen, E. M., Nishiki, K., Erecinska, M., and Wilson, D. F. (1982). Role of mitochondrial oxidative phosphorylation in regulation of coronary blood flow. *Am. J. Physiol. 243*:H159-H169.

Orrenius, S., Jewell, S. A., Bellomo, G., Thor, H., Jones, D. P., Smith, M. T. (1983). Regulation of calcium compartmentation in the hepatocyte – a critical role of glutathione. In *Functions of Glutathione. Biochemical, Physiological, Toxicological, and Clinical Aspects*. Edited by A. Larsen, S. Orrenius, A. Holmgren, and B. Mannervik. Raven Press, New York.

Ovetsky, R. M., Sprague, R. S., Stephenson, A. H., Dahms, T. E., and Lonigro, A. J. (1987). Inhibition of leukotriene synthesis does not alter the pulmonary pressor response to alveolar hypoxia. *Am. Rev. Resp. Dis. 135*: A127.

Pagliara, A. S., Hover, B. A., Ellerman, J., and Matschinsky, F. M. (1975). Iodoacetate and iodoacetamide-induced alterations of pancreatic and B-cell responses. *Endocrinology 97*:698.

Patterson, C. E., Butler, J. A., Byrne, F. D., and Rhodes, M. L. (1985). Oxidant lung injury: intervention with sulfhydryl reagents. *Lung 163*:23-32.

Peake, M. D., Harabin, A. L., Brennan, N. J., and Sylvester, J. T. (1981). Steady-state vascular responses to graded hypoxia in isolated lungs of five species. *J. Appl. Physiol. 51*:1214-1219.

Pease, R. D., and Benumof, J. L. (1982). P_aO_2 interaction on hypoxic pulmonary vasoconstriction. *J. Appl. Physiol. 53*:134-139.

Pittman, R. N., and Duling, B. R. (1973). Oxygen sensitivity of vascular smooth muscle. I. In vitro studies. *Microvasc. Res. 6*:202-211.

Plumier, L. (1904). La circulation pulmonaire chez la chien. *Arch. Int. Physiol. 1*:176-213.

Porcelli, R. J., and Bergofsky, E. H. (1973). Adrenergic receptors in pulmonary vasoconstrictor responses to gaseous and humoral agents. *J. Appl. Physiol. 34*:483-488.

Reeves, J. T., Daoud, F. S., and Estridge, M. (1972). Pulmonary hypertension caused by minute amounts of endotoxin in calves. *J. Appl. Physiol. 33*: 739-743.

Reeves, J. T., Grover, R. F., McMurtry, I., Weir, E. K. (1985). Pulmonary vascular reactivity. *Bull. Eur. Physiopathol. Resp. 21*:583-590.

Rengo, F., Trimarco, B., Ricciardelli, B., Volpe, M., Violini, R., Sacca, L., and Chiariello, M. (1979). Effects of disodium cromoglycate on hypoxic pulmonary hypertension in dogs. *J. Pharmacol. Exp. Ther. 211*:686-689.

Rister, M., and Bachner, R. L. (1976). The alteration of superoxide dismutase, catalase, glutathione peroxidase and NAD(P)H cytochrome c reduction in guinea-pig polymorphonuclear leukocytes and alveolar macrophages during hyperoxia. *J. Clin. Invest. 58*:1174-1184.

Rosen, P., and Stier, A. (1973). Kinetics of CO and O_2 complexes of rabbit liver microsomal cytochrome P-450. *Biochem. Biophys. Res. Commun. 51*: 603-611.

Rosenblum, W. I. (1983). Effects of free radical generation on mouse pial arterioles: probable role of hydroxyl radicals. *Am. J. Physiol. 245*:H139-H142.

Rosenthal, M., LaManna, J. C., Jobsis, F. F., Levasseur, J. E., Kontos, H. A., and Patterson, J. L. (1976). Effects of respiratory gases on cytochrome a in intact cerebral cortex. Is there a critical PO_2? *Brain Res. 108*:143-154.

Roth, Z., and Dikstein, S. (1982). Inhibition of ruthenium red-insensitive mitochondrial Ca^{2+} release and its pyridine nucleotide specificity. *Biochem. Biophy. Res. Commun. 105*:991-996.

Rounds, S., and McMurtry, I. F. (1981). Inhibitors or oxidative ATP production cause transient vasoconstriction and block subsequent pressor responses in rat lungs. *Circ. Res. 48*:393-400.

Rubanyi, G. M., and Vanhoutte, P. M. (1986). Oxygen-derived free radicals, endothelium and responsiveness of vascular smooth muscle. *Am. J. Physiol. 250*:H815-H821.

Said, S. I., Yoshida, T., Kitamura, S., and Vreim, C. (1974). Pulmonary alveolar hypoxia: release of prostaglandins and other humoral mediators. *Science 285*:1181-1183.

Schellenberg, R. R., and Foster, A. (1984). Differential activity of leukotrienes upon human pulmonary vein and artery. *Prostaglandins 27*:475-482.

Schmid, A., Barhanin, J., Coppola, T., Borsotto, M., and Lazdunski, M. (1986). Immunochemical analysis of subunit structures of 1,4-dihydropyridine receptors associated with voltage-dependent Ca^{2+} channels in skeletal, cardiac, and smooth muscles. *Biochemistry 25*:3492-3495.

Schuster, D. P., and Dennis, D. R. (1987). Leukotriene inhibitors do not block hypoxic pulmonary vasoconstriction in dogs. *J. Appl. Physiol. 62*:1808-1813.

Sener, A., Malaisse-Lagae, F., Dufrane, S. P., and Malaisse, W. J. (1984). The coupling of metabolic to secretory events in pancreatic islets. *Biochem. J. 220*:433-440.

Shelton, G. (1970). The effect of lung ventilation on blood flow to the lungs and body of the amphibian *Xenopus laevis. Resp. Physiol. 9*:183-196.

Shirai, M., Sada, K., and Ninomiya, I. (1986). Effects of regional alveolar hypoxia and hypercapnia on small pulmonary vessels in cats. *J. Appl. Physiol. 61*:440-448.

Sobol, B. J., Bottex, G., Emirgil, C., and Gissen, H. (1963). Gaseous diffusion from alveoli to pulmonary vessels of considerable size. *Circ. Res. 13*:71-79.

Somlyo, A. P. (1985). Excitation-contraction coupling and the ultrastructure of smooth muscle. *Circ. Res. 57*:497-507.

Stanbrook, H. S., and McMurtry, I. F. (1983). Inhibition of glycolysis potentiates hypoxic vasoconstriction in rat lungs. *J. Appl. Physiol. 55*:1467-1473.

Staub, N. C. (1963). The interdependence of pulmonary structure and function. *Anesthesiology 24*:831-854.

Sventeck, J. C., and Zambraski, E. J. (1985). Effects of 100 percent oxygen on the cardiovascular responses to vasoactive compounds in the dog. *Aviat. Space Environ. Med. 56*:972-975.

Sylvester, J. T., and McGowan, C. (1978). The effects of agents that bind to cytochrome P-450 on hypoxic pulmonary vasoconstriction. *Circ. Res. 43*:429-437.

Sylvester, J. T., Harabin, A. L., Peake, M. D., and Frank, R. S. (1980). Vasodilator and constrictor responses to hypoxia in isolated pig lungs. *J. Appl. Physiol. 49*:820-825.

Tate, R. M., Morris, H. G., Schroeder, W. R., and Repine, J. E. (1984). Oxygen metabolites stimulate thromboxane production and vasoconstriction in isolated saline-perfused rabbit lungs. *J. Clin. Invest. 74*:608-613.

Tierney, D. F., Ayers, L., and Kasuyama, R. S. (1977). Altered sensitivity to oxygen toxicity. *Am. Rev. Resp. Dis. 115*:59-65.

Toivonen, H., Hartiala, J., and Bakhle, Y. S. (1981). Effects of high oxygen tension on the metabolism of vasoactive hormones in isolated perfused rat lungs. *Acta Physiol. Scand. 111*:185-192.

Tollins, M., Weir, E. K., Chesler, E., Nelson, D. P., and From, A. H. L. (1986). Pulmonary vascular tone is increased by a voltage-dependent calcium channel potentiator. *J. Appl. Physiol. 60*:942-948.

Tucker, A., and Reeves, J. T. (1975). Nonsustained pulmonary vasoconstriction during acute hypoxia in anesthetized dogs. *Am. J. Physiol. 228*:756-761.

Tucker, A., Weir, E. K., Grover, R. F., and Reeves, J. T. (1976). Oxygen-tension-dependent pulmonary vascular responses to vasoactive agents. *Can. J. Physiol. Pharmacol. 55*:251-257.

Turrens, J. F., Freeman, B. A., and Crapo. J. D. (1982a). Hyperoxia increases H_2O_2 release by lung mitochondria and microsomes. *Arch. Biochem. Biophys. 217*:411-421.

Turrens, J. F., Freeman, B. A., Levitt, J. C., and Crapo, J. D. (1982b). The effect of hyperoxia on superoxide production by lung submitochondrial particles. *Arch. Biochem. Biophys. 217*:401-410.

Vaage, J., Bjertnaes, L., and Hauge, A. (1975). The pulmonary vasoconstrictor response to hypoxia: effects of inhibitors of prostaglandin biosynthesis. *Acta Physiol. Scand. 95*:95-101.

Vader, C. R., Mathias, M. M., and Schatte, C. L. (1981). Pulmonary prostaglandins Med. 6:101-110.

Vader, C. R., Mathias, M. M., and Schatte, C. L. (1981). Pulmonary prostaglandin metabolism during normobaric hyperoxia. *Prostaglandins Med. 6*: 101-110.

Vallieres, J., Scarpa, A., and Somlyo, A. P. (1975). Subcellular fractions of smooth muscle: isolation, substrate utilization and Ca^{2+} transport by main pulmonary artery and mesenteric vein mitochondria. *Arch. Biochem. Biophys. 170*:659-669.

Van Breeman, C., Aaronson, P., Loutzenhiser, R., and Meisheri, K. (1980). Ca^{2+} movements in smooth muscle. *Chest 78*:157-165.

Voeklel, N. F. (1986). Mechanisms of hypoxic pulmonary vasoconstriction. *Am. Rev. Resp. Dis. 133*:1186-1195.

Voelkel, N. F., McMurtry, I. F., and Reeves, J. T. (1981a). Hypoxia impairs vasodilation in the lung. *J. Clin. Invest. 67*:238-246.

Warshaw, J. B., Wilson, C. W., III, Saito, K., and Prough, R. A. (1985). The responses of glutathione and antioxidant enzymes to hyperoxia in developing lung. *Pediatr. Res. 19*:819-823.

Weir, E. K., Will, J. A., Lundquist, L. J., Eaton, J. W., and Charles, E. (1983). Diamide inhibits pulmonary vasoconstriction induced by hypoxia or prostaglandin $F_{2\alpha}$. *Proc. Soc. Exp. Biol. Med. 173*:96-103.

Weir, E. K. (1984). Acute hypoxic pulmonary hypertension. In *Pulmonary Hypertension*. Edited by E. K. Weir and J. T. Reeves. Futura, New York., pp. 251-289.

Weir, E. K., and Grover, R. F. (1978). The role of endogenous prostaglandins in the pulmonary circulation. *Anesthesiology 48*:201-212.

Weir, E. K., and Will, J. A. (1982). Oxidants: a new group of pulmonary vasodilators. *Clin. Resp. Physiol. 18*:81-85.

Weir, E. K., McMurtry, I. F., Tucker, A., Reeves, J. T., and Grover, R. F. (1976). Prostaglandin synthetase inhibitors do not decrease hypoxic pulmonary vasoconstriction. *J. Appl. Physiol. 41*:714-718.

Weir, E. K., Eaton, J. W., and Chesler, E. (1985). Redox status and pulmonary vascular reactivity. *Chest 88*:249S-252S.

Weiss, G. B. (1985). Calcium kinetics in vascular smooth muscle. *Chest 88*:220S-223S.

White, C. W., and Repine, J. E. (1985). Pulmonary antioxidant defense mechanisms. *Exp. Lung Res. 8*:81-96.

White, C. W., Mimmack, R. F., and Repine, J. E. (1986). Accumulation of lung tissue oxidized glutathione (GSSG) as a marker of oxidant induced lung injury. *Chest 89*:111S-113S.

White, R. E., and Coon, M. J. (1980). Oxygen activation by cytochrome P-450. *Ann. Rev. Biochem. 49*:315-356.

Wilson, D. F., Erecinska, M., Drown, C., and Silver, I. A. (1979). The oxygen dependence of cellular energy metabolism. *Arch. Biochem. Biophys. 195*: 485-493.

Wolin, M. S., and Burke, T. M. (1987). Mechanisms of oxygen tension and hydrogen peroxide dependent modulation in force in the pulmonary artery. *Am. Rev. Resp. Dis. 135*:A127.

Yokochi, K., Olley, P. M., Sideris, E., Hamilton, F., Huhtanen, D., and Coceani, F. (1982). Leukotriene D_4: a potent vasoconstrictor of the pulmonary and systemic circulations in the newborn lamb. In *Leukotrienes and Other Lipoxygenase Products*. Edited by B. Samuelsson and R. Padetti. Raven pp. 251-289.

Yusa, T., Crapo, J. D., and Freeman, B. A. (1984). Hyperoxia enhances lung and liver nuclear superoxide generation. *Biochim. Biophys. Acta 798*:167-174.

Zasslow, M. A., Benumof, J. L., and Trousdale, F. R. (1982). Hypoxic pulmonary vasoconstriction and the size of hypoxic compartment. *J. Appl. Physiol. 53*:626-630.

Zhu, Y. J., Kradin, R., Brandstetter, R. D., Staton, G., Moss, J., and Hales, C. A. (1983). Hypoxic pulmonary hypertension in the mast cell deficient mouse. *J. Appl. Physiol. 54*:680-686.

9

Autonomic Control of the Pulmonary Circulation

ALBERT L. HYMAN, HOWARD L. LIPPTON, COLBY W. DEMPESY, CHARLES J. FONTANA, DONALD E. RICHARDSON, RICHARD W. RIECK, and PHILIP J. KADOWITZ

Tulane University School of Medicine
New Orleans, Louisiana

I. Introduction

Although the pulmonary vascular bed is in series with the systemic bed, it conducts the entire cardiac output at a pressure less than 20% of systemic vascular pressure. The lung endeavors to preserve efficient gas exchange by maintaining this low vascular pressure as a deterrent to formation of pulmonary edema. Hence, the responses of these vessels to a variety of physiologic and pharmacologic stimuli would be expected to be dissimilar to those in the systemic circulation. An enormous number of studies have confirmed the ability of the pulmonary vessels to respond actively to physiologic stimuli such as hypoxia and changes in blood pH and to a host of humoral and exogenously administered vasoactive substances (Grover et al., 1983). However, the role of neurally mediated mechanisms in the regulation of the pulmonary vascular bed remains enigmatic. This chapter examines the evidence that the autonomic nervous system possesses the capacity to contribute to the regulation of the pulmonary circulation, and suggests that it may exercise a homeostatic role in the integrated function of the lung.

Five specific topics of inquiry, each cardinal to the thesis of autonomic regulation of the pulmonary vascular bed, are discussed.

1. Anatomic evidence of innervation of the pulmonary vascular bed with sympathetic and parasympathetic motor fibers
2. Pharmacologic evidence for the presence of subtypes of adrenergic and cholinergic receptors in pulmonary resistance vessels; these responses are changed by alterations in levels of vasoconstrictor tone in the pulmonary vascular bed
3. Response of the pulmonary vascular bed to postganglionic sympathetic nerve stimulation; these responses are altered by changes in the level of pulmonary vasomotor tone
4. Responses of the pulmonary vascular bed to parasympathetic nerve stimulation, and the effect of pulmonary vascular tone on these responses
5. The effects of stimulation of the brain on pulmonary vascular resistance, and the influence of pulmonary vascular tone on these responses

The results of our experiments, along with data accumulated from other laboratories, strongly support the concept that the central nervous system, integrated with the autonomic nervous system, has the capacity to regulate the pulmonary circulation.

II. Anatomic Evidence of Autonomic Motor Nerve Supply to the Pulmonary Vascular Bed

In many species there is abundant evidence that sympathetic and parasympathetic nerve fibers innervate pulmonary vessels (Fillenz, 1970; Hebb, 1969; Naigaishi, 1972; Verity and Bevan, 1968; von Euler and Lishajko, 1958). Using fluorescence histochemistry and stretched preparations, Fillenz (1970) demonstrated fluorescent nerve fibers in the walls of 30-300 μm intrapulmonary arteries and larger intrapulmonary veins of the dog. Kadowitz and co-workers (1976) also showed by fluorescence histochemistry that adrenergic nerves are present in intrapulmonary large and small arteries (down to 25 μm) and larger intrapulmonary veins (Fig. 1). These fluorescent preparations clearly identified the characteristic beading typical of adrenergic vasomotor nerves (Burnstock et al., 1970; Furness and Malmfors, 1974; Furness and Marshall, 1974). Furthermore, studies by Kadowitz et al. (1976) showed that chronic treatment with 5- and 6-hydroxydopamine analogs, which, like dopamine, are taken up by adrenergic terminals, removed the histochemical evidence of adrenergic innervation in intrapulmonary vessels. Electron microscopic studies further indicated that 5- and 6-hydroxydopamine increased the size and density of dense cores in small and large vesicles of adrenergic varicosities of intrapulmonary vessels. These substances, therefore, served as markers for identification of adrenergic terminals, because in glutaraldehyde-fixed tissues adrenergic varicosities contain little or no dense core (Burnstock et al., 1970). Additionally, a close correlation was established between anatomic presence of adrenergic nerves and physiologic function. Not only did these histologic markers identify the presence of sympathetic nerve supply, but they also attenuated the arterial and venous responses to sympathetic nerve stimulation by depleting norepinephrine from the adrenergic terminals (Kadowitz et al., 1976). In contrast, the responses to exogenous norepinephrine were not attenuated by these markers but were blocked by alpha adrenergic receptor antagonists. These adrenergic terminals are found in the arterial adventitia and outer third of the media, but only in the adventitia of pulmonary veins. They contain many small and a few large dense-core vesicles. Thus, hemodynamic, histochemical, and ultrastructural studies indicate that vasomotor tone in the pulmonary vascular bed can be regulated by sympathetic nerves.

Fillenz (1970) found evidence of cholinergic innervation in the ir. . a-pulmonary arteries of the dog, but none were identified in intrapulmonary veins. Additional studies (Kadowitz et al., 1976) have shown that 20-40% of the varicosities in intrapulmonary arteries of the dog contain many small agranular and a few large opaque vesicles, further suggesting the presence of cholinergic vesicles. The histologic appearance of this type of vesicle was not altered by the 5- and 6-hydroxydopamine markers. Cholinergic vesicles have not been identified in intrapulmonary veins of the dog. Moreover, the physiologic evidence that neurogenically released acetylcholine may serve to modulate release of adrenergic transmitter is supported by the anatomic evidence indicating the close proximity of adrenergic and cholinergic vesicles in intrapulmonary arterial segments. The ability of acetylcholine to inhibit the release of norepinephrine from the adrenergic terminals and modulate the increase in isometric tension in response to sympathetic stimulation has been demonstrated in isolated segments of dog intrapulmonary arteries (Vanhoutte, 1974).

The intrapulmonary arterial innervation of the cat has also been the subject of extensive study (Cech and Dolezel, 1967; Hebb, 1969; Falck, 1962; Fisher, 1965; Verity et al., 1964). In this species, too, light microscopy has demonstrated the presence of fine unmyelinated nerves in pulmonary arteries. In addition, acetylcholinesterase-containing nerves, some of which are localized in the tunica media, are known to be present in intrapulmonary arteries in cats. Studies with the Falck-Hillarp technique have revealed fluorescent nerves near the adventio-medial junction of feline intrapulmonary arteries (Cech and Colezel, 1967; Falck, 1962; Hebb, 1969). The nerve organization in this species also indicated that no more than the outer third of the tunica media is innervated (Verity and Bevan, 1968). As in the dog, the adventitia of both the small intrapulmonary arteries and veins have adrenergic vesicles (Rhodin, 1978). Further-

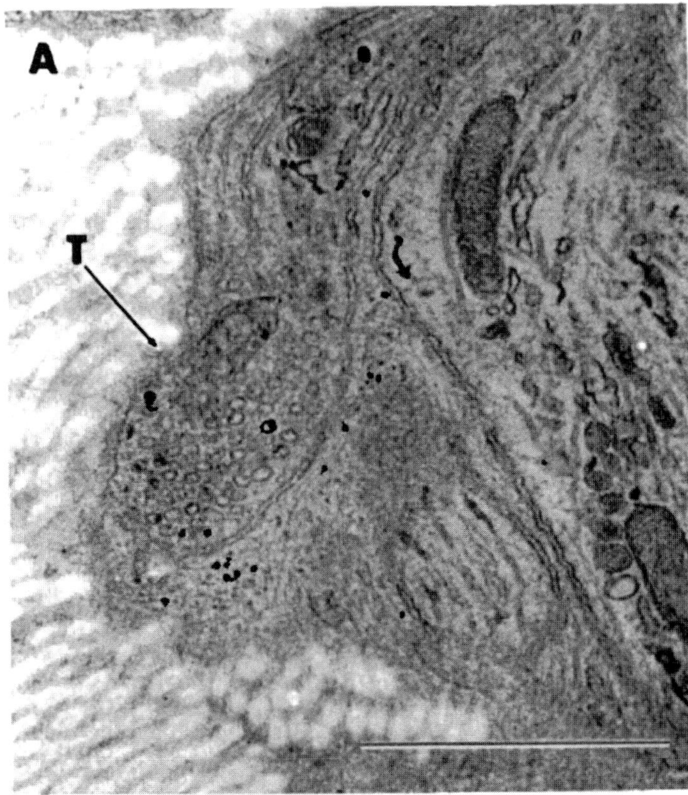

Figure 1 Electron micrographs of adventitial-medial zone of canine intrapulmonary artery. In untreated dogs nerve terminals (T) contain very few dense-core vesicles, making identification difficult (panel A). This type of appearance is common in glutaraldehyde-fixed tissues. In dogs treated with 5-hydroxydopamine, the density and size of dense-core vesicles of adrenergic (A) terminals are increased (panels B and C). Panel D is from a dog treated with 6-hydroxydopamine. SM, smooth muscle cells; C, cholinergic terminal; SC, Schwann cells. Bar in lower right-hand corner of each picture is 1 μm.

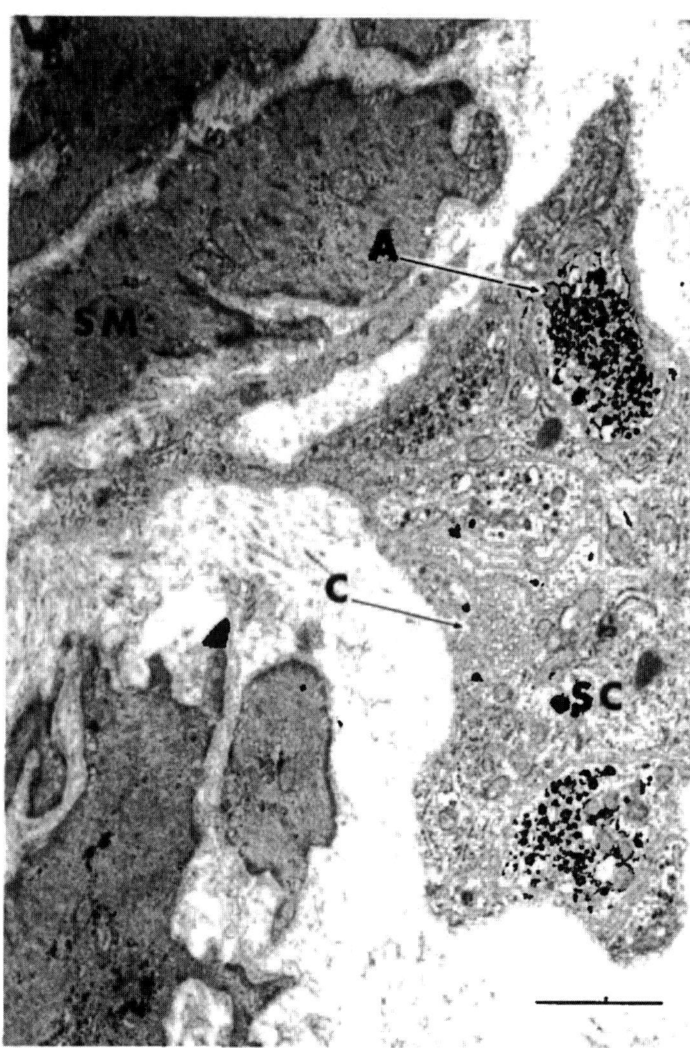

Figure 1B

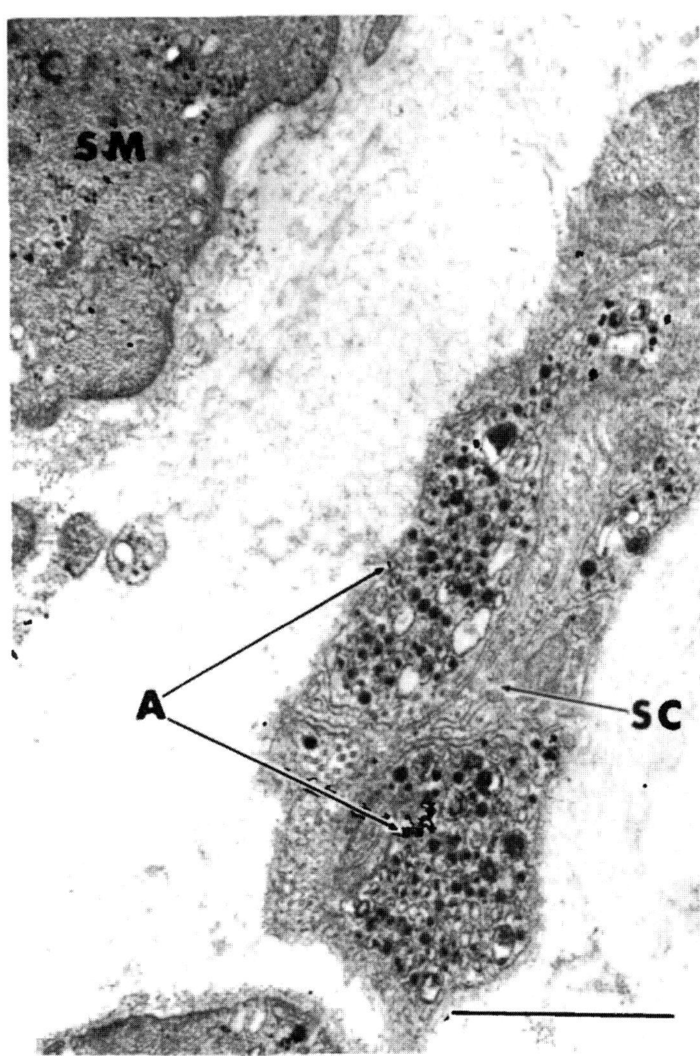

Figure 1C

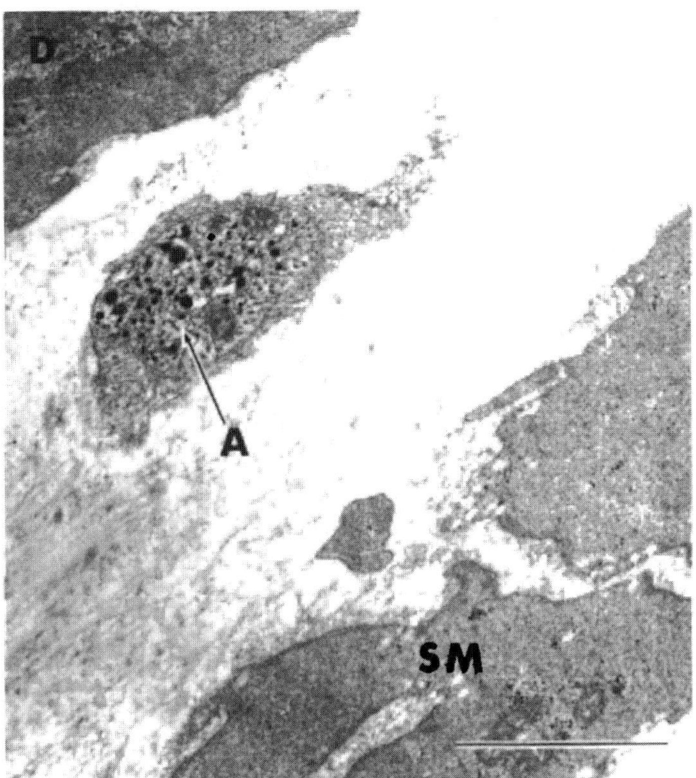

Figure 1D

more, studies using 5-hydroxydopamine in the cat have identified a periarterial plexus of nerves in the walls of pulmonary arteries that extend into the lung to innervate even small arteries having a single layer of smooth muscle cells (Knight et al., 1981). These studies further suggested that adrenergic terminals are suitably positioned to cause the release of norepinephrine and thus cause a decrease in compliance of larger arteries and an increase in resistance in smaller pulmonary arteries and veins. Medium-size and small cat arteries also contain apparent cholinergic nerves. Cholinergic terminals appear to be closely related to arterial adrenergic terminals in the cat and in this species as well may act indirectly by modulating the release of norepinephrine from the closely located adrenergic terminals.

Hebb (1969) has compared the motor innervation of several other species, including the rat, rabbit, sheep, and calf. The most complete adrenergic motor innervation is found in the rabbit, cat, sheep, and dog. In the rat, adrenergic nerve fibers were found external to the media in extrapulmonary arteries and were most clearly marked in the main pulmonary artery. None of the intrapulmonary arteries is innervated. On the other hand, rat larger pulmonary veins appear to have innervation, which may extend from the left atrium. Similarly, in the calf, the adrenergic motor nerve supply is sparse in arterial segments, but larger pulmonary veins appear to be innervated, except near the heart where nerves become sparse again. Further, Hebb (1969) has described cholinergic motor innervation in sheep, calf, pig, cat, and rabbit. In general, predominantly the larger arteries are supplied especially at the adventitia and near the vasa vasorum. No evidence of cholinergic nerves supplying intrapulmonary vessels was found in the guinea pig, except perhaps in the main lobar vein.

III. Specific Types of Adrenergic and Cholinergic Receptors in the Pulmonary Vascular Bed

It has been known for about 40 years that postjunctional alpha adrenergic receptor stimulation causes pulmonary vasoconstriction in the isolated perfused lung segment (Konzeth and Hebb, 1949). Studies of the direct effects of alpha receptor stimulation, predominantly those mediated by norepinephrine, have been obscured for the most part by concurrent passive changes induced by the drug's tendency to increase pulmonary blood flow or raise left atrial pressure. Using an intact chest technique in spontaneously breathing dogs with controlled pulmonary blood flow and left atrial pressure, Hyman (1969a) demonstrated that norepinephrine directly constricted pulmonary veins and upstream (arterial) vessels. Other investigators have subsequently used stop-flow techniques (Linehan and Dawson, 1982; Rippe et al., 1987) and have similarly identified vasoconstrictor responses to norepinephrine in both the venous and arterial segments of the pulmonary blood vessels.

Moreover, the hypothesis that all postjunctional alpha adrenoceptors are not of a single type was suggested as early as 1965 (Bevan and Osher, 1965). In the systemic vascular beds, both alpha_1 and alpha_2 postjunctional receptors for vasoconstriction have been identified in a number of species including humans (Bobik, 1982; Constantine et al., 1980; De May and Vanhoutee, 1981; Janernig et al., 1978; Langer et al., 1980; Langer and Shepperson, 1982; Ruffolo et al., 1981; Starke et al., 1974). Although only postjunctional alpha_1 receptors were identified in isolated rabbit pulmonary arterial segments (Borowski et al., 1977; Starke et al., 1974, 1975a, b), Hyman and Kadowitz (1985) identified both alpha_1 and alpha_2 adrenoceptors in the pulmonary vessels of intact spontaneously breathing cats under conditions of constant flow and left atrial pressure (Figs. 2 and 3). They showed that intralobar injections of the alpha_1

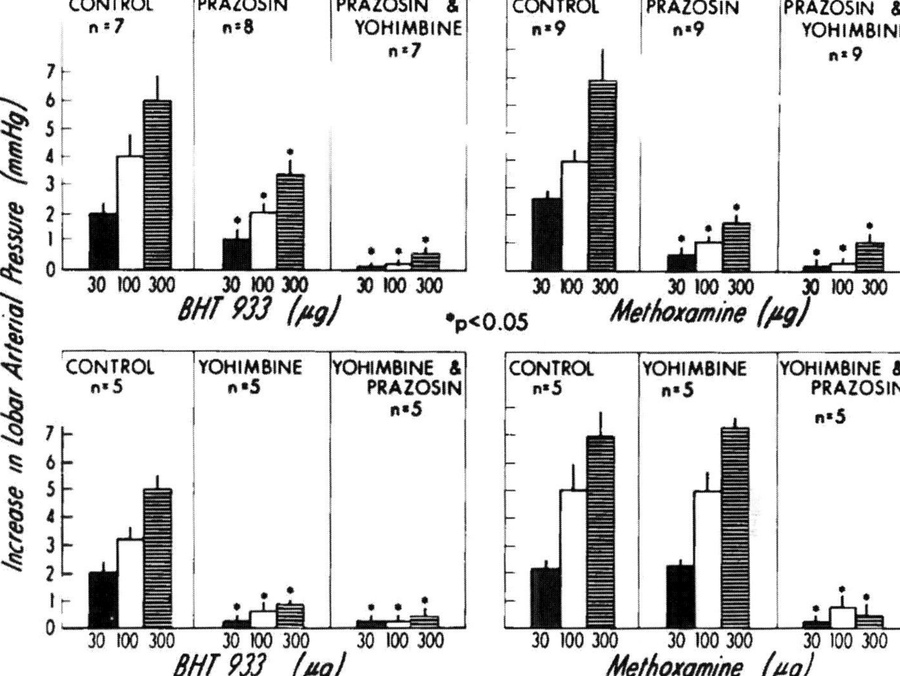

Figure 2 *Top left panels*: Effects of prazosin and of prazosin + yohimbine on increases in lobar arterial pressure in response to BHT 933. *Top right panels*: Influence of yohimbine and of yohimbine + prazosin on responses to BHT 933. *Lower left panels*: Effects of prazosin and of prazosin + yohimbine on responses to methoxamine. *Lower right panels*: Effects of yohimbine and of yohimbine + prazosin on responses to methoxamine. *n*, number of cats; *asterisk*, response is significantly different from control.

agonists phenylephrine and methoxamine and the $alpha_2$ agonists BHT 933 and UK 14304 caused pulmonary vasoconstrictor responses in a dose-related manner. In these intact cats, prazosin, a specific $alpha_1$ adrenoceptor antagonist, blocked responses to the $alpha_1$ adrenoceptor to a greater extent than responses to $alpha_2$ agonists. On the other hand, yohimbine, a specific $alpha_2$-receptor antagonist, blocked the responses to $alpha_2$ agonists without affecting responses to $alpha_1$ agonists.

After destruction of the adrenergic vesicles with 6-hydroxydopamine, this pattern of responses was unchanged, indicating that these were indeed postjunctional adrenoceptors. However, in propranolol-treated cats, the $alpha_1$ antagonist prazosin blocked the response to the $alpha_1$ agonists without altering

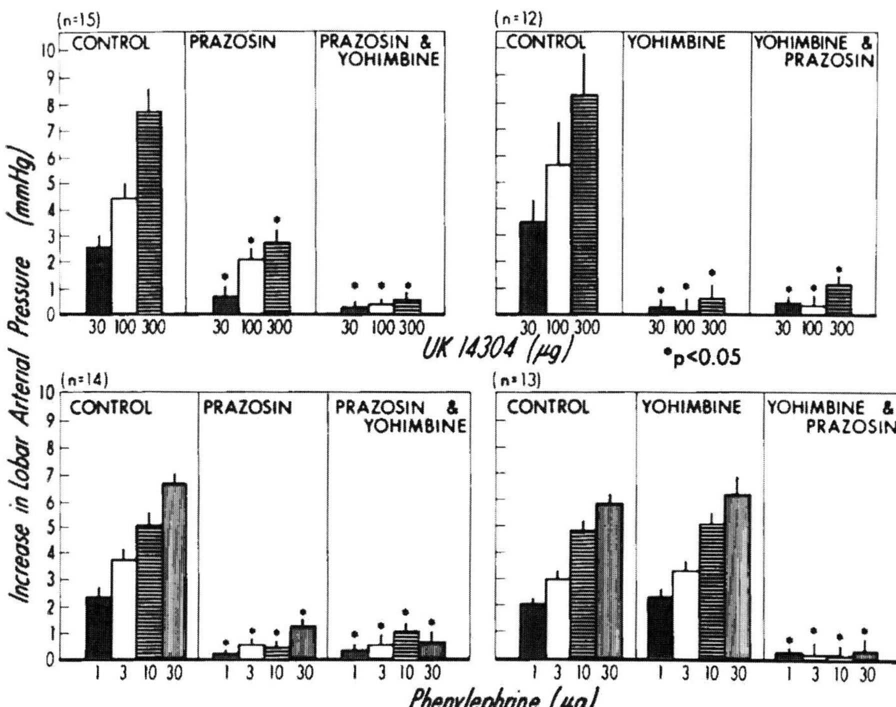

Figure 3 *Top left panels*: Effects of prazosin and of prazosin + yohimbine on increases in lobar arterial pressure in response to UK 14,304. *Top right panels*: Effects of yohimbine and of yohimbine + prazosin on responses to UK 14,304. *Lower left panels*: Influence of prazosin and of prazosin + yohimbine on responses to phenylephrine. *Lower right panels*: Effects of yohimbine and of yohimbine + prazosin on responses to phenylephrine. *n*, number of animals; *asterisk*, response is significantly different from control.

the responses to $alpha_2$ agonists, and again the integrity of the specific blocking activity of the $alpha_2$ antagonist yohimbine was preserved (Fig. 4). The studies with propranolol suggest that in the pulmonary vascular bed there is an interaction between $alpha_1$ and $beta_2$ adrenoceptors. A similar interaction has been reported in the systemic vascular bed (McGrath, 1982; Wilffert et al., 1983a, b). The nature of this interaction is unclear. Since, in that study, the blockade with prazosin was similar in 6-hydroxydopamine-treated cats and untreated cats, the interaction is not likely to be related to the influence of prazosin on prejunctional $alpha_2$ receptors.

The response to exogenous norepinephrine was blocked to a large extent by the $alpha_1$ antagonist prazosin and to a much lesser extent by the $alpha_2$

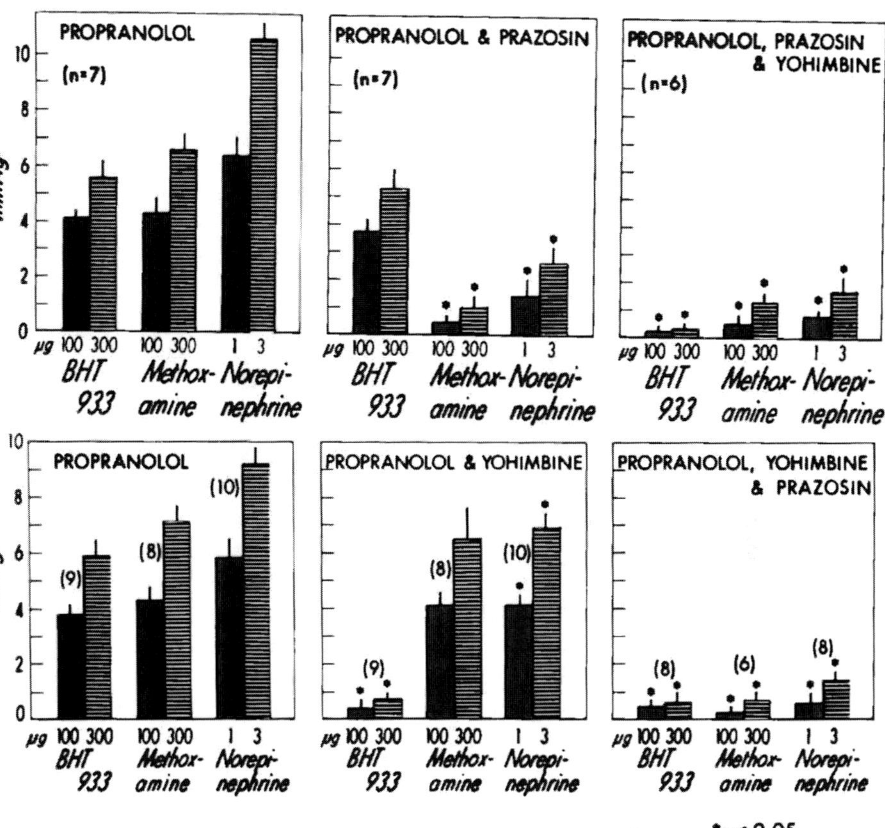

Figure 4 *Top panels*: Effects of prazosin and of prazosin + yohimbine on responses to BHT 933, methoxamine, and norepinephrine in propranolol-treated animals. *Lower panels*: Influence of yohimbine and yohimbine + prazosin on responses to BHT 933, methoxamine, and norepinephrine in propranolol-treated animals. *n*, number of cats; *asterisk*, responses were significantly different from those treated with propanolol (*left-hand panel*).

antagonist yohimbine. Hence, the responses to exogenous or humorally mediated norepinephrine are mediated largely by $alpha_1$ adrenoceptors. This predominant $alpha_1$-stimulating effect of norepinephrine in the pulmonary vascular bed differs markedly from the responses found in the systemic vascular bed, where exogenous or humorally mediated norepinephrine stimulates predominantly $alpha_2$ adrenoceptors. An explanation for the differences in receptor subtypes stimulated by norepinephrine is not clear. They may be related in part to the difference in tone in the two vascular beds, since enhancement in pulmonary vascular tone greatly increases responses to alpha$_2$ agonists but only slightly increases alpha$_1$ responses.

The importance of uptake I in the pulmonary vascular bed is further demonstrated by the effects of chemical destruction of the prejunctional adrenergic vesicles with 6-hydroxydopamine. After these vesicles are destroyed, the responses to norepinephrine and phenylephrine, which are taken up by the adrenergic vesicles (uptake I) are greatly enhanced. On the other hand, responses to methoxamine and the alpha$_2$ agonists, which are not subject to uptake I, are not enhanced by adrenergic vesicle destruction. The role of uptake II in the pulmonary vascular bed has not been established.

The difference between the studies in intact spontaneously breathing cat pulmonary vessels, which showed both alpha$_1$ and alpha$_2$ adrenoceptors in the pulmonary vascular bed (Hyman and Kadowitz, 1985), and the isolated rabbit pulmonary artery studies (Borowski et al., 1977; Starke et al., 1974-1975a, b) showing only alpha$_1$ adrenoceptors is not explained. In addition to species differences, the intact cat studies examined responses in small resistance arteries, whereas the rabbit isolated strip studies referred to large conducting arteries. Moreover, others have found uneven distribution of postjunctional alpha adrenoceptors in arterial and venous segments (de May and Vanhoutte, 1981). Still others have suggested that alpha adrenoceptors may be transformed from one subtype to the other when vessels are isolated, and this may explain different response patterns observed in vivo and in vitro (McGrath, 1982). Further, the responses to alpha$_1$ and alpha$_2$ adrenoceptor stimulation may be altered when vessels are perfused with blood or with artificial perfusates (McGrath, 1982).

At resting tone, the pulmonary vessels are, for a large part, dilated, and beta adrenoceptor mediated vasodilator responses are not readily identified. However, masked beta adrenoceptor vasodilator responses are indeed present at resting tone. This is indicated by the fact that, at resting tone, responses to amines possessing both alpha and beta adrenoceptor stimulating properties are enhanced by beta adrenoceptor blockade. This masked beta effect at resting tone has been demonstrated with norepinephrine, epinephrine, and phenylephrine (Hyman et al., 1981; Hyman and Kadowitz, 1985, 1986) but is not apparent with methoxamine, an alpha$_1$ agonist without beta receptor stimulating properties.

These beta receptor responses are blocked by a specific beta$_2$ blocking agent, ICI 118551, as well as by the nonselective beta$_{1\text{-}2}$ blocker propranolol (Hyman et al., 1981; Hyman and Kadowitz, 1985-1986) and are only weakly blocked by the specific beta$_1$ blocking agent metroprolol. Furthermore, the pulmonary vasodilator response to the specific beta$_2$ agonist albuterol was blocked by both the specific beta$_2$ antagonist ICI 118551 and the nonselective beta$_{1\text{-}2}$ antagonist propranolol. Thus, in the pulmonary vascular bed, as in the systemic bed, vasodilator responses to beta adrenoceptor stimulation are mediated by $beta_2$ adrenoceptor subtypes. This masked beta effect may be important in clinical cardiology. Patients receiving long-term nonselective beta blocking drugs for angina or hypertension may, in the natural course of their disease, develop acute myocardial infarction with hypotension and left ventricular failure. In these patients, the pulmonary vasoconstrictor response to drugs with both alpha and beta agonist effects would be expected to be greatly enhanced, a condition that may promote the tendency for pulmonary edema.

Increases in tone in the pulmonary vascular bed greatly enhance the vasoconstrictor response to $alpha_2$ agonists and the vasodilator responses to $beta_2$ agonists but only modestly enhance the vasoconstrictor responses to $alpha_1$ receptor stimulation (Hyman and Kadowitz, 1986) (Figs. 5 and 6). This altered response at high tone does not appear to be specifically mediated by any particular vasoconstricting agent, since it has been demonstrated under conditions in which tone was enhanced by U46619, a thromboxane A_2 stimulator, serotonin, angiotensin, hypoxia, acidemia, and even spontaneously arising pulmonary vasoconstriction in intact animals (Hyman and Kadowitz, 1986; Silvone et al., 1968). Thus, vasoconstrictor responses to the direct effect of clonidine-like $alpha_2$ agonists, such as UK 14304 and BHT 933, are greatly increased when pulmonary vasoconstriction is present (Hyman and Kadowtiz, 1986). The enhanced response to methoxamine, an $alpha_1$ agonist, is not as striking.

Enhancement of vasodilator responses to $beta_2$ adrenoceptor stimulation at high pulmonary vascular tone has also been identified (Hyman and Kadowitz, 1986). Those studies demonstrated that when the vasodilator responses to a $beta_{1-2}$ agonist, isoproterenol, were compared to a nonadrenergic vasodilator, nitroglycerin, at two levels of enhanced tone, the vasodilator response to the two agonists were not similarly enhanced. When tone was raised to a moderate level, vasodilator responses to the beta adrenoceptor agonist and nitroglycerin became significant and dose related. However, as tone was further increased, the vasodilator responses to the beta adrenoceptor agonist were greater than those noted at moderately elevated tone, whereas the responses to the nonspecific vasodilator nitroglycerin were not proportionately enhanced. Further evidence of the enhancement of $beta_2$ responses at elevated tone is found in the altered responses of amines with both alpha and beta agonist effects. Although phenylephrine is generally considered to be a selective $alpha_1$ adrenoceptor agonist, it has been reported that pressor responses to phenylephrine were reversed after treatment with alpha adrenoceptor blocking agents and that the decreases in systemic arterial pressure were blocked by propranolol (Lefevre et al., 1977). However, the responses to phenylephrine are different in the feline pulmonary vascular bed in that the constrictor response is reversed and a vasodilator response is unmasked at elevated tone without alpha adrenoceptor blockade (Fig. 6). The vasodilator responses to phenylephrine and to epinephrine at elevated vascular tone are blocked by propranolol, suggesting that

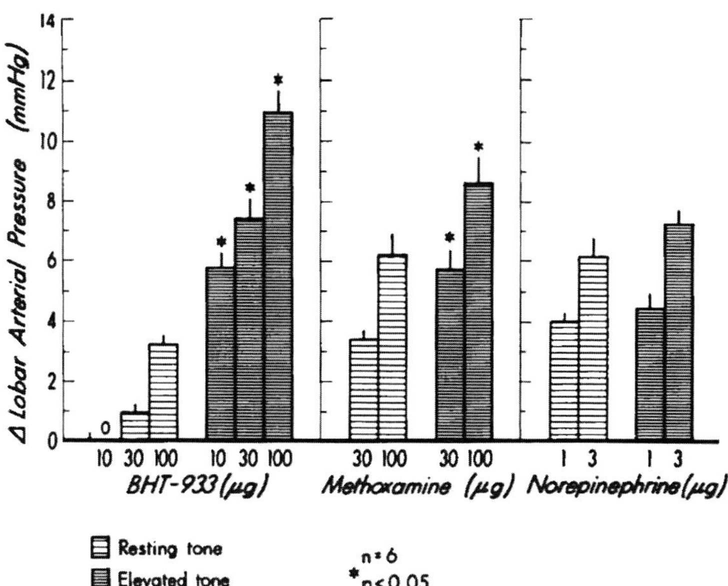

Figure 5 Comparison of increases in lobar arterial pressure in response to BHT 933, methoxamine, and norepinephrine under resting tone conditions, and when vascular tone was elevated to a high steady level by infusion of the prostaglandin endoperoxide analog U46619. *n*, number of animals; *asterisk*, responses under elevated tone conditions are significantly greater than responses under resting tone conditions.

they result from stimulation of beta adrenoceptors. Further, the vasoconstrictor responses to phenylephrine and epinephrine after beta adrenoceptor blockade at elevated tone are mediated for the most part by alpha$_1$ adrenoceptors, since they are sensitive to blockade by prazosin. In addition, after beta adrenoceptor blockade, the enhancement of vasoconstrictor responses to phenylephrine and epinephrine induced by increasing vascular tone is only moderate, like other alpha$_1$ agonist responses. It is similar to that observed with methoxamine and was unlike the enhanced responses seen with the alpha$_2$ adrenoceptor agonists. Enhancement of responses to these alpha and beta adrenoceptor agonists at elevated levels of vascular tone appear to be related largely to tone-induced changes in activity of alpha$_1$, alpha$_2$, and beta$_2$ adrenoceptors.

Norepinephrine stimulates alpha$_1$ and beta$_2$ adrenoceptors and, to a lesser extent, alpha$_2$ adrenoceptors in the pulmonay vascular bed of the cat. The vasoconstrictor response to exogenous norepinephrine is not altered by increasing pulmonary vascular tone, suggesting that the alpha and beta$_2$ stimu-

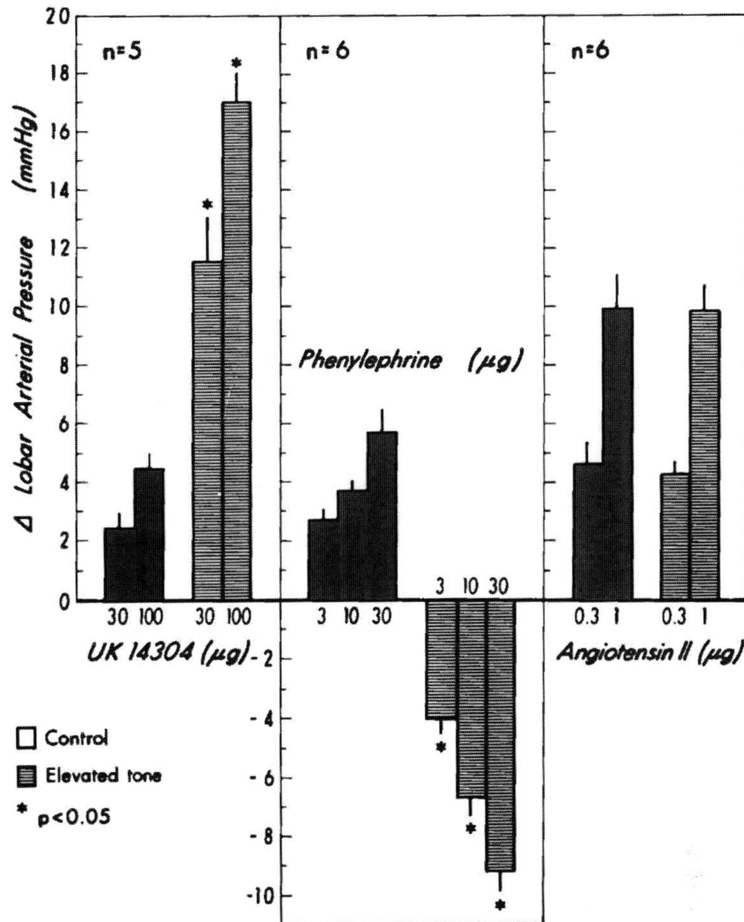

Figure 6 Influence of an elevation in vascular tone on responses to UK 14,304, phenylephrine, and angiotensin II in the feline pulmonary vascular bed. Responses were obtained under control (resting tone) conditions and when tone was elevated by intralobar infusion of U46619.

lating properties of the amine are enhanced in a balanced fashion so that the net response is not changed (Fig. 5). This hypothesis is supported by the observations that the vasoconstrictor response to norepinephrine is enhanced at high vascular tone after beta adrenoceptor blockade and that a vasodilator response equal in magnitude to the vasoconstrictor response is recorded after $alpha_1$ adrenoceptor blockade with prazosin. The smaller contribution of $alpha_2$ adrenoceptors to the norepinephrine-induced vasoconstriction at elevated tone is indicated by the observation that yohimbine attenuates the pressor response but does not reverse it (Figs. 7 and 8). Additionally, this vasodilator response is enhanced when there is combined $alpha_1$ and $alpha_2$ adrenoceptor blockade. Previous reports have also shown that the vasoconstrictor response to neurally released norepinephrine in the feline pulmonary vascular bed is modulated by concurrent $beta_2$ adrenoceptor stimulation (Hyman et al., 1981).

Epinephrine and phenylephrine are less potent vasoconstrictors than norepinephrine in the feline pulmonary vascular bed, and at baseline (low) vascular tone the alpha adrenoceptor stimulating activity with each amine is sufficient to overcome the concurrent beta adrenoceptor stimulating properties. However, at elevated vascular tone, the enhancement of the $beta_2$ adrenoceptor stimulating activity is greater than the modest effects of elevated tone on $alpha_1$ adrenoceptor responses, and the net effect seen in response to epinephrine and phenylephrine is vasodilation, whereas with norepinephrine the alpha stimulating properties predominate.

The feline pulmonary vascular bed has both postjunctional $alpha_1$ and $alpha_2$ adrenoceptors, and norepinephrine and epinephrine act, for the most part, on $alpha_1$ adrenoceptors to elicit vasoconstriction. Further, $alpha_2$ and $beta_2$ and, to a lesser extent, $alpha_1$ adrenoceptor mediated responses are enhanced when vasoconstriction is elevated. This effect is rapid in onset and reversible in nature. It is therefore possible that tone-dependent changes in adrenoceptor responses may afford an explanation for divergent vascular responses reported for agents such as epinephrine that have alpha and beta adrenoceptor stimulating properties in the pulmonary circulation.

The mechanism by which these alterations in alpha adrenoceptor responses are mediated is unclear. Since the responses to angiotensin II (Hyman and Kadowitz, 1986) and U46619 (Kadowitz et al., 1987), the thromboxane A_2 stimulator, are not altered at high tone, these alterations do not appear to reflect a purely physical change in lumen/wall ratio. They could result from an effect on alpha adrenoceptor number or sensitivity with the $alpha_2$ population affected to a greater extent than the $alpha_1$ adrenoceptor population. Further, vasoconstriction has been shown to alter the configuration of the smooth muscle cell membrane, and that contraction has caused large bulbous evaginations of the plasma membrane not seen in relaxed cells (Dingemans and Wagenvoort, 1976; Fay and Delise, 1973). Mesenteric arterioles undergo complex shape changes during vasoconstriction, and these changes could have profound implications for the control of vascular resistance (Greensmith and Duling, 1984). It is possible that such changes in vessel morphology and physical state of cell membranes (Dingemans and Wagenvoort, 1976; Fay and Delise, 1973; Greensmith and Duling, 1984) could alter alpha adrenoceptor function in the feline pulmonary vascular bed. Moreover, the mediation of the enhanced $beta_2$ adrenoceptor response at high tone is also not established. Whatever the mechanisms, these

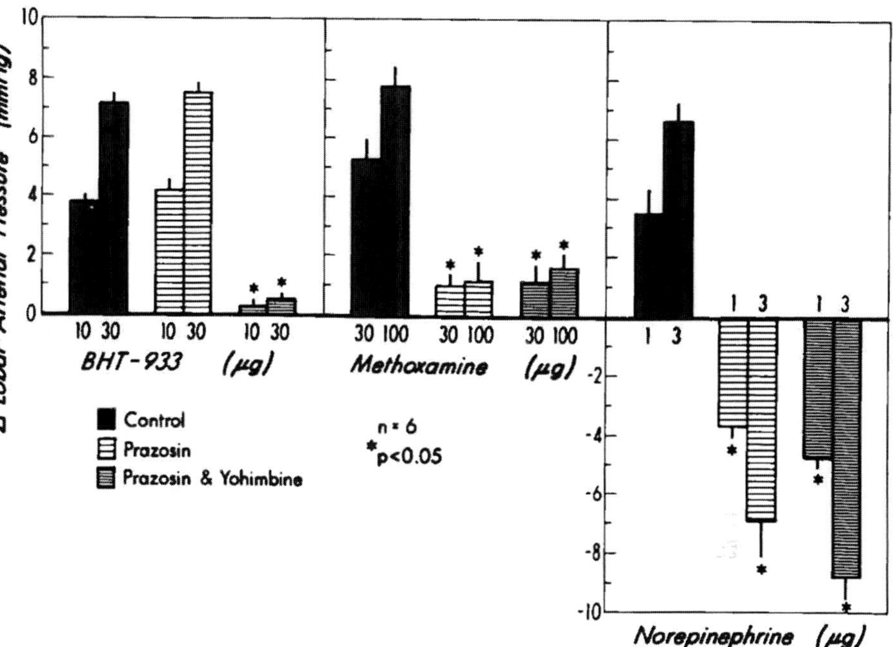

Figure 7 At elevated tone, $alpha_1$ and $alpha_2$ agonists are blocked by their selective agonists, but the response to norepinephrine is completely reversed by prazosin. This suggests that even at elevated tone the vasoconstrictor effect of norepinephrine is mediated in the main by $alpha_1$ receptors.

alterations in adrenoceptor responses are peculiar to pulmonary vessels that are actively constricted, since these responses are not seen when similar degrees of pulmonary hypertension are induced passively by increasing the pulmonary venous pressure. In the latter circumstance, vessel wall tension is greatly increased, and the vessels are distended rather than actively constricted.

IV. Responses of the Pulmonary Vascular Bed to Sympathetic and Parasympathetic Stimulation

Electrical stimulation of the sympathetic nerves has been shown to cause pulmonary vasoconstriction (Daly and Hebb, 1966; Hakim and Dawson, 1979; Kadowitz and Hyman, 1973) and a decrease in pulmonary arterial compliance (Ingram et al., 1968; Pace, 1971). Increases as great as 70% in vascular resistance have been demonstrated (Kadowitz et al., 1974, 1975). Moreover, others have found no change in small vessel tone or resistance (Ingram et al., 1968), although

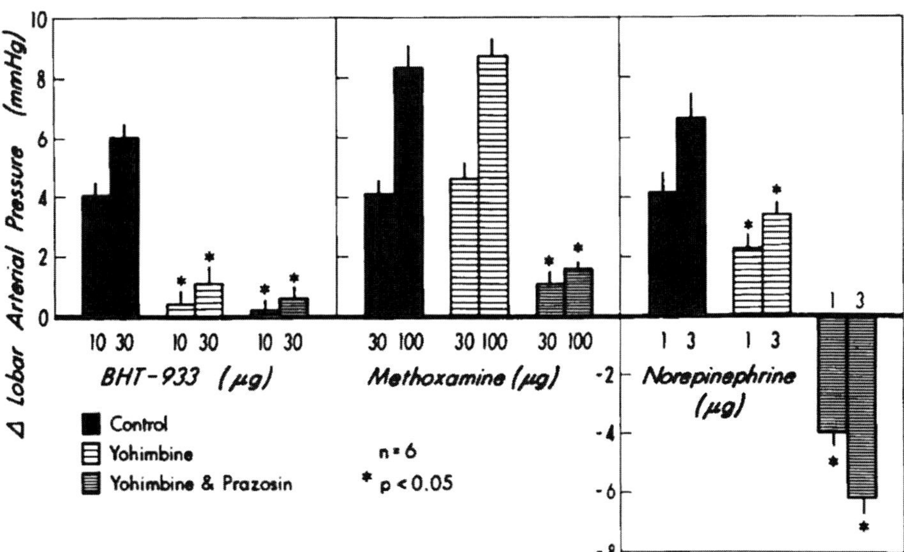

Figure 8 In contrast to Figure 7, $alpha_2$ blockade with yohimbine attenuates the vasoconstrictor response to norepinephrine, suggesting that $alpha_2$ receptor stimulation contributes to the vasoconstrictor response, but the $alpha_1$ receptor response predominates.

most recent investigations indicate that vascular resistance increases with sympathetic stimulation (Malik, 1985). The segmental distribution of the vasoconstrictor response is not entirely established. Direct measurements of pressure in intrapulmonary veins of 2.5-3.0 mm diameter have indicated that these vessels participate in the vasoconstrictor response (Kadowitz et al., 1975). Although the venous constriction is generally less intense than the arterial, some studies suggest that it may account for as much as half the total increase in pulmonary vascular tone (Kadowitz et al., 1975). On the other hand, others (Hakim and Dawson, 1979) using a stop-flow technique were unable to identify a venous component in the pulmonary vasoconstrictor response, although these vessels did constrict to exogenous norepinephrine.

Although the decrease in compliance of large pulmonary arteries and increased resistance of the smaller vessels are generally accepted as mediated by alpha adrenoceptors, the contribution of beta receptor stimulation by sympathetic nerve stimulation has received less attention (Kadowitz and Hyman, 1973; Porcelli and Bergofsky, 1973; Silvone et al., 1968). Some systemic vascular beds have been reported to dilate in response to sympathetic nerve stimulation (Greenway and Lawson, 1969; Greenway et al., 1968; Ngai et al., 1966; Pegram et al., 1976; Viveros et al., 1968), but some investigators have challenged the concept that beta adrenoceptors are innervated and that neuronally released norepinephrine can elicit vasodilation (Russell and Moran, 1980). In the normally dilated pulmonary vascular bed, $beta_2$ adrenoceptor mediated responses are masked at resting tone, so that only a vasoconstrictor response is elicited by sympathetic nerve stimulation. However, after specific $beta_2$ adrenoceptor blockade with ICI 118551, the pressor response to sympathetic nerve stimulation is enhanced (Hyman, 1986). Thus, the pressor response at resting tone is the net result of the stronger $alpha_{1-2}$ agonist effect of the neurotransmitter norepinephrine and its weaker $beta_2$ agonist effect. This masked $beta_2$ vasodilator effect was not identified in an earlier study using propranolol (Hyman et al., 1981). The reasons for this difference in response to nerve stimulation after the selective and nonselective beta blockers are unclear. Prejunctional $beta_2$ adrenoceptors have been reported to enhance norepinephrine release (Langer, 1977). Nonetheless, where pulmonary vascular tone was elevated and the alpha effect of the neurotransmitter norepinephrine was blocked with the nonselective alpha adrenoceptor blocker phenoxybenzamine, sympathetic nerve stimulation produced a pure vasodilator effect (Hyman et al., 1981). Here, the postjunctional beta2 agonist effect of the neurotransmitter norepinephrine was unmasked by blocking the alpha adrenoceptor constricting effect. These data further indicate that $beta_2$ adrenoceptors in the pulmonary vascular bed are innervated, and a masked vasodilator response can be operative.

The subtypes of alpha adrenoceptors that are stimulated by neurally released norepinephrine have received little attention. At resting tone the vasopressor response to sympathetic nerve stimulation was completely blocked by the selective $alpha_1$ antagonist prazosin and not significantly altered by the selective $alpha_2$ antagonist yohimbine (Hyman, 1986). Thus, at resting tone in the pulmonary vascular bed, the vasoconstrictor effect of sympathetic nerve stimulation is mediated primarily by $alpha_1$ adrenoceptors. This is similar to the systemic vascular bed in which the vasoconstrictor response to sympathetic nerve stimulation is also mediated by $alpha_1$ adrenoceptors (Langer, 1977). The role that pre- and postjunctional $alpha_2$ adrenoceptors may play in the response to nerve stimulation is less clearly documented. Should postjunctional $alpha_2$ adrenoceptors be present, their blockade with yohimbine could attenuate the vasoconstrictor response. However, the concurrent prejunctional $alpha_2$ blockade with yohimbine may enhance the release of norepinephrine. Hence, the failure of the $alpha_2$ antagonist yohimbine to attentuate the vasoconstrictor response to sympathetic stimulation could simply indicate that there are no postjunctional $alpha_2$ adrenoceptors. The vasoconstrictor response to exogenous specific $alpha_2$ agonists would then result from stimulation of only extrajunctional $alpha_2$ adrenoceptors. Alternatively, the failure of yohimbine to affect the response to sympathetic nerve stimulation at resting tone could be a consequence of the net effect of postjunctional $apha_2$ blockade tending to attenuate the constrictor response, balanced by the prejunctional $alpha_2$ blocking effect tending to release more norepinephrine and enhance the vasoconstrictor effect. Studies with tyramine, however, support the hypothesis that both pre- and postjunctional $alpha_2$ adrenoceptors do contribute to the response, although their roles are probably less important than that of $alpha_1$ adrenoceptors. Tyramine is an agent that releases norepinephrine from the adrenergic vesicles by mechanisms that are independent of prejunctional $alpha_2$ adrenoceptor modulation. In those studies, yohimbine did not attentuate the constrictor response to sympathetic stimulation but did attentuate the vasoconstrictor responses to exogenously administered norepinephrine and to tyramine (Hyman, 1986). This finding suggests that $alpha_2$ adrenoceptors are present in the postjunctional area. Blockade of these postjunctional $alpha_2$ adrenoceptors with yohimbine results in attentuation of the responses to norepinephrine released from the adrenergic vesicle by tyramine as well as the constrictor response to exogenous norepinephrine. Moreover, the failure of yohimbine to attentuate the constrictor response to sympathetic nerve stimulation supports the concept that at resting tone the effects or pre- and postjunctional $alpha_2$ blockade are nearly balanced. Since prazosin blocked the response, the contribution of junctional $alpha_2$ receptor responses is small. Earlier studies using isolated electrically stimulated strips of dog pulmonary artery also suggested the presence of pre- and postjunctional $alpha_2$ receptors (Constantine et al., 1980). These studies suggest differences between the pulmonary and systemic adrenergic innervation, in that the postjunctional area of pulmonary vessels contain both $alpha_1$ and $alpha_2$ as well as $beta_2$ receptors (Fig. 9).

The effects of sympathetic nerve stimulation at enhanced pulmonary vascular tone have been investigated recently in this laboratory (Hyman, 1986). Vasoconstriction of the pulmonary vascular bed was produced by a variety of interventions, including infusions of U46619, serotonin, and angiotensin, and on occasion it occurred spontaneously in cats without pretreatment. Regardless of the method of enhancing the vascular tone, sympathetic nerve stimulation for 15-30 sec under these conditions produced an initial pulmonary vasoconstrictor response lasting 20-30 sec followed by a more prolonged (30-90 sec) vasodilator response (Hyman, 1986) (Fig. 10). The vasoconstrictor response was attenuated by both the $alpha_1$ blocker prazosin and the $alpha_2$ blocker yohimbine and abolished by the administration of both. Thus, the vasoconstrictor effect of sympathetic nerve stimulation at elevated tone results from postjunctional alpha adrenoceptor stimulation. However, at elevated tone, the mediation of the alpha vasoconstrictor response appears to be somewhat different than at resting tone, since at resting tone the response appeared to be almost entirely mediated by $alpha_1$ adrenoceptors and almost completely blocked by prazosin. At elevated tone, the mediation appears to be more complex, involving an interplay between postjunctional $alpha_2$ adrenoceptors, which at high tone cause greatly

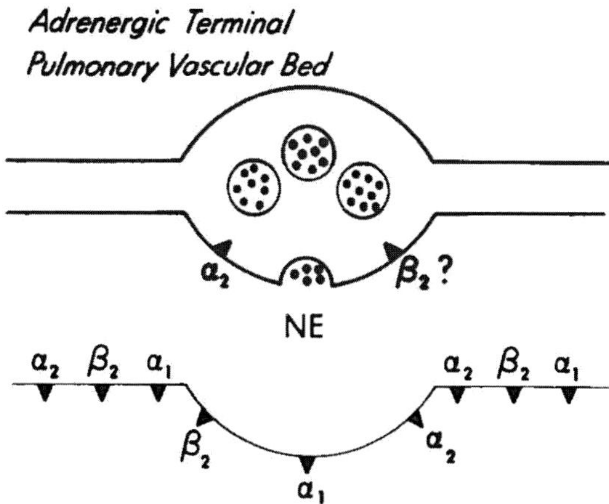

Figure 9 Diagrammatic representation of a pulmonary vascular adrenergic terminal. The data suggest the presence of prejunctional $alpha_2$ receptors and postjunctional $alpha_1$ and $alpha_2$ receptors, as well as $beta_2$ receptors. In addition, there are extrajunctional $alpha_{1-2}$ and $beta_2$ receptors.

enhanced responses; prejunctional $alpha_2$ adrenoceptors; $alpha_1$ adrenoceptors, whose responses are not as greatly enhanced; and $beta_2$ postjunctional adrenoceptors, which at high tone also cause greatly enhanced dilator responses. Thus, attenuation of the vasoconstrictor response at enhanced tone by the $alpha_2$ antagonist yohimbine may represent a reflection of greatly enhanced responses to postjunctional $alpha_2$ adrenoceptors at elevated tone, and perhaps prejunctional $alpha_2$ blockade.

The pulmonary vasodilation that succeeds the vasoconstrictor response during sympathetic nerve stimulation at elevated tone is blocked both by the $beta_2$ specific antagonist ICI 118551 and propranolol, confirming again that the $beta_2$ adrenoceptors in the pulmonary vascular bed are innervated. Since at elevated tone the initial $apha_{1-2}$ mediated vasoconstrictor response is enhanced by $beta_2$ blockade and the succeeding vasodilator response is enhanced by $alpha_{1-2}$ blockade, those studies again indicate that the response to sympathetic nerve stimulation in the pulmonary vascular bed results from the net effect of opposing alpha and beta adrenoceptor stimulation. At resting tone, the response to sympathetic stimulation is predominantly mediated by $alpha_1$ adrenoceptors. At elevated tone, $beta_2$ and $alpha_2$ responses are greatly enhanced, and here a biphasic response results from neurogenic stimulation of $alpha_1$, $alpha_2$, and $beta_2$ adrenoceptors.

V. Effects of Parasympathetic Nerve Stimulation on Pulmonary Vascular Resistance

A large number of investigations have established that the pulmonary vascular bed responds to muscarinic receptor stimulation (Feeley et al., 1963; Hyman,

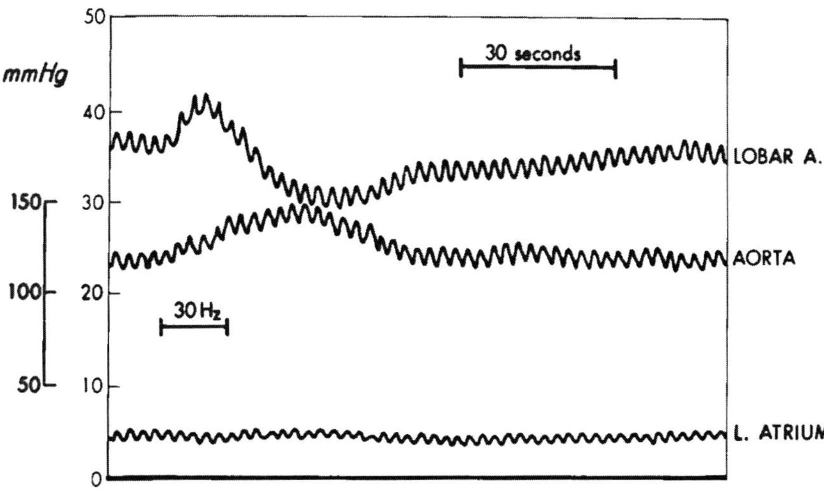

Figure 10 Tracing of lobar arterial pressor response to sympathetic nerve stimulation. Lobar arterial flow is held constant. The initial vasoconstrictor response is followed by a longer vasodilator response. Elevated tone was maintained by continuous infusion of U46619.

1969b; Rudolph et al., 1959). However, the responses to acetylcholine have varied from vasoconstriction in some studies to vasodilation in others. Studies of infusions of acetylcholine have also shown pulmonary venoconstriction in intact (Hyman, 1969b) and open-chest (Feeley et al., 1963) dogs. Indeed, at low tone, the pulmonary arterial pressor effect appears to be contributed to by pulmonary venous constriction and a combination of active pulmonary arterial constriction and passively mediated effects resulting from segmental displacement of blood from the pulmonary veins to the arterial segment (Feeley et al., 1963; Hyman, 1969b). In other studies, however, acetylcholine induced a vasodilator response (Alcock et al., 1935; Rose, 1957). Rudolph and co-workers (1959) proposed that the level of tone in the pulmonary vascular bed may be a critical factor in determining the response to acetylcholine. Indeed, in the dog with controlled flow at low tone, acetylcholine caused constriction, but at high tone with uncontrolled flow this agent caused a vasodepressor response. Subsequent studies with controlled flow and left atrial pressure have also emphasized the critical nature of pulmonary vascular tone in determining the response to acetylcholine. Under conditions of controlled flow, at very low pressures (10-12 mmHg) and constant flow at physiologic levels in intact cats, acetylcholine causes a dose-related pressor response (Hyman and Kadowitz, 1987). Small increases in pressure (around 3-5 mmHg), which may occur spontaneously during the course of the experiment, reverse the response. Mild hypertension, when induced by breathing 10% O_2, completely reverses the response, and vasodilation is seen, except at the higher dose (30 μg) of acetylcholine where the response becomes biphasic, depressor-pressor. At even higher levels of tone induced by infusion of U46619 (perfusion pressures, about 30 mmHg), the response is reversed, and acetylcholine in even the higher doses causes a profound vasodilation. When tone is elevated, infusions of nitroglycerin quickly return the pulmonary vessels to low tone and revert their response back to vasoconstrictor (Fig. 11). Since both types of responses are completely blocked by atropine, these responses are both due to muscarinic receptor stimulation. However, mediation of the divergent responses to stimulation of this pulmonary muscarinic receptor at various levels of tone are unclear. The muscarinic-1 subtype antagonist pirenzepine (50 μg/kg) blocks the pressor response, but not the vasodilator response, suggesting that subtypes of muscarinic receptors may be involved. On the other hand, the muscarinic-2 blocker gallamine, in doses up to 10 mg/kg, does not attenuate the pressor or depressor response. Alternatively, the reversal at high tone may suggest that endothelium-derived relaxing factor (Furchgott and Zawadski, 1980) may be more active at high tone in the pulmonary vascular bed. Additional studies are necessary to explain the mediation of this tone dependency.

There is species difference in pulmonary vascular responses to acetylcholine. In the rabbit, at low pulmonary vascular tone acetylcholine is also a vasoconstrictor, but at high tone it is a vasodilator only at very low doses. As the dose is increased at high tone, the initial vasodilator response decreases, and vasoconstriction becomes the predominant response. The vasoconstrictor response in the rabbit, but not the cat, is mediated in part by cyclooxygenase-derived products of archidonic acid, but the dilator response is not. As in the cat, all responses are blocked by atropine, and only the constrictor response is blocked by pirenzepine. A previous report has also shown that in the rabbit the pressor response is mediated in part by cholinergic receptor activation of the arachidonic cascade (Hassan et al., 1986).

Parasympathetic nerve stimulation via the cervical vagosympathetic nerve causes pulmonary vasodilation when tone is enhanced by hypoxia or other vasoconstricting stimuli in cats (Nandiwada et al., 1983). However, this dilation is seen only after the sympathetic neurotransmitter is blocked (Fig. 12). The response is enhanced by physostigmine and blocked by atropine. Little if any response is seen under these conditions at resting tone.

The role of the endothelium-derived relaxing factor (EDRF) in mediating vasodilator responses to parasympathetic nerve stimulation is also unclear. Since the cholinergic vesicles release acetylcholine into the adventitia during parasympathetic stimulation, this neurotransmitter must pass through the media before reaching the endothelium to stimulate release of EDRF. Furthermore, at low vascular tone acetylcholine introduced through the lumen cases vasoconstriction.

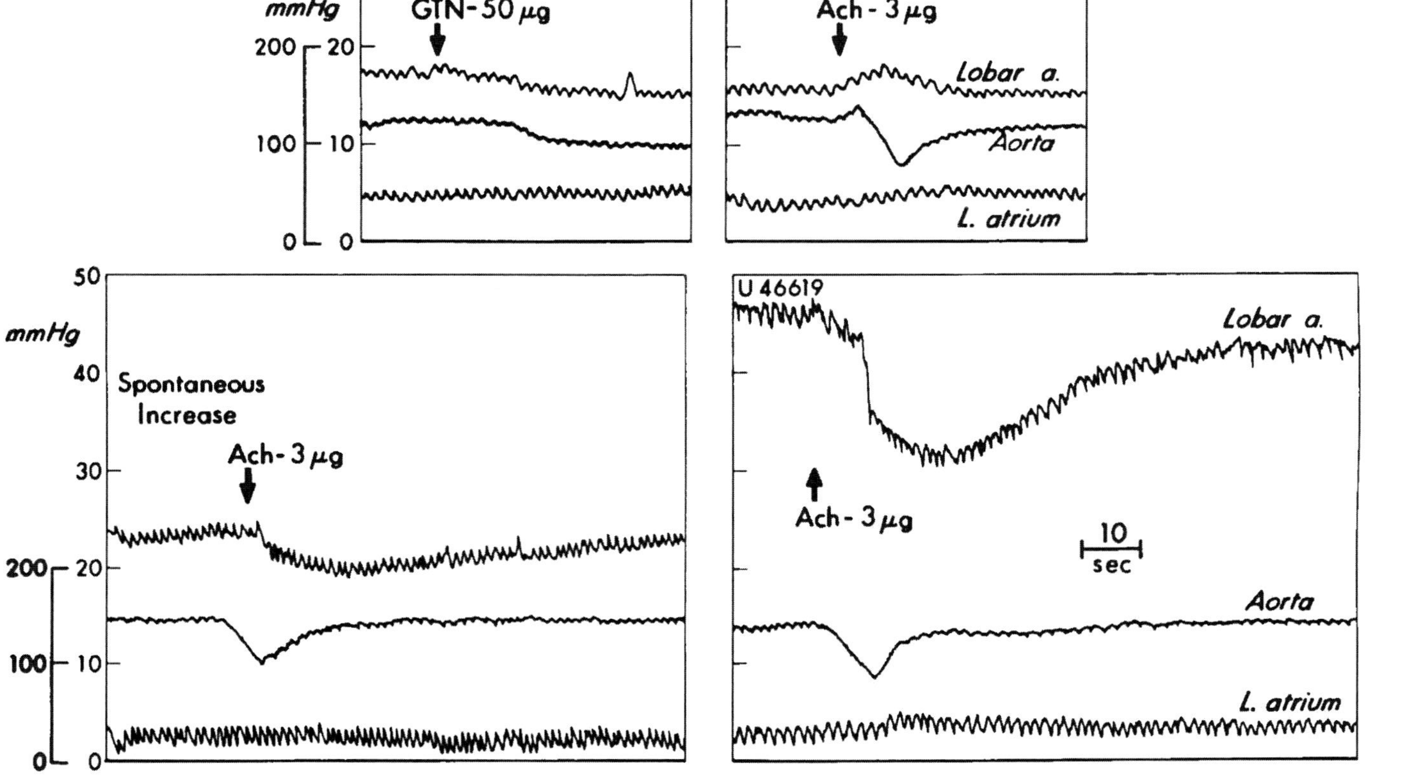

Figure 11 The spontaneous increase in pulmonary vascular tone is decreased by a bolus injection of 50 µg nitroglycerin. At lower tone, acetylcholine induces vasoconstriction. As tone again increases, either spontaneously or with U46619, the same dose of acetylcholine now induces vasodilation.

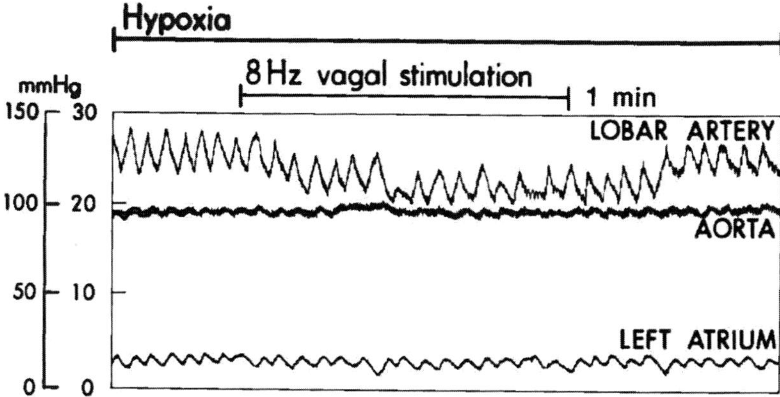

Figure 12 Records from an experiment illustrating the effect of vagal stimulation at 8 Hz on lobar arterial pressure when lobar vascular resistance had been increased by ventilation with 10% O_2 in nitrogen. When the FL_{O2} was decreased from 0.21 to 0.10, lobar arterial pressure was increased from 18 to 28 mmHg in this animal.

VI. The Effects of Stimulation of the Brain on Pulmonary Vascular Resistance

The Cushing reflex in response to increased cerebrospinal pressure has been extensively studied, but the pulmonary vascular responses are inconsistent. This may result in part from concurrent acute systemic hypertension and heart failure, decreased left ventricular diastolic compliance, and greatly increased left atrial pressure. These changes passively distend pulmonary vessels and obscure any reflex vasoconstriction. Indeed, even when pulmonary vasoconstriction is identified (Hessler and Cassin, 1977; Marion and Dawson, 1980), the actual contribution of intrinsic pulmonary adrenergic nerves is unclear (Lloyd, 1973; Marion et al., 1979). Bloodborne catecholamines released from adrenal glands during brain stimulation from increased cerebrospinal fluid pressure may induce a humorally mediated pulmonary vasoconstriction in the dog (Marion et al., 1979). These observations seem to have been mediated at low pulmonary vascular tone. Presumably, in the dog as well as the cat, epinephrine and norepinephrine both cause vasoconstriction at low tone.

The pulmonary vascular responses to electrical stimulation of discrete areas of the brain are poorly understood. Electrical stimulation of the hypothalamic integrative area for the defense reaction caused small increases in calculated pulmonary vascular resistance and pulmonary blood flow in open-chest dogs (Anderson and Brown, 1967). In contrast, other investigators found that stimulation of the hypothalamic defense area stiffened large pulmonary arteries with little or no effect on pulmonary vascular resistance in open-chest dogs with constant flow perfusion (Szidon and Fishman, 1981).

Recent work in our laboratory has focused on the effects of electrical stimulation of two separate areas of the brain, a discrete area of the forebrain and the C_1 area of the medulla in intact-chest cats (Hyman, 1986) (Fig. 13). The septal nuclei in the forebrain consist of the dorsal aspect, which includes the lateral septal nucleus, and a ventral aspect, which includes a medial septal nucleus (Krayniak et al., 1980). Although the locations of the tracts from these nuclei to the medullary area are not established, it is generally believed that the dorsal aspect projects through the diagonal band of Broca to the medial preoptic-hypothalamic region and then to the habenula via the stria medullaris. The ventral aspect projects mainly through the horizontal limb of the diagonal band of Broca to the lateral preoptic-hypothalamic region by way of the medial forebrain bundle and continues to the ventral tegmentum.

Stimulation in this diagonal band area caused an abrupt increase in aortic pressure, often of 75-125 mmHg. Small inconsistent responses were observed at resting pulmonary vascular tone, but when the tone was actively increased by any of several methods there was an abrupt pulmonary vasoconstrictor response persisting for 20-30 sec followed by a marked prolonged (204 min) vasodilator response. The entire response was blocked by freezing or severing the spinal cord, suggesting a pathway from the forebrain through the spinal cord that can regulate vasomotor tone in the pulmonary vascular bed. By increasing the extracorporeal delay from the time blood is withdrawn from the femoral artery to the time it is pump-perfused into the hemodynamically separated lobar artery, the vasodilator response could be separated into an early and a late vasodilator component (Fig. 14). The early constrictor-dilator response was not blocked by conventional pharmacologic blocking agents, including histamine, opiate, prostaglandin, peptide, and autonomic blockers. The mediation of this intial response is unclear. However, the later dilator response was blocked by the specific $beta_2$ blocking agent ICI 118551. In addition, circulating blood epinephrine levels rose 10-15-fold during stimulation. Since epinephrine is a potent vasodilator in the cat pulmonary vascular bed at high tone, the delayed prolonged vasodilator response appears to be mediated by circulating epineprhine, probably derived from the adrenal medulla. This prolonged vasodilator response may serve to protect the lung from severe pulmonary congestion induced by the intense systemic vasoconstriction displacing blood into the pulmonary circulation. Others have also attributed the pulmonary vasoconstrictor response in the dog during increased intercranial pressure to circulating catecholamines (Marion and Dawson, 1980). The inconsistent pulmonary vascular resistance changes identified with dog hypothalamic stimulation may have been related in part to the fact that these responses were studied only at low resting pulmonary vascular tone. Moreover, the site of simulation and the animal species were different.

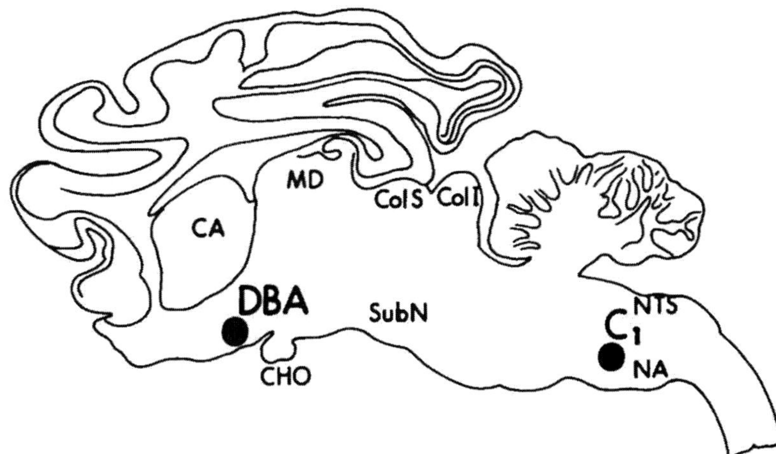

Figure 13 Parasaggital section of cat brain, showing position of diagonal band area (DBA), caudate nucleus (CA), medial dorsal nucleus of thalamus (MD), superior and inferior collulici (Col S, Col I), the C_1 area, the nucleus of the tractus solitarius (NTS), and nucleus ambiguus (NA).

In contrast, electrical stimulation in the medullary vasomotor regulatory center in the C_1 region also causes a pulmonary vascular response when tone is elevated (Hyman, 1986). Here, there is an abrupt vasoconstrictor response lasting 15-30 sec followed by a longer vasodilator response (45-90 sec). This response is quite similar to that observed with sympathetic nerve stimulation at elevated pulmonary vascular tone. Indeed, the initial vasoconstrictor response is mediated by alpha adrenoceptors and is blocked by phenoxybenzamine and phentolamine. After blockade of the alpha adrenoceptors, the vasodilator response is enhanced. The beta 2 specific antagonist ICI 118551 and propranolol block the vasodilator response and concurrently enhance the vasoconstrictor response. These responses appear to be mediated directly through the sympathetic nervous system.

The prolonged secondary vasodilator response consistently seen on stimulation of the forebrain area appears only randomly with stimulation of the C_1 area, suggesting random concurrent stimulation of fibers of passage. However, the randomly occurring delayed, prolonged vasodilator response is consistently blocked by $beta_2$ agonists. Although the early vasoconstrictor-vasodilator response observed with stimulation of C_1 nuclei is not accompanied by elevated circulating epinephrine levels, circulating epinephrine levels are greatly increased when the randomly occurring late, prolonged vasodilator response is observed.

In summary, the pulmonary vascular bed is richly innervated with adrenergic and cholinergic nerve terminals. These vessels respond to sympathetic and

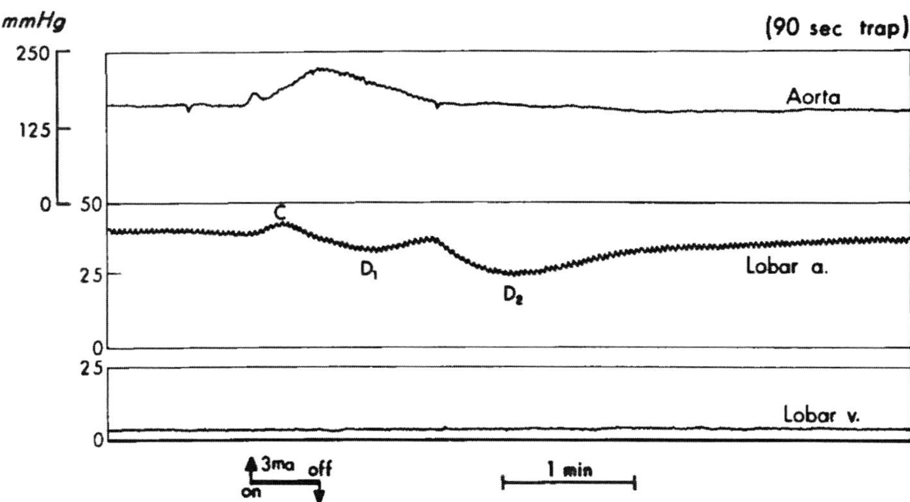

Figure 14 Tracings from an experiment illustrating responses to forebrain stimulation when the length (volume) of the perfusion circuit was extended to give a delay (trap) time of 90 sec. With the long delay in the circuit, the secondary vasodilator component was separated into two components. The first dilator component was labeled D1, and the second larger component was labeled D2.

parasympathetic nerve stimulation and to stimulation of discrete areas of the brain. The pulmonary resistance vessels contain $alpha_1$ and $alpha_2$ adrenoceptors, $beta_2$ adrenoceptors, and muscarinic adrenoceptors, all of which are innervated. The responses of these receptors to stimulation depends on the level of tone in the vessels at the time of stimulation. At low resting pulmonary vascular tone, $alpha_{1-2}$ and muscarinic adrenoceptor stimulation causes vasoconstriction, and $beta_2$ adrenoceptor stimulation causes vasodilation, which is masked. Sympathetic nerve stimulation causes vasoconstriction, and this response is enhanced by $beta_2$ antagonists. These responses are mediated largely by $alpha_1$-type adrenoceptors, and $alpha_2$ adrenoceptors play a smaller role. This is similar to the systemic vascular bed. Exogenous norepinephrine causes pulmonary vasoconstriction, mediated largely by $alpha_1$ adrenoceptors. In the systemic bed, exogenous norepinephrine stimulates predominantly $alpha_2$ adrenoceptors. It seems provident that circulating norepinephrine stimulates $alpha_1$ adrenoceptors in the pulmonary bed, since at elevated tone the vasoconstrictor response to stimulation of these receptors is not as great as those to stimulation of $alpha_2$ responses. Inconsistent responses to stimulation of the parasympathetic nerves and electrode stimulation of the brain are observed at resting tone.

When tone is increased in the pulmonary vascular bed, responses to $alpha_2$ and $beta_2$ adrenoceptor stimulation are greatly increased, and muscarinic receptor responses to exogenous acetylcholine are reversed, becoming vasodilator responses. The response to exogenous norepinephrine is enhanced only after beta blockade. Sympathetic nerve responses become biphasic, revealing the effects of both alpha and beta adrenoceptor stimulation, and parasympathetic nerve stimulation causes a vasodilator response. Stimulation of discrete areas of the forebrain causes an early constrictor-dilator response in the pulmonary vessels, which is mediated intrinsically, and a humorally mediated prolonged vasodilator response. The latter response is blocked by $beta_2$ antagonists and is concurrent with tenfold increases in circulating epinephrine blood levels. Stimulation of the C_1 area of the medulla causes an early constrictor-dilator response, which is sympathetically mediated and is similar to sympathetic nerve stimulation and elevated tone.

Our knowledge of lung function has advanced a long way from the rather unsuspecting idea that the lung possesses a purely passive vascular bed regulated entirely by the systemic circulation and devoid of intrinsic vasomotor mechanisms. Presently, firm evidence exists that the pulmonary vascular bed is capable of responding to neural regulation, but many questions remain to be clarified. Although electrical and chemical stimulation can induce these responses, the physiologic significance of this capacity to respond is not understood. The role served by neural mechanisms in attempting to maintain low pressure in the pulmonary vascular bed is not established. Moreover, the role of neural regulation in maintaining oxygenation, coordinating lung ventilation and perfusion, and serving as a buffer against disturbances caused by pulmonary responses to vasoactive agents introduced from the systemic bed needs to be unraveled. The possibility that the responses to nerve stimulation in the brain can be lateralized is untested. The large body of evidence indicating the potential of neural regullation, both centrally and peripherally, speaks against this function remaining in the body as a vestigial structure.

References

Alcock, P., Berry, J. L., and Daly, I. de B. (1935). The actions of drugs on the pulmonary circulation. *Quart. J. Exp. Physiol. Cog. Med. Sci. 25*:369-391.

Anderson, F. L., and Brown, A. M. (1967). Pulmonary vasoconstriction elicited by stimulation of the hypothalamic integrative area for the defense reaction. *Circ. Res. 21*:747-756.

Bevan, J. A., and Osher, J. V. (1965). Relative sensitivity of some large blood vessels of the rabbit to sympathomimetic amines. *J. Pharmacol. Exp. Ther. 150*:370-374.

Bobik, A. (1982). Identification of alpha adrenoreceptor subtypes in dog arteries by [^{3}H] yohimbine and [^{3}H] prazosin. *Life Sci. 30*:219-228.

Borowski, E., Starke, K. Ehrl, H., and Endo, T. (1977). A comparison of pre- and postsynaptic effect of α-adrenolytic drugs in the pulmonary artery of the rabbit. *Neuroscience 2*:285-296.

Burnstock, G., Gaunow, B., and Iwayama, T. (1970). Sympathetic innervation of the vascular smooth muscle in normal and hypertensive animals. *Circ. Res.* 26/27(II):5-21.

Cech, S., and Dolezel, I (1967). Monoaimergic innervation of the pulmonary vessels in various laboratory animals (rat, rabbit, cat). *Experientia 23*: 114-115.

Constantine, J. W., Gunnell, D., and Weeks, R. A. (1980). Alpha 1 and 2 vascular receptors in the dog. *Eur. J. Pharmacol. 66*:281-286.

Daly, I. de B., and Hebb, C. (1966). *Pulmonary and Bronchial Vascular Systems.* Williams and Wilkins, Baltimore, MD.

DeMay, J., and Vanhoutte, P. M. (1981). Uneven distribution of postjunctional alpha 1- and alpha 2-like adrenoceptors in the canine arterial and venous smooth muscle. *Circ. Res. 48*:875-884.

Dingemans, K. P., and Wagenvoort, C. A. (1976). Ultrastructural study of contraction of pulmonary vascular smooth muscle. *Lab. Invest. 35*:205 212.

Euler, U. S. von and Lishajko, I. (1958). Catecholamines in the vascular wall. *Acta Physiol. Scand. 42*:333-341.

Falck, B. (1962). Observations on the possibilities of the cellular localization of monoamines by fluorescent method. *Acta Physiol. Scand. 56*:1-26.

Fay, F. S., and Delise, C. M. (1973). Contraction of isolated smooth muscle cells – structural changes. *Proc. Natl. Acad. Sci. USA 70*:641-645.

Feeley, J. W., Lee, T. D., and Milnor, W. R. (1963). Active and passive components of pulmonary vascular responses to vasoactive drugs in the dog. *Am. J. Physiol. 205*:1193-1199.

Fillenz, M. (1970). Innervation of pulmonary and bronchial blood vessels of the dog. *J. Anat. 106*:449-461.

Fisher, A. W. F. (1965). The intrinsic innervation of the pulmonary vessels. *Acta Anat. 60*:481-496.

Furchgott, F. R., and Zawadski, J. V. (1980). The obligatory role of endothelial cells in the relaxation of arterial smooth muscle by acetylcholine. *Nature (Lond.)* 288:373-376.

Furness, J. B., and Marshall, J. M. (1974). Correlation of the directly observed responses of the mesenteric vessels of the rat to nerve stimulation and noradrenaline with the distribution of adrenergic nerves. *J. Physiol. (Lond.)* 239:75-88.

Furness, J. B., and Malmfors, T. (1974). Aspects of the arrangement of the adrenergic innervation in the guinea-pig as revealed by the fluorescence histochemical method applied to stretched air-dried preparations. *Histochemie 25*:297-309.

Greensmith, J. E., and Duling, B. R. (1984). Morphology of the constricted arteriolar wall: physiological implications. *Am. J. Physiol. 247*: *(Heart Circ. Physiol. 16)*:H687-H698.

Greenway, C. V., and Lawson, A. E. (1969). Beta adrenoceptors in the hepatic artery of the anesthetized cat. *Can. J. Physiol. Pharmacol. 47*:415-419.

Greenway, C. V., Lawson, A. E., and Stark, R. D. (1968). Vascular responses of the spleen to nerve stimulation during normal and reduced blood flow. *J. Physiol. (Lond.)* 194:421-433.

Grover, R. F., Wagner, W. W., McMurty, I. F., and Reeves, J. T. (1983). The pulmonary circulation. In *Handbook of Physiology*. Sect. 2 *The Cardiovascular System*. Edited by J. T. Shepherd, and F. Abboud. American Physiologic Society, Bethesda, MD, pp. 103-136.

Hakim, T. S., and Dawson, C. A. (1979). Sympathetic nerve stimulation and vascular resistance in pump-perfused dog lung lobe. *Proc. Soc. Exp. Biol. Med. 160*:38-41.

Hassan, A., Kasher, El, and Catravas, J. D. (1986). Prostanoid mediation of pulmonary vascular response to acetylcholine in rabbits. *Am. J. Physiol. 251 (Heart Circ. Physiol. 20)*:H808-H814.

Hebb, C. (1969). Motor innervation of the pulmonary blood vessels of mammals. In *Pulmonary Circulation and Interstitial Space*. Edited by A. P. Fishman, and H. H. Hecht. University of Chicago Press, Chicago.

Hessler, J. R., and Cassin, S. (1977). Effects of increased intracranial pressure in pulmonary vascular resistance in fetal and neonatal goats. *Am. J. Physiol. 232 (Heart Circ. Physiol.)*H671-H675.

Hyman, A. L. (1969a). The direct effect of norepinephrine and of angiotensin on the pulmonary veins of intact dogs. *J. Pharmacol. Exp. Ther. 165*:87-96.

Hyman, A. L. (1969b). The direct effects of vasoactive agents on pulmonary veins. Studies of responses to acetylcholine, serotonin, histamine, and isoproterenol in intact dogs. *J. Pharmacol. Exp. Ther. 168*:96-105.

Hyman, A. L. (1986). The Dickinson W. Richards Memorial Lecture. Neural control of the pulmonary vascular bed. *Circulation 74*(II):IID.

Hyman, A. L., and Kadowitz, P. J. (1985). Evidence for the existence of postjunctional alpha 1 and 2 adrenoceptors in cat pulmonary vascular bed. *Am. J. Physiol. 249*:H391-H398.

Hyman, A. L., and Kadowitz, P. J. (1986). Enhancement of alpha and beta adrenoceptor responses by elevations in vascular tone in the pulmonary circulation. *Am. J. Physiol. 250*: *(Heart Circ. Physiol.)*H1109-H1116.

Hyman, A. L., and Kadowitz, P. J. (1988). Tone-dependent responses to acetylcholine in the feline pulmonary vascular bed. *J. Appl. Physiol.* (in press).

Hyman, A. L., Nandiwada, P., Knight, D. S., and Kadowitz, P. J. (1981). Pulmonary vasodilator responses to catecholamines and sympathetic nerve stimulation in the cat. Evidence that vascular beta-2 adrenoceptors are innervated. *Circ. Res. 48*:407-415.

Ingram, R. H., Szidon, J. P., Skalak, P., and Fishman, A. P. (1968). Effects of sympathetic nerve stimulation on the pulmonary arterial tree of the isolated lobe perfused in situ. *Circ. Res. 22*:801-815.

Janernig, R. A., Moulds, R. F. W., and Shaw, J. (1978). The action of prazosin in human vascular preparations. *Arch. Int. Pharmacodyn. Ther. 231*: 81-89.

Kadowitz, P. J., and Hyman, A. L. (1973). Effect of sympathetic nerve stimulation on pulmonary vascular resistance in the dog. *Circ. Res. 32*:221-227.

Kadowitz, P. J., Joiner, P. D., and Hyman, A. L. (1974). Effects of sympathetic nerve stimulation on pulmonary vascular resistance in intact spontaneously breathing dogs. *Proc. Soc. Exp. Biol. Med. 147*:68-71.

Kadowitz, P. J., Joiner, P. D., and Hyman, A. L. (1975). Influences of sympathetic stimulation and vasoactive substances on canine pulmonary veins. *J. Clin. Invest. 56*:354-365.

Kadowitz, P. J., Knight, D. S., Hibbs, R. G., Ellison, J. P., Joiner, P. D., Brody, M. J., and Hyman, A. L. (1976). Influence of 5- and 6-hydroxydopamine on adrenergic transmission and nerve terminal morphology in the canine pulmonary vascular bed. *Circ. Res. 39*:191-199.

Kadowitz, P. J., Waring, P. H., Hyman, A. L., and Nandiwada, P. A. (1987). Influence of OKY-1581 on responses to arachidonic acid in the feline pulmonary vascular bed. *Prost. Leuk. Med.* (submitted).

Knight, D. S., Ellison, J. P., Hibbs, R. G., Hyman, A. L., and Kadowitz, P. J (1981). The light and electron microscopic study of the innervation of pulmonary vascular bed. *Prost. Leuk. Med. 31*:117-122.

Konzeth, H., and Hebb, C. O. (1949). Vaso- and bronchomotor actions of norepinephrine and of adrenaline in the isolated perfused lungs of dogs. *Arch. Int. Pharmacodyn. Ther. 73*:210-224.

Krayniak, P., Weiner, S., and Siegel, A. (1980). An analysis of the efferent connections of the septal area in the cat. *Brain Res. 180*:15-29.

Langer, S. Z. (1977). Presynaptic receptors and their role in regulation of transmitter release. *Brit. J. Pharmacol. 60*:481-497.

Langer, S. Z., and Shepperson, N. B. (1982). Postjunctional alpha 1-2 adrenoceptors, preferential innervation of alpha 1 adrenoceptors and role of neuronal uptake. *J. Cardiovasc. Pharmacol. 4*:S8-S13.

Langer, S. Z., Massingham, R., and Shepperson, N. B. (1980). Presence of post-synaptic alpha 2 adrenoceptors of predeominantly extrasynaptic location in vascular smooth muscle of the dog hind limb. *Clin. Sci. 59*:225A-228A.

Lefevre, F., Fenord, S., and Cavero, J. (1977). Vascular beta adrenoceptor stimulating properties of phenylephrine. *Eur. J. Pharmacol. 43*:85-88.

Linehan, J. H., and Dawson, C. A. (1982). A three compartment model of the pulmonary vasculature: effects of vasoconstriction. *J. Appl. Physiol. 53*: 158-168.

Lloyd, T. C., Jr. (1973). Effects of increased cerebrospinal fluid pressure on pulmonary vascular resistance. *J. Appl. Physiol. 35*:332-335.

McGrath, J. C. (1982). Evidence for more than one type of postjunctional alpha adrenoceptor. *Biochem. Pharmacol. 31*:467-484.

Malik, A. B. (1985). Mechanisms of neurogenic edema. *Circ. Res. 57*:1-18.

Marion, M. B., and Dawson, C. A. (1980). Pulmonary venoconstriction caused by elevated cerebrospinal fluid pressure in the dog. *J. Appl. Physiol.: Resp. Environ. Exercise Physiol. 49*:73-78.

Marion, M. B., Hakim, T. S., and Dawson, C. A. (1979). Pulmonary hemodynamic responses to elevated cerebrospinal pressure in the dog. *J. Appl. Physiol. 46*:84-88.

Naigaishi, C. (1972). *Functional Anatomy and Histoloy of the Lung*. University Park Press, pp. 180-243, Baltimore.

Nandiwada, P., Hyman, A. L., and Kadowitz, P. J. (1983). Pulmonary vasodilator response to vagal stimulation and acetylcholine in the cat. *Circ. Res. 53*:86-95.

Ngai, S. H., Rosell, S., and Wallenberg, L. R. (1966). Nervous regulation of blood flow in adipose tissue of the dog. *Acta Physiol. Scand. 68*:397-403.

Pace, J. B. (1971). Sympathetic control of pulmonary vascular impedance in anesthetized dogs. *Circ. Res. 29*:555-568.

Pegram, B. L., Bevan, R. D., and Bevan, J. A. (1976). Facial vein of the rabbit. Neurogenic vasodilation mediated by beta adrenergic receptors. *Circ. Res. 39*:854-860.

Porcelli, R. J., and Bergofsky, E. (1973). Adrenergic receptors in pulmonary vasoconstrictor responses to gaseous and humoral agents. *J. Appl. Physiol. 34*:483-488.

Rhodin, J. A. G. (1978). Microscopic anatomy of the pulmonary vascular bed of the cat lung. *Microvasc. Res. 160*:193-199.

Rippe, B., Parker, J. C., Townsley, M. I., Mortellaro, N. A., and Taylor, A. E. (1987). Segmental vascular resistances and compliance in dog lungs. *J. Appl. Physiol. 62*:1206-1215.

Rose, J. C. (1957). Active constriction and dilation in pulmonary circulation in response to acetylcholine. *Proc. Soc. Exp. Biol. Med. 94*:734-737.

Rudolph, A. M., Kurland, M. D., Auld, P. A. M., and Paul, M. H. (1959). Effects of vasodilator drugs on normal and serotonin constricted pulmonary vessels in the dog. *Am. J. Physiol. 197*:617-623.

Ruffolo, R. R., Waddell, J. E., and Yaden, E. L. (1981). Postsynaptic alpha adrenergic receptor subtypes differentiated by yohimbine in tissues from the rat. Existence of alpha-2 adrenergic receptors in rat aorta. *J. Pharmacol. Exp. Ther. 217*:235-240.

Russell, M. P., and Moran, N. C. (1980). Evidence of a lack of innervation of α-2 adrenoceptors in blood vessels of the gracilis muscle of the dog. *Circ. Res. 46*:344-352.

Silvone, E. D., Inoue, T., and Grover, R. F. (1968). Comparison of hypoxia, pH and sympathomimetic drugs on bovine pulmonary vasculature. *J. Appl. Physiol. 24*:355-365.

Starke, K. H., Montel, H., Gayk, W., and Merker, R. (1974). Comparison of the effects of clonidine on pre- and postsynaptic adrenoceptors in the rabbit pulmonary artery. *Naunyn-Schmiedeberg's Arch. Pharmacol. 285*:133-150.

Starke, K., Borowski, E., and Endo, T. (1975a). Preferential blockade of presynaptic alpha adrenoceptors by yohimbine. *Eur. J. Pharmacol. 34*:385-388.

Starke, K., Endo, T., and Taube, H. D. (1975b). Relative pre- and postsynaptic potencies of alpha adrenoceptor agonists in the rabbit pulmonary artery. *Naunyn-Schmiedeberg's Arch. Pharmacol. 291*:55-78.

Szidon, J. P., and Fishman, A. P. (1981). Participation of the pulmonary circulation in the defense reaction. *Am. J. Physiol. 220*:364-370.

Vanhoutte, P. M. (1974). Inhibition by acetylcholine of adrenergic transmission in vascular smooth muscle. *Circ. Res. 34*:317-326.

Verity, M. A., and Bevan, J. A. (1968). Fine structural study of the teriminal effector plexus; neuromuscular and intermuscular relationships in the pulmonary artery. *J. Anata. 103*:49-63.

Verity, M. A., Hughes, T., and Bevan, J. A. (1964). Innervation of the pulmonary artery bifurcation of the cat. *Am. J. Anat. 116*:75-90.

Viveros, O. H., Garlick, D. G., and Renkin, E. M. (1968). Sympathetic beta adrenergic vasodilation in skeletal muscle of dogs. *Am. J. Physiol. 215*:1218-1225.

Wilffert, B. M., Gauw, A. M., Timmermans, P. B. M. W. M., and Van Zwieten, P. A. (1983a). Interaction between beta-2 adrenoceptor mediated vasodilation and alpha-2 adrenoceptor mediated vasoconstriction in the pithed normotensive rat. *J. Cardiovasc. Pharmacol. 5*:822-828.

Wilffert, B. M., Gauw, A. M., Timmermans, P. B. M. W. M., and Van Zwieten, P. A. (1983b). Interaction between beta-2 adrenoceptor mediated vasodilation and alpha-1 adrenoceptor mediated vasoconstriction in the pithed normotensive rat. *J. Cardiovasc. Pharmacol. 5*:829-835.

10

Right Ventricular Function in Pulmonary Hypertension

JOHN T. REEVES
and BERTRON M. GROVES

University of Colorado
Health Sciences Center
Denver, Colorado

DARYA TURKEVICH

University of Colorado
School of Medicine
Denver, Colorado

DOUGLASS A. MORRISON

University of Colorado
Health Sciences Center and
Denver VA Medical Center
Denver, Colorado

JOHN A. TRAPP

University of Colorado
College of Engineering and
Applied Science
Denver, Colorado

I. Introduction

In the normal adult, the right ventricle and the left ventricle are in series. If the right ventricle does not pump enough blood to meet the body's demand, the result is a limited cardiac output, no matter how healthy the left ventricle might be. At rest, the normal right ventricular systolic pressure is quite low compared to that of the left ventricle. However, relatively small increments in the resistance against which the right ventricle must work may be accompanied by reductions in the fraction of blood ejected (Brent et al., 1982, 1983). Furthermore, nearly all forms of heart or lung disease are complicated at some point in their natural history by pulmonary hypertension (Reeves and Groves, 1984), which may limit the flow of blood to the left heart. A further complication of the pulmonary hypertension is overt right heart failure, which is accompanied by particularly severe morbidity and mortality. Thus an understanding of right heart function in health and disease is of great importance. Even so, the normal and abnormal right heart have had relatively little study, and we hope that this chapter will encourage further inquiry.

II. Approach

Our approach will be to document, in general, the magnitude of circulatory impairment attributable to the right heart in pulmonary hypertension. We will then consider, against the background of normal function, the abnormal features of right heart function in pulmonary hypertension and will attempt to consider how the abnormalities may have arisen. Finally we will consider function of the right ventricle in chronic obstructive pulmonary disease, one of the most common causes of pulmonary hypertension.

Factors that can load the right heart and impair function include an increase in lung blood flow, a decrease in compliance of the large pulmonary arteries, and an increase in pulmonary vascular resistance. All elevate pulmonary artery pressure, yet they may not be equivalent stresses. First, consider increased blood flow. There is considerable increase in pulmonary arterial pressure during upright exercise, which may be sustained for several hours daily in the case of the endurance runner or manual laborer. However, impaired right heart function attributable to exercise has not been described. In persons with large left-to-right shunts, the right ventricle functions well as long as the pulmonary vascular resistance remains low (Konstam et al., 1983). The presence of a low pulmonary vascular resistance minimizes the load on the right ventricle by optimally matching output impedance of the pump to the input impedance of the pulmonary vascular system (Milnor, 1983). Second, consider compliance changes in the large pulmonary vessels. Decreased arterial compliance, of itself, seems unlikely to cause major impairment of right heart function. For example, aging decreases compliance of the large pulmonary and systemic arteries (Gonza et al., 1974) but does not, of itself, appear to cause clinical heart disease. Finally, consider increased resistance. Increased pulmonary vascular resistance does lead to impaired right heart function and is associated with symptoms and death, such as is seen in pulmonary emboli or primary pulmonary hypertension. How resistance loads the right heart may be complex. Increased resistance causes increased pressure, and increased pressure decreases vascular compliance, which may further increase the load on the ventricle. Thus, the increase in resistance may initiate an adverse series of events. If so, one must inquire how increasing the pulmonary vascular resistance results in impaired right ventricular function.

III. Lung Vessel Resistance and Right Heart Function in Humans

Ventricular contractility is probably best assessed by considering pressure-volume relationships at end-systole and end-diastole (Sagawa, 1978; Ross, 1983; Elzinga and Westerhof, 1979). Such information is not available for the right ventricle in normal humans or in patients with pulmonary hypertension. A cruder estimate of right ventricular function can be obtained from a simple measurement of stroke volume or cardiac output. Below we relate published data of cardiac output and pulmonary resistance from patients who have isolated pulmonary vascular diseases, such as primary pulmonary hypertension. Increments in lung vascular resistance are associated with reductions in the resting stroke volume (Fig. 1A). Because the heart rate does not completely compensate for the reduced stroke volume, minute volume, i.e., cardiac output, is also reduced (Fig. 1B). In the flow-pressure plot of Figure 1B, we show pressure versus cardiac output, in order to determine how flow varies as pressure increases. The results suggest that a doubling of pressure to a mean of only 30 mmHg may be associated with a somewhat decreased flow, although few measurements in this range are reported. The lines of constant total pulmonary resistance drawn through the origin suggest that resistance increases of two- to fourfold are associated with a low forward flow. Yet another estimate of right ventricular function is the right ventricular ejection fraction. The concept that high pulmonary resistance affects the ability of the right ventricle to eject blood is supported by improved ejection fractions in patients who have had reduction in resistance following surgical correction of mitral stenosis. The right ventricular ejection fraction was inversely related both to pulmonary arterial pressure and to resistance (Cohen et al., 1985).

If pump function is reduced at rest, then the additional stress of exercise should confirm the abnormal function. Unfortunately, there are few data available for a comparison relating arteriovenous oxygen difference to oxygen uptake. The data that are available indicate an increased oxygen extraction to very near maximal values for small oxygen uptakes (Fig. 2), suggesting a marked limitation of exercise cardiac output. To determine how the right heart functions with only minimal pulmonary vascular disease, we need measurements at rest and during exercise in individuals having only slightly increased resistances.

Normally the left ventricle increases stroke volume when end-diastolic volume is increased, as indicated by the Frank-Starling relationship. The right ventricle also obeys this relationship. How the right ventricle increases output with raised filling pressure is thus a measure of pump function. In patients with varying degrees of lung vessel disease, the right ventricular stroke volumes were low for the filling pressures measured (Fig. 3). In particular, when the filling pressures were elevated in the most severely affected patients, the very low stroke volumes suggested a failure of the Frank-Starling mechanism.

Right ventricular function may be rather sensitive to chronically imposed increases in resistance, as indicated by the following: Small increments in resistance at rest are associated with decreased output; increase in output with exercise is impaired; and, increments in right atrial pressure are not accompanied by appropriate increments in stroke volume. Although right heart output func-

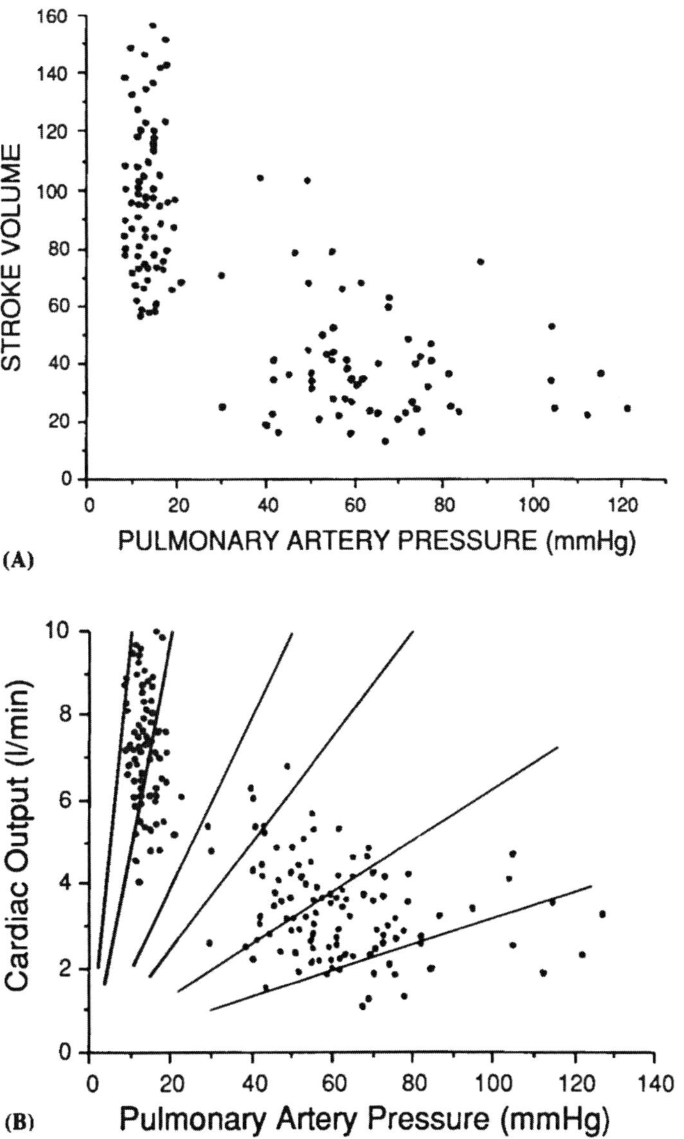

Figure 1 Relation of flow to mean pulmonary arterial pressure at rest in normal subjects and in patients with isolated pulmonary vascular disease (Data from: Berkenboom et al., 1982; Camerini et al., 1980; Douglas, 1983; Honey et al., 1980; Horowitz et al., 1981; Ikram et al., 1982; Jenkins and Page, 1981; Konstam et al., 1983; Leirer et al., 1983; Lupi-Herrera et al., 1982; Malcic and Richter, 1985; Packer et al., 1982; Rich et al., 1982, 1985; Rubin et al., 1980, 1983; Rubino and Schroeder, 1979; Ruskin and Hutter, 1979; and Wise, 1983). (A) Relation of stroke volume to pressure. (B) Relation of cardiac output to pressure. Shown, drawn through the origin, are lines of constant total pulmonary resistance in units (pulmonary arterial pressure/flow).

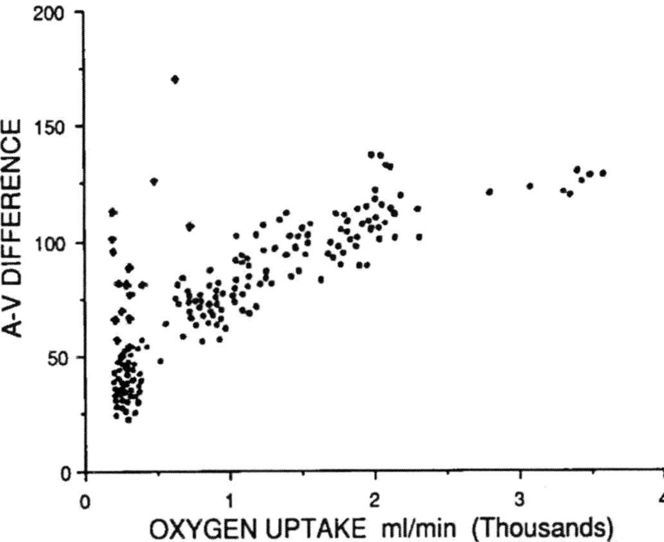

Figure 2 Relation of arteriovenous oxygen difference to oxygen uptake at rest and during exercise in normal subjects from the literature (●) and patients with pulmonary hypertension (+). Patients with pulmonary hypertension have widened arteriovenous oxygen differences, i.e., lower cardiac outputs, for a given oxygen uptake. (Data from Reeves et al., 1961, 1987; Benegard et al., 1960; Lupi-Herrera et al., 1982; and Gurtner et al., 1975).

tion is impaired, reported resistance values more than 10 times normal indicate a remarkable adaptation in right heart pump function. Unfortunately, the adaptation is not sufficient to restore normal output.

IV. Lung Vessel Resistance and Right Heart Function In Vitro

While the patient studies indicate that increased pulmonary vascular resistance impairs right heart function, the mechanisms must be evaluated in animal studies, where ionotropy (basic contractile state), filling pressure (preload), and arterial pressure (afterload) can be controlled. Afterload has two components: increased resistance and decreased compliance. The isolated heart studied by Elzinga et al. (1980) nicely sheds light on the nature of the imposed load that adversely affects right heart function. Elzinga and co-workers attached isolated cat hearts to their model of the pulmonary vascular system, in which they could vary, independently, the peripheral resistance and the compliance. Their meas-

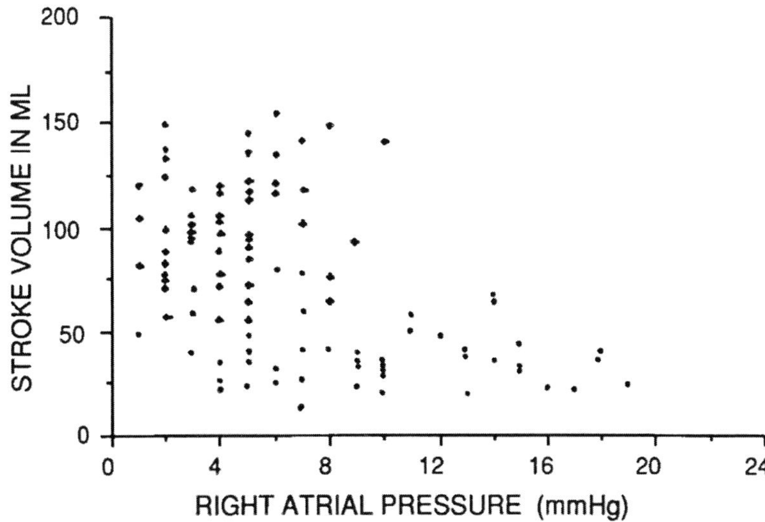

Figure 3 Relation of stroke volume to right atrial pressure at rest and during exercise in normal subjects (+) from this laboratory and from the literature and in patients with pulmonary hypertension (•). (Sources as in Figure 2).

urements of right ventricular and pulmonary arterial pressure and pulmonary arterial flow under normal conditions (low vascular resistance and high compliance) yielded pressure values and flow contours that in some respects resembled those seen normally (Fig. 4). When the peripheral resistance was nearly quadrupled without changing compliance, the pressure in the right ventricle rose and the flow fell (Fig. 4), as was seen in the human patient population. Elzinga et al. (1980) also reported that a mere doubling of resistance decreased flow. A reduction in flow that was relatively greater than the increase in pressure was consistent with their concept that the isolated heart normally functions at maximum power output. A deviation from the normal load caused a reduction in power output (van den Horn et al., 1985). Thus, the experiment suggested that right heart function was sensitive to small increments in resistance, a finding supported by the human studies.

V. High Resistance Plus Low Compliance and Right Heart Function

When the resistance alone was increased, the pulmonary arterial pulse pressure became more narrow (Fig. 4), which is not what is seen in pulmonary hyper-

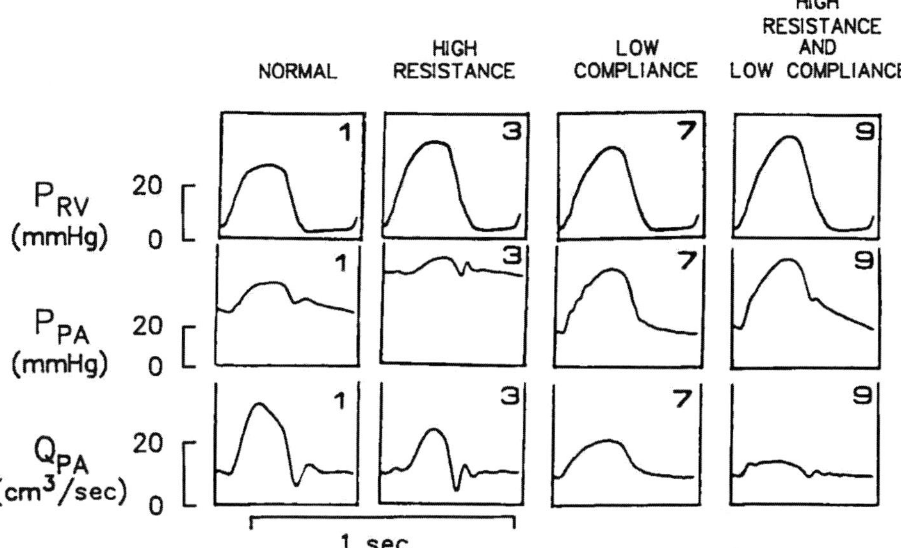

Figure 4 Measurements during representative cardiac cycles at 120 beats/min from the isolated cat heart preparation of Elzinga et al. (1900). The rows indicate right ventricular pressure (PRV), pulmonary arterial pressure (PPA), and pulmonary arterial flow velocity (QPA). The columns from left to right are: low resistance and high compliance (normal), resistance increased to 4 times normal and high compliance (High R), resistance normal but compliance reduced to 1/16 normal (Low CC), and resistance increased to 4 times normal plus compliance reduced to 1/16 normal (High R, LowC). Increased resistance or decreased compliance each increase the load on the right ventricle. The combined effects of the two depress flow more than either alone. (Used with permission.)

tensive patients (Fig. 5). Rather, in clinical pulmonary hypertension, pulmonary arterial pulse pressure is usually increased. In humans with chronically increased pulmonary vascular resistance, pulmonary hypertension is accompanied by increased turgidity and thickness of the walls of the large pulmonary arteries. Both increased pressure within the lumen and the increased wall thickness stiffen the walls, causing a decrease in compliance in the large pulmonary arteries (Milnor and Bertram, 1978).

One wonders whether a compliance decrease further loads the right ventricle. Therefore, it becomes important to know the effects both of increased resistance and of decreased compliance on right heart function. When both were present, the findings more closely resembled those seen in the patient population (Fig. 4). That is, there was a marked reduction in flow accompanied by right

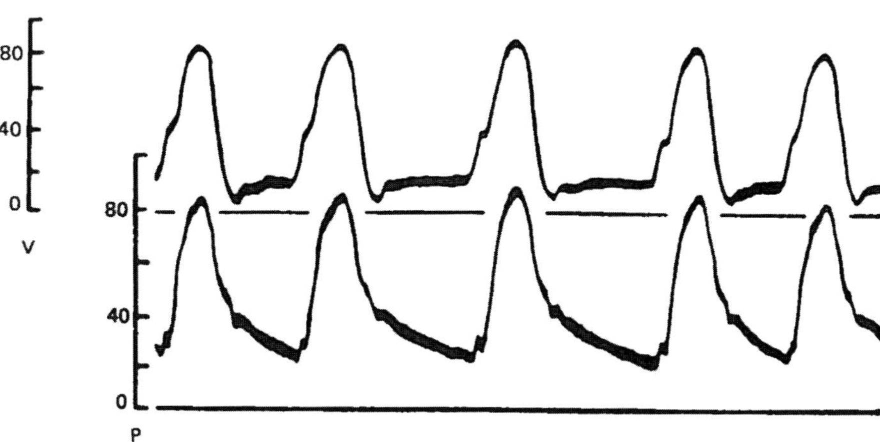

Figure 5 Redrawn pressure tracings from the pulmonary artery and right ventricle from the first human being to have pulmonary arterial pressure measured (Cournand et al., 1945). The patient had pulmonary hypertension from rheumatic heart disease. The right ventricular pressure contour (upper panel, V scale) showed a sharp initial upstroke, followed by a short plateau and a late systolic pressure rise. The pulmonary arterial pressure contour (lower panel, P scale) shows a wide pulse pressure. (Used with permission).

ventricular hypertension and an increase in the pulse pressure in the main pulmonary artery. These findings suggested that a reduction in compliance, when added to the increase in resistance, caused a further decrease in flow. The implication was that the low compliance imposed an additional load to the right ventricle.

VI. Lung Vessel Compliance and Right Heart Function

The decreased vascular compliance itself deserved examination. When, in their model, Elzinga et al. (1980) decreased compliance by a factor of 16 without increasing the resistance, they saw a reduction in flow that was not as great as when resistance increased fourfold. There was an increase in right ventricular systolic pressure. The pulmonary arterial diastolic pressure, however, remained low, resulting in a large increase in pulmonary arterial pulse pressure. These results confirmed that decreased compliance of the large pulmonary arterial vessels contributed to some extent to the loading of the ventricle. It is also probably responsible for the large pulse pressure seen in the pulmonary hypertensive patient.

The increase in systolic pressure and the increase in pulse pressure also occur in the systemic circulation of aged persons with stiffened vessels and patients with systemic hypertension. Increased amplitude was one of the features of the hypertensive pulse in early clinical descriptions, along with a late peak and the absence of the normal diastolic wave (O'Rourke, 1985). Presumably, as compliance decreases and wave speed increases, the first reflected wave returns earlier, augmenting the pressure in late systole rather than in early diastole (O'Rourke, 1985). Similarly, left ventricular hypertrophy in hypertensive subjects related to systolic pressure and arterial pulse wave velocity even at constant diastolic pressure, suggesting that decreased compliance contributes independently to the left ventricular systolic load (Bouthier et al., 1985).

VII. Late Systolic Loading of the Right Ventricle

Examination of Figure 4 suggests that the reduction of compliance in the isolated heart model not only increased the right ventricular pressure but also altered the shape of the pressure curve. The peak pressure occurred later in systole. The contour is of interest in that late peaking of pressure is also a characteristic of persons with pulmonary hypertension. The first human being for whom measurement of pulmonary arterial pressure was reported had pulmonary hypertension and a right ventricular pressure contour (Fig. 5; See also Cournand et al., 1945) characterized by a pressure plateau in early systole and a subsequent late systolic pressure rise. Utilizing high fidelity catheter recordings in the right ventricle in humans without pulmonary hypertension, we have noted that the pressure contour resembles a square wave (Fig. 6A). But when there is pulmonary hypertension, the right ventricular pressure has a shoulder followed by a secondary pressure rise (Fig. 6A). This contour is not observed in pulmonary valvular stenosis. With obstruction at the level of the pulmonary valve, there is right ventricular hypertension, but the right ventricular contour does not have the shoulder and the secondary pressure rise; rather it has a smooth single peak (Fig. 6B). In our experience, only when there is obstruction well distal to the pulmonary valve does the right ventricular pressure assume this peculiar contour. This suggests that a load is imposed on the ventricle late in systole and the ventricle responds to that load by increasing pressure. The magnitude of the late pressure rise in some individuals accounts for 30-40% of the total systolic pressure. If the late pressure rise does reflect an increased load on the ventricle, it is a load of some magnitude and therefore may be of importance.

The question arises, therefore, whether a load suddenly imposed during ejection can alter the ventricular pressure contour within the beat. In the disorder of asymmetric septal hypertrophy, for example, the left ventricular

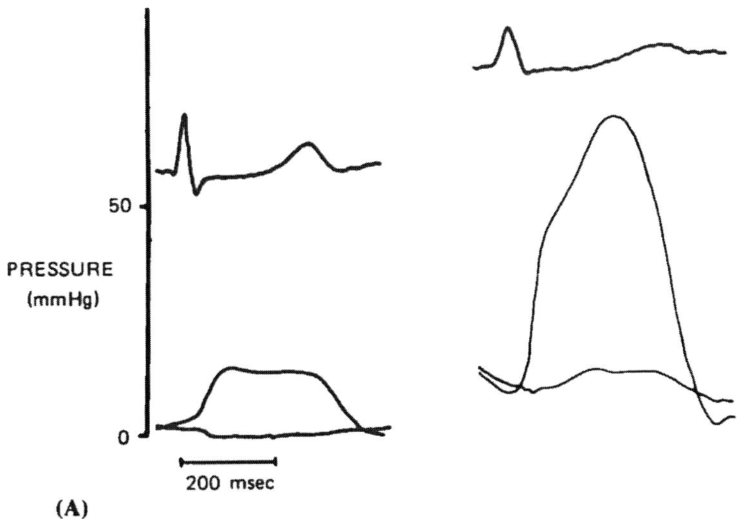

(A)

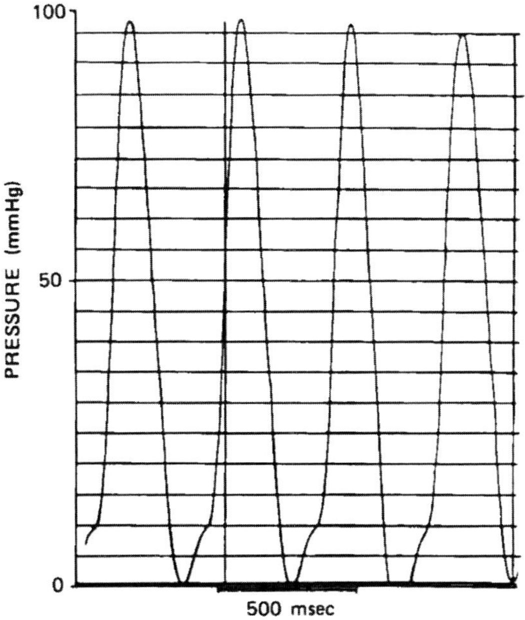

(B)

cavity pressure rises to a normal plateau during the initial part of ejection. However, in midsystole the septum bulges into the left ventricular outflow tract, causing partial obstruction during ejection. As outflow obstruction develops, the left ventricle develops an additional increase in pressure in late systole. That the left ventricular pressure can respond quickly to an imposed load has been confirmed by Hori et al. (1985). These authors found that imposing an impedance on the left ventricle early in systole caused an early increase in the left ventricular pressure (Fig. 7). When they imposed the impedance later in systole, the pressure rose late in systole, producing a contour in the left ventricle similar to that seen in the right ventricle during pulmonary hypertension. Thus, imposition of an extra load during the course of ejection will deform the ventricular pressure contour.

It seems that during the course of a single myocardial contraction the left ventricle can "perceive" a change in load and respond to the change. No change in the power output of the ventricle would necessarily be required if flow generation decreased while pressure generation increased.

Assuming that the right ventricle functions like the left ventricle, these observations have led us to consider that the secondary pressure rise seen in the pulmonary hypertensive patient results from a late systolic load that is imposed on the right ventricle. We have considered that the pressure contour results from the presence of abnormal pulmonary circulation, because loading the ventricle with a fixed obstruction at the outlet valve is not associated with the shoulder and the late pressure rise. Since the in vitro experiments of Elzinga et al. (1980) (Fig. 4) showed an increase in the late peak in response to decrease compliance, we speculate that the reduced compliance may be largely responsible for the late load on the ventricle.

If the late load on the ventricle adversely affects function, then one would expect that flow would not rise as the pressure increases late in systole. The in vitro model shows that pressure and flow contours become quite dissimilar when there is increased resistance and decreased compliance. In the model, the flow was maximal early in systole but had decreased in later systole when the pressure was maximal. With normal hemodynamics, pressure and flow contours look very much alike. The model suggested that the late load on the ventricle was as-

---

Figure 6 High fidelity right ventricular pressure tracings using a Millar catheter in patients undergoing cardiac catheterization. (A) Pulmonary arterial and right atrial pressures from patients without and with pulmonary hypertension. The ventricular contours differ. With pulmonary hypertension the ventricular contour shows a shoulder in early systole followed by a late systolic pressure rise. (From Reeves et al., 1985.) (B) Right ventricular pressure from a patient with congenital valvular pulmonic stenosis. The shoulder and late pressure rise are absent.

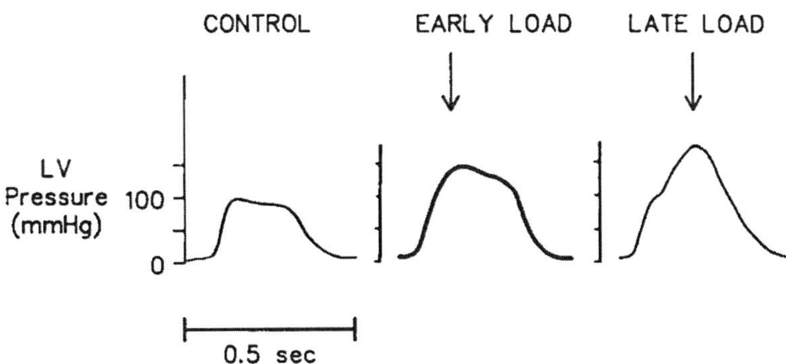

Figure 7 Left ventricular pressure response to imposition of a sudden load during systole. Left, a normal pressure. Middle, the pressure contour in response to sudden partial occlusion of the ascending aorta early in systole. Right, the pressure contour in response to sudden partial occlusion of the ascending aorta in late systole. Ventricular pressure rises quickly in response to loads imposed during systole. (From Hori et al., 1985, with permission.)

sociated with impaired output, specifically at the time when the load was maximal.

One wants to know whether the isolated heart model provides insight into the pathophysiology of human pulmonary hypertension. Available data suggest that the flow patterns from the model do resemble those observed in pulmonary hypertensive subjects. Velocity of blood flow at the pulmonary valve or in the proximal pulmonary artery has been estimated using a variety of ultrasound methods, including contrast echocardiography (Zieher et al., 1986) and Doppler (Kitabatake et al., 1983; Zieher et al., 1986). In normal subjects, maximal flow velocity occurs in mid-systole, while in pulmonary hypertensive subjects the velocity peaks early (Fig. 8). Doppler measurements have confirmed that the peak velocity of blood flow occurs earlier the greater the elevation of the pulmonary vascular resistance (Kitabatake et al., 1983). Thus the pressure peaks later than the flow in hypertensive subjects, and the flow may be falling while the pressure is rising. In the model of Elzinga et al. the situation of increased resistance with decreased compliance appears to approximate these findings in human pulmonary hypertensive disease. The combination of increased resistance and decreased compliance acts to impose an additional late load on the right ventricle. In addition, a late systolic augmentation of a simulated arterial pulse can be produced passively, by the early return of a reflected wave (O'Rourke, 1985).

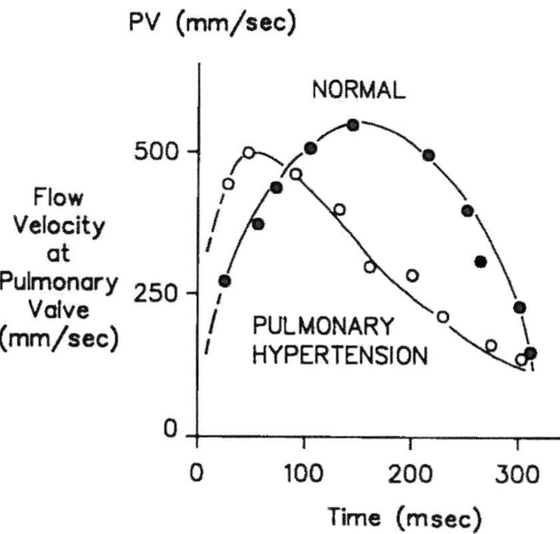

Figure 8 Relation of flow velocity at the pulmonary valve to time after pulmonic valve opening in a normal patient and in a patient with pulmonary hypertension. In the patient with pulmonary hypertension, the peak velocity was achieved earlier. (From Zieher et al. 1986, with permission.)

VIII. Pulmonary Hypertension and Coronary Blood Flow

One mechanism by which the development of pulmonary hypertension could impair right heart function is by interfering with the nutrient blood flow to the right ventricle. Both left and right coronary arteries arise from the root of the aorta. Because the left ventricle generates the systolic pressure in the aortic root, blood cannot flow through the left ventricular myocardial layers that are generating the pressure. Therefore coronary flow to the left ventricle is near zero during systole and occurs largely during diastole (Gregg et al., 1965). Under normal conditions the aortic pressure is always higher than the right ventricular pressure, and therefore blood flow to the right ventricle can be continuous. However, if the pressure rises on the right side of the heart but not in the aorta, then the pressure gradient for coronary perfusion and hence coronary flow to the right heart would decrease. The dog has been convenient for study because the right ventricle is largely supplied from the right coronary artery, and the left ventricle is supplied from the left coronary artery. (In humans, the right coronary artery supplies varying amounts of left ventricular tissue.) Coronary flow to the right ventricle in the dog continued throughout the cardiac cycle (Fig. 9A). The capacity for high systolic flow in the right coronary artery was well illustrated

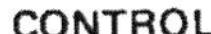

PEAK REACTIVE HYPEREMIA

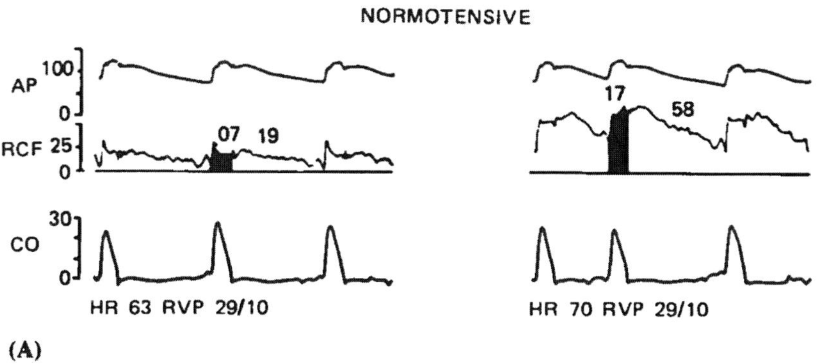

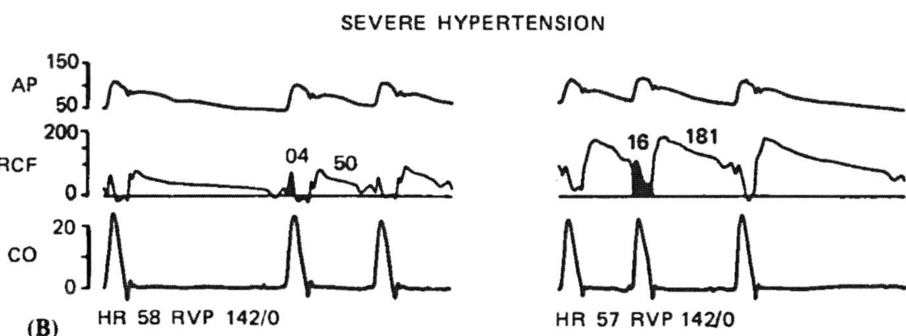

Figure 9 Measurements relating to right coronary arterial flow in unanesthetized dogs. Left, control measurements; right, measurements (reactive hyperemia) following release after occlusion of the right coronary artery. (A) Measurements in a normal dog. (B) Measurements in a dog with severe congenital pulmonary valvular stenosis. In each panel, from top to bottom, are arterial pressure measured in the aorta (AP), right coronary arterial flow (RCF), and cardiac output (CO) measured above the aortic valve. Heart rate and right ventricular pressure are noted beneath each tracing. (From Lowensohn et al., 1976, used with permission.)

during reactive hyperemia following release of a temporarily occluded right coronary artery. However, in dogs with congenital pulmonic stenosis and chronic elevation of right ventricular systolic pressure, the right coronary flow pattern was more phasic (Fig. 9B). Flow was virtually absent during systole, and thus right coronary flow assumed the pattern normally seen for the left coronary artery. The systolic flow remained below diastolic flow during reactive hyperemia. Total right coronary flow was increased such that the flow per 100% g of tissue was almost that of the normotensive dogs. However, given the high work load required by the hypertensive ventricle, the flow was not adequate. Thus, in dogs with severe right ventricular hypertension from congenital pulmonic stenosis, the authors observed electrocardiographic S-T changes, implying myocardial ischemia. Findings at post-mortem included subendocardial ischemia, fibrosis, and right ventricular infarction. The inner layers of the ventricle were most severely affected (Lowensohn et al., 1976).

Detailed investigation of coronary flow to the right ventricular muscle layers in acute pulmonary hypertension showed ischemia of the subendocardial layers of the right ventricular free wall and the right side of the interventricular septum (Gold and Bache, 1982). These findings are consistent with the concepts developed from the left ventricle that the tension developed and the oxygen required by the myocardium are greatest in the subendocardial layers. The hypoperfusion and ischemia occurred even though coronary vasodilator reserve had not been exhausted in these areas (Gold and Bache, 1982). Clearly, with elevated pressure, systolic coronary flow to the right heart becomes small relative to demand, total coronary flow is inadequate, and right heart myocardial damage occurs.

These findings in the dog have a counterpart in human beings with pulmonary hypertension. Right ventricular infarction has been described in children with congenital pulmonic valvular stenosis (Fransiosi and Blanc, 1968). In persons with moderate pulmonary hypertension, exercise may induce near-systemic or even suprasystemic pulmonary arterial pressures. Angina during exercise is frequent in pulmonary hypertensive patients and is poorly understood. At postmortem, right heart infarctions have been reported in persons with pulmonary hypertension and normal coronary arteries (Horan et al., 1981; Carlson et al., 1985).

IX. Pulmonary Hypertension and Left Heart Function

Normally, the left ventricle is the dominant heart pump. The right ventricle is a thin muscle that is wrapped around one third of the circumference of the thick-walled, cone-shaped left ventricle. Its weight is only one-third to one-fourth that of the left. Abnormal right ventricular function has been considered to reflect largely abnormal left ventricular function (Berger et al., 1979). Some investigators have even proposed that the right ventricle is unnecessary for normal overall heart function at rest (Guiha et al., 1974). In the open-chest dog, acute destruction of the right ventricular free wall was associated with relatively well maintained stroke volume and right atrial pressure until the pulmonary arterial pressure was raised (Brooks et al., 1971). Probably the septum and the undamaged portions of the free wall were able to compensate as long as there was no additional stress on the right ventricle (Geiran et al., 1984). In humans, the outcome after right ventricular infarction depends mostly on the extent of additional left ventricular infarction, the latter elevating the right ventricular afterload. It is probable that when stresses are placed on the right ventricle, its essential contribution to circulatory function becomes apparent.

The right ventricle has been likened to a bellows, which has a relatively large surface area/volume ratio. Bellows are well suited to deliver large and/or variable volumes at low pressures. For example, in open-chest dogs, the sudden opening of an arteriovenous shunt increased the stroke volume, largely by virtue of the changed configuration of the right ventricular chamber (Molaug et al., 1982). The implication has been that the design of the right ventricle allows it to function as a volume, rather than a pressure pump. However, while the most effective wall movement to eject blood from a bellows-like pump would seem to be the movement of the free wall toward the septum, such movement is actually small. Rather the ventricle empties largely by moving the tricuspid valve toward the apex (Fig. 10; see also Meier et al., 1980). Thus the right ventricle shortens, while the left ventricular free wall moves toward the septum with little shortening from apex to base. It may be too simplistic to consider the right ventricle as a bellows-like volume pump. Rather, Elzinga et al (1980) and Piene (1986 have pointed out that each ventricular pump should be considered adequate for the load that is normally placed on it. Further, the right heart (Maugham et al., 1979) functions like the left heart (Ross, 1983; Sagawa, 1978) in that the end-systolic and end-diastolic pressure-volume curves are linear, they change with contractile state, and they provide a description of myocardial function.

The two ventricles function as a unit, and the layers of muscle are continuous from one ventricle to the other (Armour and Randall, 1970; Armour et al., 1970). When the volume in one chamber increases, the volume and function of the other chamber is affected (Elzinga et al., 1974). For example, when the volume of the left ventricle was increased acutely, the septum moved toward the right ventricle, increasing the curvature both in the septum and in the right ventricular free wall. Resistance to right ventricular filling was increased, and both end-diastolic and end-systolic pressures also increased, probably as a result of the increased wall tension (Santamore et al., 1976b). When the septum was made acutely ischemic, the bulging became less, but the increase in right ventricular pressure became greater. When the free wall of the left ventricle was cut along its major axis, the right ventricle was no longer able to develop the usual amount of force, indicating that structural damage to the left ventricular free wall resulted in subsequent inability of the right ventricle to develop force (Santamore et al., 1976a). There were similar but smaller effects of increasing right ventricular pressure on left ventricular function (Maugham 1979). Normally

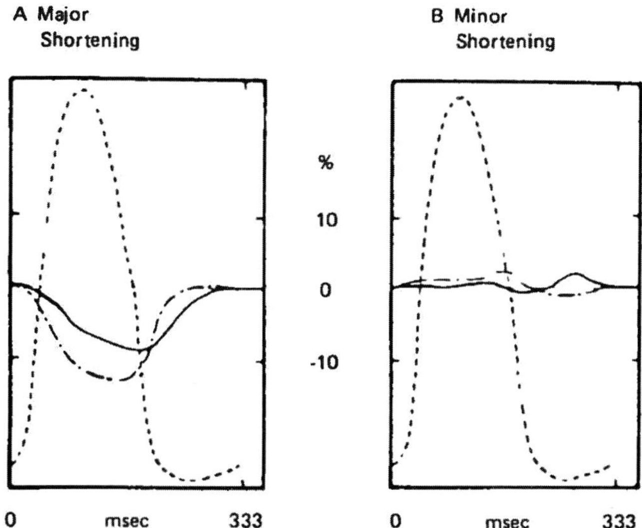

Figure 10 Shortening of myocardial segments with time during right ventricular systole. The right ventricular pressure curve is shown as a dotted line. The unbroken line is shortening in a segment at the conus of the right ventricle. The broken line is shortening in a segment at the mid ventricular level. (A) Shortening in segments parallel to the major axis of the right ventricle. (B) Shortening in segments parallel to the minor axis of the right ventricle. (From Meier et al. 1980, used with permission.)

these are minor changes that contribute to fluctuations in pressure and flow with respiration or changes in posture. However, when right ventricular volumes were considerably above normal, left ventricular function was impaired. In patients with primary pulmonary hypertension, the left ventricular prejection period is prolonged and the ejection period is shortened, suggesting that right ventricular hypertension has affected left ventricular systolic function (Leirer).

When the right ventricular pressure exceeds that in the left ventricle during systole, the left ventricular pressure also increases (Fig. 11) (Elzinga et al., 1980). Also, these authors point out that any movement of the septum to the left will increase the volume in the right heart and contribute to a drop in left ventricular pressure and output. The magnitude of the septal movement, for example from right to left with high pressures in the right ventricle, will depend on the pressure gradient from the hypertensive right ventricle to the left ventricle and on the compliance of the septal wall (Little et al., 1984). Thus when the septum is fibrotic or hypertrophied the movement might be expected to be

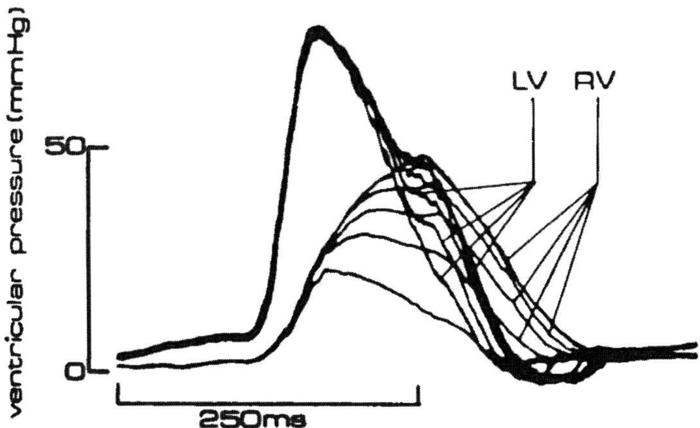

Figure 11 Deformation of the left ventricular pressure by elevated right ventricular pressure. (From Elzinga et al., 1974, with permission.)

less. The encroachment of the right side on the left may become severe (Fig. 12). The magnitude of such deformation has even been used to estimate the pressure in the right ventricular cavity (Watanabe, 1984; King et al., 1983). When the compression of the left ventricle by the right becomes severe, then the filling of the left ventricle is impaired. The mitral valve remains open throughout diastole, giving the echocardiographic appearance of mitral valvular stenosis. Also, with severe pulmonary hypertension, septal curvature is reversed and the left ventricle becomes the flattened structure. Since, as noted above, left ventricular contraction is adapted to a conical shape, such geometric distortion could also contribute to impairment of systolic function. One might even consider that, during exercise, the diastolic and systolic pressures in the right heart become so great relative to the left heart that left-aided stroke volume might not be maintained. Failure of left-aided stroke volume as a result of compression of the left side by the right side is one possible cause of syncope in the pulmonary hypertensive patient.

X. Right Heart Function in Chronic Obstructive Lung Disease

Perhaps the largest single class of persons with pulmonary hypertension is composed of patients with chronic obstructive pulmonary disease. In them, increasing evidence suggests that impairment of right heart function impairs exercise performance (Mahler et al., 1984; Matthay et al., 1980; Morrison et al.,

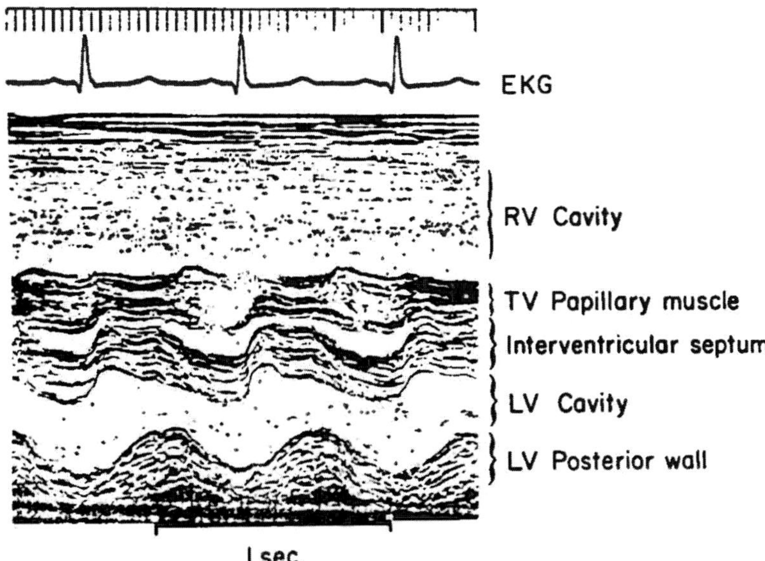

Figure 12 M-mode echocardiogram showing flattening of the cavity of the left ventricle in a patient with pulmonary hypertension.

1987). There are several factors that combine to place stress on the right heart. These include increased peripheral resistance, arterial hypoxemia, increased blood volume, and tricuspid valvular insufficiency. The obstructive pulmonary disease population has also been relatively widely studied, particularly using radionuclide scan techniques. From these patients we may gain some insight as to factors determining right heart function in lung disease in particular and in pulmonary hypertension in general. Although pulmonary hypertension is an important stress on right heart function, patients with lung disease can also have a variety of other stresses on their right heart function.

For example, as noted before, pulmonary hypertension increases right heart oxygen demand and reduces oxygen supply. In obstructive lung disease the problem of supply and demand is augmented during exercise because exercise markedly increases the pulmonary arterial pressure. Exercise also augments the hypoxemia, which further reduces the availability of oxygen. Increased respiratory effort in obstructive lung disease may also increase intrathoracic pressure, which impairs venous return, limits cardiac output, and could contribute to the poor myocardial oxygen supply. We have recently studied a patient with obstructive lung disease who, during low-level exercise, developed anginal chest pain, ischemic ST-segment depression, and ECG signs of "right heart strain." At cardiac catheterization, the patient had normal coronary arteries, but he developed severe pulmonary hypertension with exercise and by ventriculogram had augmentation of right heart dilatation. We considered that the combination of several factors contributed to induce right ventricular ischemia and failure (Morrison, D. A., Klien, C., Friefeld, B., Welsh, C. in preparation).

Overall circulatory impairment manifested by low resting and exercise cardiac outputs has been described in some patients with chronic obstructive pulmonary disease (Filley, 1968). Even with these patients with output values within the low normal range, recent data have indicated that right and left ventricular ejection fractions measured at maximum effort were depressed, which suggested the presence of myocardial dysfunction (Morrison et al., 1987). The right ventricular but not the left ventricular ejection fraction was related to the exercise level the patient could achieve, raising the possibility that function of the right but not the left ventricle was a determinant of maximum oxygen transport in these patients. Even at rest, right ventricular ejection fraction has been shown to decrease with increasing pulmonary artery pressure and resistance (Brent et al., 1982).

One expects the right ventricle to be more severely affected than the left given the increased load on the right ventricle and the many factors that can adversely affect right ventricular performance. It is difficult to determine the extent to which the right ventricle limits oxygen transport because chronic lung disease impacts on several links in the oxygen transport chain and because right ventricular function has traditionally been difficult to assess.

XI. Future Directions

The crucial location of the right ventricle and its potential importance for the circulation in chronic lung disease emphasize the need for continuing study. Potentially needed are measurements relating the contractile state of the right ventricle to the work load it faces. One needs to know how the intrathoracic pressure and local pressures around the heart, particularly during exercise in obstructed patients, influence intracardiac pressures and cardiac performance. We need to know how coronary perfusion of the right ventricle in humans is affected by increments in right ventricular pressure. The role of hypercapnia and its influence on increasing the total and central blood volume need to be studied in relation to right heart function. Also, more work needs to be done on patients earlier in the natural history of this disease, in order to better separate cause from effect as related to oxygen transport and cardiac function. Clearly we have far to go in our understanding of the function of the right heart in pulmonary hypertensive states.

Acknowledgment

This work was supported by NHLBI grant NIH 14895 and a grant from the Colorado Heart Association.

References

Anzola, J. (1956). Right ventricular contraction. *Am. J. Physiol. 184*:567-571.

Armour, J. A., and Randall, J. C. (1970). Structural basis for cardiac function. *Am. J. Physiol. 218*:1517-1723.

Armour, J. A., Pace, J. B., and Randall, W. C. (1970). Interrelationship of architecture and function of the right ventricle. *Am. J. Physiol. 218*:174-179.

Benegard, S., Holmgren, A., and Jonsson, B. (1960). The effect of body position on the circulation at rest and during exercise, with special reference to the influence on the stroke volume. *Acta Physiol. Scand. 49*:279-298.

Berger, H. J., Johnstone, D. E., Sands, J. M., Gottschalk, A., and Zaret, B. L. (1979). Response of right ventricular ejection fraction to upright bicycle exercise in coronary artery disease. *Circulation 60*:1292-1300.

Berkenboom, G., Sobolski, J., and Stoupel, E. (1982). Failure of nifedipine treatment in primary pulmonary hypertension. *Br. Heart J. 47*:511.l.

Bloomfield, R. A., Lauson, H. D., Cournand, A., E. S. Breed, E. S., and Richards, D. W., Jr. (1946). Recording of right heart and pressures in normal subjects and in patients with chronic pulmonary disease and various types of cardio circulatory disease. *J. Clin. Invest. 25*:639-664.

Bouthier, J. D., de Luca, N., Safar, M. E., and Simon, A. Ch. (1985). Cardiac hypertrophy and arterial distensibility in essential hypertension. *Am. Heart J. 109*:1345-1352.

Brent, B. N., Berger, H. J., Matthay, R. A., Mahler, D., Pytlik, L., and Zaret, B. L. (1982). Physiologic correlates of right ventricular ejection fraction in chronic obstructive pulmonary disease: a combined radionuclide and hemodynamic study. *Am. J. Cardiol. 50*:255-262.

Brent, B. N., Berger, H. J., Matthay, R. A., Mahler, D., Pytlik, L., and Zaret, B. L. (1983). Contrasting acute effects of vasodilators (nitroglycerine, nitroprusside, and hydralazine) on right ventricular performance in patients with chronic obstructive pulmonary disease and pulmonary hypertension: a combined radionuclide-hemodynamic study. *Am. J. Cardio. 51*:1681-1689.

Brooks, H., Kirk, E. S., Vokonas, P. S., Urschel, C. W., and Sonnenblick, E. H. (1971). Performance of the right ventricle under stress: relation to right coronary flow. *J. Clin. Invest. 50*:2176-2183.

Burrows, B., Kettel, L. S., Niden, A. H., et al. (1972). Patterns of cardiovascular dysfunction in chronic obstructive lung disease. *New Engl. J. Med. 286*:912-918.

Camerini, F., Alberti, E., Klugmann, S., and Salvi, A. (1980). Primary pulmonnary hypertension: effects of nifedipine. *Br. Heart J. 44*:352-356.

Carlson, E. B., Reimer, K. A., Rankin, J. S., Peter, R. H., McCormack, K. M., and Alexander, L. G. (1985). Right ventricular subendocardial infarction in a patient with pulmonary hypertension, right ventricular hypertrophy, and normal coronary arteries. *Clin. Cardiol. 8*:499-502.

Cohen, M., Horowitz, S. F., Machac, J., Mindich, B. P., and Fuster, V. (1985). Response of the right ventricle to exercise in isolated mitral stenosis. *Am. J. Cardiol.* 55:1054-1058.

Cournand, A., Bloomfield, R. A., and Lauson, H. D. (1945). Double lumen catheter for intravenous and intracardiac blood sampling and pressure recording. *Proc. Soc. Exp. Biol. Med. 60*:73-75.

Degaute, J. P., Domenighetti, G., Naeije, R., Vincent, J. L., Treyvaud, D., and Perret, C. I. (1981). Oxygen delivery in acute exacerbation of chronic obstructive pulmonary disease. *Am. Rev. Resp. Dis. 124*:26-30.

Douglas, J. S. (1983). Hemodynamic effects of nifedipine in primary pulmonary hypertension. *J. Am. Coll. Cardiol. 2*:174-179.

Elzinga, G., and Westerhof, N. (1979). How to quantify pump function of the heart. *Circ. Res. 44*:303-308.

Elzinga, G., Grondelle, R. van, Westerhof, N., and Bos, G. C. van den (1974). Ventricular interference. *Am. J. Physiol. 226*(5):941-947.

Elzinga, G., Piene, H., and Jong, J. P. de (1980). Left and right ventricular pump function and consequence of having two pumps in one heart. *Circ. Res. 46*:564-574.

Filley, G. F., Beckwitt, H. J., Reeves, J. T., and Mitchell, R. S. (1968). Chronic obstructive pulmonary disease: Oxygen transport in two clinical types. *Am. J. Med. 44*:26-38.

Fransiosi, R. A., and Blanc, W. A. (1968). Myocardial infarcts in infants and children I: a necropsy study in congential heart disease. *J. Pediatr. 73*:309-319.

Geiran, O., Molaug, M., and Kiil, F. (1984). Compensatory cardiac mechanisms evoked by acute occlusion of the right coronary artery in dogs. *Acta Physiol. Scand. 120*:185-195.

Gold, F. L., and Bache, R. J. (1982). Transmural right ventricular blood flow during acute pulmonary artery hypertension in the sedated dog. *Circ. Res. 51*:196-204.

Gonza, E. R., Marble, A. E., Shaw, A., and Holland, J. G. (1974). Age related changes in the mechanics of the aorta and pulmonary artery in man. *J. Appl. Physiol. 36*:407-411.

Gregg, D. E., Khouri, E. M., and Rayford, C. R. (1965). Systemic and coronary energetics in the resting unanesthetized dog. *Circ. Res. 16*:102-113.

Guiha, N. H., Limas, C. J., and Cohn, J. N. (1974). Predominant right ventricular dysfunction after right ventricular destruction in the dog. *Am. J. Cardiol. 33*:254-258.

Gurtner, H. P., Walser, P., and Fassler, B. (1975). Normal values for pulmonary hemodynamics at rest and during exercise in man. *Prog. Resp. Res. 9*:295-315.

Honey, M., Cotter, M., Davies, N., and Denison, D. (1980). Clinical and haemodynamic effects of diazoxide in primary pulmonary hypertension. *Thorax 35*:269-276.

Horan, L. G., Flowers, N. C., and Havelda, C. J. (1981). Relation between right ventricular mass and cavity size: an analysis of 1500 human hearts. *Circ. 64*:135-138.

Hori, M., Inoue, M., Kitakaze, M., Tsujioka, K., Fukunami, M., Nakajima, S., Kitabake, A., and Abe, H. (1985). Loading sequence is a major determinant of afterload-dependent relaxation in intact canine heart. *Am. J. Physiol. 249*:H747-H754.

Horn, G. J., van den, Westerhof, N., and Elzinga, G. (1985). Optimal power generation by the left ventricle. *Circ. Res. 56*:252-261.

Horowitz, J. D., Brennan, J. B., Oliver, L. E., Harding, D., Goble, A. J., and Louis, W. J. (1981). Effects of captopril (SQ 14,225) in a patient with primary pulmonary hypertension. *Postgrad. Med. J. 57*:115-116.

Ikram, H., Maslowski, A. H., Nichols, M. G., Espiner, E. A., and Hull, F. T. L. (1982). Haemodynamic and hormonal effect of captopril in primary pulmonary hypertension. *Brit. Heart J. 48*:541-545.

Jenkins, R. M., and Page, M. McB. (1981). Remission of primary pulmonary hypertension during treatment with diazoxide. *Brit. Med. J. 282*:1118.

Kawakami, Y., Kishi, F., Yamamoto, H., and Miyamot, K. (1983). Relation of oxygen delivery, mixed venous oxygenation, and pulmonary hemodynamics to prognosis in chronic obstructive pulmonary disease. *New Eng. J. Med. 308*:1045-1049.

King, M. E., Braun, H., Goldblatt, A., Liberthson, R., and Weyman, A. E. (1983). Interventricular septal configuration as a predictor of ventricular systolic hypertension in children: a cross-sectional echocardiographic study. *Circulation 68*:68-75.

Kitabatake, A., Inoue, M., Asao, M., Masuyama, T., Tanouchi, J., Morita, T., Mishima, M., Uematsu, M., Shimazu, T., Hori, M., and Abe, H. (1983). Noninvasive evaluation of pulmonary hypertension by a pulsed Doppler technique. *Circulation 68*:302-309.

Konstam, M. A., Idoine, J., Wynne, J., Grossman, W., Cohn, L., Beck, J. R., Kozlowski, J., and Holman, B. L. (1983). Right ventricular function in adults with pulmonary hypertension with and without atrial septal defect *Amer. J. Cardiol. 51*:1144-1149.

Leier, C. V., Bambach, D., Nelson, S., Hermiller, J. B., Huss, P., Magorien, R. D., and Unverfeth, D. V. (1983). Captopril in primary pulmonary hypertension. *Circulation 67*:155-161.

Leier, C. V., Sahar, D., Hermiller, J. B., and Unverferth, D. V. (1985). Combining left ventricular systolic time intervals and M-mode echocardiography in the evaluation of primary pulmonary hypertension in women. *Clin. Cardiol. 8*:166-172.

Little, W. C., Badke, F. R., and O'Rourke, R. A. (1984). Effect of right ventricular pressure on the end-diastolic left ventricular pressure-volume relationship before and after chronic right ventricular pressure overload in dogs without pericardia. *Circ. Res. 54*:719-730.

Lowensohn, H. S., Khouri, E. M., Gregg, D. E., Pyle, R. L., and Patternson, R. E. (1976). Phasic right coronary blood flow in conscious dogs with normal and elevated right ventricular pressures. *Circ. Res. 39*:760-766.

Lupi-Herrera, E., Sandoval, J., Seoane, M., and Bialostozky, D. (1982). The role of hydralazine therapy for pulmonary arterial hypertension of unknown cause. *Circulation 65*:645-653.

MacNee, W., Prince, K., Flenley, D. C., and Muir, A. L. (1985). Effects of pulmonary hypertension on right ventricular performance in chronic bronchitis and emphysema. *Prog. Resp. Dis. 20*:108-116.

Maddahi, J., Berman, D. S., Matsuoka, D. T., Waxman, A. D., Forrester, J. S., and Swan, H. J. C. (1980). Right ventricular ejection fraction during exercise in normal subjects and in coronary artery disease patients: assessment by multiplegated equilibrium scintigraphy. *Circulation 62*:133-140.

Mahler, D. A., Brent, B. N., Loke, J., Zaret, B. L., and Matthay, R. A. (1984). Right ventricular performance and central circulatory hemodynamics during upright exercise in patients with chronic obstructive disease. *Am. Rev. Resp. Dis. 130*:772-779.

Malcic, I., and Richter, D. (1985). Verapamil in primary pulmonary hypertension. *Brit. Heart J. 53*:345-347.

Marmor, A. T., Mijiritesky, Y., Plich, M., Frenkel, A., and Front, D. (1986). Improved radionuclide method for assessment of pulmonary artery pressure in COPD. *Chest 89*:64-69.

Matthay, R. A., Berger, H. J., Davies, R. A., Loke, J., Mahler, D. A., Gottschalk, A., and Zaret, B. L. (1980). Radionuclide assessment of right and left ventricular exercise performance in chronic obstructive pulmonary disease. *Ann. Int. Med. 93*:234-239.

Maugham, W. L., Shoukas, A. A., Sagawa, K., and Weisfeldt, M. L. (1979). Instantaneous pressure-volume relationship of the canine right ventricle. *Circ. Res. 44*:309-315.

Meier, G. D., Bove, A. A., Santamore, W. P., and Lynch, P. R. (1980). Contractile function in canine right ventricle. *Am. J. Physiol. 239*:H794-H804.

Melot, C., Naeiji, R., Mols, P., Vandenbossche, J. -L., and Denolin, H. (1983). Effects of nifedipine on ventilation/perfusion matching in primary pulmonary hypertension. *Chest 83*:203-207.

Milnor, W. R. (1983). *Hemodynamics*. Williams and Wilkins, New York.

Milnor, W. R., and Bertram, C. D. (1978). The relation between arterial viscoelasticity and wave propagation in the canine femoral artery. *Circ. Res. 43*: 870-879.

Mithoefer, J. C., Ramirez, C., and Cook, W. (1978). The effect of mixed venous oxygenation on arterial blood in chronic obstructive pulmonary disease. *Am. Rev. Resp. Dis. 117*:259-264.

Molaug, M., Geiran, O., Stokland, O., Thorvaldson, J., and Ilebekk, A. (1982). Dynamics of intraventricular septum and free ventricular walls during blood volume expansion and selective right ventricular volume loading in dogs. *Acta Physiol. Scand. 116*:245-256.

Morrison, D. A., Goldman, S., and Henry, R. (1983). The effect of pulmonary hypertension on systolic function of the right ventricle. *Chest 84*:250-257.

Morrison, D. A., Henry, R., and Goldman, S. (1986). Preliminary study of the effects of low flow oxygen on oxygen delivery and right ventricular dysfunction in chronic lung disease. *Am. Rev. Resp. Dis. 133*:390-395.

Morrison, D. A., Adcock, K., Collins, C. M., Goldman, S., Cladwell, J. H., and Schwarz, M. I. (1987). Right ventricular dysfunction and the exercise limitation of chronic obstructive pulmonary disease. *J. Am. Coll. Cardiol., 9*:1219-1229.

Morrison, D. A., Ovitt, T., and Hammermeister, K. (1988). The effect of tricuspid regurgitation on the right ventricular ejection fraction-pulmonary artery pressure relationship. In Press. *Am. J. Cardiol.*

O'Rourke, M. F. (1985). Basic concepts for the understanding of large arteries in hypertension. *J. Cardiovasc. Pharmacol. 7*:S14-S21.

Packer, M., Greenberg, B., Massie, B., and Dash, H. (1982). Deleterious effects of hydralazine in patients with pulmonary hypertension. *New Engl. J. Med. 306*:1326-1331.

Packer, M., Medina, N., Yshak, M., and Wiener, I. (1984). Detrimental effects of verapamil in patients with primary pulmonary hypertension. *Br. Heart J. 52*:106-111.

Piene, H. (1986). Pulmonary arterial impedance and right heart function. *Physiol. Rev. 66*:606-652.

Poderoso, J. J., Biancolini, C. A., Del Bosco, C. G., Cataalano, H. N., Peralta, J. G., Goldenberg, D. B. I., and Suarez, L. D. (1983). Captopril versus hydralazine in primary pulmonary hypertension. *J. Clin. Pharmacol. 23*:563-566.

Reeves, J. T., and Groves, B. M. (1984). Approach to the patient with pulmonary hypertension. In *Pulmonary Hypertension*, Chap. 1. Edited by E. K. Weir and J. T. Reeves. Futura, Mt. Kisco, NY, pp. 1-44.

Reeves, J. T., Grover, R. F., Filley, G. F., and Blount, S. G., Jr. (1961). Circulatory changes in man during mild supine exercise. *J. Appl. Physiol. 16*:279-282.

Reeves, J. T., Turkevich, D., and Morrison, D. A. (1985). Noninvasive detection of pulmonary hypertension. *Semin. Resp. Med. 7*:147-159.

Reeves, J. T., Dempsey, J. A., and Grover, R. F. (1987). Pulmonary circulation during exercise, This volume.

Rich, S., Martinez, J., Lam, W., and Rose, K. M. (1982). Captopril as treatment for patients with primary pulmonary hypertension. *Br. Heart J. 48*:272-277.

Rich, S., Brundage, B. H., and Levy, P. S. (1985). The effect of vasodilator therapy on the clinical outcome of patients with primary pulmonary hypertension. *Circulation 71*:1191-1196.

Ross, J. (1983). Cardiac function and myocardial contractility: a perspective. *J. Am. Coll. Cardiol. 1*:52-62.

Rubin, L. J., and Peter, R. S. (1980). Oral hydralazine therapy for primary pulmonary hypertension. *New Engl. J. Med. 302*:69-73.

Rubin, L. J., Nicod, P., Hillis, L. D., and Firth, B. G. (1983). Treatment of primary pulmonary hypertension with nifedipine. *Ann. Int. Med. 99*:433-438.

Rubino, J., and Schroeder, J. S. (1979). Diazoxide in treatment of primary pulmonary hypertension. *Br. Heart J. 42*:362-363.

Ruskin, J. N., and Hutter, A. M. (1979). Primary pulmonary hypertension treated with oral phentolamine. *Ann. Int. Med. 90*:772-774.

Sagawa, K. (1978). The pressure-volume diagram revisited. *Circ. Res. 43*:677-687.

Santamore, W. P., Lynch, P. R., Heckman, J. L., Bove, A. A., and Meier, G. D (1976a). Left ventricular effects on right ventricular developed pressure. *J. Appl. Physiol. 41*:925-930.

Santamore, W. P., Lynch, P. R., Meier, G., Heckman, J. L., and Bove, A. A. (1976b). Myocardial interaction between the ventricles. *J. Appl. Physiol. 41*:362-368.

Shimada, R., Takeshita, A., and Nakamura, M. (1984). Noninvasive assessment of right ventricular systolic pressure in atrial septal defect: Analysis of the end-systolic configuration of the ventricular septum by 2-dimensional echocardiography. *Am. J. Cardiol. 53*:1117-1123.

Tenney, S. M., and Mithoeffer, J. C. (1982). The relationship of mixed venous oxygenation to oxygen transport: with special reference to adaptation to high altitude and pulmonary disease. *Am. Rev. Resp. Dis. 125*:474-479.

Wade, W. G. (1959). The pathogenesis of infarction of the right ventricle. *Br. Heart J. 21*:545-554.

Wang, S. W. S., Pohl, J. E. F., Rowlands, D. J., and Wade, E. G. (1978). Diazoxide in treatment of primary pulmonary hypertension. *Br. Heart J. 40*:572-574.

Watanabe, K. (1984). Evaluation of right ventricular pressure by two-dimensional echocardiography. *Jap. Heart. J. 25*:523-531.

Wise, J. R. (1983). Nifedipine in the treatment of primary pulmonary hypertension. *Am. Heart J. 105*:693-694.

Zieher, A. M., Bonzel, T., Wollschlaeger, H., Hohnloeser, S., Hust, M. H., and Just, H. (1986). Noninvasive evaluation of pulmonary hypertension by quantitative contrast M-mode echocardiography. *Am. Heart J. 111*:297-306.

Part II

PATHOPHYSIOLOGY

11

Etiologic Mechanisms in Persistent Pulmonary Hypertension of the Newborn

KURT R. STENMARK, STEVEN H. ABMAN, and FRANK J. ACCURSO

University of Colorado
Health Sciences Center
Denver, Colorado

I. Introduction

Persistent pulmonary hypertension of the newborn (PPHN) is a significant problem which complicates a wide variety of neonatal cardiorespiratory disorders, including hyaline membrane disease, asphyxia, meconium aspiration syndrome, sepsis, congenital diaphragmatic hernia, and also idiopathically ("persistent fetal circulation"), (Levin et al., 1976). Published reports have estimated its incidence as high as 1 in 1000 live births, with mortality ranging between 20 and 50% (Heymann and Hoffman, 1984). We recently reviewed the records of infants admitted to the nursery of the Childrens Hospital, Denver, for the interval August 1984 to July 1985 (Quissel, 1987). Sixty-three of 628 admissions (all outborn, requiring transport to TCH), or approximately 10% of admissions, had pulmonary hypertension as the primary problem on admission. The etiologies were multiple and included respiratory distress syndrome (23/63 patients) aspiration (13/63), congenital anomalies (12/63), and primary or idiopathic cases (13/63). Despite the diversity of clinical settings associated with PPHN, these disorders are related by common clinical and physiologic abnormalities. As has been described elsewhere (Drummond et al., 1977; Fox and Durara, 1983; Fox et al., 1977; Goetzman and Riemenschneider, 1980), the infants showed severe hypoxemia, echocardiographic evidence of pulmonary hypertension, and right-to-left shunting through the foramen ovale and ductus arterisus. The pulmonary hypertension often did not regress despite hyperoxic hyperventilation and vasodilator therapy, as has been reported (Rabinovitch, 1985; Kulik and Lock 1984). Of the 63 infants, 13 (21%) died and 25 went on to develop bronchopulmonary dysplasia (defined by an oxygen requirement and radiographic lung changes after 30 days of life). Cost analysis for the time spent in the level III ICN showed an average cost of $1500/day, a cost nearly double that of even the small premature infant <1000 g with RDS (Hernandez et al., 1986). Conservative estimates place the cost at greater than $4 million for these 63 infants.

The mechanisms that control high pulmonary vascular resistance in the fetus and that allow a rapid decrease in this resistance during normal adaptation to extrauterine life are not known. A better understanding of these mechanisms will provide insight into the problem of neonatal pulmonary hypertension where the pulmonary vasculature fails to adapt to extrauterine life. This chapter will explore changes that take place in the fetus that could be associated with neonatal pulmonary hypertension. The alternative but not necessarily exclusive hypothesis, that structural abnormalities and pulmonary hypertension often develop rapidly and viciously in the neonatal period, will also be explored.

II. Fetal Pulmonary Circulation and Persistent Pulmonary Hypertension of the Newborn

Although there are many differences between the various neonatal disorders that are included in the syndrome of PPHN, common characteristics include the presence of marked pulmonary hypertension, an abnormal pulmonary vasoreactivity, and, in infants dying with PPHN, marked structural alterations in the pulmonary vascular bed. The clinical observations of elevated pulmonary artery pressure and the presence of right-to-left shunting across the foramen ovale and ductus arteriosus parallel the normal physiology of the fetus, leading to the notion that PPHN might represent the failure of the fetal pulmonary circulation to undergo a normal adaptation to postnatal conditions and that mechanisms maintaining the high pulmonary vascular resistance in the fetus persist after birth (Gersony et al., 1969). Experimental and clinical studies have suggested that intrauterine events may be important determinants of its pathogenesis. Supportive evidence includes the timing of onset of abnormal vasoreactivity within the first several hours of birth, the severity of histologic findings in infants dying within the first few days of life (Haworth and Reid, 1976; Murphy et al., 1981), and animal models suggesting that in utero stimuli such as hypoxia (Goldberg et al., 1971) and hypertension (Levin et al., 1978a) can cause smooth muscle thickening of small pulmonary arteries. Thus, on the basis of these ob-

observations, a better understanding of the normal and abnormal fetal pulmonary circulation may provide insight into the pathogenesis and pathophysiology of PPHN. Several questions regarding mechanisms maintaining high pulmonary vascular resistance and responses to vasodilating stimuli in the normal fetus and responses to intrauterine "injury," including hypoxia and hypertension, will be discussed in this section.

A. Normal Fetal Pulmonary Circulation

Part of the difficulty in studying fetal pulmonary vascular responses to abnormal stresses such as hypoxia and hypertension is that mechanisms controlling the normal fetal and transitional circulations are incompletely understood. The high fetal pulmonary vascular resistance is likely related, at least in part, to the low arterial oxygen tension in the normally oxygenated fetus (Dawes et al., 1953). Although increasing fetal PO_2 to 55 torr may suffice to increase pulmonary blood flow to levels achieved at birth (Morin et al., 1984), several studies have demonstrated striking increases with mechanical ventilation of the fetal lung without increasing fetal PO_2 (Cassin et al., 1964; Rudolph et al., 1986). Thus, the relative contributions of increased PO_2 and ventilation remain unclear. Whether the response of fetal pulmonary blood flow to increases in PO_2 and the onset of breathing (ventilation) is direct or partially mediated through the release of vasoactive mediators is not completely understood. (Refer to Section V of this chapter)

Although many investigators have studied the responses of the normal fetus to various pharamcologic or mechanical stimuli, most studies have been directed toward identifying agents that are either dilators or constrictors. Few studies have examined other important aspects of fetal pulmonary vasoreactivity, such as the responses to more prolonged stimuli or responses following injury. In the neonatal lamb, for example, Lock and co-workers have demonstrated altered pulmonary vascular reactivity to adrenergic stimuli following acute hypoxia (Lock et al., 1981) and have shown striking differences between the acute and chronic responses to indomethacin administration (Lock et al., 1980). Such variables as vascular tone, time- and dose-dependent responses, age of the animal, and other factors are critical determinants in understanding vasoreactivity and the control of the fetal pulmonary circulation. For example, although it has been well known that even small increases in fetal PO_2 can vasodilate the pulmonary vascular bed of late-gestation animals (Dawes and Mott, 1962), this response has been recently demonstrated to be time dependent (Accurso et al., 1986b). That is, although increasing fetal PO_2 by 5 torr doubles pulmonary blood flow during the first hour of O_2 exposure, pulmonary blood flow steadily declines toward baseline values, despite maintaining constant elevation of fetal PO_2 (Fig. 1). The fetal pulmonary circulation therefore adapts to the sustained vasodilating stimulus of oxygen.

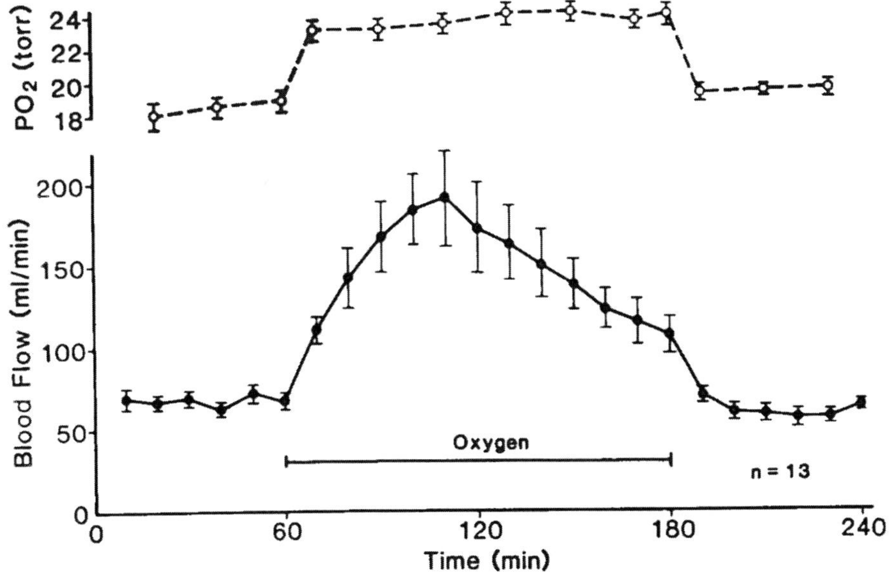
PO2 (torr)
24
22
20
18
Blood Flow (ml/min)
200
150
100
50
0
Oxygen
n = 13
0
60
120
180
240
Time (min)

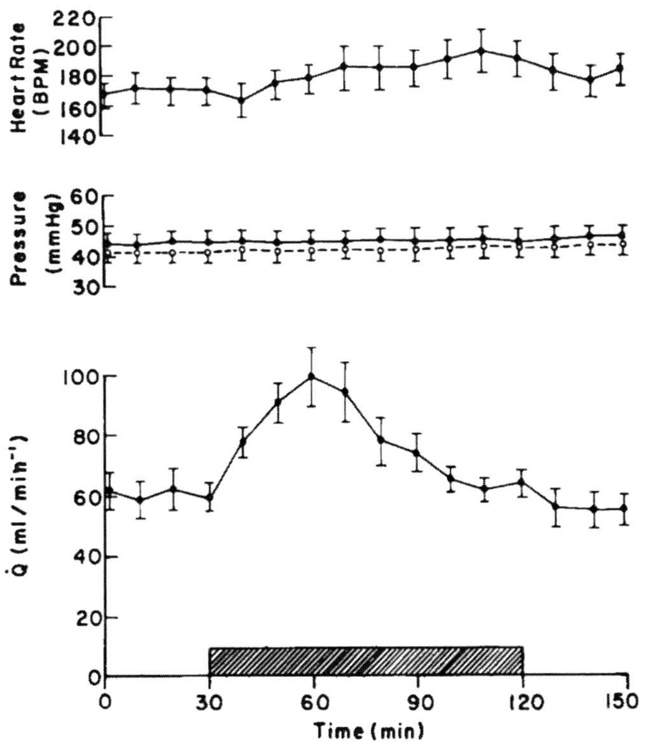
Heart Rate (BPM)
220
200
180
160
140
Pressure (mmHg)
60
50
40
30
Q̇ (ml/min⁻¹)
100
80
60
40
20
0
0
30
60
90
120
150
Time (min)

Further study has demonstrated that this "adaptation" or time dependency of a vasodilating stimulus is not unique to oxygen. That is, pulmonary vasodilation in response to the local infusion of several pharmacologic stimuli, including tolazoline (Fig. 1; Abman et al., 1986); acetylcholine, histamine, and bradykinin (Accurso et al., 1987); and prostaglandins I_2, E_1, and D_2 (Abman et al, 1985), is not sustained over a 2-hr study period. In addition, acute increases in fetal pulmonary blood flow secondary to partial compression of the ductus arteriosus and subsequent elevation of pulmonary arterial pressure are not sustained over 2 hr (Abman and Accurso, 1987). With each stimulus, subsequent exposure to the same or different stimuli following a brief recovery period shows a blunted vasodilating response (Accurso et al., 1987; Abman and Accurso, 1987). Although the mechanisms is not understood, these studies suggest the the responses of the normal fetal pulmonary circulation to vasodilating stimuli are characterized by time dependence and that mechanisms exist in the fetus that oppose vasodilation. From a teleological standpoint, mechanisms that oppose vasodilation in the fetus may be important in redirecting flow from the lung to other fetal organs or in protecting the developing lung from deleterious effects of increased flow. In addition, it can be speculated that the persistence or accentuation of these mechanisms may contribute to the failure to sustain the drop in pulmonary vascular resistance at birth.

B. Responses of the Fetal Pulmonary Circulation to Intrauterine Stress

Although adult animal models of chronic pulmonary hypertension in response to monocrotaline (Meyrick and Reid, 1979a), chronic hypoxia (Meyrick and Reid, 1978), endotoxin (Meyrick and Brigham, 1986), hyperoxia (Jones et al. 1984), and other stimuli have examined the complex relationships between structure and function of the pulmonary circulation, few studies have examined the response of the fetal pulmonary circulation to injury. Understanding the functional and structural characteristics of PPHN will demand improved understanding of vasoreactivity and remodeling in utero and in the immediate newborn period (Fig. 2). The injury in PPHN occurs at a time of rapid growth and differentiation of the lung, further adding to the complexity of the potential impact of injury to the normal processing governing pulmonary vascular develop-

Figure 1 Time-dependent responses of the fetal pulmonary circulation to vasodilating stimuli. *Top*: Response of left pulmonary artery blood flow to increases in PO_2 in chronically prepared fetal lambs. PO_2, as measured from main pulmonary artery blood was increased by administering 100% O_2 to ewes for 2-hr study periods (Accurso et al., 1986). *Bottom*: Response of left pulmonary artery blood flow to the local infusion of tolazoline for 90 min. (Abman et al., 1986).

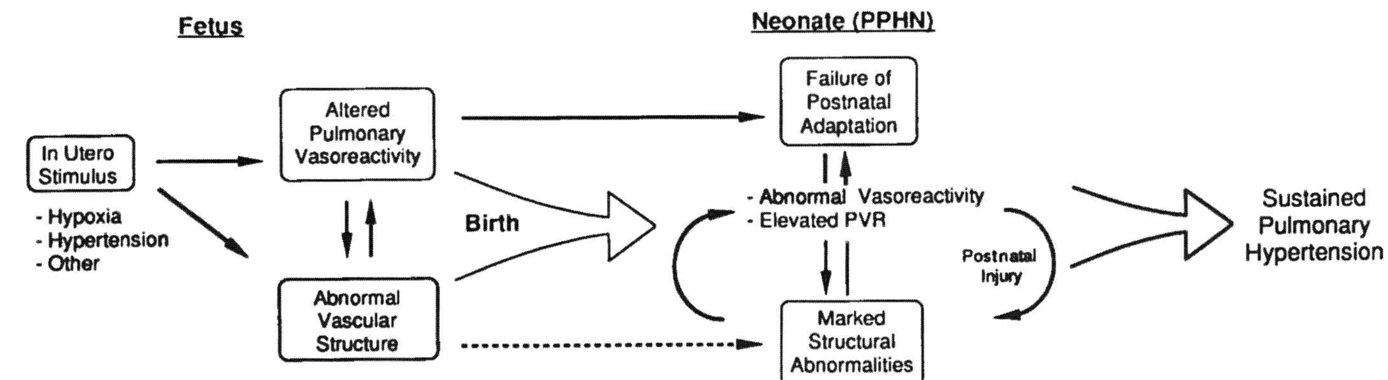

Figure 2 Schematic representation of the pathogenesis of PPHN. It is hypothesized that intrauterine stimuli, such as hypoxia and hypertension, can alter fetal pulmonary vasoreactivity with or without changes in vascular structure. With increased severity or duration of the intrauterine stimulus, or from the persistent hypertension itself, structural changes appear. Additional hemodynamic stresses associated with delivery may superimpose an acute hypoxic stress, further altering vasoreactivity during the transitional period (birth). The presence of an abnormal vasoreactivity (failure to achieve or sustain pulmonary vasodilation) may then lead to further hypertensive injury, causing more structural changes. In addition, attempts to treat the abnormal vasoreactivity may add further injury (hyperoxia, barotrauma, other). This postnatal injury may then lead to sustained pulmonary hypertension.

ment. The perinatal lung may respond to injury with a more marked cellular (proliferative) response than the adult lung allowing for the possibility that some of the pulmonary vascular remodeling seen at autopsy in human infants dying with PPHN even during the first days of life could either be substantially compounded by or the result of postnatal injury (sustained hypertension, hyperoxia, hypoxia, barotrauma, or other) (see below). Thus, postnatal therapy may substantially influence outcome (Wung, 1985), as the initial abnormality of vasoreactivity can be converted to fixed hypertension with postnatal injury. Several studies have examined the link between intrauterine stresses, such as hypoxia and hypertension, and changes in fetal or neonatal structure or vascular reactivity (Table 1). Consideration of fetal pulmonary vascular reactivity, as well as structure, is particularly important in light of the observation that some infants with PPHN demonstrate a "maladaptation," or abnormal vasoreactivity with pulmonary vessels that are (presumably) structurally normal (Rudolph, 1980). These infants initially fail to achieve or sustain a drop in pulmonary vascular resistance at birth but later show clinical recovery. Maladaptation may represent an intrauterine injury to the pulmonary circulation that is severe enough to produce altered vasoreactivity but not of sufficient severity or duration to produce structural changes (Fig. 2).

Experimental and clinical studies suggest that perinatal hypoxia may play an important role in the pathophysiology of PPHN. However, mechanisms linking hypoxia with this syndrome are not clear. Acute hypoxia causes pulmonary vasoconstriction in the fetal lamb (Cohn et al., 1974; Peeters et al. 1979). In addition, prolonged exposure to acute hypoxia can alter fetal pulmonary vasoreactivity (Abman and Accurso, 1987). As shown in Figure 3, 2 hr of hypoxia leads to sustained increases in fetal pulmonary vascular resistance. Interestingly, the rise in pulmonary artery pressure and fall in pulmonary blood flow persist for at least 1 hr following the correction of fetal hypoxia and in the absence of acidemia. This persistent elevation of pulmonary vascular resistance was not seen following briefer (30 min) exposure to hypoxia. Furthermore, the posthypoxia period is characterized by a blunted vasodilating response to small increases in fetal PO_2 (Fig. 4), suggesting that prolonged episodes of acute hypoxia can decrease responsiveness to vasodilating stimuli, and may help clarify mechanisms linking acute hypoxia with the "maladaptation" form of PPHN.

Chronic hypoxia in neonatal and adult animals produces pulmonary vascular remodeling and hypertension, but whether chronic hypoxia leads to structural changes of the fetal pulmonary circulation is controversial. Goldberg et al. (1971) found that intrauterine hypoxia led to increased thickening of pulmonary vascular smooth muscle in neonatal rats. Reid's laboratory, however, reported no change in vascular smooth muscle thickening or extension following chronic intrauterine hypoxia in rats (Geggel, 1986a) and guinea pigs (Murphy, 1986). They suggested that the histologic changes reported by Goldberg et al.

Table 1 Fetal Models of Persistent Pulmonary Hypertension

Study	Species	Experimental Design	Results	
			Physiology	Histology
A. Intrauterine hypoxia				
S. J. Goldberg et al. (1971)	Rat	Chronic hypoxia administered to late gestation pregnant animal	–	Increased smooth muscle in small pulmonary arteries
Geggel (1986a)	Rat	Chronic hypoxia administered to late gestation pregnant animal	–	No change with hypoxia
Murphy (1986)	Guinea pig	Chronic hypoxia administered to late gestation pregnant animal	Pulmonary and systemic artery pressures not different at birth	No change with hypoxia
Gersony et al. (1976)	Sheep	Induced maternal hypotension in late gestation animals; delivered fetus 24 hours later	Greater right-to-left shunting in study animals	–
Drummond (1980)	Sheep	Placental embolization produced chronic hypoxia in 3 fetuses	Higher PA pressure than in single control animal	–
Soifer (1983)	Sheep	Chronic partial umbilical cord compression	Sustained elevation of PVR following acute hypoxia at 1-2 hr of life	–

B. Intrauterine hypertension				
Ruiz et al. (1972)	Sheep	Ligation of ductus arteriosus (DA) in late gestation fetus	Three animals had abnormal vector cardiograms	Increased smooth muscle and adventitial changes of small pulmonary arteries.
Levin et al. (1986b)	Sheep	Six fetal lambs made hypertensive by renal artery; umbilical artery or DA occlusion	Pulmonary arterial pressures increased to between 70 and 100 mmHg	Increased smooth muscle thickening of 5th generation pulmonary artery
Abman & Accurso (1987)	Sheep	Serial hemodynamics measurements with partial DA occlusion acute/chronic	Acute/chronic hypertension caused transsient rise in flow altered P-Q relationship and decreased vasodilation with increased PO_2	Increased smooth muscle and adventitial thickening of small pulmonary arteries
C. Prostaglandin synthesis inhibition				
Harker et al. (1981)	Rat	Indomethacin administered to pregnant animals in late gestation	–	Increased smooth muscle of small pulmonary arteries
Levin et al. (1979)	Sheep	Indomethacin administered to pregnant animals in late gestation	Pulmonary artery pressure increased	Increased smooth muscle of small pulmonary arteries
deMello et al. (1987)	Guinea pig	Indomethacin administered to pregnant animals in late gestation	Pulmonary artery pressure at birth not different from controls	No change

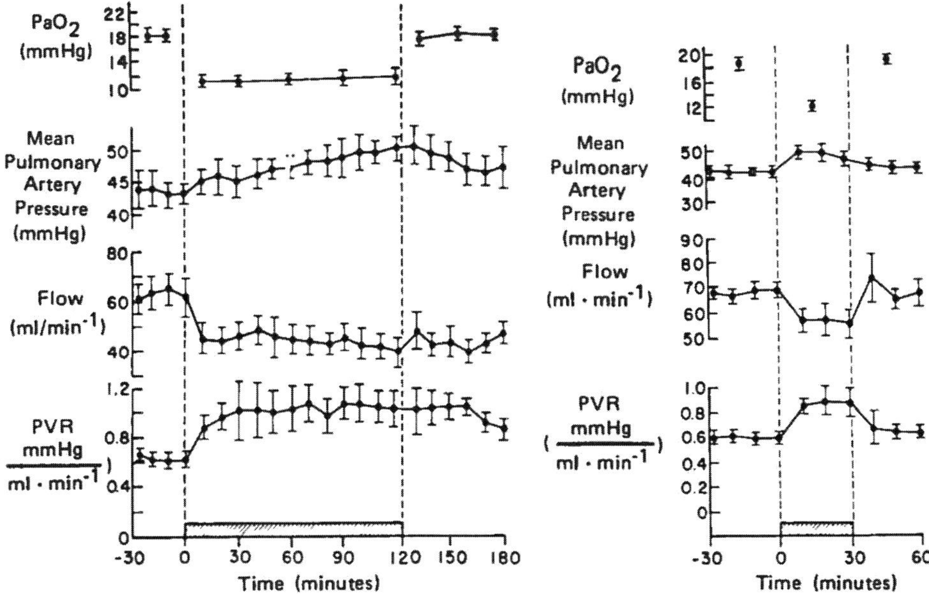

Figure 3 Hemodynamic response to 2 hr (left) or 30 min (right) of hypoxia in chronically prepared fetal lambs. Hypoxia was induced by the administering hypoxic gas (10-12% Fi_{O2}) to the ewe. As shown, despite the correction of fetal hypoxemia during the posthypoxia period, pulmonary vascular resistance (PVR) remains elevated following 2 hr but not 30 min exposure to hypoxia.

reflect differences in lung fixation technique. Since these studies were done in small animals, however, there is no information on fetal hemodynamics or blood gas tensions. In the guinea pig but not in the rat study, the hypoxic animals were growth retarded, suggesting some effect of intrauterine hypoxia at least with the guinea pigs. Murphy et al. (1986) reported neonatal pulmonary and systemic arterial pressures, oxygen consumption, and cardiac output (by the Fick method) following hypoxia. In comparison with control animals, pulmonary and systemic arterial pressures were not different, but oxygen consumption and cardiac output were much lower in the hypoxia group.

In general, although intrauterine growth retardation has been associated with chronic hypoxia, PPHN is not commonly found in growth-retarded human newborns. This suggests the intriguing possibility that chronic hypoxia may not be an important causal factor in the pathogenesis of PPHN, but rather, the association of PPHN with perinatal hypoxia may reflect intrauterine stress from other causes, which then lead to acute hypoxia at the time of delivery.

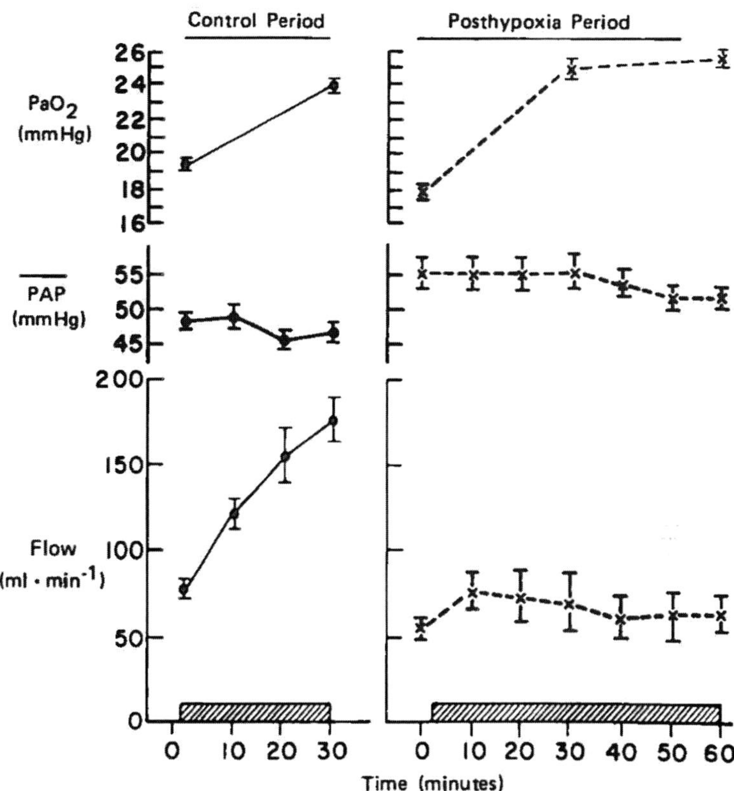

Figure 4 The response of fetal pulmonary blood flow to increased fetal PO_2 is blunted during the posthypoxia period, following 2 hr of hypoxia. The left panel shows the response to increased PO_2 during the control period; the right panel illustrates the response to the same increase in PO_2 during the posthypoxia period.

Studies of sheep have suggested that hypoxia induced by placental embolization (Drummond, 1978), maternal hypotension (Gersony et al., 1976), or partial compression of the umbilical cord (Soifer et al., 1983) may alter neonatal pulmonary vascular resistance. However, structural changes in these models were not reported. Soifer et al. (1983) have reported preliminary results in fetal sheep made chronically hypoxic through partial compression of the umbilical cord. They found an abnormal recovery from hypoxia following cesarean section delivery after 2 weeks of intrauterine hypoxia, suggesting altered postnatal pulmonary vasoreactivity following in utero hypoxia. However, arterial PO_2 and pulmonary arterial pressure were not different from control animals, and there was no right-to-left shunting. In three animals, Drummond and Bissonette (1978) found that chronic embolization of the placenta with production of fetal hypoxia and mild respiratory acidemia led to an increase in pulmonary arterial pressure following delivery as compared to a control animal. The precise nature of the fetal insult is difficult to judge in this study as no fetal hemodynamic data are presented. Gersony et al. (1976) induced maternal hypotension pharmacologically and found that a day following delivery newborn lambs exhibited increased pulmonary arterial pressures and increased right-to-left atrial and ductal shunting. This study suggested that a manipulation as brief as a 90-min period of maternal hypotension may alter pulmonary vascular adaptation after birth. However, since neither fetal blood gas tensions nor hemodynamic measurements were made, the precise nature and severity of the fetal insult is difficult to assess.

Hypoxia in the fetus is a complex stimulus, as the response includes pulmonary and systemic hypertension as well as a decrease in pulmonary blood flow. Evidence has been presented that pulmonary hypertension without hypoxia produces structural abnormalities in the fetal pulmonary circulation. Levin et al. produced pulmonary hypertension in fetal sheep through renal artery constriction (four animals), partial occlusion of the ductus arteriosus (one animal), and occlusion of an umbilical artery (one animal). Pulmonary blood flow and fetal and transitional pulmonary vasoreactivity were not studied, making the functional significance of the in utero pulmonary hypertension unclear.

To determine the effects of acute (2 hr) and chronic (3-10 days) pulmonary hypertension on fetal pulmonary vascular reactivity, the hemodynamic response to partial occlusion of the ductus arteriosus in chronically instrumented fetal lambs has been studied (Abman and Accurso, 1988). Acute partial compression of the ductus increased fetal pulmonary arterial pressure from 47 ± 1 to 61 ± 1 mmHg, with left pulmonary arterial blood flow concomitantly increasing from 75 ± to 150 ± 20 ml/min. Despite maintaining a constant pulmonary arterial pressure, flow steadily declined and was not different from baseline at 2 hr. As characterized by assessments of pressure-flow relationships before and after acute occlusion, and by the vasodilating response to increases in fetal PO_2, pulmonary vasoreactivity was decreased. These physiological changes persisted with chronic occlusion. At autopsy, small pulmonary arteries in the hypertensive animals appeared to have smooth muscle and perivascular adventitial thickening in comparison with control animals (Fig. 5). These findings suggest that acute and chronic hypertension can alter fetal pulmonary vasoreactivity and provide some preliminary data that intrauterine hypertension can induce structural changes in the pulmonary vessels that parallel human PPHN.

As discussed below, several lines of experimental evidence suggest that arachidonic acid metabolites are important in the fetal or transitional pulmonary circulation. The clinical observation that PPHN has been reported in association with maternal ingestion of cyclooxygenase inhibitors adds further interest to these experimental observations (Manchester et al., 1976; Levin et al., 1978a). It is unclear, however, whether these effects were due to closure of the ductus arteriosus or direct action (constriction) of fetal pulmonary arteries. Following chronic administration of indomethacin to late-gestation pregnant rats, Harker et al. (1980) found increased smooth muscle thickness of small pulmonary arteries and a high stillbirth rate. In a similar study with sheep, Levin et al. (1979) reported elevation of fetal pulmonary arterial pressure and thickening of the pulmonary vascular smooth muscle in fifth-generation vessels. Pulmonary blood flow was not measured in these studies. In contrast to these findings, a recent study reported no changes in muscularization of the pulmonary circulation following chronic indomethacin administration to pregnant guinea pigs (deMello et al., 1987). Since there were no hemodynamic measurements it is hard to quantitate the effects of indomethacin or the severity of pulmonary hypertension caused by its administration or to demonstrate that there was a sustained effect on the ductus or pulmonary artery to aorta gradient.

In summary, a complex array of factors can potentially modulate pulmonary vascular tone during fetal life. The intrauterine history of the pulmonary circulation appears to be important in determining the success or failure of the transition of the pulmonary circulation at birth. Greater insight into the biochemical and physiological mechanisms altering the perinatal pulmonary circulation may lead to greater success in understanding the pathogenesis, pathophysiology, and treatment of PPHN.

III. Neonatal Pulmonary Hypertension: Role and Mechanisms of Structural Changes in the Pulmonary Circulation

The newborn human and certain species of newborn animals, when given the proper stimulus, rapidly develop virulent pulmonary hypertension accompanied by remarkable vascular morphologic changes that may be unique to the newborn period of life. A number of excellent studies have provided descriptions of the normal vasculature of the newborn lung, the location of the smooth muscle, the pattern of growth of vessel and parenchyma after birth, and the extension of muscle into the new and lengthening vessels (Naeye, 1961; Haworth and Hislop, 1981; Meyrick and Reid, 1982; Reeves and Leathers, 1967; Hislop and Reid, 1978; Rendeas et al., 1978). In comparison to normals, infants dying of pulmonary hypertension show an increase in peripheral lung arterial muscularization, with greater extension of mature muscle cells into the more peripheral (intraacinar) arteries than normal (Murphy et al., 1981; Haworth and Reid, 1976). The larger arteries, greater than 150 μm in diameter, usually but not

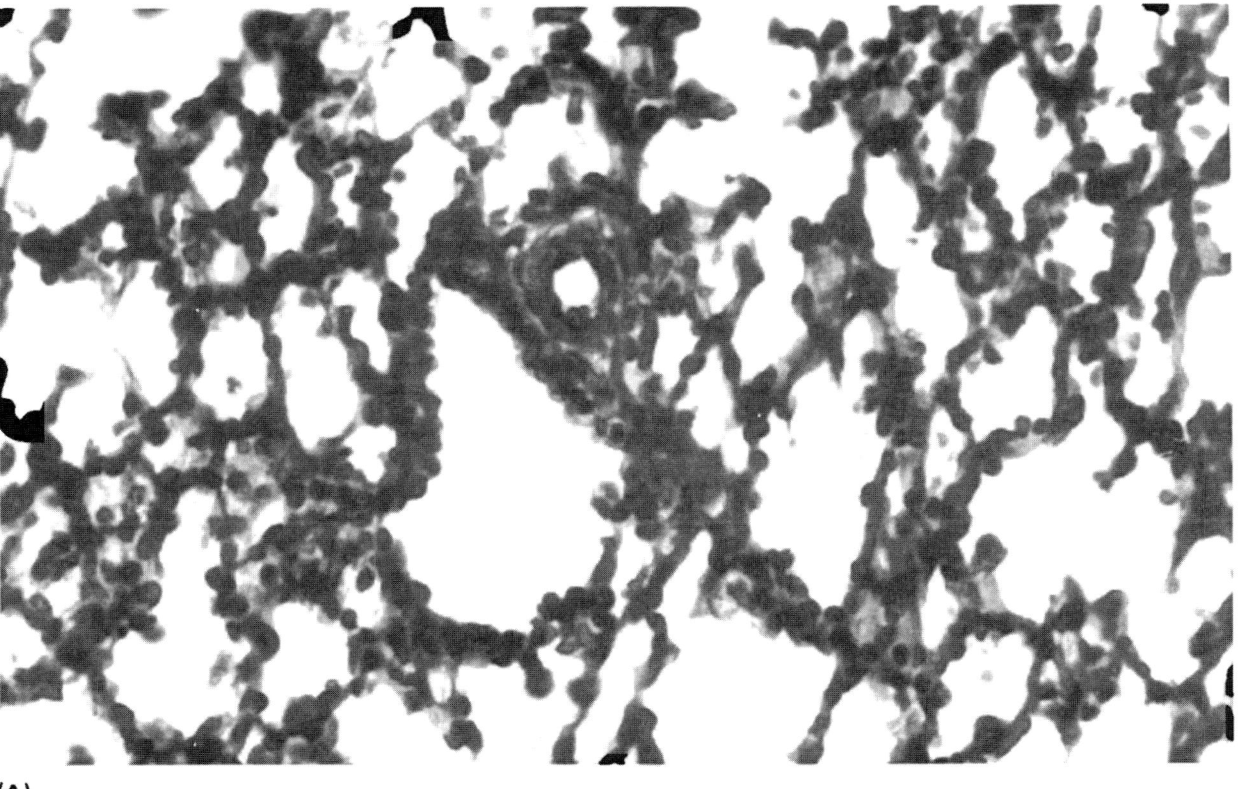

(A)

Figure 5 Histologic changes following chronic partial occlusion of the ductus arteriosus in a late gestation fetal animal. Partial occlusion was maintained for 7 days, with a mean pulmonary arterial pressure of 70 mmHg (normal 50 mmHg). Comparison made with a control animal of similar gestational age. (A) Control; (B) Chronic occlusion. occlusion.

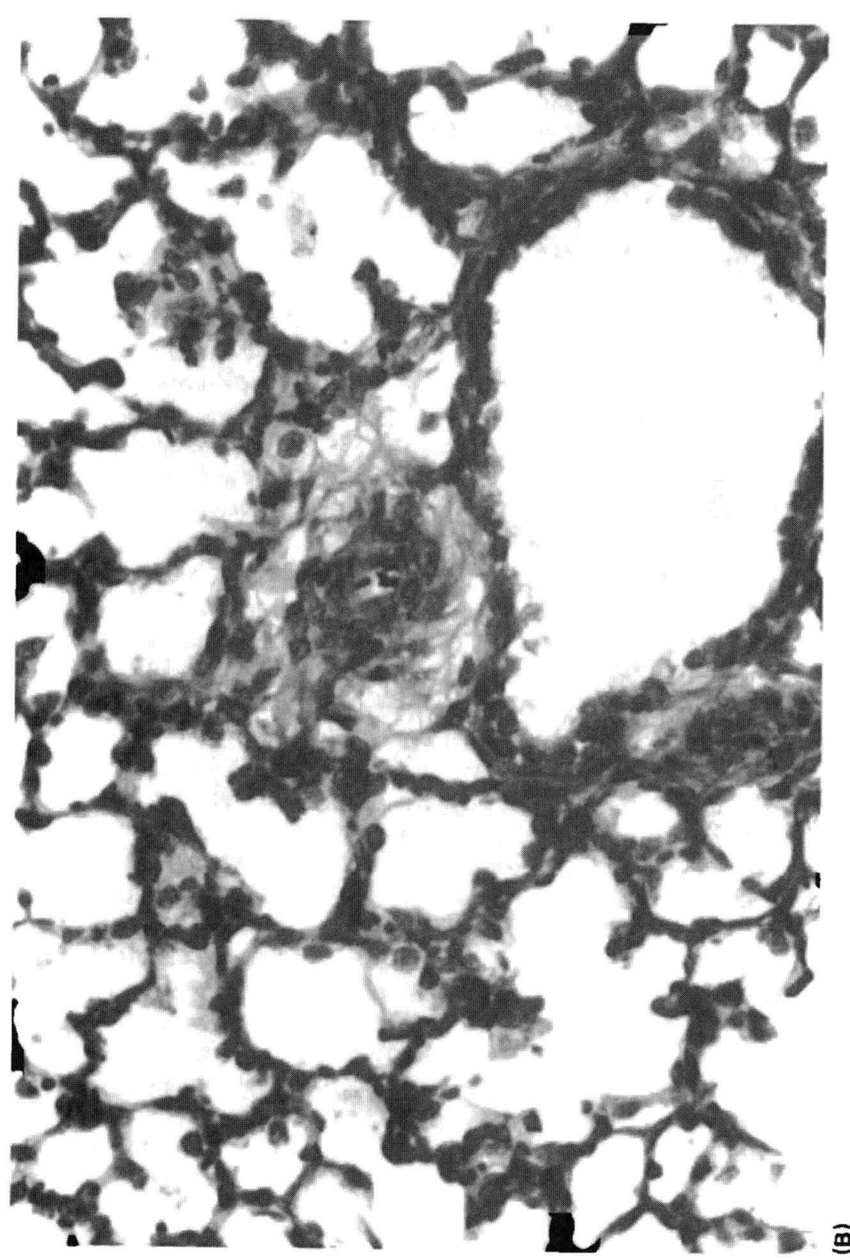
(B)

always have increased muscle. There is encroachment on the lumen by smooth muscle cells and by swollen, enlarged, endothelial cells. Marked abnormalities in the adventitia have also been commented upon (Murphy et al., 1981). Our review (in progress) of autopsies of infants dying with severe neonatal pulmonary hypertension has shown right ventricular hypertrophy, patency of the foramen ovale and ductus arteriosus, and histologically luminal narrowing, medial hypertrophy, and marked adventitial thickening (Fig. 6).

Increased muscularity and luminal narrowing will potentiate the pulmonary vascular obstruction and hypertension, contributing to a vicious cycle. As stated above, one view is that there is excessive growth of muscle in utero, which after birth initiates the vicious circle of maintained pulmonary arterial pressure, leading to further vascular changes. On the other hand, the structural abnormalities observed may be due initially to failure of the vessels to adapt normally to extrauterine life and subsequently to postnatal development of muscle and adventitia in response to the presence of pulmonary hypertension. It has recently been shown that newborn calves exposed to hypoxia radidly develop suprasystemic pulmonay hypertension (Stenmark et al., 1987a). The calves demonstrated severe hypoxemia, right-to-left shunting of blood through the foramen ovale and ductus arteriosus, and a lack of reversibility to oxygen breathing – characteristics very similar to those of the human newborn with pulmonary hypertension. Morphometric analysis of the lung vessels showed that the arterioles had decreased luminal diameters, increased medial thickness, and distal muscularization. Most striking, however, were the changes in the adventitia. The adventitia was markedly thickened and demonstrated evidence of cellular proliferation and extreme extracellular matrix deposition (Fig. 7).

Allen and Haworth (1986) have used newborn pigs exposed to hypoxia to show by light and electron microscopy a retention of fetal characteristics of the pulmonary endothelial and smooth muscle cells. The smooth muscle had an increase in myofilament volume density. Connective tissue was increased mainly by collagen, elastin, and ground substance. They found that only 3 days of hypoxia prevented the normal postnatal regression of the arterial changes. The stimulation of myofilaments and connective tissue persisted, suggesting the potential for excessive contraction in abnormally stiff arteries.

Extrauterine hypoxia-induced changes may indeed occur very rapidly. Sobin et al.(1983) demonstrated increased fibroblasts in the arterial wall 8 hr after initiating hypoxia, and by 24 hr the number had tripled. Various lung cell types are increased with hypoxia (Niedenzu et al., 1981; Voelkel et al., 1977), with particularly early metabolic activity in the adventitia (Meyrick and Reid, 1979b). Thus the possibility that rapid changes can take place in the lung arteries in postnatal life should be considered. The following sections examine mechanisms controlling both cellular and extracellular matrix proliferation in pulmonary hypertension.

A. Cellular Proliferation

As stated above, in both infants with persistent pulmonary hypertension and animal models of pulmonary hypertension, there is both extension of smooth muscle into smaller, more peripheral arteries and thickening of the media and adventitia of previously muscularized arteries. This requires proliferation of smooth muscle cells and fibroblasts and/or their precursors. However, little is known of the mechanisms that regulate proliferation of pulmonary vascular cells.

The endothelium is thought by many to play a key role in the regulation of smooth muscle cell growth. For example, bovine aortic endothelial cells were the first proliferative diploid cell found to secrete mitogenic activity for smooth muscle cells and fibroblasts (Gajdusek and Schwartz 1984). Endothelial cells from many species and sites have since been shown to constituitively secrete growth factors for connective tissue cells. The levels of mitogen secreted are sufficiently high that smooth muscle cells cocultured with endothelial cells in the absence of exogenous mitogens proliferate as if in the presence of high serum concentrations. At least two major growth-promoting factors have been identified in conditioned media from uninjured endothelial cells in culture. These are platelet-derived growth factor (PGDF) (DiCorleto, 1984) and fibroblast growth factor (FGF) (DiCorleto et al., 1983; Gajdusek et al., 1980). At least one other, as yet unidentified, growth factor (Gajdusek et al., 1980) also has been reported to be produced by endothelial cells. Perhaps equally as important as the mitogenic activity expressed by endothelial cells is the recent description of an endothelial cell-produced heparin-like inhibitor of smooth muscle cell proliferation (Gajdusek et al., 1980; Castellot et al., 1981). This factor, under normal conditions, could prevent or limit abnormal proliferation of smooth muscle cells. With endothelial injury, it is possible that a decreased production of this inhibitor could lead to smooth muscle cell proliferation. These findings are of particular relevance to the possible factors controlling lung vascular proliferation because they suggest that vascular proliferation could be regulated by factors that are produced and act locally within the lung.

Of great interest is the fact that cultured endothelial cells can be stimulated by several exogenous factors to produce growth factors. Bacterial endotoxin and phorbol esters have been shown to stimulate production of PDGF (Fox and DiCorleto, 1984). Hypoxia, which has been shown to negatively influence smooth muscle cell growth directly (Benitz et al., 1986a), appears to be capable of stimulating smooth muscle proliferation either by stimulating the production of a mitogenic factor from endothelial cells (Vender et al., 1984) or by decreasing the production of the heparin-like inhibitor (Humphries et al., 1986), or both. In any case, these studies indicate that pulmonary vascular injury may result in the aberrant production of paracrine growth factors by the endothelium.

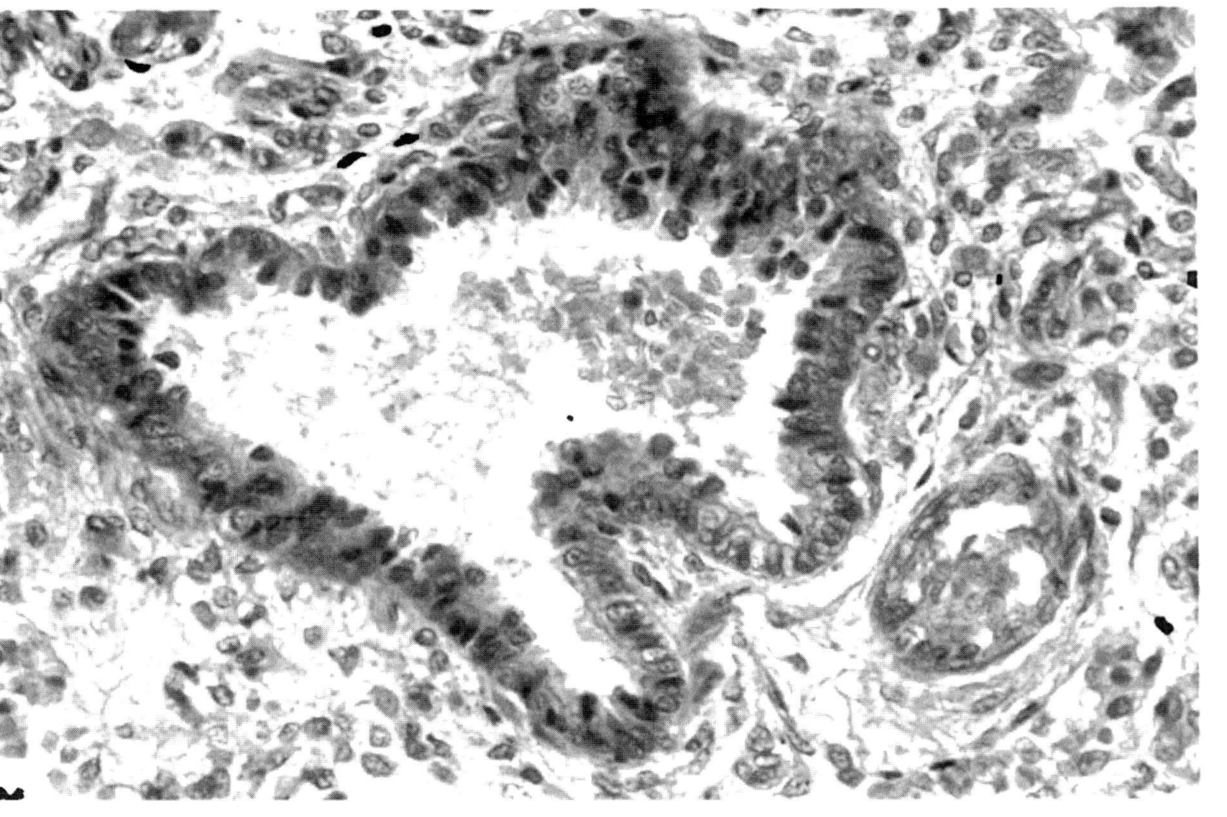

Figure 6 (A) Photomicrograph of a small pulmonary artery and accompanying airway in a 5-day-old infant dying with respiratory distress syndrome and no evidence or suspicion of pulmonary hypertension. The vessel shown demonstrates a single medial layer of smooth muscle cells with little adventitia being observed.

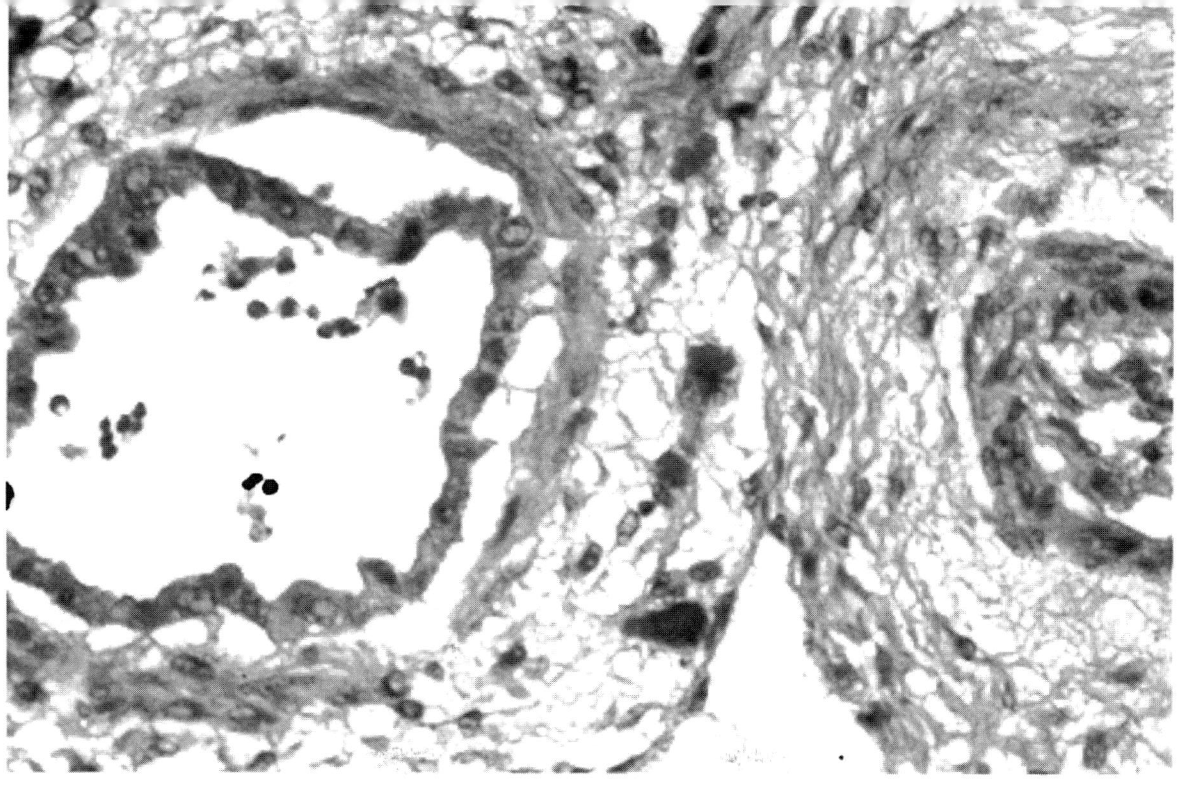

(B) Photomicrograph of a small pulmonary artery and accompanying airway in a 6-day-old infant dying with severe pulmonary hypertension. The vessel shown demonstrates luminal narrowing with swollen endothelial cells, medial thickening, and marked adventitial thickening. The adventitia demonstrates an increase in cellularity as well as a significant increase in what appeared to be collagen.

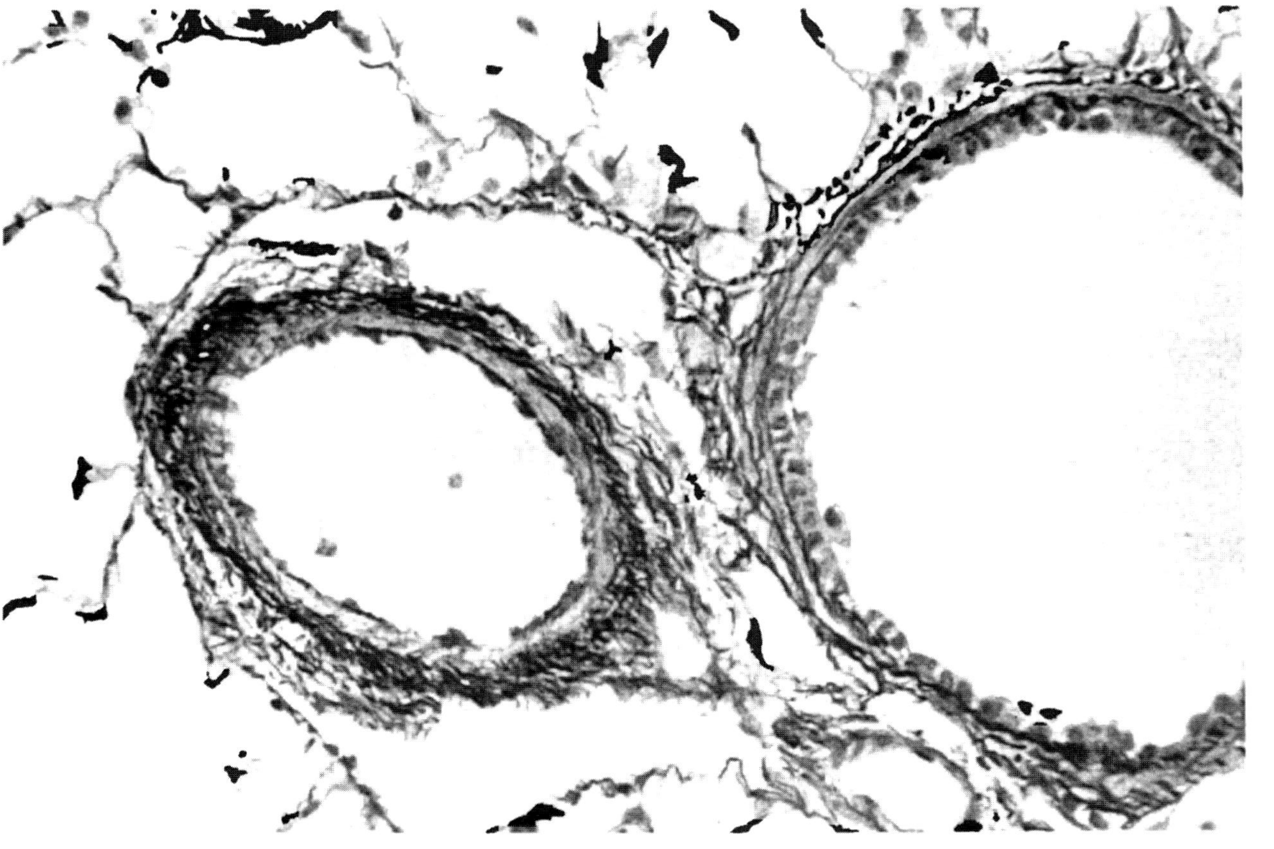

Figure 7 (A) Photomicrograph of a muscular pulmonary artery and the accompanying airway in a 17-day-old calf born and living at 1500 m. The mean pulmonary artery pressure measured was 27 mmHg. (Luna stain, 500 X.)

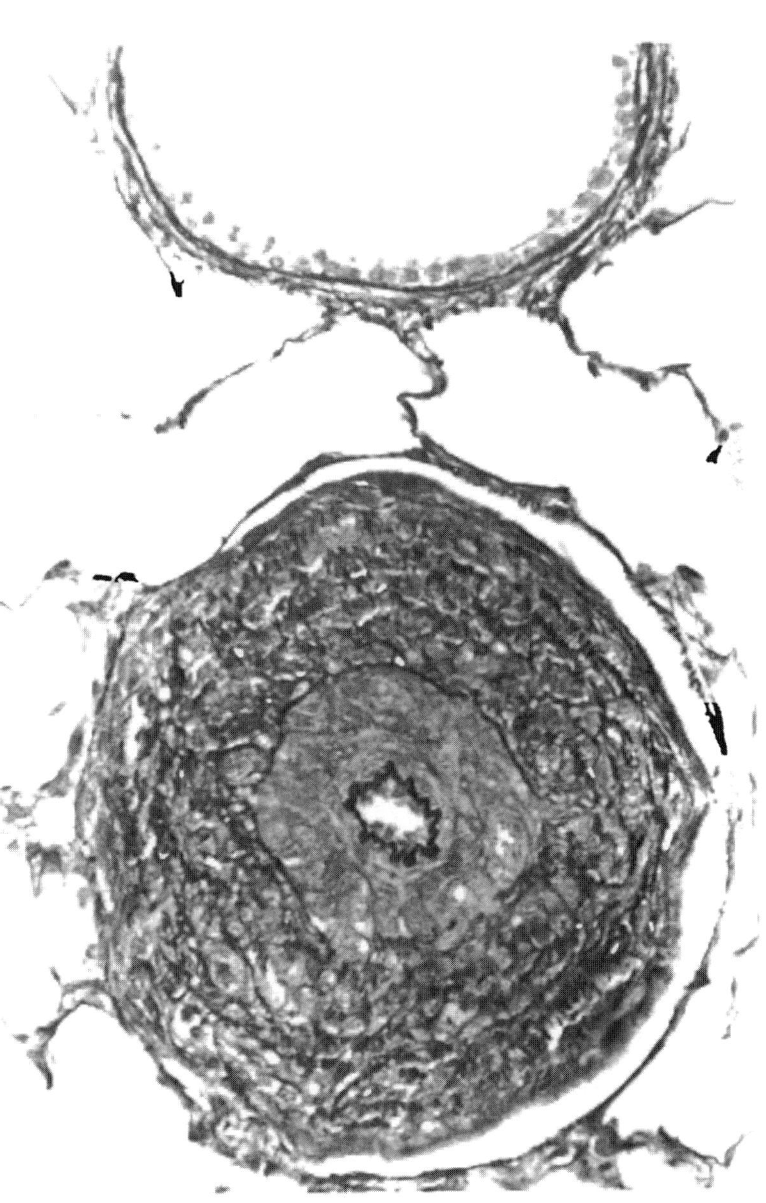

(B) Photomicrograph of a muscular pulmonary artery and accompanying airway in a 17-day-old calf after 15 days at 4300 m. Mean pulmonary arterial pressure was 98 mmHg. Pulmonary arterial pressure remained suprasystemic with 100% oxygen breathing. Luminal narrowing, medial hypertrophy, and marked adventitial thickening are present. Note also disruption of the external elastic lamina. Collagen and elastin content of the adventitia are increased (Luna stain, 500X).

Alternatively, and/or perhaps additively (Fig. 8), there is a possibility that endothelial injury could lead to the permeation of plasma proteins into the vessel wall. Vascular leak presents many possible mechanisms for altering cellular phenotypes. The extravasation of blood components into the tissue compartment, for example, could expose medial and adventitial cells to specific modifiers, such as peptide mitogens and differentiation factors, that might contribute to the genesis of vascular remodeling (Ross, 1986). That plasma factors may gain access to the vascular wall and be associated with vascular proliferation is suggested by literature relating to atherosclerosis, where protein accumulation has been reported in the aortas of many species (Jorgensen et al., 1972; Packham et al., 1967; Goldberg et al., 1980). Maximal accumulation corresponds to sites where early proliferation is noted. Ross (1986) has summarized data indicating that smooth muscle multiplication can occur even though the endothelium remains intact. Thus in the systemic circulation, the entry of plasma factors into the vessel wall with or without endothelial integrity may allow growth factors, including platelet-derived growth factor, to stimulate proliferation. Increased permeation of plasma into the pulmonary artery vessel wall in pulmonary hypertension has also been noted and suggested to have a potential role in structural remodeling (Jaenke and Alexander, 1973) (Fig. 9). Hypoxia, which has been reported to increase lung water and protein leak, either by damaging the endothelial barrier and/or increasing microvascular pressure, could be a critical factor in his process by providing the driving force to push blood or endothelial cell-derived factors into the vascular tissue.

Thus, many factors and injuries appear capable of stimulating vascular smooth muscle proliferation. Can this process be interrupted? Interestingly, heparin has been demonstrated to inhibit proliferation of smooth muscle cells from systemic arteries of mature animals both in vivo and in vitro (Hoover et al., 1980; Guyton et al., 1980). More recently, Benitz (1986) has shown that heparin specifically and reversibly inhibited proliferation of fetal pulmonary vascular smooth muscle cells in vitro. Hales and co-workers have reported that heparin attenuated the hypoxia-induced vascular proliferation in mice and guinea pigs (Hales et al., 1983; Hassovin et al., 1986), although others have not found quite so dramatic effects (Geggel, 1986c). In chronically hypoxic newborn calves, Fasules (1987a) has shown that heparin attenuates the degree of pulmonary vascular medial and advential thickening. However, the protective or ameliorative effects of heparin on pulmonary vascular remodeling in pulmonary hypertension are not universal, as heparin failed to attenuate the vascular changes induced by monocrotaline (Fasules, 1987b).

In summary, it appears that interactions between endothelial cells, smooth muscle cells and fibroblasts mediated by both autocrine, paracrine, and perhaps plasma factors are important in regulating the phenotypic state of the pulmonary the vascular bed. Under certain injury conditions, rapid changes in the phenotype of various pulmonary vascular cells can take place (Fig. 8).

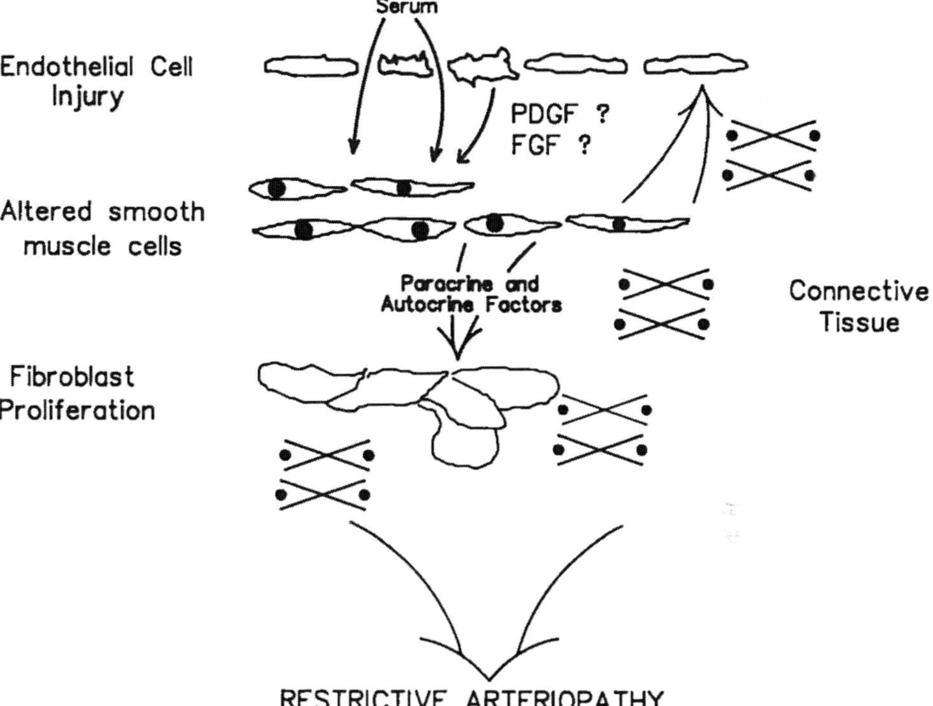

Figure 8 Schematic representation of the hypothetical possibilities involved in the pathogenesis of the vascular changes observed in pulmonary hypertension. Endothelial injury (following hypoxia, high pressure, or other stimuli) may lead to release of growth or differentiation factors from the endothelium, which cause a phenotypic alteration in connecting tissue cells. Alternatively, or perhaps additionally, leak of plasma factors into the medial area of the vessel could be associated with a phenotypic change in the smooth muscle cell. These altered smooth muscle cells increase production of various connective tissue proteins and also begin to secrete autocrine or paracrine factors that can influence further the phenotype of the SMC and cause significant changes in the fibroblasts and endothelial cells in the vessel wall. One such paracrine factor, SMEF, has been shown to increase elastin production by both fibroblasts and endothelial cells. Thus, the SMC could play a critical role in the vascular remodeling seen in pulmonary hypertension.

B. Extracellular Matrix Proliferation

The structural changes observed in neonatal humans, calves, piglets, and rats with pulmonary hypertension support the hypothesis that components of the

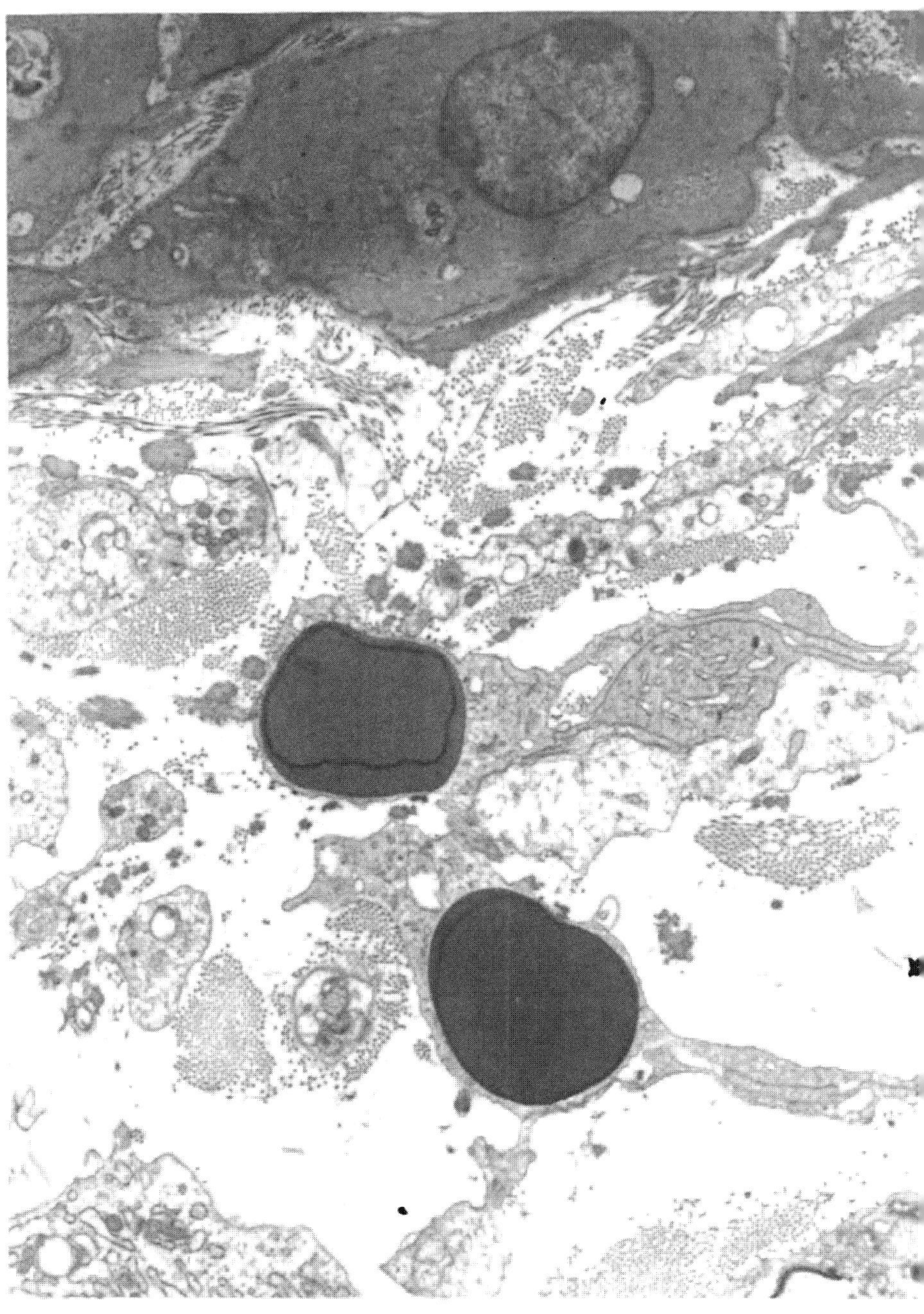

extracellular matrix, i.e., collagen and elastin, play an important role in the hypertensive process.

Increases in pulmonary arterial collagen have been noted both in chronic hypoxic pulmonary hypertension (Kerr et al., 1984), and in monocrataline-induced pulmonary hypertension (Kameji et al., 1980). Vascular collagen is also increased in experimental systemic hypertension (Franklin et al., 1982; Iwatsuki et al., 1972). A potentially important role for connective tissue in hypoxic pulmonary hypertension is suggested by the work of Kerr et al. (1984), where the antifibrotic agent B-aminoproprionitrile (BAPN), an inhibitor of collagen and elastin cross-linkage, reduced the right ventricular systolic pressure, pulmonary arterial wall thickness, and hydroxyproline content in hypoxic rats. Poiani et al. (1986) also showed that adult rats progressively increased their pulmonary vascular collagen during 3 days exposure to hypoxia. The changes were reversible. They felt that the accumulation of collagen may be due to both an increase in synthesis and a decrease in degradation. Their conclusion was that the induction and regression of hypoxic pulmonary hypertension was accompanied by changes in collagen metabolism.

To investigate cellular stimuli that might elicit changes in pulmonary arterial connective tissue production, the synthesis of collagen and elastin in blood vessels of animals with pulmonary hypertension has been studied. Elastin, the extracellular matrix protein responsible for elastic recoil of arteries, is synthesized during development by smooth muscle cells. Normally, this highly cross-linked protein is localized principally in the medial layer of the vessel, but in pulmonary hypertension striking increases in elastin can be observed in the adventitia (Fig. 10). Because elastin production in normal vascular tissue is associated with medial smooth muscle cells, the onset of elastin synthesis in other cell types provides a convenient marker for identifying phenotypic alterations in the diseased vessel. Mecham et al. (1987) and Stemmark et al. (1987b) found elastin synthesis in newborn calves with severe pulmonary artery hypertension to be approximately fourfold higher in the pulmonary artery from pulmonary hypertensive animals than in controls (Fig. 11). Northern blot analysis of RNA extracted from the tissues and hybridized with a cDNA probe for elastin demonstrated a similar increase in elastin specific mRNA in pulmonary hypertensive calves, suggesting that vascular elastin synthesis is regulated by pretranslational events. No changes in either elastin synthesis or elastin levels

---

Figure 9 Electronmicrograph of the adventitia of a small pulmonary artery from a newborn calf with severe pulmonary hypertension. Note the presence of fibroblasts (F) with dense endoplasmic reticulum, collagen (C), and erythrocytes (E). Extravasation of other erythocytes appears to have taken place in vivo because of the thin cellular layer surrounding the cells. (Original magnification, X 8100.)

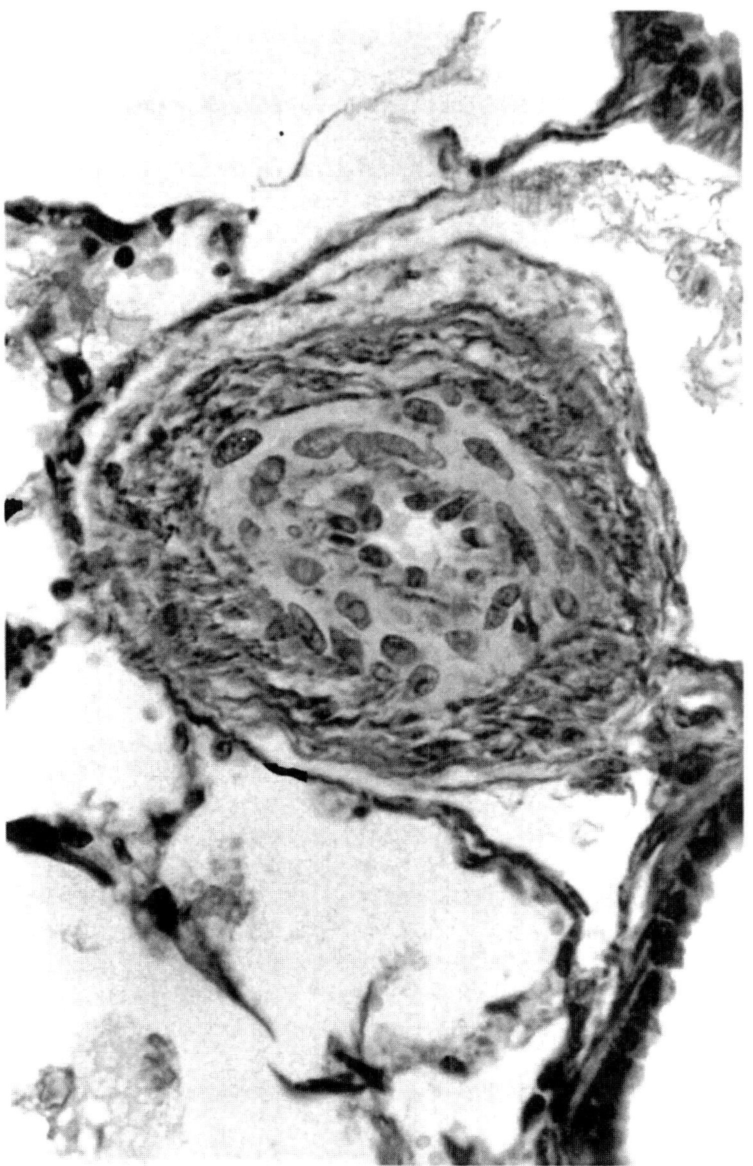

Figure 10 Photomicrograph of a small pulmonary artery from a neonatal pulmonary hypertensive calf, demonstrating a thickened hypercellular adventitia that stains positive for elastin. Immunohistochemistry was done with monoclonal antibodies to bovine alpha-elastin. (Original magnification, X 125.)

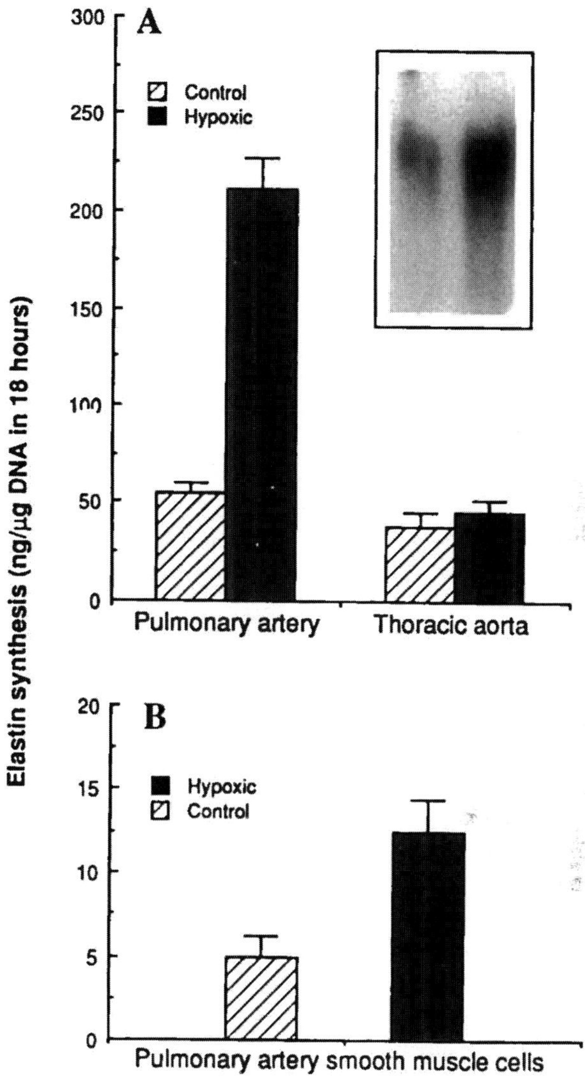

Figure 11 (A) Elastin production and elastin mRNA levels in the lobar pulmonary artery and thoracic aorta of a control and hypoxic, pulmonary hypertensive neonatal calf. Values are expressed as nanograms of alpha-elastin equivalents per microgram of DNA. Insert: Northern blot analysis of elastin mRNA levels in pulmonary artery tissue. Left lane, control; right lane, hypertensive animal. (B) Elastin production by pulmonary artery medial SMCs from control and hypoxic, hypertensive animals.

by pretranslational events. No changes in either elastin synthesis or elastin levels were observed in thoracic aorta from the same animals, implying that hypoxia per se does not affect elastin metabolism. These findings are very similar to those observed in the pulmonary hypertensive rat (Yohn et al., 1987). Cultured smooth muscle cells from pulmonary hypertensive calves produced twice as much elastin per microgram DNA as control smooth muscle cells (Fig. 11). Cultured fibroblasts from pulmonary hypertensive calves produced four to five times as much elastin as control calves. The variations in elastin production appear to reflect stable phenotypes, since relative differences persisted vitro through numerous population doubling.

Little is known about the stimuli leading to acquisition of the elastin phenotype by pulmonary artery cells. Previous findings that the smooth muscle cell could influence elastin synthesis in cultured endothelial cells (Mecham et al., 1983) suggested the possibility that the elastin phenotype is influenced in the diseased vessel by specific factors released locally by activated smooth muscle cells. An elastogenic factor was apparently produced by the smooth muscle cells of the pulmonary hypertensive artery. This factor, termed smooth muscle-derived elastogenic factor (SMEF), was found to act at a transcriptional level both as an enhancer of elastin synthesis and as a differentiation factor, inducing expression of the elastin phenotype in responsive cells (Mecham et al., 1987). Further SMEF was shown to alter cell surface receptors as well, an important finding because cell surface modulation could have important physiological consequences by altering receptor-mediated responses such as cell movement or the ability of the cell to respond metabolically to external stimuli. Riley's group has presented evidence to suggest that the endothelium is important in the acute rise in elastin and collagen synthesis that occurs with increased wall tension (Riley, D.J., personal communication).

The structural changes observed in both human infants and neonatal animals with severe pulmonary hypertension affect all layers of the vascular wall. The question should be asked, how do these morphologic changes affect the function of the vessel? The large and small vessels, together with the right heart, of course, consititute a system that must somehow function even in the presence of pulmonary hypertension if the individual is to survive. Changes in the small vessels will clearly change resistance, while changes in the large conducting arteries will affect compliance in the system. In the neonate the pulmonary trunk normally contains layers of elastin, and this is retained in pulmonary hypertension existing from early life (Heath et al., 1959). Szarek and Evans (1987) have recently demonstrated that the mechanical properties of large and small vessels are altered differentially in chronic hypoxia. Active tension is reduced in both large and small vessels despite the existence of hypertension. In large vessels, wall stiffness is unchanged, but in small vessels wall stiffness is increased, perhaps an important component of the maintenance of the hypertension. Further, vaso-

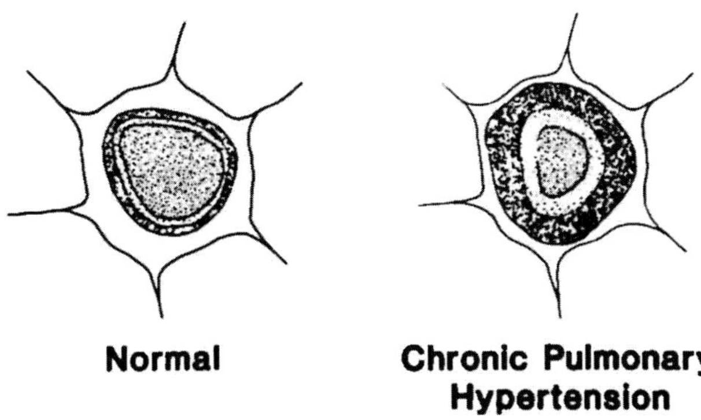

Figure 12 Schematic representation demonstrating the concept that not only do the medial and adventitial thickening observed in neonatal pulmonary hypertension cause luminal narrowing, which increases pulmonary vascular resistance, but also this "restrictive sheath" could significantly limit the ability of the vessel to vasodilate.

dilation is impaired in both hypoxid (Stenmark et al. 1987a) and hyperoxic (Coflesky and Evans, 1987) models of neonatal pulmonary hypertension. Though clearly many factors could be involved, structural changes in the media and adventita could form a restrictive sleeve around the vessel leading to impairment of vasodilation (Fig. 12).

In summary, neonatal models of pulmonary hypertension may provide insight into some of the mechanisms by which severe pulmonary hypertension comes about rapidly and is not easily or quickly reversed. Furthermore, the findings that (1) pulmonary artery endothelial cells produce a smooth muscle mitogen and/or fail to produce an inhibitor in response to hypoxia and (2) pulmonary artery smooth muscle cells in severe hypoxic pulmonary hypertension generate one or more factors that affect both the secretory and responsive properties of surrounding cells will provide a direction for further research into molecular and cellular mechanisms controlling growth, differentiation, and vascular responsiveness in diseased vessels.

IV. Vascular Reactivity Changes in Persistent Pulmonary Hypertension

In the newborn, the pulmonary arteries are relatively thick walled, which may account for an augmented reactivity such as an increased pressor response to hypoxia (James and Rowe 1957; Rudolph and Yuan, 1966). An augmented proliferative potential normally present but induced or stimulated by injury could set the stage for rapid distal muscularization, increased medial and adventitial thickening, and endothelial proliferation. Perhaps the combined abilities of lung vessels in newborns to vasoconstrict and proliferate cause the frequent severe pulmonary hypertensive syndromes seen in the neonate.

A feature of severe neonatal pulmonary hypertension syndromes is a frequently refractory state to vasodilators. Numerous possibilities exist to explain this state. Damage to endothelial cells could decrease their production of vasodilator substances (Ryan and Ryan, 1977; Said, 1982). Arteries that have thick walls may constrict but not relax, and their very mass may partially occlude the lumen of the vessel. Elastin and collagen that is rapidly laid down may also reduce the capacity to relax. The metabolic activity of the newborn vessels may be different from that expected in older individuals. For example, prostaglandin D_2 is a dilator in the fetal goat but a constrictor later in adult life (Cassin et al., 1981). These factors all contribute to the severity of the pulmonary hypertensive problem in the newborn, and potential mechanisms are explored in the following paragraphs.

A. Endothelial Injury and Neonatal Pulmonary Hypertension

Although hypoxia has been speculated to be important or etiologically involved in many cases of persistent pulmonary hypertension, the underlying cause or signal for vasoconstriction or the persistent elevation of pulmonary vascular resistance in most cases remains unknown. The reports of endothelial cell injury in various types of human and experimental pulmonary hypertension (Rabinovitch et al., 1986; Meyrick and Reid, 1983) and the potential role of endothelium-derived mediators in controlling vascular smooth muscle tone raise the possibility that abnormal endothelial cell function could promote vasoconstriction either by interfering with production or action of a dilator or by inducing the production of a constrictor.

Present evidence demonstrates that the vascular endothelium is not simply a passive, nonthrombotic interface between blood and vessel wall but instead plays a dynamic role in controlling processes such as hemostasis, inflammation, and vascular permeability. There is also increasing evidence that the endothelium plays an important, active role in vasoregulation. Endothelial cells inactivate, activate, and produce several substances that can alter vascular tone (Ryan and Ryan, 1977; Griffith et al., 1984). For example, the inactivation of 5-hydroxytryptamine, norepinephrine, bradykinin, enkephalins, acetylcholine, ATP, ADP, and certain prostaglandins takes place at the endothelial cell level. Furthermore, endothelial cells are also involved in the activation of angiotensin I to angiotensin II and in the production of prostacyclin (PGI_2), a probable potent determinant of pulmonary vascular reactivity under a variety of conditions (Grover et al., 1983; Hyman et al., 1982). Abnormal metabolism of vasoactive substances has been reported in many forms of pulmonary hypertension (Meyrick and Reid, 1983). The neonate may be particularly prone to endotehlial metabolic dysfunction (Davidson and Stalcup, 1984).

Another aspect of endothelial cell function that has received considerable recent attention is the generation of nonprostaglandin substances that either mediate or modulate the in vitro responses of vascular smooth muscle to various stimuli. Initial work by Furchgott (1983), which has been confirmed and extended by many others (Peach et al., 1985; Vanhoutee and Miller, 1985), suggests that the endothelium plays an obligatory role in the relaxation of isolated systemic and pulmonary arteries caused by endogenous substances such as acetylcholine, bradykinin, histamine (H_1), 5-hydroxytryptamine, substance P, VIP, thrombin, ATP, ADP, and platelet activating factor through the generation of endothelial cell-derived relaxing factor. In contrast, relaxations, elicited by endogenous vasodilators such as PGI_2, adenosine, and atrial natriuretic factor and by exogenous agents like calcium channel blockers (nifedipine), nitroprusside, and isoproterenol, are not obligatorily dependent on endothelial cells but instead are due to direct actions on the smooth muscle. There is further evidence to suggest that constrictor agents such as norepinephrine and angiotensin II also stimulate endothelial cells to release a relaxing factor (other than or in addition to PGI_2) that modulates the direct vasoconstriction (Furhgott, 1984). Thus, the response to a given vasoconstrictor may depend on a balance between its effects on endothelial and smooth muscle cells.

The chemical nature of EDRF has not been established. However, current evidence (Furchgott, 1984; Diamond and Chu, 1983) suggests that its direct action on systemic and pulmonary vascular smooth muscle mimics that of the nitrites and leads to the activation of guanylate cyclase, increased levels of cyclic GMP, and protein phosphorylation and dephosphorylation of the myosin light chain.

In addition to endothelial production of the potent vasodilators PGI_2 and EDRF, there is evidence for endothelial generation of vasoconstrictor signals. Anoxia has been shown to augment the contractile responses of isolated arteries and veins to norepinephrine (DeMey and Vanhoutte, 1982). This augmentation was reduced or arrested after removal of the endothelium. Further experiments by Vanhoutte and Miller (1985) suggest that both anoxia and hypoxia induce the release of a vasoconstrictor substance (rather than inhibit the production of a relaxing factor). Endothelium-dependent hypoxic contraction of unstimulated porcine pulmonary arteries has also been reported. In addition, O'Brien (1984) and Agricola and co-workers (1985) have detected the production of a vasoconstrictor peptide by both systemic and pulmonary artery endothelial cells in culture. It is not known if endothelial cells in vivo produce this vasoconstrictor under either physiological or pathological conditions.

In summary, evidence suggests that pulmonary vascular reactivity to a variety of stimuli may be determined in part by signals arising from the endothelium. Injury to the endothelium may thus induce changes in receptor-dependent activation of endothelial cells, in the endothelial capacity to release mediators, and in the responsiveness of smooth muscle to mediators. Any one or all of these changes could have significant effects on vasoregulation in the pulmonary circulation.

B. Structural Changes and Alterations of Vascular Reactivity

The altered wall structure observed in pulmonary hypertension itself may alter reactivity (Park et al., 1977). For example, pulmonary artery but not aortic helical strips from altitude-exposed pulmonary hypertensive animals had increased contractility to prostaglandin $F_{2\alpha}$ and decreased response to angiotensin II. Emery et al. (1981) concluded that both mechanical and reactive properties of the lung vascular bed were altered by chronic exposure to hypoxia. The contractions of the pulmonary vasculature in the isolated lung were increased by hypoxia, angiotensin II, and ATP. Vasodilatation in response to isoproterenol and adenosine was greater in chronically hypoxic rats than in controls. Bee and Wach (1983) found that lungs isolated from immature rats exposed chronically to hypoxia were more reactive than lungs from similarly exposed mature rats. However, McMurtry et al. (1978) have shown that lungs from chronically hypoxic rats show depressed acute hypoxic responses. Davies et al. (1985) suggested that newly muscularized arteries have decreased responses to norepinephrine. In rats given monocrotaline, the response to contractile agonists was increased early in the injury but was decreased later after pulmonary hypertension had developed. Dilation to ACh and isoproterenol was also reduced later (Altiere et al., 1986). Systemic arteries from the spontaneously hypertensive rat also show diminished relaxation (Cohen and Berkowitz 1976). Thus evidence from many investigations in adult animals indicates that structural changes in the walls of pulmonary arteries alter the reactivity of those arteries.

Experiments in neonatal pulmonary hypertensive animals have also demonstrated altered reactivity. Tucker and co-workers have demonstrated heightened reactivity to pressor agents including hypoxia, PGI_2, and angiotensin (Tucker et al., 1987). Impaired vasodilation to vasodilators including oxygen, nitroprusside, and prostacyclin has been demonstrated in severe chronic neonatal pulmonary hypertension in calves (Orton et al., 1987). In contrast, normal newborn calves made acutely hypoxic respond well to tolazoline (Tucker et al., 1984). These results suggest that the structurally altered bed behaves much differently from the normal bed. Yet most pharmacological information has come from normal animals following an acute intervention. These observations could explain the

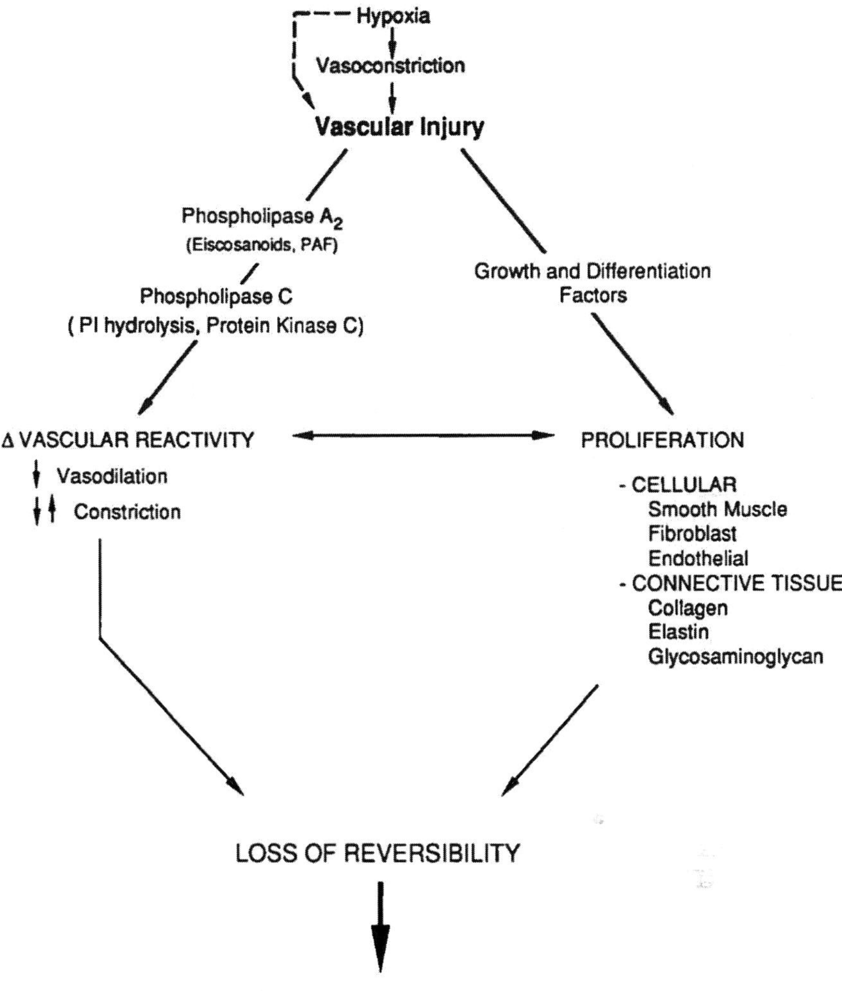

Figure 13 Diagram illustrating the hypothetical interrelationship between changes in vascular reactivity and vascular proliferation following vasular injury. Both pathways appear to be related and important in the physiological and pharmacological abnormalities noted in severe pulmonary hypertension.

failure of vasodilators in the human condition, where the pulmonary vascular remodeling has taken place.

To summarize, it appears that structural, biochemical, and metabolic changes can all occur in pulmonary hypertensive vessels. Consideration must be given to the fact that the pulmonary hypertensive process is accompanied by altered reactivity to constrictors and dilators and that responses in the acutely stressed pulmonary vascular bed are not necessarily akin to those observed when remodeling of the bed has taken place. A schematic representation of how reactivity and proliferative changes are related to pulmonary hypertension is shown in Figure 13.

V. Role of Mediators in the Pulmonary Hypertensive Process of the Newborn

As discussed above, many factors can affect pulmonary vascular resistance in the fetus and newborn and thereby modulate pulmonary blood flow. Recent clinical and experimental evidence supports a role for vasoactive mediators in modulating the vascular tone of both the fetus and the newborn. Most recent work focuses on the lipid mediators, and this work is discussed.

The main clinical features in infants with PPHN are pulmonary hypertension, hypoxemia, pulmonary edema, and bronchoconstriction. These features would seem to correlate with some of the known actions of eicosanoids (especially thromboxane and the sulfidopeptide-containing leukotrienes) and platelet activating factor (PAF) as shown in Table 2.

These clinical findings, the demonstrated potent actions of lipid mediators, and the finding that certain stimuli, including hypoxia, can lead to the simultaneous release of precursors which if metabolized could produce prostaglandins, leukotrienes, and platelet activating factors (Chilton and Murphy, 1986) support the hypothesis illustrated in Figure 14. One could speculate that in the fetus vasoconstrictor substances predominate. With birth, under normal circumstances, vasodilators would be produced, leading to a decrease in pulmonary vascular tone. In PPHN, an abnormal persistence of constrictors or an inability to produce vasodilators may be related to syndrome.

Work in animal models supports this hypothesis. First, there is increasing evidence to suggest that prostacyclin plays an important physiological role in causing postnatal pulmonary vasodilation. Lung distension or mechanical stimulation of the lungs leads to prostacyclin production (Leffler et al., 1980). Treatment of the fetus with indomethacin before ventilation blocked prostacyclin production and decreased the pulmonary vasodilatation seen with ventilation of the lungs (Leffler et al., 1978). Chronic treatment with cyclooxygenase blockers is associated with an increased incidence of persistent pulmonary hypertension syndromes (Levin et al., 1978a). Other mechanisms may also be involved in the stimulation of prostacyclin. For example, both bradykinin and angiotensin II, which increase in concentration immediately after birth, stimulatate prostacyclin production.

Table 2 Comparison of PPHN with Actions of Eiocosanoids and PAF

Features of PPHN	Lung actions of eicosanoids	Actions of PAF
Pulmonary hypertension	Smooth muscle constriction[c,k,p]	Smooth muscle constriction[c,k,p]
Pulmonary edema	Vascular permeability[c,k,m]	Vascular permeability[c,k,m]
Airway resistance	Bronchoconstriction[k]	Bronchoconstriction[k]
	Produced by lung cells[g-i]	Produced by lung-associated cells[m]
	Produced by pulmonary vascular tissue[j]	
	Hypoxemia	

[a]Hanna et al., 1981. [b]Yokochi et al., 1982. [c]Voelkel et al., 1982. [d]Casey 1982. [e]Daheln 1981, [f]Weiss 1982. [g]Sirois 1985. [h]Farmer 1975. [i]Fleisch 1982. [j]Piper and Levine, 1986. [k]Hamasaki 1984. [l]Heffner 1983. [m]Gillespie and Bowdy, 1986. [m]Chang et al., 1987.

The potential role of lipid mediators in maintaining high fetal pulmonary vascular resistance has been suggested by several studies. Soifer et al. (1984) reported that the tracheal fluid of fetal sheep contained leukotrienes. Leukotrienes are potent pulmonary vasoconstrictors in the fetus. Moreover it has been demonstrated that both a leukotriene receptor antagonist (FPL 55712) and a synthesis inhibitor (U 60 257) decrease fetal pulmonary vascular resistance and increase pulmonary blood flow and in addition inhibit hypoxic vasoconstriction in the neonatal lamb (Schreiber et al., 1985; LeBidois et al, 1986; Soifer et al., 1986). Leffler, however, has not found a role for the leukotrienes in the pressor response to hypoxia in neonatal piglets (Leffler et al., 1984). Experimental work in the group B streptococcal sepsis model of neonatal pulmonary hypertension also suggests that lipid mediators may be mechanistically involved in the pulmonary hypertensive process. Infusion of GBS or its extracellular toxin causes an initial period of marked pulmonary hypertension followed by a later phase characterized by increased vascular permeability and increased pulmonary vascular resistance. The initial phase of pulmonary hypertension is associated with a marked rise in thromboxane. Cyclooxygenase inhibition (Rojas, 1983; Runkle, 1984) prevents both the rise in thromboxane and the deleterious hemodynamic

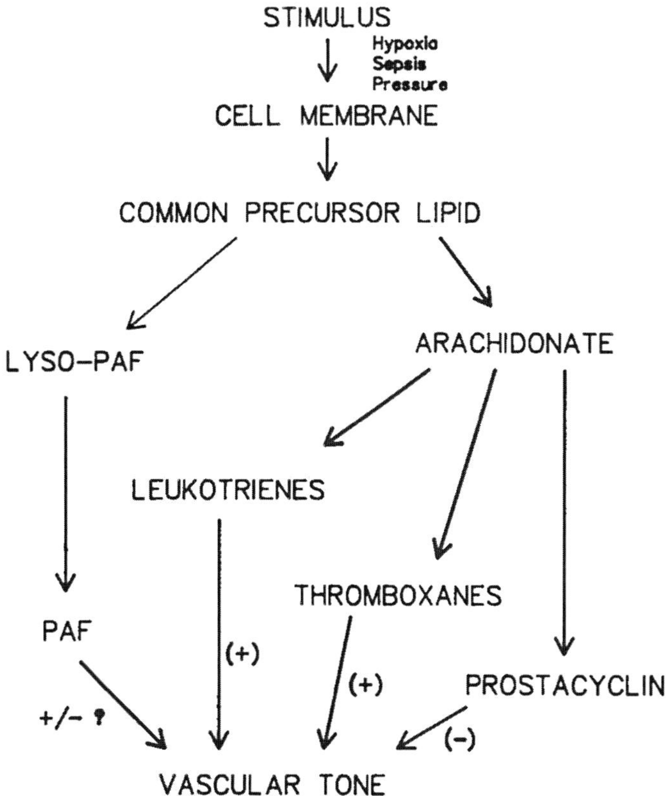

Figure 14 Schema showing how a specific stimulus could hypothetically lead to the production of lipid mediators having potentially significant effects on vascular tone.

effects of GBS infusion. The early phase of pulmonary hypertension was also modified by a leukotriene receptor antagonist (Goldberg, 1986). The late phase of increased vascular permeability and pulmonary hypertension is not inhibited by indomethacin but is prevented by steroids (Rojas, 1986). Furthermore, at least in adult sheep, the late phase is associated with a rise in 5- and 12-hydro-oxyeicosatetraenoic acid concentrations, major by-products of the lipooxygenase enzymes.

The role of PAF must also be considered. Recent evidence suggests that PAF is released during acute alveolar hypoxia (Prevost et al., 1984). That PAF is a potent pulmonary inflammatory mediator is also clear (Levi et al., 1984). The effects of PAF on the pulmonary circulation, however, are unclear. Gillespie has recently suggested that PAF depresses pulmonary vascular responsiveness to certain pressor stimuli (Gillespie and Bowdy, 1986). McMurtry and Morris (1986) have also demonstrated that low doses of PAF caused inhibition of the hypoxic pressor response both in vivo and in vitro. Further, Accurso and co-workers (1986a) demonstrated that PAF is a very potent vasodilator in the ovine fetus. On the other hand, chronic infusion of PAF into the rabbit has been associated with the development of pulmonary hypertension (Ohar et al., 1986).

In human studies, the presence of leukotrienes C_4 and D_4 has been demonstrated in the airway lavage of infants with severe persistent pulmonary hypertension but not in the airway lavage of infants without pulmonary hypertension (Stenmark et al., 1983). Further, higher plasma thromboxane levels have been documented in infants with PPHN than in controls (Hammerman et al., 1987).

In summary, it seems possible that regulation of the perinatal pulmonary circulation reflects a balance between humoral mediators producing active pulmonary vasoconstriction and those leading to pulmonary vasodilatation. In the hypoxic environment of the fetus, constrictors dominate. In the normal newborn, the increase in pulmonary blood flow could reflect a shift to a predominance of dilators, though the exact stimulus for this remains unknown. The infant with pulmonary hypertension may demonstrate a shift to a more fetal type of pattern.

References

Abman, S. H., and Accurso, F. J. (1988). Acute and chronic fetal pulmonary hypertension alters pulmonary vasoreactivity. *Chest 93*:117-118.

Abman, S. H., Wilkening, R. B., and Accurso, F. J. (1985). Temporal response of the fetal pulmonary circulation to local infusion of arachidonic acid and prostaglandins. *ARRD 131*:A255.

Abman, S. H., Accurso, F. J., Ward, R. M., and Wilkening, R. B. (1986). Adaptation of fetal pulmonary blood flow to local infusion of tolazoline. *Pediatr. Res. 20*:1131-1135.

Abman, S. H., Accurso, F. J., Wilkening, R. B., and Meschia, G. (1987). Persistent fetal pulmonary hypoperfusion following acute hypoxia. *Am. J. Physiol. 253*:H941-H948, 1987.

Accurso, F., Abman, S., Wilkening, R. B., Worthen, S., and Henson, P. M. (1986a). Exogenous platelet activating factor produces pulmonary vasodilatation in the ovine fetus. *Am. Rev. Resp. Dis. 133*:A11.

Accurso, F. J., Alpert, B., Wilkening, R. B., Petersen, R. C., and Meschia, G. (1986b). Time-dependent response of fetal pulmonary blood flow to an increase in fetal oxygen tension. *Resp. Physiol. 63*:43-52.

Accurso, F. J., Abman, S. H., and Wilkening, R. B. (1988). Densitization of the fetal pulmonary circulation to vasodilatory stimuli. *Chest 93*:1845.

Agricola, K. M., Rubanyi, G., Paul, R. J., and Highsmith, R. F. (1985). Characterization of a potent coronary artery vasoconstrictor produced by endothelial cells in culture. *Am. J. Physiol. 248*:C550-C556.

Allen, K., and Haworth, S. G. (1986). Impaired adaptation of intrapulmonary arteries to extrauterine life in newborn pigs exposed to hypoxia: an ultrastructural study. *J. Pathol. 150*:205-212.

Altiere, R. J., Olson, J. W., and Gillespie, M. N. (1986). Altered pulmonary vascular smooth muscle responsiveness in monocrotaline-induced pulmonary hypertension. *J. Pharmacol. Exp. Ther. 236*:390-395.

Bee, D., and Wach, R. A. (1983). Hypoxic pulmonary vasoconstriction in chronically hypoxic rats. *Resp. Physiol. 56*:91-101.

Benitz, W. E., Coulson, J. D., Lessler, D. S., and Bernfield, M. (1986a). Hypoxia inhibits proliferation of fetal pulmonary arterial smooth muscle cells in vitro. *Pediatr. Res. 20*:966.

Benitz, W. E., Lessler, D. S., Coulson, J. D., and Bernfield, M. (1986b). Heparin inhibits proliferation in the absence of platelet derived growth factor. *J. Cell Physiol. 121*:1.

Casey, L., Clarke, J., Fletcher, J., and Ramwell, P. (1982). Cardiovascular respiratory and hematologic effects of leukotriene D_4 in primates. In *Leukotrienes and other Lipoxygenase Products*. Edited by B. Samuelsson and R. Paoletti. Raven Press, New York, pp. 201-210.

Cassin, S., Dawes, G. S., and Mott, J. C. (1964). The vascular resistance of the fetal and newly ventilated lung of the lamb. *J. Physiol. 171*:61.

Cassin, S., Tod, M., Philips, J., Frislinger, J., Jordon, J., and Gibbs, C. (1981). Effects of PGD_2 on perinatal circulation. *Am. J. Physiol. 240*:H755-H760.

Castellot, J. J., Addonizio, M. L., Rosenberg, R. D., and Karnovsky, M. J. (1981). Cultured endothelial cells produce a heparaine like inhibitor of smooth muscle cell growth. *J. Cell Biol. 90*:372.

Chang, S., Feddersen, C. O., Henson, P. M., and Voeklel, N. F. (1987). Platelet-activating factor mediated hemodynamic changes and lung injury in endotoxin-treated rats. *J. Clin. Invest. 79*:1498-1509.

Chilton, F. H., and Murphy, R. C. (1986). Remodeling of arachidonate-containing phosphoglycerides within the human neutrophil. *J. Biol. Chem. 261*:7771-7777.

Coflesky, J. T., and Evans, J. N. (1987). Changes in pulmonary vascular reactivity following acute lung injury: response of neonatal rats to hyperoxia. *Am. Rev. Resp. Dis. 135*:A132.

Cohen, M. L., and Berkowitz, B. A. (1976). Decreased vascular relaxation in hypertension. *J. Pharmacol. Exp. Ther. 196*:396-406.

Cohn, H. E., Sacks, E. J., Heymann, M. A., and Rudolph, A. M. (1974). Cardiovascular responses to hypoxemia and acidemia in fetal lambs. *Am. J. Obstet. Gynecol. 120*:817.

Daheln, S. E., Bork, J., and Hedquist, P. (1981). Leukotrienes promote plasma leakage and leukocyte adherence in postcapillary venules: in vivo effects of relevance to acute inflammatory response. *Proc. Natl. Acad. Sci. USA 78*:3887-3891.

Davidson, D., and Stalcup, S. A. (1984). Role of angiotensin converting enzyme activity in the circulatory adjustments at birth in sheep. *Am. Rev. Resp. Dis. 129*:A340.

Davies, P., Maddalo, F., and Reid, L. (1985). Effects of chronic hypoxia on structure and reactivity of rat lung microvessels. *J. Appl. Physiol. 58*(3): 795-801.

Dawes, G. S., and Mott, J. C. (1962). The vascular tone of the fetal lung. *J. Physiol. (Lond.) 164*:465-477.

Dawes, G. S., Mott, J. C., and Widdicombe, J. G. (1953). Changes in the lung of the newborn lamb. *J. Physiol. 121*:541.

deMello, D., Murphy, J., Aronovitz, M., Davies, P., and Reid, L. (1987). Effects of indomethacin in utero on the pulmonary vasculature of the newborn guinea pig. *Fed. Proc. 46*:4679.

DeMey, J. G., and Vanhoutte, P. M. (1982). Heterogeneous behavior of the canine arterial and venous wall: importance of endothelium. *Circ. Res. 51*: 439-447.

Diamond, J., and Chu, E. B. (1983). Possible role for cyclic GMP in endotheliumm-dependent relaxation of rabbit aorta by acetylcholine. Comparison with nitroglyercin. *Res. Commun. Chem. Path. Pharmacol. 41*:369-375.

DiCorleto, P. E. (1984). Cultured endothelial cells produce multiple growth factors for connective tissue cells. *Exp. Cell Res. 153*:167.

DiCorleto, P. E., Gajdusek, C. M., Schwartz, S. M., and Ross, R. (1983). Biochemical properties of the endothelium derived growth factor: comparison to other growth factors. *J. Cell Physiol. 114*:339.

Drummond, W. H., Peckman, G. J., and Fox, W. W. (1977). The clinical profile of the newborn with persistent pulmonary hypertension. *Clin. Pediatr. 16*: 335-341.

Drummond, W. H., and Bissonnette, J. M. (1978). Persistent pulmonary hypertension in the neonate: Development of an animal model. *Am. J. Obstet. Gynecol. 131*:761-763.

Emery, C. J., Bee, D., and Barer, G. R. (1981). Mechanical properties and reactivity of vessels in isolated perfused lungs of chronically hypoxic rats. *Clin. Sci. 61*:569-580.

Farmer, J. B., Richards, I. M., Sheard, P., and Woods, A. M. (1975). Mediators of passive lung anaphylaxis in the rat. *Br. J. Pharacol.* *55*:57-64.

Fasules, J., Stenmark, K. R., Henson, J., Voelkel, N. F., Tucker, A., and Reeves, J. T. (1987). Heparin attenuates pulmonary vascular thickening in chronically hypoxic neonatal calves. *Am. Rev. Resp. Dis.* *135*:A129.

Fasules, J. W., Stenmark, K. R., Henson, P. M., Voelkel, N. F., and Reeves, J. T. (1987b). Neither anticoagulant nor nonanticoagulant heparin affect monocrotaline lung injury. *J. Appl. Physiol.* *62*:816-820.

Fleisch, J. H., Haisch, K. D., and Paethe, S. M. (1982). Slow reacting substance of anaphylaxis (SRS-A) release from guinea pig lung parenchyma during antigen- or ionophore-induced contraction. *J. Pharmacol. Exp. Ther.* *221*: 146-151.

Fox, P. L., and DiCorleto, P. E. (1984). Regulation of production of a platelet derived growth factor-like protein by cultured bovine aortic endothelial cells. *J. Cell Physiol.* *121*:298-308.

Fox, W. W., and Durara, S. (1983). Persistent pulmonary hypertension in the neonate: diagnosis and management. *J. Pediatr.* *103*:505-514.

Fox, W. W., Gewitz, M. H., Dinwiddie, R., Drummond, W. H., and Peckham, G. J. (1977). Pulmonary hypertension in the perinatal aspiration syndromes. *Pediatrics* *59*:205-211.

Franklin, T. J., Morris, W. P., and Loveday, B. F. (1982). Effects of inhibitors of collagen maturation on hypertension in rats. *Blood Vessels* *19*:217-225.

Furchgott, R. F. (1983). Role of endothelium in responses of vascular smooth muscle. *Circ. Res.* *53*:557-573.

Furchgott, R. F. (1984). The role of endothelium in the responses of vascular smooth muscle to drugs. *Ann. Rev. Pharmacol. Toxicol.* *24*:175-197.

Gajdusek, C. M., and Schwartz, S. M. (1984). Comparison of intracellular and extracellular nitrogenic activity. *J. Cell Physiol.* *121*:316.

Gajdusek, C., DiCorleto, P. E., Ross, R., and Schwartz, S. M. (1980). An endothelial cell derived growth factor. *J. Cell Biol.* *85*:467.

Geggel, R. L., Aronovitz, B. S., and Reid, L. M. (1986a). Effects of chronic in utero hypoxemia on rat neonatal pulmonary arterial structure. *J. Pediatr.* *108*:756-759.

Geggel, R. L., Aronovitz, M. J., and Reid, L. M. (1986b). Effects of chronic in utero hypoxemia on rat neonatal pulmonary arterial structure. *Pediatr. Res.* *20*:A368.

Geggel, R. L., Hu, L. M., and Reid, L. (1986c). Effect of heparin during chronic hypoxia; a hemodynamic study including acute hypoxic challenge. *Fed. Proc.* *45*:A4585.

Gersony, W. M., Duc, C. V., and Sinclair, J. D. (1969). "PEG" syndrome (persistence of the fetal circulation). *Circulation* *3*:40.

Gersony, W. M., Morishima, H. O., and Daniel, S. (1976). The hemodynamic effects of intrauterine hypoxia: an experimental model in newborn lambs. *J. Pediatr. 89*:631.

Gillespie, M. N., and Bowdy, B. D. (1986). Impact of platelet activating factor on vascular responsiveness in isolated rat lungs. *Am. Soc. Pharmacol. Exp. Ther. 236*:396-402.

Goetzman, B. W., and Reimenschneider, T. A. (1980). Persistence of the fetal circulation. *Pediatr. Rev. 2*:37-40.

Goldberg, I. D., Stemerman, M. B., and Handin, R. I. (1980). Vascular permeation of platelet factor 4 after endothelial injury. *Science 209*:611-612.

Goldberg, R. N., Suguihara, C., Steitfeld, M. M., Runkle, B., and Bancalari, E. (1985). Effects of leukotriene antagonist FPL57231 on the early hemodynamic manifestations of group B BETA streptococcal sepsis (GBS) in piglets. *Pediatr. Res. 19*:342A.

Goldberg, S. J., Levy, R. A., and Siassi, B. (1971). Effects of maternal hypoxia and hyperoxia upon the neonatal pulmonary vasculature. *Pediatrics 48*: 528.

Griffith, T. M., Edwards, D. H., Lewis, M. J., Newby, A. C., and Henderson, A. H. (1984). The nature of endothelium-derived vascular relaxant factor. *Nature 308*:645-647.

Grover, R. F., Wagner, W. W., Jr., McMurtry, I. F., and Reeves, J. T. (1983). Pulmonary circulation. In *The Handbook of Physiology. Sect. 2, The Cardiovascular System*. Vol. III. Edited by J. T. Shepherd and F. M. Abboud, Am. Physiol. Soc. Bethesda, MD, Chap. 4, pp. 103-127.

Guyton, J. R., Rosenberg, R. D., Clowes, A. W., and Karnovsky, M. J. (1980). Inhibition of rat arterial smooth muscle cell proliferation by heparin: in vivo studies with anticoagulant and nonanticoagulant heparin. *Circ. Res. 46*:625.

Hales, C. A., Kradin, R. L., Brandstetter, R. P. and Zhu, Y. (1983). Impairment of hypoxic pulmonary artery remodeling by heparin in mice. *Am. Rev. Resp. Dis. 128*:747-751.

Hamasaki, Y., Mojarad, M., Saga, T., Tai, H. H., and Said, S. I. (1984). Platelet activating factor raises airway and vascular pressures and induces edema in lungs perfused with platelet free solution. *Am. Rev. Resp. Dis. 29*:742-746.

Hammerman, C., Lass, N., Strates, E., Komar, K., and Bui, K. C. (1987). Prostonoids in neonates with persistent pulmonary hypertension. *J. Pediatr. 110*:470-471.

Hanna, C. J., Bach, M. K., Pane, P. D., and Schellenberg, R. R. (1981). Slow-reacting substances (leukotrienes) contract human airway and pulmonary vascular smooth muscle in vitro. *Nature 290*:343-344.

Harker, L. C., Kirkpatrick, S. E., and Friedman, W. F. (1981). Effects of indomethacin on fetal rat lungs: a possible cause of persistent fetal circulation (PFC). *Pediatr. Res. 15*:147.

Hassovin, P., Kradin, R., Thompson, T., and Hales, C. (1986). Effect of heparin on hypoxic pulmonary hypertension and vascular remodeling. *Am. Rev. Resp. Dis. 133*:A228.

Haworth, S. G., and Hislop, A. (1981). Adaptation of the pulmonary circulation to extra uterine life in the pig and its relevance to the human infant. *Cardiovasc. Res. 15*:108-119.

Haworth, S. G., and Reid, L. (1976). Persistent fetal circulation: newly recognized structural features. *J. Pediatr. 88*:614-620.

Heath, D., DuShane, J. W., Wood, E. H., and Edwards, J. E. (1959). The structure of the pulmonary trunk at different ages and in cases of pulmonary hypertension and pulmonary stenosis. *J. Pathol. Bacteriol. 77*:443-456.

Heffner, J. E., Shoemaker, S. A., Canham, E. M., Patel, M., McMurtry, I. F., Morris, H. E., and Repine, J. E. (1983). Acetyl glyceryl either phosphorylcholine stimulated human platelets cause pulmonary hypertension and edema in isolated rabbit lungs. *J. Clin. Invest. 71*:351-357.

Hernandez, J. A., Offuh, J., and Butterfield, L. J. (1986). The cost of care of the less-than-1000-gram infant. *Clin. Perinatol. 13*:461.

Heymann, M. A., and Hoffman, J. I. C. (1984). Persistent pulmonary hypertension syndromes in the newborn. In *Pulmonary Hypertension*. Edited by E. K. Weir and J. T. Reeves. Futura, New York. Chap. 2, pp. 45-71.

Hislop, A., and Reid, L. (1978) Formation of the pulmonary vasculature. In *Development of the Lung*. Edited by W. A. Hodson, Marcel Dekker, New York, p. 52.

Hoover, R. L., Rosenberg, R., Haering, W., and Karnovsky, M. J. (1980). Inhibition of rat arterial smooth muscle proliferation by heparin II: in vitro studies. *Circ. Res. 47*:578-583.

Humphries, D. E., Lee, S. L., Fanburg, B. L., and Silbert, J. E. (1986). Effects of hypoxia and hyperoxia on proteoglycon production by bovine pulmonary artery endothelial cells. *J. Physiol. 126*:249.

Hyman, A. L., Spannhake, W., and Kadowitz, P. J. (1982). Pharmacology of the pulmonary circulation. In *Progress in Cardiology*. Vol. 11. Edited by R. N. Yu and J. F. Goodwin. Lea and Febiger, Philadelphia, pp. 107-130.

Iwatsuki, K., Cardinale, G. J., Spector, S., and Udenfriend, S. (1972). Reduction of blood pressure and vascular collagen in hypertensive rats by B-aminopropionitrile. *Proc. Natl. Acad. Sci. USA 74*:360-362.

Jaenke, R. S., and Alexander, A. F. (1973). Fine structural alterations of bovine peripheral pulmonary arteries in hypoxia-induced hypertension. *Am. J. Pathol. 73*:377-398.

James, L. S., and Rowe, R. D. (1957). The pattern of response of pulmonary and systemic arterial pressures in newborn and older infants to short periods of hypoxia. *J. Pediatr. 51*:5.

Jones, R., Zapel, W. M., and Reid, L. (1984). Pulmonary artery remodeling and pulmonary hypertension after exposure to hyperoxia for 7 days. *Am. J. Pathol. 117*:273-285.

Jorgensen, L., Packham, M., Rowsell, H. C., and Mustard, J. F. (1972). Deposition of formed elements of blood on the intima and signs of intimal injury in the aorta of rabbit, pig and man. *Lab. Invest. 27*:341.

Kameji, R., Otsuka, H., and Hayashi, Y. (1980). Increase of collagen synthesis in pulmonary arteries of monocrotoline treated rats. *Experientia (Basel) 36*:441-442.

Kerr, J. S., Riley, D. J., Frank, M. M., Trelstad, R. L., and Frankel, H. M. (1984). Reduction of chronic hypoxic pulmonary hypertension in the rat by B-aminopropionitrile. *J. Appl. Physiol: Resp. Environ. Exercise Physiol. 57*(6):1760-1766.

Kulik, T. J., and Lock, J. E. (1984). Pulmonary vasodilator therapy in persistent pulmonary hypertension of the newborn. *Clin. Perinatal. 11*:693-701.

LeBidois, J., Soifer, S. J., and Heymann, M. A. (1986). Inibition of leukotriene synthesis increases pulmonary blood flow in fetal lambs. *Pediatr. Res. 20*: 434A.

Leffler, C. W., Mitchell, J. A., and Green, R. S. (1984). Cardiovascular effects of leukotrienes in neonatal piglets. *Circ. Res. 55*:780-787.

Leffler, C. W., Tyler, T. L., and Cassin, S. (1978). Effect of indomethacin on pulmonary vascular response to ventilation of fetal goats. *Am. J. Physiol. 234*:H346-H351.

Leffler, C. W., Hessler, J. R., and Terragno, N. A. (1980). Ventilation induced release of protoglandin-like material from fetal lungs. *Am. J. Physiol. 238*: 282-286.

Levi, R., Burke, J. A., Guo, Z. G., Hattori, Y., Hoppens, C. M., McManus, L. M., Hanahan, D. J., and Pickard, R. N. (1984). Acetyl glyceryl ether phosphorylcholine (AGEPC), a putative mediator of cardiac anaphylaxis in the guinea pig. *Circ. Res. 54*:117-124.

Levin, D. L., Heymann, M. A., Kitterman, J. A., Gregory, G. A., Phibbs, R. H. and Rudolph, A. M. (1976). Persistent pulmonary hypertension of the newborn infant. *J. Pediatr. 89*:626-630.

Levin, D. L. (1980). Effects of inhibition of prostaglandin synthesis on fetal development, oxygenation, and the fetal circulation. *Semin. Perinatol. 4*: 35-44.

Levin, D. L., Fixler, D. E., Morris, F. C., and Tyson, J. (1978a). Morphologic analysis of the pulmonary vascular bed ininfants exposed in utero to prostaglandin synthetase inhibitors. *J. Pediatr. 92*:478-483.

Levin, D. L., Hyman, A. I., and Heymann, M. A. (1978b). Fetal hypertension and the development of increased pulmonary vascular smooth muscle:

a possible mechanism for persistent pulmonary hypertension of the newborn infant. *J. Pediatr. 92*:265.

Levin, D. L., Mills, L. J., and Parkey, M. (1979). Constriction of the fetal ductus arteriosus after administration of indomethacin to the pregnant ewe. *J. Pediatr. 94*:647-650.

Levin, D. L., Weinberg, A. G., and Perkin, R. M. (1983). Pulmonary microthrombi syndrome in newborn infants with unresponsive persistent pulmonary hypertension. *J. Pediatr. 102*:299.

Lister, G. (Chairman) (1986). Persistent Pulmonary Hypertension of the Neonate. Symposium American Thoracic Society. *Am. Rev. Resp. Dis. 134*; 834-835.

Lock, J. E., Olley, P. M., and Coceani, F. (1979). Use of prostacyclin in persistent fetal circulation. *Lancet 2*:1343.

Lock, J. E., Olley, P. M., and Soldin, S. (1980). Indomethacin-induced pulmonary vasoconstriction in the conscious newborn lamb. *Am. J. Physiol. 238*:H639-H651.

Lock, J. E., Olley, P. M., and Coceani, F. (1981). Enhanced beta-adrenergic receptor responsiveness in the hypoxic neonatal pulmonary circulation. *Am. J. Physiol. 240*:H697.

McMurtry, I. F., and Morris, K. G. (1986). Platelet activating factor causes pulmonary vasodilation in the rat. *Am. Rev. Resp. Dis. 133*:A227.

McMurtry, I. F., Petrun, M. D., and Reeves, J. T. (1978). Lungs from chronically hypoxic rats have decreased pressor response to acute hypoxia. *Am. J. Physiol. 235*:H104-H109.

Manchester, D., Mangolis, H. A., and Sheldon, R. E. (1976). Possible association between maternal indomethacin therapy and primary pulmonarv hpertension of the newborn. *Am. J. Obst. Gynecol. 126*:467-469.

Mecham, R. P., Madaras, J., McDonald, J. A., and Ryan, U. (1983). Elastin production by cultured calf pulmonary artery endothelial cells. *J. Cell Physiol. 116*:282-288.

Mecham, R. P., Whitehouse, L. A., Wrenn, D. S., Parks, W. C., Griffin, G. L., Senior, R. W., Crouch, E. C., Voelkel, N. F., and Stenmark, K. R. (1987). Smooth muscle-mediated connective tissue remodeling in pulmonary hypertension. *Science 237*:423-426.

Meyrick, B., and Brigham, K. L. (1986). Repeated *E. coli* endotoxin-induced pulmonary inflammation causes chronic pulmonary hypertension in sheep. *Lab. Invest. 55*:164-176.

Meyrick, B., and Reid, L. (1978). Effect of continued hypoxia on rat pulmonary arterial circulation. *Lab. Invest. 38*:188.

Meyrick, B., and Reid, L. (1979a) Development of pulmonary arterial changes in rats fed with *crotolaria spectabilas*. *Am. J. Pathol. 94*:37.

Meyrick, B., and Reid, L. (1982). Normal postnatal development of the media of the rat hilar pulmonary artery and its remodeling by chronic hypoxia. *Lab. Invest.* *46*:505-516.

Meyrick, B., and Reid, L. (1983). Pulmonary hypertension. Anatomic and physiologic correlates. *Clin. Chest Med.* *4*:199-217.

Morin, F. C., Egan, E. A., and Lundgren, C. E. G. (1984). Response of the pulmonary vasculature of the fetal lamb to hyperbaric oxygenation. *Pediatr. Res.* *18*:399A.

Meyrick, B., and Reid, L. (1979b). Hypoxia and incorporation of ^{3}H-thymidine by cells of the rat pulmonary arteries and alveolar wall. *Am. J. Pathol.* *96*: 51-70.

Murphy, J. D., Rabinovitch, M., Goldstein, J. D., and Reid, L. M. (1981). The structural basis of persistent pulmonary hypertension of the newborn infant. *J. Pediatr.* *98*:962-967.

Murphy, J. D., Aronovitz, M. J., and Reid, L. M. (1986). Effects of chronic in utero hypoxia on the pulmonary vasculature of the newborn guinea pig. *Pediatr. Res.* *20*:292-295.

Naeye, R. L. (1961). Arterial changes during the perinatal period. *Arch. Pathol.* *71*:121-128.

Niedenzu, C., Grasedyck, K., Voelkel, N. F., Bittmann, S., and Lindner, J. (1981). Proliferation of lung cells in chronically hypoxic rats. *Int. Arch. Occup. Environ. Health* *4*:185-193.

O'Brien, R. F., Seton, M. P., Makarski, J. S., Center, D. M., Rounds, S. (1984). Thiourea causes endothelial cells in tissue culture to produce neutrophil chemattractant activity. *Am. Rev. Resp. Dis.* *130*:103-109.

Ohar, J. A., Pyle, J. A., Hyers, T. M., and Webster, R. O. (1986). AGEPC-induced pulmonary vascular injury – a rabbit model of pulmonary hypertension. *Am. Rev. Resp. Dis.* *133*:A159.

Orton, E. C., Stenmark, K. R., Tucker, A., and Reeves, J. T. (1987). Acetylcholine causes selective pulmonary vasodilation in severe chronic neonatal pulmonary hypertension in calves. *Fed. Proc.* *46*:4627.

Packham, M. A., Rowsell, H. C., Jorgensen, L., and Mustard, J. F. (1967). Localized protein accumulation in the wall of the aorta. *Exp. Mol. Pathol.* 7:214-232.

Park, M. K., Zakheim, R. M., Mattioli, L., and Sunderson, J. (1977). Altered reactivity of rat pulmonary arterial smooth muscle to vasoactive agents in hypoxia. *Proc. Soc. Exp. Biol. Med.* *155*:274-277.

Peach, M. J., Singer, H. A., and Loeb, A. L. (1985). Mechanisms of endothelium-dependent vascular smooth muscle relaxation. *Biochem. Pharmacol.* *34*:1867-1874.

Peters, L. L. H., Sheldon, R. E., Jones, M. D., Makowski, E. L., and Meshia, G.

(1979). Blood flow to fetal organs as a function of arterial oxygen content. *Am. J. Obst. Gynecol. 135*:637-646.

Piper, P. J., and Levene, S. (1986). Generation of leukotrienes from fetal and neonatal porcine blood vessels. *Biol. Neonate 49*:109-112.

Poiani, G. J., Chae, C. V., Tozzi, C. A., Ruppert, C. L., and Riley, D. J. (1986). Collagen synthesis and proteinase activity in the hypertensive pulmonary artery of the rat. *Am. Rev. Resp. Dis. 133*:A228.

Prevost, M. C., Cariven, C., Simon, M. F., Chap, H., and Douste-Blazy, L. (1984). Platelet activating factor (PAF acether) is released into rat pulmonary alveolar fluid as a consequence of hypoxia. *Biochem. Biophys. Res. Commun. 119*:58-63.

Rabinovitch, M. (1985). Morphology of the developing pulmonary bed: Pharmacologic implications. *Pediat. Pharmacol. 5*:31-48.

Rabinovitch, M., Bothwell, T., Hayakawa, B. N., Williams, W. G., Trusler, G. A., Rowe, R. D., Olley, P. M., and Cutz, E. (1986). Pulmonary artery endothelial abnormalities in patients with congenital heart defects and pulmonary hypertension. *Lab. Invest. 55*:632-653.

Reeves, J. T., and Leathers, J. E. (1967). Postnatal development of pulmonary and bronchial arterial circulations in the calf and the effects of chronic hypoxia. *Anat. Rec. 157*:641-656.

Rendeas, A., Branthwaite, M., and Reid, L. (1978). Growth of pulmonary circulation in normal pig structural analysis and cardiopulmonary function. *J. Appl. Physiol. 45*:806-817.

Rojas, J., Larsson, L. E., Ogletree, M. L., Brigham, K. L., and Stahlman, M. T. (1983). Effects of cyclooxygenase inhibition on the response to Group B streptococcal toxin in sheep. *Pediatr. Res. 17*:107-110.

Rojas, J., Palme, C., Ogletree, M. L., Hellerqvist, C. G., Brigham, K. L., and Stahlman, M. T. (1984). Effects of methylprednisolone on the response to Group B streptococcal toxin in sheep. *Pediatr. Res. 18*:1141-1144.

Ross, R. (1986). The pathogenesis of atherosclerosis – an update. *New Engl. J. Med. 314*:488-500.

Rubanyi, G. M., and Vanhoutte, P. M. (1985). Hypoxia releases a vasoconstrictor substance from the canine vascular endothelium. *J. Physiol. 364*: 45-56.

Rudolph, A. M. (1980). High pulmonary vascular resistance after birth: pathophysiologic considerations and etiologic classification. *Clin. Pediatr. 19*: 585-590.

Rudolph, A. M., and Yuan, S. (1966). Response of the pulmonary vasculature to hypoxia and H^+ ion concentration changes. *J. Clin. Invest. 45*:399-411.

Rudolph, A. M., Teitel, D. F., Iwamoto, H. S., and Gleason, C. A. (1986). Ventilation is more important than oxygenation in reducing pulmonary vascular resistance at birth. *Pediatr. Res. 20*:439A.

Ruiz, V., Piasecki, G. J., and Baloglik, K., Polanksy, B. J., Jackson, B. T. (1972). An experimental model for fetal pulmonary hypertension. *Am. J. Surg. 123*:468-471.

Runkle, B., Goldberg, R. N., Streitfeld, M. M., Clark, M. R., Buron E., Setzer, E. S., and Bancalari, E. (1984). Cardiovascular changes in group B streptococcal sepsis in the piglet: response to indomethacin and relationship to prostacyclin and thromboxane A_2. *Pediatr. Res. 18*:874-878.

Ryan, J. W., and Ryan, U. S. (1977). Pulmonary endothelial cells. *Fed. Proc. 36*: 2683-2691.

Ryan, U. S., and Ryan, J. W. (1977). Correlations between the fine structure in the alveolar-capillary unit and its metabolic activities. In *Metabolic Functions of the Lung*. Edited by J. R. and Y. S. Bankle. Vol 4: *Lung Biology in Health and Disease*. Edited by C. Lenfant. Marcel Dekker, New York.

Said, S. I. (1982). Metabolic functions of the pulmonary circulation. *Circ. Res. 50*:325-333.

Schreiber, M. D., Heymann, M. A., and Soifer, S. J. (1985). Leukotriene inhibition prevents and reverses hypoxic pulmonary vasoconstriction in newborn lambs. *Pediatr. Res. 19*:437-441.

Sirois, P., Brousseau, Y., Chagnon, M., Gentile, J., Gladu, M., Salari, H., and Borgeat, P. (1985). Metabolism of leukotrienes by adult and fetal human lungs. *Exp. Lung Res. 9*:17-30.

Sobin, S. S., Tremer, H. M., Hardy, J. D., and Chiodi, H. P. (1983). Changes in arteriole in acute and chronic hypoxic pulmonary hypertension and recovery in rat. *J. Appl. Physiol. 55*(5):1445-1455.

Soifer, S. J., Kaslow, D., and Heymann, M. A. (1983). Prolonged intrauterine hypoxia produces pulmonary hypotension in the newborn lamb. *Pediatr. Res. 17*:336A.

Soifer, S. J., Loitz, R., Roman, C., and Heymann, M. A. (1984). Do leukotrienes control pulmonary blood flow in the fetal lamb? *Pediatr. Res. 18*:347A.

Soifer, S. J., Schreiber, M. D., Frantz, E. G., and Heyman, M. A. (1986). Inhibition of leukotriene synthesis attenuates hypoxia induced pulmonary vasoconstriction in newborn lambs. *Pediatr. Res. 20*:441A.

Stenmark, K. R., James, S. L., Voelkel, N. F., Toews, W. H., Reeves, J. T., and Murphy, R. C. (1983). Leukotriene C_4 and D_4 in neonates with hypoxemia and pulmonary hypertension. *New Engl. J. Med. 309*:77-80.

Stenmark, K. R., Fasules, J., Voelkel, N. F., Henson, J., Tucker, A., Hyde, D. M., Wison, H., and Reeves, J. T. (1987a). Severe pulmonary hypertension and arterial adventitial changes in newborn calves at 4300m. *J. Appl. Physiol. 62*:821-831.

Stenmark, K. R., Reeves, J. T., Voelkel, N. F., Crouch, E. C., and Mecham, R. P. (1987b). Altered pulmonary vascular elastin metabolism in severe hypoxic pulmonary hypertension. *Fed. Proc. 46*:A1168.

Szarek, J. L., and Evans, J. N. (1987). Mechanical properties of rat pulmonary arteries in hypoxia induced pulmonary hypertension. *Am. Rev. Resp. Dis. 135*:A131.

Tucker, A., Greenlees, K. J., and Gotshall, R. W. (1984). Pulmonary systemic vascular responses to tolazoline in neonatal and mature calves. *Pediatr. Pharmacol. 4*:115-128.

Tucker, A., Alberts, M. K., Andersen, K. K., and Wilke, W. L. (1987). Vascular reactivity in lungs isolated from rats exposed from both to moderate altitude and/or lead. *Fed. Proc. 46*:4516.

Vanhoutte, P. M., and Miller, V. M. (1985). Heterogeneity of endothelium-dependent responses in mammalian blood vessels. *J. Cardiovasc. Pharmacol.* 7:S120S23.

Vender, R. L., Kwock, L., and Friedman, M. (1984). Hypoxic pulmonary endothelium increases pulmonary artery smooth muscle cell number in vitro. *Am. Rev. Resp. Dis. 129*:A343.

Voelkel, N. F.,Wiegers, U., Sill, V., and Trautmann, J. (1977). A kinetic study of lung DNA-synthesis during simulated chronic high-altitude hypoxia. *Thorax 32*:578-581.

Voelkel, N. F., Worthen, S., Reeves, J. T., Henson, P. M., and Murphy, R. C. (1982). Non-immunological production of leukotrienes induced by platelet activating factor. *Science 218*:286-289.

Weiss, J. W., Drasen, J. M., Coles, N. et al. (1982). Bronchoconstrictor effects of leukotriene C in humans. *Science 216*:196-198.

Wung, J. T., James, L. S., Kilchevsky, E., and James, E. (1985). Managment of infants with severe respiratory failure and persistence of the fetal circulation, without hyperventilation. *Pediatrics 76*:488-494.

Yohn, S. E., Poiani, G. J., Tozzi, C. A., Belsky, S. A., Deak, S. B., Yu, S. Y., and Riley, D. J. (1987). Elastin synthesis in the hypertensive pulmonary artery of the rat. *Am. Rev. Resp. Dis. 135*:A130.

Yokochi, K., Olley, P. M. Sideris, E., Hamilton, F., Huhtanen, D., and Coceani, F. (1982). Leukotriene D_4: a potent vasoconstrictor of the pulmonary and systemic circulations in the newborn lamb. In *Leukotrienes and other Lipoxygenase Products*. Edited by B. Samuelsson and R. Paoletti. Raven Press, New York, pp. 211-214.

12

Pulmonary Circulatory Control in Lung Injury

SHARON I. S. ROUNDS*

Boston University School of Medicine
Boston, Massachusetts

I. Introduction

Pulmonary hypertension is a frequent finding in both acute and chronic lung diseases, and it has been reported that the presence of pulmonary hypertension denotes a poorer prognosis in diseases as diverse as adult respiratory distress syndrome (ARDS) (Sibbald et al., 1978; Vito et al., 1974) and chronic obstructive lung disease (Burrows et al., 1972). With the advent of potent vasodilator agents that can reduce pulmonary vascular resistance, there has been increasing interest in whether morbidity and mortality can be improved by ameliorating pulmonary hypertension (Reeves et al., 1986).

In studies of the pathogenesis of pulmonary hypertension after lung injury, there is increasing evidence that pulmonary vascular reactivity to pressor stimuli can also be altered, even in the absence of concomitant pulmonary hypertension. Changes in vascular reactivity could also affect the consequences of lung injury. Increased vascular reactivity may predispose to sustained pulmonary hypertension (Hill et al., 1984), while decreased vascular reactivity to hypoxia

---

*Present affiliation: Brown University, Providence VA Medical Center, Providence, Rhode Island.

may exacerbate mismatch of ventilation and perfusion and thereby worsen hypoxemia (Dantzker and Bower, 1981).

In this review, the causes and consequences of pulmonary hypertension and altered vascular reactivity after lung injury will be considered. The focus is on ARDS in humans and on animal models of acute injury resulting in increased permeability edema. In addition, evidence for altered vascular reactivity in chronic lung diseases will be considered, as well as the potential role for altered vascular reactivity as a precipitating event in the pathogenesis of sustained pulmonary hypertenson.

II. Acute Lung Injury

A. Adult Respiratory Distress Syndrome

The disease ARDS is a syndrome of acute respiratory failure, characterized by increased permeability pulmonary edema that results in refractory hypoxemia, decreased lung compliance, and bilateral diffuse alveolar infiltrates on chest radiograph. The syndrome may be precipitated by a variety of insults or events and frequently results in death (Ashbaugh et al., 1967). Several authors have reported the presence of pulmonary hypertension in individuals with ARDS, as outlined in Table 1. The degree of elevation of pulmonary arterial (PA) pressure or arteriolar resistance (PVR) is generally modest. Although it has been stated that the absence of pulmonary hypertension might cause doubt regarding the diagnosis of ARDS (Zapol et al., 1985), pulmonary hypertension was not invariably present in at least three reported series (Brigham et al., 1983; Sibbald et al., 1978; Vito et al., 1974).

There are multiple potential causes for pulmonary hypertension in patients with ARDS, including ventilation with positive end-expiratory pressure (PEEP); vasoconstriction in response to hypoxia or circulating vasoactive mediators; and vascular obstruction by swollen microvascular endothelium, clot, or inflammatory cell aggregates (Zapol et al., 1985). Although PEEP may influence PA pressures (Cassidy et al., 1978), Zapol and Snider (1977) found that discontinuation of PEEP did not ablate pulmonary hypertension in 10 patients with ARDS. Pulmonary vasoconstriction in response to alveolar hypoxia is an important mechanism of acute and chronic pulmonary hypertension (Fishman, 1976) and can be exacerbated by acidemia or hypercarbia (Enson et al., 1964). However, the studies summarized in Table 1 showed no apparent relationship between PaO_2, PaO_2/FIO_2, or PA-$PaDO_2$ and PA pressures. In addition, Fugueras et al., (1976) reported that acidemia and hypercarbia did not correlate with pulmonary hypertension in a series of 75 patients critically ill from a variety of causes. However, vasoconstriction, perhaps in response to vasoactive mediators, has been noted in other reports. Weigelt and coauthors found that the vasodilator nitroprusside significantly lowered PA pressure and PVR in nine patients with ARDS (Weigelt et al., 1982). Zapol et al. (1985) reported that isopro-

Table 1 Pulmonary Hypertension in Patients with ARDS[a]

Study	Number of Patients	Patient group[b]	Ppa, mmHg	PVR, mmHg.min/L	Qs/Qt, %	PA-PaO_2, mmHg	PaO_2,[c] mmHg	PaO_2/FIO_2	Mortality	Reference
1	14	–	26±7 (11-41)	8.8±7.2 (1.6-30)	–	306±103 (114-503)	228±143 (43-493)	259±114 (72-493)	4/14	Brigham et al., 1983
2	30	–	32±8	4.7±2.0	–	–	–	–	24/30	Zapol and Snider 1977
3	9	–	26±2	1.8±0.2	36±5	–	67±8	–	–	Weigelt et al., 1982
4	11	a	32±8	6.0±1.3	54±9	–	47±12	–	9/11	Lamy et al., 1976
	13	b	38±5	5.5±1.3	45±9	–	60±17	–	10/13	
	21	c	31±13	4.6±1.5	40±7	–	66±15	–	11/21	
5	16	a	31±7	3.1±1.5	–	–	87±36	–	15/16	Greene et al., 1981
	13	b	26±8	2.1±1.6	–	–	91±21	–	6/13	
	11	c	28±6	1.8±1.1	–	–	95±34	–	4/11	
6	14	d	15±3	2.6±2.8	–	–	–	232±87	–	Sibbald et al., 1978
	37	e	27±7	4.2±2.1	–	–	–	178±71	10/37	
7	14	f	28±7	–	25±5	396±34	–	–	3/14	Sibbald et al., 1981
	5	g	38±7	–	31±3	432±50	–	–	5/5	
8	17	h	23±10	–	29±17	–	–	–	17/17	Vito et al., 1974
	8	i	12±5	–	28±16	–	–	–	0/8	

[a]Data are mean ± SD; range in parentheses, if available.

[b]Patient group definititions: a, severe; b, moderate; c, severe respiratory failure; d, low Ppa; e, high Ppa; f, responders; g, nonresponders to corticosteroids; h, deaths; i, survivors. See original references for details.

[c]PaO_2 on a variety of levels of F_IO_2 and PEEP. *Source*: Data adapted from references noted.

terenol infusion reduced PVR and that nitroprusside reduced both PVR and PA pressures in 15 patients studied early in the course of ARDS. However, these authors also reported failure of vasodilators to relieve pulmonary hypertension during the late stages of severe ARDS, and they hypothesized that vascular obstruction might also play a role (Zapol et al., 1985). This hypothesis is supported by studies showing pulmonary artery filling defects detected by bedside balloon occlusion angiography (Greene et al., 1981) and by postmortem examination revealing obstruction of vessels by thromboemboli, leukocytes, swollen endothelium, and fibrocellular intimal proliferation (Tomashefski et al., 1983). In addition, when ARDS was of prolonged duration (greater than 10 days), vascular remodeling was seen on postmortem examination with extension of smooth muscle into normally nonmuscular arteries and increasing medial thickness of muscular arteries (Tomashefski et al., 1983; Snow et al., 1982). Thus, the causes of pulmonary hypertension in ARDS include vasoconstriction, possibly more important in the early phases of the disease, and vascular obstruction, which becomes more prominent with prolonged duration of illness. To our knowledge, there have been no studies in humans with ARDS of pulmonary vascular responsiveness to vasoconstrictor stimuli such as alveolar hypoxia or circulating vasoactive mediators. Thus, the role of altered vascular reactivity in the development of pulmonary hypertension in this disease remains unknown.

Examination of the data summarized in Table 1 reveals no apparent correlation of mean PA pressure or PVR with shunt fraction or various measures of the severity of impairment of oxygenation. This lack of correlation of pulmonary hypertension with shunt fraction is graphically illustrated in Figure 1. Thus, the magnitude of pulmonary hypertension does not appear to be a marker for the severity of respiratory failure.

Some authors have reported improved survival in patients with ARDS in whom pulmonary hypertension was not present. Vito and coauthors found that survivors of ARDS associated with sepsis had normal PA pressures, while nonsurvivors had significantly higher pressures (Table 1, study 8; Vito et al., 1974). Similarly, Sibbald et al. (1978) reported significantly higher mortality in septic patients with widened differences (greater than 5 mmHg) between PA diastolic and capillary wedge pressures (Table 1, study 6). Sibbald and colleagues also reported that patients with ARDS due to sepsis who responded to corticosteroid therapy with decreased albumin clearance into bronchial secretions had lower PA pressures than nonresponders both before and after therapy and less mortality (Table 1, study 7; Sibbald et al., 1981). Other studies summarized in Table 1 fail to demonstrate an apparent correlation between the degree of pulmonary hypertension and mortality. Available data relating PA pressure and mortality are graphically illustrated in Figure 2. Indeed, in a prospective study of 88 patients with ARDS from a variety of causes, PA pressures measured on the day of entry into the study did not predict subsequent mortality (Fowler et al., 1985).

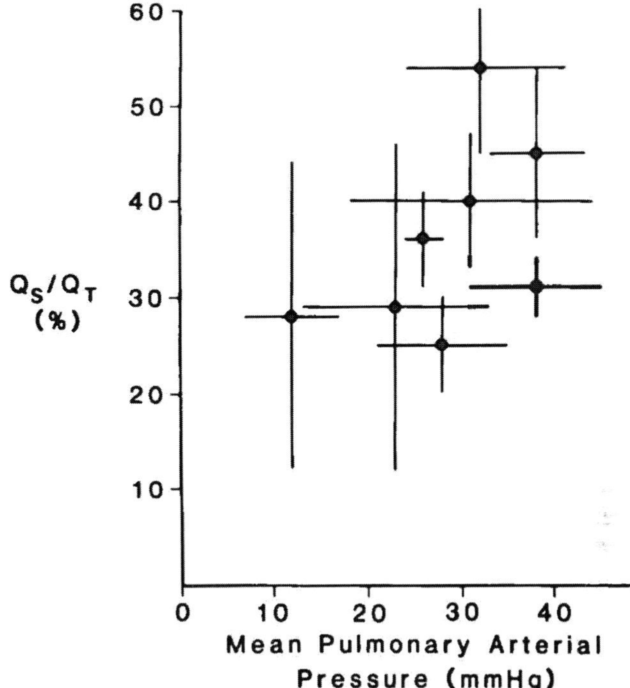

Figure 1 In the series listed in Table 1, there is no apparent correlation of mean pulmonary arterial pressure ($\bar{P}pa$) with shunt fraction (QS/QT). Data are mean ± SD.

This is not surprising, since other studies have shown that sepsis is an important cause of mortality in ARDS, outweighing even respiratory failure as a direct cause of death (Bell et al., 1983; Montgomery et al., 1985). Thus pulmonary hypertension does not appear to be associated with mortality in patients with ARDS, and the clinical significance of this finding remains unclear.

Although the presence of pulmonary hypertension does not appear to be related to the magnitude of hypoxemia or to mortality in ARDS, studies in animals suggest that abnormalities in pulmonary vascular control could affect the extent of edema and the adequacy of gas exchange in acute lung injury. For example, studies of acid aspiration pneumonia in isolated dog lungs, summarized by Permutt (1985), showed significant positive correlation between PA pressure and the extent of edema, as assessed by rate and lung weight gain. When PA pressure was reduced by infusion of vasodilators, the rate of weight gain was decreased (Permutt, 1985). Similarly, others have demonstrated that alveolar hy-

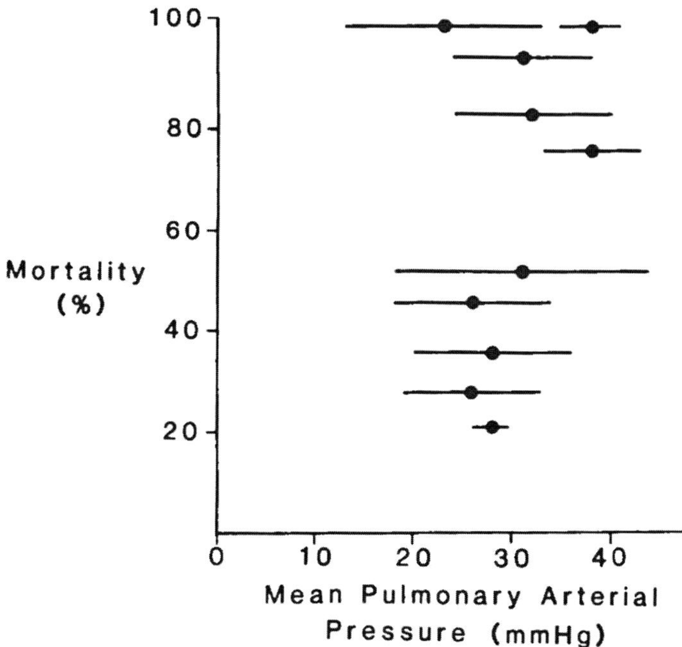

Figure 2 Mortality from ARDS did not correlate with mean pulmonary arterial pressure in the series listed in Table 1.

poxia sufficient to double PVR increased lung lymph flow or lung weight, presumably by increasing the pulmonary transvascular gradient of hydraulic pressure and thereby increasing filtration of fluid into the lungs (Bressack and Bland, 1980; Mitzner and Sylvester, 1981). Thus, increases in PA pressure can exacerbate the degree of edema formation. However, the clinical significance of this phenomenon is not clear since Brigham et al. (1983) found that increases in extravascular lung water, assessed with a multiple tracer technique, did not correlate with mortality or PA-PaO_2 in 14 patients with ARDS.

The adequacy of gas exchange in acute lung injury is in part dependent on the preservation of hypoxic pulmonary vasoconstriction, a reflex mechanism that would serve to divert blood flow away from nonventilated alveoli, thus optimizing ventilation-perfusion matching (Fishman, 1976). The presence of pulmonary hypertension has been shown to blunt the hypoxic pressure response (Benumof and Wahrenbrock, 1975), and depressed hypoxic pressor responses have been described in some animal models of acute lung injury (see below, Newman et al., 1983). Depression of the hypoxic pressor response might be expected to exacerbate shunting and hypoxemia. In support of this, Zapol et al.

(1985) and Weigelt et al. (1982) found that infusion of nitroprusside, an agent that inhibits hypoxic vasoconstriction (Pace, 1978), into patients with ARDS increased shunt fraction and decreased PaO_2. In addition, Brigham et al. (1983) reported that in patients with ARDS, lung vascular [^{14}C]urea permeability surface area correlated with PA-PaO_2 and was significantly lower in survivors. These authors interpreted the lower permeability surface area in survivors as reflective of decreased perfused vascular area and suggested that it reflected reduced perfusion of edematous areas that could aid in optimizing ventilation-perfusion matching.

In summary, pulmonary hypertension has been reported to be present frequently in humans with ARDS. Although there is no clear relation between pulmonary hypertension with mortality or the adequacy of gas exchange, it is clear that abnormal pulmonary circulatory control can influence both the extent of edema formation and the adequacy of gas exchange.

B. Acute Lung Injury—Animal Models

Pulmonary Hypertension in Acute Lung Injury

In the past several years there has been a great deal of experimental work on ARDS utilizing animal models. Dogs and sheep have been frequently studied due to ease of catheterization and ability to monitor lung lymph flow and protein content, a measure of lung vascular fluid flux and permeability. These studies have largely focused on unraveling the pathogenesis of the increased permeability pulmonary edema characteristic of this disorder, and the insights gained are outlined in revent reviews (Brigham and Meyrick, 1986; Heffner et al., 1987; Tate and Repine, 1983). Since many of these studies utilized catheterized, intact animals or isolated, perfused lungs, information can also be gleaned from them regarding the pathogenesis of abnormalities in pulmonary circulatory control.

Pulmonary hypertension, manifested by increased PA pressure and vascular resistance, has been described in many animal models of acute lung injury, including those due to embolization with air (Ohkuda et al., 1981), glass beads (Mlczoch et al., 1978), autologous clot (Utsunomiya et al., 1981), or thrombin infusion (Johnson et al., 1982); antiplatelet antibody (Snapper et al., 1984); endotoxin (Brigham et al., 1979); oleic acid (Julien et al., 1986); platelet activating factor (Voelkel et al., 1982); phorbal myristate acetate (Shasby et al. 1982); splanchnic artery occlusion (Pilati and Maron, 1985); zymosan-activated plasma (Perkowski et al., 1983); H_2O_2 (Tate et al., 1984); and the organic peroxide *tert*-butyl hydroperoxide (Gurtner et al., 1983). However, pulmonary hypertension is not an inevitable accompaniment of acute lung injury since it was not observed in sheep injured with alpha-naphthylthiourea (ANTU) (Rutili et al., 1982) or hyperoxia (Newman et al., 1983), despite increased microvascular permeability as manifested by increased lung lymph protein flow. Species differences have been reported in the association of pulmonary hypertension with increased permeability edema. For example, ethchlorvynol caused transient pulmonary hypertension in sheep (Glauser et al., 1982) but not in dogs (Fairman et al., 1981); and hydrogen peroxide caused increased perfusion pressures in lungs isolated from rabbits (Tate et al., 1984) but not in lungs isolated from rats (Burghuber et al., 1984).

The time course of pulmonary hypertension with acute lung injury is variable. In most models, such as those caused by endotoxin (Brigham et al., 1979), oleic acid (Julien et al., 1986), thrombin infusion (Johnson et al., 1982), or phorbal myristate acetate (Loyd et al., 1983), there is an immediate increase in PA pressures and PVR, followed by decreases to more modest levels that are sustained over several hours and accompanied by increased vascular permeability. In others, such as glass bead emboli (Johnson and Malik, 1982), the pulmonary hypertension is sustained at high levels.

As in the case of ARDS in humans, there are several possible causes of pulmonary hypertension seen in animal models of acute lung injury: vasoconstriction of pre- or postcapillary vessels; vascular obstruction by clot, foreign bodies, or inflammatory cell aggregates; compression of vessels; vascular obstruction by clot, foreign bodies, or inflammatory cell aggregates; compression of vessels by perivascular edema; and hypoxic vasoconstriction. Evidence for vasoconstriction includes the diminution in hypertension seen with time in many models, as noted above. Also, vasodilators, such as prostacyclin in the case of endotoxin (Demling et al., 1981b) or thrombin infusion (Perlman et al., 1986) and nitroprusside or isoproterenol in the case of acid aspiration (Miuus et al., 1985) or oleic acid (Prewitt and Wood, 1981), have been reported to be effective in preventing pulmonary hypertension. Finally, evidence for the effect of vasoactive mediators includes the decreases in pulmonary hypertension in some models (see below) by treatment of animals with inhibitors of synthesis or antagonists of arachidonic acid metabolites. The contribution of vascular obstruction can be inferred from studies demonstrating large and small vessel thrombosis (Tomashefski et al., 1983; Jones et al., 1985), platelet sequestration (Spragg et al., 1982), leukocyte aggregates (Meyrick and Brigham, 1983), and endothelial cell blebbing or swelling (Meyrick et al., 1972; O'Brien et al., 1985). Severe edema formation due to increased permeability (Boiteau et al., 1986) or hydrostatic pressure (Ngeow and Mitzner, 1983) can also contribute to pulmonary hypertension. The contribution of hypoxic vasoconstriction depends upon the degree of hypoxia and the maintenance of normal responsiveness of the pulmonary circulation to hypoxia (see below).

The site of vasoconstriction after acute lung injury may differ among models. In hydrostatic edema, increased PA pressure was due to increases in both capillary and upstream extraalveolar vessels (Ngeow and Mitzner, 1983).

There is evidence for venous constriction after oleic acid-induced injury (Hofman and Ehrhart, 1983; Boiteau et al., 1986). Hypoxia causes predominantly arteriolar constriction (Nagaska et al., 1984), and vasoactive mediators may cause either arteriolar or venous constriction (Brody and Stemmer, 1968).

Considerable evidence has accrued supporting a role for the potent pulmonary vasoconstrictor thromboxane A_2 (TxA_2) as a mediator of the early phase of pulmonary hypertension, but not of subsequent increases in vascular permeability. This has been observed in several models (summarized in Table 2), such as after enotoxin (Huttemeier et al., 1982), thrombin infusion (Garcia-Szabo et al., 1984), platelet activating factor (Heffner et al., 1983), and autologous clot (Utsunomiya et al., 1982b). In the case of endotoxin, pulmonary hypertension was prevented or meliorated by pretreatment with inhibitors of cyclooxygenase (Weir et al., 1976; Hales et al., 1981; Snapper et al., 1983b) or thromboxane synthetase (Casey et al., 1982; Kubo and Kobayashi, 1985; Watkins et al., 1982; Winn et al., 1983; Huttemeier et al., 1982). In addition, concomitant with the early phase of pulmonary hypertension and similarly inhibited, there are increases in blood and lung lymph concentrations of thromboxane B_2 (TxB_2), the stable metabolite of TxA_2 (Hales et al., 1981; Demling et al., 1981a). However, TxA_2 is likely not the only factor responsible for this response, since the hypertension has been reported to be decreased but not totally prevented despite prevention of increased TxB_2 concentrations (Ahmed et al., 1986). Also, cyclooxygenase metabolites of arachidonic acid do not appear to be important mediators of pulmonary hypertension in all models of acute lung injury. For example, pulmonary hypertension after oleic acid has been reported to be unaffected by pretreatment of sheep with either indomethacin (Olanoff et al., 1984) or ibuprofen (Julien et al., 1986). It should be noted that studies using pharmacologic inhibitors should be interpreted with caution since these agents may not be specific in their actions and effects may vary with dosage.

Lipoxygenase products of arachidonic acid metabolism might also play a role in pulmonary hypertension seen after acute lung injury (Table 2), since the lipoxygenase end-organ receptor antagonist FPL-57231 completely blocked pulmonary hypertension seen after endotoxin (Ahmed et al., 1986), and diethylcarbamazine, a phospholipase A_2 inhibitor, prevented pulmonary hypertension seen after platelet activating factor (Kenzora et al., 1984; Voelkel et al., 1982). The lipoxygenase product leukotriene C_4,D_4 is also a potent pulmonary vasoconstrictor (Voelkel et al., 1984; Hand et al., 1981). Another 5-lipoxygenase product, 5-hydroxy-6,8,11,14-eicosatetraenoic acid, was increased in lung lymph after endotoxin (Ogletree et al., 1982). The cellular source of vasoconstrictor cyclooxygenase or lipoxygenase metabolites of arachidonic acid metabolites is as yet unknown. Potential sources include polymorphonuclear leukocytes (Lewis and Austen, 1984), platelets (Goetzl, 1980), and cells of the vascular wall (Piper and Galton, 1984).

Table 2 Mechanisms of Pulmonary Hypertension in Some Animals Models of Acute Lung Injury – Effects on Pulmonary Hypertension of Pharmacologic Inhibition of Arachidonic Acid Metabolism[a]

		Enzyme inhibited		
Cause[b]	Species	Cyclooxygenase	Thromboxane synthetase	Lipoxygenase
Acid aspiration	Dog	–	N (Huval et al., 1983a)	–
Autologous clot	Dog	D (Utsunomiya, 1982a)	D (Utsunomiya, 1982a)	–
Antiplatelet antibodies	Sheep	P (Snapper et al., 1984)	–	–
Endotoxin	Sheep	D (Snapper et al., 1983b)	D (Kubo and Kobayaski, 1985; Watkins et al., 1982; Huttemeier et al., 1982)	P (Ahmed et al., 1986)
	Goat	–	P (Winn et al., 1983)	–
	Dog	P (Weir et al., 1976; Hales et al., 1981)	P (Hales et al., 1981)	–
	Baboon	–	P (Casey et al., 1982)	–

	Pig	D (Olson et al., 1985)		
Glass beads	Dog	D (Mlczoch et al., 1978)	–	–
H_2O_2	Rabbit	D (Tate et al., 1984)	–	–
	Rat	N (Burghuber, 1984)	–	D (Burghuber, 1984)
Mesenteric ischemia	Dog	P (Wilkerson, 1977)	–	–
Oleic acid	Sheep	N (Julien et al., 1986; Olanoff et al., 1984)	–	–
PAF	Dog	–	–	P (Kenzora et 1984)
	Rabbit	–	P (Heffner et al., 1983)	
	Rat	D (Voelkel et al, 1982)	–	P (Voelkel et al., 1982)

Table 2 (continued)

Cause[b]	Species	Enzyme inhibited		
		Cyclooxygenase	Thromboxane synthetase	Lipoxygenase
Thrombin	Sheep	N (Johnson and Malik, 1985)	D (Garcia-Szabo et al., 1983, 1984)	–
ZAP	Sheep	D (Fountain et al., 1980; Perkowski et al., 1983)	–	–

[a]N, no effect; D, decreased; P, prevented.
[b]PAF, platelet-activating factor; ZAP, zymosan-activated plasma.

Another vasoconstrictor mediator that may contribute to pulmonary hypertension due to autologous clot is serotonin (5-hydroxytryptamine) (Hechtman et al., 1984). Pretreatment of animals with the serotonin antagonist cyproheptadine (Utsonomiya et al., 1981) prevented, and ketanserin, a serotonin receptor antagonist (Huval et al., 1983b), reversed pulmonary hypertension after autologous clot infusion. Moreover, autologous clot infusion caused plasma levels of 5-hydroxytryptamine to increase (Utsonomiya et al., 1981). In clinical trials, ketanserin decreased physiologic shunt and PA pressure in patients with early (4 days or less), but not with late, ARDS associated with a variety of etiologies (Huval et al., 1984). Acute lung injury may result in decreased uptake of 5-hydroxytryptamine by pulmonary endothelium in animal models (Block and Fisher, 1977; Block and Schoen, 1981) and in humans with ARDS (Gillis et al., 1986). In addition, platelets, an important source of 5-hydroxytryptamine, were found to be sequestered in the pulmonary circulation of patients with acute respiratory failure (Schneider et al., 1980). These results suggest that 5-hydroxytryptamine might be an important mediator of abnormalities in pulmonary circulatory control in ARDS.

Considerable effort has been devoted to determining the roles of leukocytes and platelets in the development of increased permeability edema (summarized in Table 3 and reviewed by Heffner et al., 1987; Tate and Repine, 1983; Brigham and Meyrick, 1986). These studies have usually entailed depletion of circulating leukocytes by bone marrow depression with antimetabolities, platelet depletion with antiplatelet antibody, or perfusion of isolated organs with cell-free perfusate. In interpreting these studies, it should be kept in mind that it is possible that residual, marginated leukocytes or platelets within the circulation of either intact animals or isolated lungs might be sufficient to release potent vasoactive mediators. Although neutropenia attenuated increased vascular permeability in the air emboli (Flick et al., 1981), endotoxin (Heflin and Brigham, 1981), and thrombin infusion models (Tahamont and Malik, 1983), little or no effect on early pulmonary hypertension was noted. In addition, endotoxin-induced leukopenia did not correlate with the magnitude of pulmonary hypertension (Snapper et al., 1983a). Also, hydroxyurea-induced neutropenia had no effect on vascular permeability or on pulmonary hypertension seen after oleic acid (Julien et al., 1986) or phorbal myristate acetate (Dyer and Snapper, 1986). In contrast, in the case of glass bead emboli (Johnson and Malik, 1982) and in one study of endotoxin-induced (Huttemeier et al., 1982) injury, the magnitude of pulmonary hypertension was decreased by leukocyte depletion. In addition, complement activation by infusion of zymosan-activated plasma caused marked granulocyte aggregation within pulmonary capillaries and pulmonary hypertension, although changes in vascular permeability were small (Fountain et al., 1980; Meyrick and Brigham, 1984). In some studies, inhibition of TxA_2 synthesis by cyclooxygenase inhibitors prevented the pulmonary hypertensive

Table 3 Mechanisms of Pulmonary Hypertension in Some Animal Models of Acute Lung Injury – Effect on Pulmonary Hypertension of Depletion of Leukocytes, Platelets, or Fibrinogen[a]

Cause[b]	Species	Substance Depleted		
		Leukocytes	Platelets	Fibrongen
Air emboli	Sheep	N (Flick et al., 1981)	–	–
Endotoxin	Sheep	N (Heflin and Brigham, 1981)	N (Snapper et al., 1984)	–
		D (Huttemeier et al., 1982)	–	–
	Dog	–	P (Bredenberg et al., 1980)	–
Glass beads	Sheep	N (Flick et al., 1981)	D (Binder, 1979)	D (Binder et al., 1979)
	Dog	D (Mlczoch et al., 1978)	–	–

Oleic acid	Sheep	N (Julien et al., 1986)	N (Julien et al., 1986)	–
PMA	Sheep	N (Dyer and Snapper, 1986)	–	–
	Rabbit	N (Shasby et al., 1982)	–	–
Thrombin	Sheep	N (Tahamont and Malik, 1983)	N (Tahamont and Malik, 1983)	D (Johnson et al., 1983)
ZAP	Sheep	–	N (McDonald et al., 1983)	–

[a]N, no effect; D, decreased; P, prevented.
[b]PMA, phorbal myristate acetate; ZAP, zymosan-activated plasma.

response to zymosan-activated plasma (Fountain et al., 1980; McDonald et al., 1983). These results suggest that when there is sufficient leukocyte sequestration within the lung, pulmonary hypertension may result from vascular obstruction or vasoactive mediator (e.g., TxA_2 release from leukocytes, even when changes in vascular permeability are less severe. However, Johnson et al. (1984) reported no differences in lung leukocyte sequestration among sheep that responded or did not respond to complement activation induced by cobra venom factor. Thus, although leukocytes may potentiate the increased permeability aspect of some models of lung injury, the role of these cells in the pulmonary hypertensive response is variable and may depend upon the degree of leukocyte sequestration.

Platelet depletion prevented pulmonary hypertension in one study of endotoxin-induced injury in dogs (Bredenberg et al., 1980) and decreased it after glass bead emboli (Mlczoch et al., 1978) but had little or no effect on pulmonary hypertension in other studies of injury due to endotoxin (Snapper et al., 1984), oleic acid (Julien et al., 1986), thrombin infusion (Tahamont and Malik, 1983), or zymosan-activated plasma (McDonald et al., 1983). Platelet deposition within the lung accompanied lung injury after oleic acid (Spragg et al., 1982), endotoxin (Hechtman et al., 1978), hemorrhagic shock (Martin et al., 1981), and acid aspiration (Utsunomiya et al., 1982a). Thus, normal circulating levels of platelets do not appear to be necessary for pulmonary hypertension after all forms of acute lung injury, although platelet entrapment may occur. These studies do not exclude a role for potent vasoactive mediators released from residual platelets, such as TxA_2 or 5-hydroxytryptamine (see above), or interactions between platelets and leukocytes (Heffner et al., 1987).

Thrombosis of both small and larger pulmonary vessels is frequently found in lungs of patients who died with ARDS (Bone et al., 1976; Jones et al., 1985; Blaisdell and Schlobohm, 1973) and was the most frequent pathologic finding in the series of 22 patients reported by Tomashefski et al. (1983). Saldeen reported a possibly important role for fibrinogen, fibrin, or their degradation products in the pathogenesis of ARDS (Saldeen, 1976). They found extensive fibrin deposition in lungs following trauma or orthopedic surgery, and the extent of deposition correlated with respiratory impairment. In addition, activation of intravascular coagulation has been reported in patients with ARDS (Carvalho, 1985). Thus, the clotting cascade has been implicated in the development of ARDS and has been assessed in animal models (Table 3). Johnson et al. (1983) found that fibrinogen depletion prevented both the pulmonary hypertension and increased permeability seen after thrombin infusion in sheep, but that inhibition of fibrinolysis did not alter the pulmonary hypertension, although vascular permeability did decrease (see Chapter 13). However, neither heparin anticoagulation nor fibrinogen depletion altered the pulmonary hypertension seen after glass bead emboli (Binder et al., 1979). Heparin anticoagulation also did not prevent pulmonary hypertension after air emboli (Flick et al., 1983), nor was there evidence of activation of the clotting cascade (O'Brodovich et al., 1983). Differences in the effect on pulmonary hypertension of fibrinogen depletion in these models may relate to the nature of the infused substance, with the clotting cascade playing a larger role in the case of thrombin infusion but not after vascular obstruction by air or glass beads.

Since activated neutrophils are capable of releasing toxic oxygen metabolites, such as H_2O_2 and superoxide anion, and because neutrophils appear to participate in the development of increased permeability edema (Tate and Repine, 1983), it is possible that oxidants also play a role in pulmonary hypertension (see Table 4). In support of this, Tate and colleagues observed that perfusion of isolated rabbit lungs with purine plus xanthine oxidase caused vasoconstriction, which was inhibited by catalase (Tate et al., 1982) and associated with TxB_2 release into lung effluent (Tate et al., 1982). These results suggested that H_2O_2 might stimulate vasoconstriction via TxA_2 production. In addition the organic peroxide *tert*-butyl hydroperoxide also stimulated vasoconstriction in isolated rabbit lungs (Gurtner et al., 1983). In vivo investigations of the role of oxidants have assessed the effect of agents that dissipate oxidants, such as superoxide dismutase (SOD) and catalase. SOD did not prevent the pulmonary hypertensive response to endotoxin (Traber et al., 1985) or air emboli (Flick et al., 1983). The combination of SOD and the vehicle ficoll did decrease the pulmonary hypertension seen after thrombin infusion, but Ficoll alone nearly completely inhibited the response (Johnson et al., 1986). The reasons for this inhibition by ficoll are as yet unclear but may relate to effects on neutrophil function. Nevertheless, superoxide anion per se does not appear to be responsible for pulmonary hypertension in these models of lung injury. On the other hand, catalase, which consumes H_2O_2, did ameliorate pulmonary hypertension caused by endotoxin in sheep (Milligan et al., 1985) and prevented pressor responses to H_2O_2 in isolated rabbit lungs (Tate et al., 1984). Thus, H_2O_2 may mediate some of the pulmonary hypertensive response, perhaps via TxA_2 production.

Corticosteroids, in particular high doses of methylprednisolone, have been examined for ability to ameliorate acute lung injury because of reports of efficacy in humans (Sibbald et al., 1981). Methylprednisolone only slightly decreased pulmonary hypertension after endotoxin (Brigham et al., 1981). However, the combination of nonsteroidal and steroidal anti-inflammatory agents was very effective in preventing pulmonary hypertension after endotoxin (Begley et al., 1984; Olson et al., 1985) as well as release of arachidonic acid metabolites (Ogletree et al., 1986). Methylprednisolone did not affect pulmonary hypertension caused by oleic acid in sheep (Julien et al., 1986) but did prevent increased PA pressures in isolated, perfused lobes of dog lung (Broe et al., 1981; Hofman and Ehrhart, 1983). The reason for these conflicting results is not clear, but differences in species or type of preparation may play a role.

Table 4 Mechanisms of Pulmonary Hypertension in Some Animal Models of Acute Lung Injury – Effects on Pulmonary Hypertension of Steriods or Oxidant Scavengers[a]

Cause	Species	Steriods	Oxidant Scavengers: Superoxide Dismutase	Oxidant Scavengers: Catalase
Acid Aspiration	Dog	P (Toung et al., 1976)	–	–
Air emboli	Sheep	–	N (Flick et al., 1983)	–
Endotoxin	Sheep	D[b] (Begley et al., 1984)	N (Traber et al., 1985)	P (Milligan et al., 1985)
	Pig	D (Olson et al., 1985)	–	–
H_2O_2	Rabbit	–	N (Tate et al., 1984)	P (Tate et al., 1984)
Oleic acid	Sheep	N (Julien et al., 1986)	–	–
	Dog	P (Broe et al., 1981)	–	–
Thrombin	Sheep	–	N (Johnson et al., 1986)	–
ZAP	Sheep	–	N (Perkowski et al., 1983)	–

[a]N, no effect; D, decreased; P, prevented; ZAP, zymosan-activated plasma.
[b]Combination of methylprednisolone plus meclofenamate prevented pulmonary hypertension.

The recently described peptidergic substance endothelial cell-derived vasoconstrictor is among the myriad of potential vasoconstrictor mediators of pulmonary hypertension that may be relevant to acute lung injury. This substance is produced by cultured endothelial cells (O'Brien et al., 1987; Hickey et al., 1985; Gillespie et al., 1986a). In addition, anoxia caused contraction of vascular rings with intact endothelium (Rubanyi and Vanhoutte, 1985), an effect that may be caused by the same agent. Since acute lung injury is frequently associated with endothelial cell dysfunction, it is tempting to speculate that this endothelial cell-derived factor may play a role in pulmonary hypertension.

In summary, pulmonary hypertension has been observed as a consequence of many, but not all, animal models of acute lung injury. Vasoconstriction occurs in the early phase of injury, but vascular obstruction and edema formation are also likely to contribute to increases in PVR, particularly later in the course. Evidence is available that TxA_2, lipoxygenase products, and serotonin are chemical mediators of vasoconstriction. Oxidants may play a role by stimulating TxA_2 release. Depletion of blood cells such as leukocytes and platelets or inhibition of clot formation does not uniformly prevent pulmonary hypertension.

Effects of Acute Lung Injury on Vascular Reactivity

Vascular reactivity to hypoxia and circulating vasoactive mediators has been assessed in a few models of acute lung injury (Table 5). Changes in vascular reactivity are important since decreased reactivity to hypoxia could exacerbate V/Q mismatching and thereby increase hypoxemia. For example, vasodilator drug infusion increased shunt fraction in dogs with pneumococcal pneumonia (Goldzimer et al., 1974), presumably via inhibition of hypoxic vasoconstriction (Hiser et al., 1975). Other investigators have suggested that failure of hypoxic vasoconstriction is in part responsible for hypoxemia seen in pneumococcal pneumonia (Light et al., 1981). On the other hand, increased vasoconstriction responses to vasoactive mediators might precipitate or exacerbate pulmonary hypertension (see below).

Animal models of acute lung injury in which vascular reactivity has been found to be depressed include those caused by endotoxin (Hales et al., 1981; Hutchison et al., 1985; Reeves and Grover, 1974; Weir et al., 1976), hyperoxia (Newman et al., 1981, 1983), H_2O_2 (Burghuber et al., 1984), and platelet activating factor (Gillespie and Bowdy, 1986). In the case of endotoxin, Reeves and Grover (1974) demonstrated some years ago that, in dogs, endotoxin caused loss of pulmonary pressor responses to hypoxia and to $PGF_{2\alpha}$ but not to serotonin. In subsequent studies, Weir et al. (1976) found that pretreatment with the cyclooxygenase inhibitors meclofenamate or indomethacin prevented loss of hypoxic vasoconstriction but that platelet depletion with antiplatelet serum had no

Table 5 Effect of Acute Lung Injury on Vascular Reactivity

Cause[a]	Species	Vascular reactivity		Reference
		Increased	Decreased	
ANTU	Rat	+		Hill and Rounds, 1983
Endotoxin	Dog		+	Reeves and Grover, 1974; Weir et al., 1976; Hales et al., 1981
	Sheep		+	Hutchison et al., 1985
Hyperoxia	Rat		+	Newman et al., 1981
	Sheep		+	Newman et al., 1983
H_2O_2	Rat		+	Burghuber et al., 1984
Monocrotoline	Rat	+		Hilliker and Roth, 1985; Gillespie et al., 1986b
PAF	Rat		+	Gillespie and Bowdy 1986

[a]ANTU, alpha-naphthylthiourea; PAF, platelet-activating factor.

effect. These results suggested that some cyclooxygenase product might be responsible for loss of vasoreactivity. Hales and colleagues (1981) subsequently found that low doses of endotoxin in dogs caused loss of pressor responses to hypoxia, angiotensin II, and $PGF_{2\alpha}$ without pulmonary hypertension and that higher doses caused pulmonary hypertension plus loss of hypoxic vasoconstriction. In these studies both doses of endotoxin also increased blood concentrations of both TxB_2 and 6-keto $PGF_{1\alpha}$, the stable prostacyclin metabolite, but not of $PGF_{2\alpha}$. Both loss of vasoreactivity and increases in prostanoid concentrations were prevented by pretreatment of animals with indomethacin. Thus, loss of vasoreactivity was related to a cyclooxygenase metabolite, such as prostacyclin, and did not appear to be due to the pulmonary hypertensive response to endotoxin. However, Hutchison and colleagues (1985) found that, in endotoxin-treated sheep, blunting of hypoxic vasoconstriction was not reversed by meclofenamate given 4.5 hr after endotoxin. In addition, there was no correlation between lung lymph levels of TxB_2 or 6-keto-$PGF_{1\alpha}$ and the degree of blunting of hypoxic pressor responses. In summary, endotoxin causes loss of vasoreactivity independent of pulmonary hypertension, and both abnormalities in pulmonary circulatory control are prevented by cyclooxytenase inhibitors and associated with increased circulating and lung lymph prostanoid levels. However, once the acute injury is established, neither is reversed by subsequent treatment with meclofenamate.

Hyperoxia might be expected to alter pulmonary vascular reactivity via oxidant production. Indeed, Newman et al. (1981) found that exposure of rats to 100% oxygen for 48 hr resulted in blunting of pressor responses to hypoxia but not to angiotensin II, as assessed in isolated, perfused lungs. This blunting was reversed by addition of meclofenamate to perfusate, suggesting that it was due to a cyclooxygenase product. Subsequent studies in intact sheep (Newman et al., 1983) and rabbits and lambs (Raj et al., 1985) showed that oxygen breathing for 72-96 hr caused increased lung vascular permeability that was not neutrophil dependent (Raj et al., 1985) and not associated with pulmonary hypertension. As was the case in rats, oxygen breathing caused loss of hypoxic pressor responses in sheep, and pressor responses to a vasoconstrictor PGH_2 analog were also lost (Newman et al., 1983). Meclofenamate treatment of sheep failed to restore hypoxic pressor responses in oxygen-breathing sheep, and there were no changes in lung lymph prostacyclin or thromboxane metabolites after hyperoxic exposure. A preliminary report relates that newborn lambs exposed to hyperoxia also lose pressor responses to both hypoxia and intravenous lipid injections (Teague et al., 1986). Thus, hyperoxic lung injury causes loss of pulmonary vasoreactivity in the absence of pulmonary hypertension. The relation of this effect to prostanoid metabolites is not clear and may be affected by species differences.

A specific oxidant, H_2O_2, was examined for effects on vascular reactivity by Burghuber et al. (1984). They found that H_2O_2 produced by glucose and glucose oxidase in cell-free perfusates of isolated rat lungs caused loss of reactivity to hypoxia and blunting of responses to angiotensin II. This effect was prevented by catalase, but not by indomethacin, despite doses of indomethacin sufficient to inhibit H_2O_2-stimulated increases in lung effluent TxB_2, $PGF_{2\alpha}$, and 6-keto-$PGF_{1\alpha}$. Thus, although TxA_2 may mediate pulmonary hypertension caused by H_2O_2 (see above and Tate et al., 1984) these arachidonic acid metabolites did not appear to be responsible for vasoreactivity changes, and the cause of this effect remains unclear.

Platelet activating factor that been found to cause acute lung injury and pulmonary hypertension (Kenzora et al., 1984; Bessin et al., 1983; Halonen et al., 1980; Lichey et al., 1984), which was inhibited by imidazole (Heffner et al., 1983) or diethylcarbamazine (Voelkel et al., 1982), However, the effects of this agent on pulmonary circulatory control may be dose related in that McMurtry and Morris (1986) found that low doses acted as vasodilators in preconstricted intact rats, isolated rat lungs, and pulmonary artery rings and that this effect was not prevented by meclofenamate. Similarly, Gillespie and Bowdy (1986) reported that the vasoconstrictor effect of platelet activating factor was seen only at high doses. These investigators also reported that high doses of the agent blunted pressor responses to hypoxia and angiotensin II, but not to KC1 (Gillespie and Bowdy, 1986). Thus, the effects of platelet activating factor are dose related, with higher doses causing vasoconstriction, perhaps via arachidonic acid metabolites, and blunting of vascular reactivity. Lower doses, on the other hand, act as pulmonary vasodilators.

Vascular reactivity has been found to be increased in two models of acute lung injury—those due to alpha-naphthylthiourea (ANTU) (Hill and Rounds, 1983) and monocrotoline (Hilliker and Roth, 1985; Gillespie et al., 1986). In the cause of ANTU lung injury, pulmonary hypertension was not seen in intact animals (Rutili et al., 1982), except when related to vehicle (Havill et al., 1982), although the agent did cause increased permeability edema. Studies done in our laboratory (Hill and Rounds, 1983) showed that blood-perfused lungs isolated from rats treated with ANTU 4 hr previously had enhanced pressor responses to hypoxia and to angiotensin II (Fig. 3). This effect was not reversed by meclofenamate and seemed to be related to endothelial cell injury, as assessed by increased permeability edema and depressed conversion of circulating angiotensin I to angiotensin II, a metabolic function of pulmonary endothelial cells (O'Brien et al., 1985). These results led us to hypothesize that endothelial cell injury resulting in enhanced vascular reactivity might eventually result in pulmonary hypertension (see below).

The pyrrolizidine alkaloid monocrotoline also causes endothelial cell injury with increased permeability edema (Sugita et al., 1983; Miller et al..

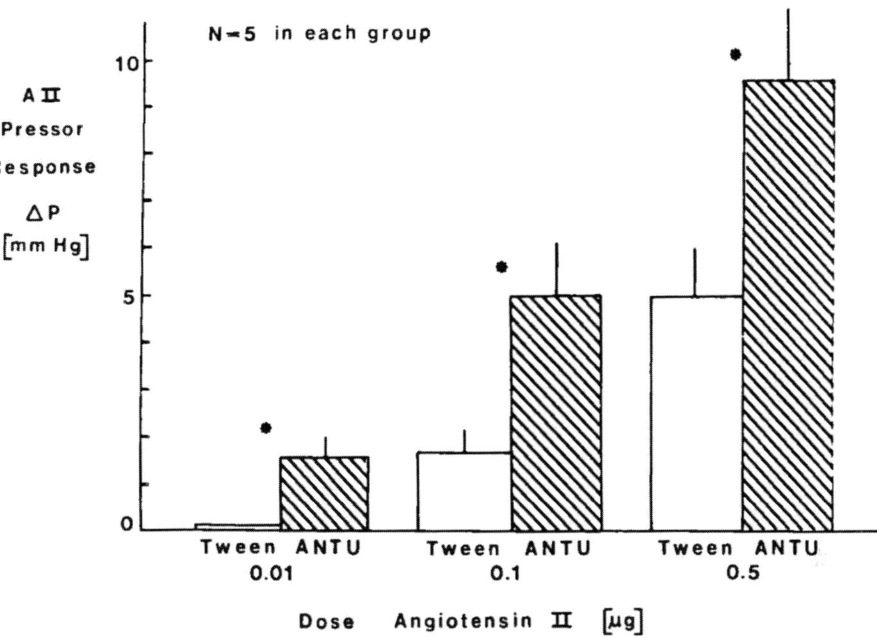

Figure 3 Pressor responses (baseline to peak mean pulmonary arterial pressure, ΔP, mmHg) to intraarterial bolus injections of angiotensin II in lungs isolated from rats pretreated with Tween 80 (vehicle) or alpha-naphthylthiourea (ANTU). Data are means ± SE. *Significant difference at $p < 0.05$. (Reprinted from Hill and Rounds, 1983.)

1978) and depression of endothelial metabolic functions (Hilliker et al., 1982). This acute injury is followed in 7-14 days by the development of sustained pulmonary hypertension (Meyrick et al., 1980; Bruner et al., 1983). Czer et al. (1986) found that within 5 min of injection of monocrotoline into dogs, pulmonary hypertension was seen that consists of an early peak followed by a fall. After 1-2 hr, PA pressures and PVR increased again and the hypertension was sustained for at least 6 hr. This effect was prevented by infusion of prostacyclin, suggesting that the initial pulmonary hypertension is due to vasoconstriction. Several investigators have shown increased pulmonary vascular reactivity to a variety of stimuli, at times before right ventricular hypertrophy or increased medial thickness of vessels has occurred (Hilliker and Roth, 1985) and as early as 4 days after monocrotoline injury (Gillespie et al., 1986b). In addition, Altiere and co-workers (1986) found that main pulmonary arteries isolated from rats treated 4 days previously with monocrotoline had enhanced contractile responses to KC1, angiotensin II, and norepinephrine. Arteries isolated after 7 or 14 days had depressed contractile responses, but after 14 days there was depression of relaxant responses to acetylcholine. Thus, vascular responsiveness to vasoconstrictors is increased in the early stages of monocrotoline lung injury when pulmonary hypertension due to vasoconstriction is present, while response to vasodilators may be depressed at later time points. The mechanism of these effects remains to be explored.

In summary, acute lung injury can cause depression or enhancement of vascular reactivity, depending on the cause of injury. The consequences of decreased reactivity may be to worsen V/Q matching and exacerbate hypoxemia, while increased reactivity to vasoconstrictor influences may be an early phase in the development of pulmonary hypertension. The mechanisms of these effects on vascular reactivity are as yet unclear, but prostacyclin production may play a role in depression of reactivity in some models, such as endotoxin or hyperoxia. Whether platelets or leukocytes are contributory is not known. Endothelial cell dysfunction or injury may accompany changes in vascular reactivity, raising the question of whether endothelial cell injury initiates the process resulting in altered vascular reactivity. In this regard, it is tempting to speculate that changes in endothelial cell-derived relaxing factor (EDRF) (reviewed by Vanhoutte et al., 1986; see also Chapter 18) might play a role in changing vascular reactivity with acute lung injury. However, Fedderson et al. (1986) reported that vasodilator responses to acetylcholine were preserved in isolated rat lungs, despite endothelial cell injury due to ANTU or hyperoxia. Further studies are required to elucidate the role, if any, of EDRF in the development of altered vascular reactivity after acute lung injury.

III. Pulmonary Circulatory Control in Chronic Lung Injury

Pulmonary hypertension is a frequent finding in numerous chronic lung disease. The presence of pulmonary hypertension correlates with increased mortality in patients with chronic obstructive lung disease (Burrows et al., 1972). However, considerably less is known regarding pulmonary circulatory control in chronic lung injury. Factors that may contribute to secondary pulmonary hypertension include intimal fibrosis, thrombosis (Wagnevoort, 1980), and vascular remodeling due to chronic hypoxia (Hislop and Reid, 1976). It is beyond the scope of this review to consider anatomic factors contributing to secondary pulmonary hypertension, but attention will be paid to effects of chronic lung injury on pulmonary vascular reactivity. It should be noted that in lung injuries accompanied by significant vascular smooth muscle proliferation, increases in the magnitude of pressor responses may be due to increased muscle mass and not necessarily to altered sensitivity to vasoconstrictor stimuli.

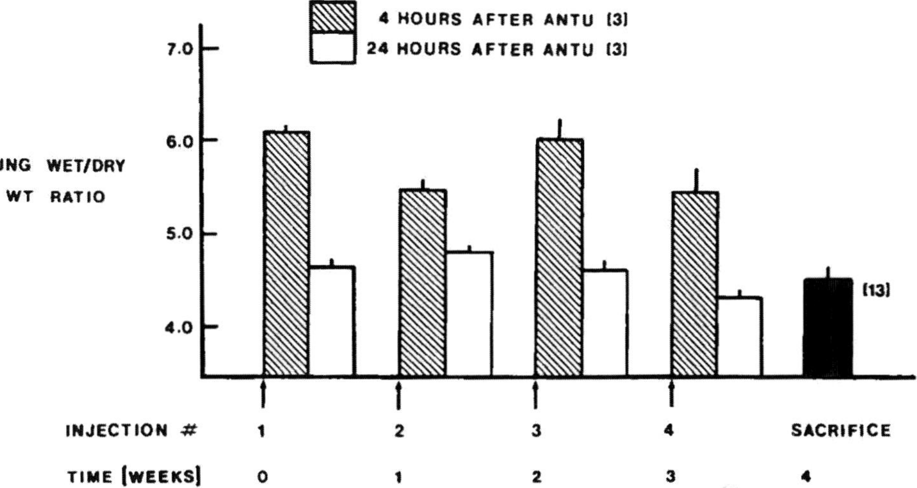

Figure 4 Wet-to-dry weight ratios of lungs 4 hr (hatched bars) and 24 hr (open bars) after four weekly intraperitoneal injections of alpha-naphthylthiourea (ANTU) (10 mg/kg body weight). Lungs from three rats were weighed at each time after each weekly injection. Solid bar is wet-to-dry lung weight ratio in 13 rats sacrificed 1 week after fourth injection. Data are means ± SE. *Significant difference at $p < 0.05$. (Reprinted from Hill et al., 1984).

A. Chronic Lung Injury in Humans

That vasoconstriction contributes to pulmonary hypertension in patients with chronic obstructive lung disease can be inferred from reports of immediate decreases in PA pressure and PVR in response to oxygen administration (Fishman et al., 1952) or vasodilators (Abraham et al., 1969). In addition, acute hypoxia can further increase PA pressures in individuals with chronic obstructive lung disease (Abraham et al., 1967; Westcott et al., 1951; Fishman et al., 1952). However, not all individuals have immediate decreases in PA pressures in response to hypoxia (Fowler and Read, 1963). It has been suggested that responders to oxygen, with intact hypoxic pressor responses, may have better survival (Ashutosh et al., 1983). Variability in preservation of hypoxic vasoconstriction and hyperoxic vasodilatation has also been reported in patients with a variety of interstitial lung diseases, including interstitial fibrosis, sarcoidosis (Weitzenblum et al., 1983), and extrinsic allergic alveolitis (Lupi-Herrera et al., 1981). The reasons for differences in hypoxic vasoconstriction are not clear but do not appear to relate to severity of lung disease or pulmonary hypertension. The existence of variability in pressor responses suggests intraindividual differences in sensitivity to hypoxia, the cause of which is unknown.

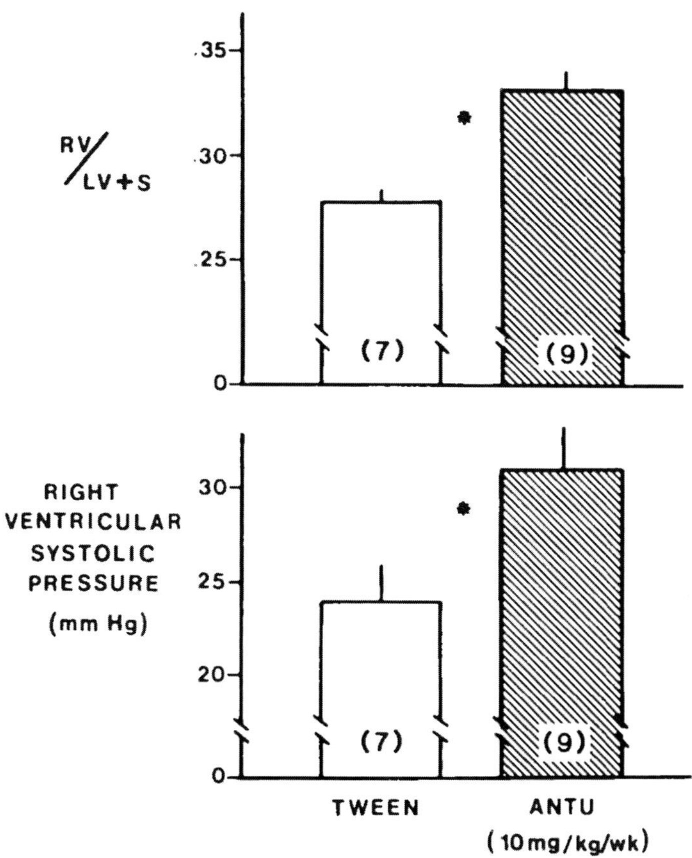

Figure 5 Upper panel, ratios of weights of right ventricle (RV) to left ventricle plus septum (LV + S). Lower panel, right ventricular systolic pressures in rats, obtained 1 week after four weekly injections of Tween 80 (vehicle) or alpha-naphthylthiourea (ANTU, 10 mg/kg body weight). Data are means ± SE. Numbers in parentheses are numbers of animals. *Significant difference at $p<0.05$. (Reprinted from Hill et al., 1984.)

B. Chronic Lung Injury in Animals

Pulmonary vascular reactivity has been studied in a few animal models of chronic lung injury. We found that repeated lung injury due to four weekly ANTU injections in rats caused recurrent increased permeability pulmonary edema (Fig. 4) and sustained pulmonary hypertension, manifested by right ventricular hypertrophy and right ventricular systolic hypertension (Fig. 5; Hill et al., 1984). Fedderson et al. (1986) have subsequently confirmed this finding.

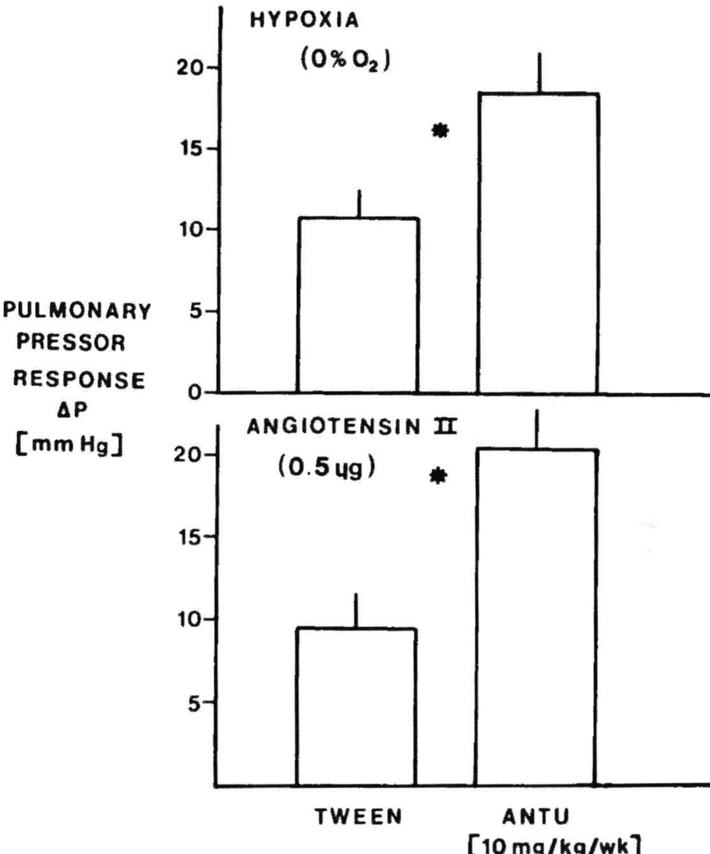

Figure 6 Pulmonary pressor responses (baseline to peak mean pulmonary arterial pressure, Δ P, mmHg) were obtained in isolated, blood-perfused lungs in response to hypoxia and angiotensin II. Lungs were isolated 1 week after four weekly injections of apha-naphthylthiourea (ANTU, 10 mg/kg body weight) or Tween 80 (vehicle). Data are means ± SE. *Significant difference at $p<0.05$. (Reprinted from Hill et al., 1984.)

The magnitude of maximal pressor responses to hypoxia and angiotensin II were increased (Fig. 6). but there was no evidence of medial hypertrophy of pulmonary arterioles. These findings led us to suggest that the enhanced vascular reactivity seen after acute ANTU lung injury (see above) caused sustained vasoconstriction and pulmonary hypertension. It is tempting to speculate that endothelial cell injury somehow precipitated this chain of events culminating in pulmonary hypertension.

Pulmonary vascular reactivity has also been found to be increased in sheep with chronic lung injury due to repeated indomethacin infusion (Meyrick et al., 1985) and following thoracic irradiation (Perkett et al., 1986). Both of these models manifested pulmonary hypertension, but as in the case of ANTU, structural changes were minimal and consisted of reduced diameter of intraacinar arteries. The relative paucity of vascular remodeling suggested that sustained vasoconstriction was important in the development of pulmonary hypertension in these models also.

On the other hand, Meyrick and Brigham (1986) reported that while repeated endotoxin infusion over 10-14 weeks caused pulmonary hypertension in sheep, vascular reactivity to PGH_2 and to hypoxia was decreased between 4 and 8 weeks, at a time when pulmonary hypertension was manifest. Thus, repeated lung injury does not invariably enhance vascular reactivity. The reasons for these differences are not known, but one possible explanation might relate to the more intense accumulation of inflammatory cells in the pulmonary vasculature of sheep subjected to repeated endotoxin infusions as compared to animals treated with ANTU (Hill et al., 1984), indomethacin (Meyrick et al., 1985), or irradiation (Perkett et al., 1986).

IV. Summary and Conclusion

Abnormalities in pulmonary circulatory control are frequent findings in both acute and chronic lung injuries. In acute lung injury resulting in increased permeability edema, pulmonary hypertension is of a modest degree and does not necessarily imply a worse prognosis. Both vasoconstriction and vascular obstruction contribute to the development of pulmonary hypertension in acute injury, with the former probably more important in the early stages of the injury. Studies in animal models have implicated arachidonic acid metabolites, especially TxA_2, as potential vasoconstrictor agents in the early phases of injury, although other vasoactive mediators, such as 5-hydroxytryptamine or lipoxygenase products, may also play a role. Although evidence has accumulated that leukocytes, fibrinogen, and platelets may contribute to the development of increased permeability in some injuries, the role of these cells in the hypertensive response is not clear. Variable effects on vascular reactivity have been found in models of acute injury, with oxidants and endotoxin causing depression but ANTU and monocrotoline causing enhancement. Although pulmonary hypertension is a frequent finding in chronic lung injuries, less is known about the effects of chronic injury on vascular reactivity and the causes of any changes. Since vascular reactivity has been found to be increased in several models without significant vascular remodeling, it may be that enhancement of vasoconstriction can predispose to the development of sustained pulmonary hypertension.

Much remains to be learned about pulmonary circulatory control in lung injury. The relation between pulmonary hypertension and mortality and between vascular reactivity and gas exchange needs to be further explored in ARDS. The contribution of vasoconstriction to pulmonary hypertension in later phases of lung injury is unclear. Understanding of these issues could guide potential use of vasodilators as therapy. The role of enchanced vascular reactivity in the development of sustained pulmonary hypertension needs to be further explored. Such studies may increase insight into the pathogenesis of primary pulmonary hypertension, a disease or group of diseases of unknown cause and high mortality.

Acknowledgments

This work was supported by a grant from the NHLBI, HL 34009. The author thanks Faith Barnard for help with literature searches, Lisa Derby for editorial aid, and Charles Vaccaro for art work.

References

Abraham, A. S., Hedworth-Whitty, R. B., and Bishop, J. M. (1967). Effects of acute hypoxia and hypervolaemia singly and together, upon the pulmonary circulation in patients with chronic bronchitis. *Clin. Sci. 33*:371-380.

Abraham, A. S., Cole, R. B., Green, I. D., Hedworth-Whitty, R. B., Clarke, S. W., and Bishop, J. M. (1969). Factors contributing to the reversibile pulmonary hypertension of patients with acute respiratory failure studied by serial observations during recovery. *Circ. Res. 24*:51-60.

Ahmed, T., Wasserman, M. A., Muccitelli, R., Tucker, S., Gazeroglu, H., and Marchette, B. (1986). Endotoxin-induced changes in pulmonary hemodynamics and respiratory mechanics: Role of lipoxygenase and cyclooxygenase products. *Am. Rev. Resp. Dis. 134*:1149-1157.

Altiere, R. J., Olson, J. W., and Gillespie, M. N. (1986). Altered pulmonary vascular smooth muscle responsiveness in monocrotoline-induced pulmonary hypertension. *J. Pharmacol. Exp. Therp. 236*:390-395.

Ashbaugh, D. G., Bigelow, D. B., and Petty, T. L. (1967). Acute respiratory distress in adults. *Lancet 2*:319-323.

Ashutosh, K., Mead, G., and Dunsky, M. (1983). Early effects of oxygen administration and prognosis in chronic obstructive pulmonary disease and cor pulmonale. *Am. Rev. Resp. Dis. 127*:399-404.

Begley, C. J., Ogletree, M. L., Meyrick, B. O., and Brigham, K. L. (1984). Modification of pulmonary responses to endotoxemia in awake sheep by steroidal and nonsteroidal anti-inflammatory agents. *Am. Rev. Resp. Dis. 130*: 1140-1146.

Bell, R. C., Coalson, J. J., Smith, J. D., and Johanson, W. G. (1983). Multiple organ system failure and infection in adult respiratory distress syndrome. *Ann. Int. Med. 99*:293-298.

Benumof, J. L., and Wahrenbrock, E. A. (1975). Blunted hypoxic pulmonary vasoconstriction by increased lung vascular pressures. *J. Appl. Physiol. 38*: 846-850.

Bessin, P., Bonnet, J., Apffel, D., Soulard, C., Desgroux, L., Pelas, I., and Benviste, J. (1983). Acute circulatory collapse caused by platelet-activating factor (PAF-acether) in dogs. *Eur. J. Pharmacol. 86*:403-413.

Binder, A. S., Nakahara, K., Ohkuda, K., Kageler, W., and Staub, N. C. (1979). Effect of heparin or fibrinogen depletion on lung fluid balance in sheep after emboli. *J. Appl. Physiol. 47*:213-219.

Blaisdell, F. W., and Schlobohm, R. M. (1973). The respiratory distress syndrome: a review. *Surgery 74*:251-262.

Block, E. R., and Fisher, A. B. (1977). Depression of serotonin clearance by rat lungs curing oxygen exposure. *J. Appl. Physiol. 42*:33-38.

Block, E. R., and Schoen, F. J. (1981). Effect of alpha naphthylthiourea on uptake of 5-hydroxytryptamine from the pulmonary circulation. *Am. Rev. Resp. Dis. 123*:69-73.

Boiteau, P., Ducas, J., Schick, Girling, L., and Prewitt, R. M. (1986). Pulmonary vascular pressure-flow relationship in canine oleic acid pulmonary edema. *J. Appl. Physiol. 251*:H1163-H1170.

Bone, R. C., Francis, P. B., and Pierce, A. K. (1976). Intravascular coagulation associated with the adult respiratory distress syndrome. *Am. J. Med. 61*: 585-589.

Bredenberg, C. E., Taylor, G. A., and Webb, W. R. (1980). The effect of thrombocytopenia on the pulmonary and systemic hemodynamics of canine endotoxin shock. *Surgery 87*:59-68.

Bressack, M. A., and Bland, R. D. (1980). Alveolar hypoxia increases lung fluid filtration in unanesthetized newborn lambs. *Circ. Res. 46*:111-116.

Brigham, K. L., and Meyrick, B. (1986). State of the art: endotoxin and lung injury. *Am. Rev. Resp. Dis. 133*:913-927.

Brigham, K. L., Bowers, R. E., and Haynes, J. (1979). Increased sheep lung vascular permeability caused by *Escherichia coli* endotoxin. *Circ. Res. 45*: 292-297.

Brigham, K. L., Bowers, R. E., and McKeen, C. R. (1981). Methylprednisolone prevention of increased lung vascular permeability following endotoxemia in sheep. *J. Clin. Invest. 67*:1103-1110.

Brigham, K. L., Kariman, K., Harris, T. R., Snapper, J. R., Bernard, G. R., and Young, S. L. (1983). Correlation of oxygenation with vascular permeability-surface area, but not with lung water in humans with acute respiratory failure and pulmonary edema. *J. Clin. Invest. 72*:339-349.

Brody, J. S., and Stemmler, E. J. (1968). Differential reactivity in the pulmonary circulation. *J. Clin. Invest. 47*:800-808.

Broe, P. J., Toung, T. J. K., Margolis, S., Permutt, S., and Cameron, J. L. (1981). Pulmonary injury caused by free fatty acid: evaluation of steroid and albumin therapy. *Surgery 89*:582-587.

Bruner, L. H., Hilliker, K. S., and Roth, R. A. (1983). Pulmonary hypertension and ECG changes from monocrotoline pyrrole in the rat. *Am. J. Physiol. 245*:H300-H306.

Burghuber, O., Mathias, M. M., McMurtry, I. F., Reeves, J. T., and Voelkel, N. (1984). Lung edema due to hydrogen peroxide is independent of cyclooxygenase products. *J. Appl. Physiol. 56*:900-905.

Burrows, B., Kettel, L. J., Niden, A. H., Rabinowitz, M., and Diener, C. F. (1972). Patterns of cardiovascular dysfunction in chronic obstructive lung disease. *New Engl. J. Med. 286*:912-918.

Carvalho, A. C. A. (1985). Blood alterations in ARDS. In *Acute Respiratory Failure*. Edited by W. M. Zapol and K. J. Falke. Marcel Dekker, New York. pp. 303-346.

Casey, L. C., Fletcher, J. R., Zmudka, M. I., and Ramwell, P. W. (1982). Prevention of endotoxin-induced pulmonary hypertension in primates by the use of a selective thromboxane synthetase inhibitor, OXY 1581. *J. Exp. Pharmacol. Ther. 222*:441-446.

Cassidy, S. S., Robertson, C. H., Pierce, A. K., and Johnson, R. L. (1978). Cardiovascular effects of positive end-expiratory pressure in dogs. *J. Appl. Physiol. 44*:743-750.

Czer, G. T., Marsh, J., Konopka, R., and Moser, K. M. (1986). Low-dose PGI_2 prevents monocrotoline-induced thromboxane production and lung injury. *J. Appl. Physiol. 60*:464-471.

Dantzker, D. R., and Bower, J. S. (1981). Pulmonary vascular tone improves VA/Q matching in obliterative pulmonary hypertension. *J. Appl. Physiol. 51*:607-613.

Demling, R. H., Smith, M., Gunther, R., Flynn, J. T., and Gee, M. H. (1981a). Pulmonary injury and prostaglandin production during endotoxemia in conscious sheep. *Am. J. Physiol. 240*:H348-H353.

Demling, R. H., Smith, M., Gunther, R., Gee, M., and Flynn, J. (1981b). The effect of prostacyclin infusion on endotoxin-induced lung injury. *Surgery 89*:257-263.

Dyer, E. L., and Snapper, J. R. (1986). Role of circulating granulocytes in sheep lung injury produced by phorbal myristate acetate. *J. Appl. Physiol. 60*:576-589.

Enson, Y., Giuntini, C. Lewis, M. L., Morris, T. Q., Ferrer, M. I., and Harvey, R. M. (1964). The influence of hydrogen ion concentration and hypoxia on the pulmonary circulation. *J. Clin. Invest. 43*:1146-1162.

Fairman, R. P., Glauser, F. L., and Falls, R. (1981). Increases in lung lymph and albumin clearance with ethclorvynol. *J. Appl. Physiol.* *50*:1151-1155.

Fedderson, C. O., McMurtry, I. F., Henson, P., and Voelkel, N. F. (1986). Acetylcholine-induced pulmonary vasodilation in lung vascular injury. *Am. Rev. Resp. Dis.* *133*:197-204.

Figueras, J., Stein, L., Diez, V., Weil, M. H., and Shubin, H. (1976). Relationship between pulmonary hemodynamics and arterial pH and carbon dioxide tension in critically ill patients. *Chest* *70*:466-472.

Fishman, A. P. (1976). Hypoxia on the pulmonary circulation: how and where it acts. *Circ. Res.* *38*:221-231.

Fishman, A. P., McClement, J., Himmelstein, A., and Cournand, A. (1952). Effects of acute anoxia on the circulation and respiration in patients with chronic pulmonary disease studied during the "steady state." *J. Clin. Invest.* *31*:770-781.

Flick, M. R., Perel, A., and Staub, N. C. (1981). Leukocytes are required for increased lung microvascular permeability after microembolization in sheep. *Circ. Res.* *48*:344-351.

Flick, M. R., Hoeffel, J. M., and Staub, N. C. (1983). Superoxide dismutase with heparin prevents increased lung vascular permeability during air emboli in sheep. *J. Appl. Physiol.* *55*:1284-1291.

Fountain, S. W., Martin, B. A., Musclow, C. E., and Cooper, J. D. (1980). Pulmonary leukostasis and its relationship to pulmonary dysfunction in sheep and rabbits. *Circ. Res.* *46*:175-180.

Fowler, K. T., and Read, J. (1963). Effect of alveolar hypoxia on zonal distribution of pulmonary blood flow. *J. Appl. Physiol.* *18*:244-250.

Fowler, A. A., Hamman, R. F., Zerbe, G. O., Benson, K. N., and Hyers, T. M. (1985). Adult respiratory distress syndrome: prognosis after onset. *Am. Rev. Resp. Dis.* *132*:472-478.

Garcia-Szabo, R. R., Peterson, M. B., Watkins, W. D., Bizios, R., Kong, D. L., and Malik, A. B. (1983). Throboxane generation after thrombin: protective effect of thromboxane synthetase inhibition on lung fluid balance. *Circ. Res.* *53*:214-222.

Garcia-Szabo, R., Kern, D. F., and Malik, A. B. (1984). Pulmonary vascular response to thrombin: effects of thromboxane synthetase inhibition with OKY-046 and OKY-1581. *Prostaglandins* *28*:851-866.

Gillespie, M. N., and Bowdy, B. D. (1986). Impact of platelet activating factor on vascular responsiveness in isolated rat lungs. *J. Pharmacol. Exp. Ther.* *236*:396-402.

Gillespie, M. N., Owasoyo, J. O., McMurtry, I. F., and O'Brien, R. F. (1986a). Sustained coronary vasoconstriction provoked by a peptidergic substance released from endothelial cells in culture. *J. Pharmacol. Exp. Ther.* *236*: 339-343.

Gillespie, M. N., Olson, J. W., Reinsel, C. N., O'Connor, W. N., and Altiere, R. J. (1986b). Vascular hyperresponsiveness in perfused lungs from monocrotoline-treated rats. *J. Appl. Physiol. 251*:H109-H114.

Gillis, C. N., Pitt, B. R., Wiedeman, H. P., and Hammond, G. L. (1986). Depressed prostaglandin E_1 and 5-hydroxytryptamine removal in patients with adult respiratory distress syndrome. *Am. Rev. Resp. Dis. 134*:739-744.

Glauser, F. L., Fairman, R. P., Millen, J. E., and Falls, R. K. (1982). Indomethacin blunts ethclorvynol-induced pulmonary hypertension but not pulmonary edema. *J. Appl. Physiol. 53*:563-566.

Goetzl, E. J. (1980). Mediators of immediate hypersensitivity derived from arachidonic acid. *New Engl. J. Med. 303*:822-825.

Goldzimer, E. L., Konopka, R. G., and Moser, K. M. (1974). Reversal of the perfusion defect in experimental canine lobar pneumococcal pneumonia. *J. Appl. Physiol. 37*:85-91.

Greene, R., Zapol, W. M., Snider, M. T., Reid, L., Snow, R., O'Connell, R. S., and Novelline, R. A. (1981). Early bedside detection of pulmonary vascular occlusion during acute respiratory failure. *Am. Rev. Resp. Dis. 124*: 593-601.

Gurtner, G. H., Knoblauch, A., Smith, P. L., Sies, H., and Adkinson, N. F. (1983). Oxidant- and lipid-induced pulmonary vasoconstriction mediated by arachidonic acid metabolites. *J. Appl. Physiol. 55*:949-954.

Hales, C. A., Sonne, L., Peterson, M., Kong, D., Miller, M., and Watkins, W. D. (1981). Role of thromboxane and prostacyclin in pulmonary vasomotor changes after endotoxin in dogs. *J. Clin. Invest. 68*:497-505.

Halonen, M., Palmer, J. D., Lohman, C., McManus, L. M., and Pinckard, R. N. (1980). Respiratory and circulatory alterations induced by acetyl glyceryl ether phosphorycholine, a mediator of IgE anaphylaxis in the rabbit. *Am. Rev. Resp. Dis. 122*:915-924.

Hand, J. M., Will, J. A., and Buckner, C. K. (1981). Effects of leukotrienes on isolated guinea-pig pulmonary arteries. *Eur. J. Pharmacol. 76*:439-442.

Havill, A. M., Gee, M. H., Washburne, J. D., Premkumer, A., Ottoviano, K., Flynn, J. T., and Spath, J. A. (1982). alpha-Naphthylthiourea produces dose-dependent lung vascular injury in sheep. *J. Appl. Physiol. 243*:H505-H511.

Hechtman, H. B., Lonergan, E. A., Staunton, P. B., Dennis, R. C., and Shepro, D. (1978). Pulmonary entrapment of platelets during acute respiratory failure. *Surgery 83*:277-283.

Hechtman, H. B., Valeri, R., and Shepro, D. (1984). Role of humoral mediators in adult respiratory distress syndrome. *Chest 86*:623-627.

Heffner, J. E., Shoemaker, S. A., Canham, E. M., Patel, M., McMurtry, I. F., Morris, H. G., and Repine, J. E. (1983). Acetyl glyceryl ether phosphorylcholine-stimulated human platelets cause pulmonary hypertension and edema in isolated rabbit lungs. *J. Clin. Invest. 71*:351-357.

Heffner, J. E., Sahn, S. A., and Repine, J. E. (1987). The role of platelets in the adult respiratory distress syndrome: culprits or bystanders? *Am. Rev. Resp. Dis. 135*:482-492.

Heflin, A. C., and Brigham, K. L. (1981). Prevention by granulocyte depletion of increased vascular permeability of sheep lung following endotoxemia. *J. Clin. Invest. 68*:1253-1260.

Hickey, K. A., Rubanyi, G., Paul, R. J., and Highsmith, R. F. (1985). Characterization of a coronary vasocontrictor produced by cultured endothelial cells. *Am. J. Physiol. 248*:C550-C556.

Hill, N. S., and Rounds, S. (1983). Vascular reactivity is increased in rat lungs injured with α-naphthylthiourea. *J. Appl. Physiol. 54*:1693-1701.

Hill, N. S., O'Brien, R. F., and Rounds, S. (1984). Repeated lung injury due to α-naphthylthiourea causes right ventricular hypertrophy in rats. *J. Appl. Physiol. 56*:388-396.

Hilliker, K. S., and Roth, R. A. (1985). Increased vascular responsiveness in lungs of rats with pulmonary hypertension induced by monocrotoline. *Am. Rev. Resp. Dis. 131*:46-50.

Hilliker, K. S., Bell, T. G., and Roth, R. A. (1982). Pneumotoxicity and thrombocytopenia after single injection of monocrotoline. *Am. J. Physiol. 242*: H573-H579.

Hiser, W., Penman, R. W., and Reeves, J. T. (1975). Preservation of hypoxic pulmonary pressor response in canine pneumoccal pneumonia. *Am. Rev. Resp. Dis. 112*:817-822.

Hislop, A., and Reid, L. (1976). New findings in pulmonary arteries of rats with hypoxia-induced pulmonary hypertension. *Brit. J. Exp. Pathol. 57*:542-554.

Hofman, W. F., and Erhart, I. C. (1983). Methylprednisolone prevents venous resistance increase in oleic acid lung injury. *J. Appl. Physiol. 54*:926-933.

Hutchison, A. R., Ogletree, M. L., Snapper, J. R., and Brigham, K. L. (1985). Effect of endotoxemia on hypoxic pulmonary vasoconstriction in unanesthetized sheep. *J. Appl. Physiol. 58*:1463-1468.

Huttemeier, P. C., Watkins, W. D., Peterson, M. B., and Zapol, W. M. (1982). Acute pulmonary hypertension and lung thromboxane release after endotoxin infusion in normal and leukopenic sheep. *Circ. Res. 50*:688-694.

Huval, W. V., Dunham, B. M., Lelcuk, S., Valeri, C. R., Shepro, D., and Hechtman, H. M. (1983a). Thromboxane mediation of cardiovascular dysfunction following aspiration. *Surgery 94*:259-265.

Huval, W. V., Mathieson, M. A., Stemp, L. I., Dunham, B. M., Jones, A. G., Shepro, D., and Hechtman, H. B. (1983b). Therapeutic benefits of 5-hydroxytryptamine inhibition following pulmonary embolism. *Ann. Surgery 197*:220-225.

Huval, W. V., Lelcuk, S., Shepro, D., and Hechtman, H. B. (1984). Role of serotonin in patients with acute respiratory failure. *Ann. Surgery 300*:166-172.

Johnson, A., and Malik, A. B. (1982). Pulmonary edema after glass bead microembolization: protective effect of granulocytopenia. *J. Appl. Physiol. 52*: 155-161.

Johnson, A., and Malik, A. B. (1985). Pulmonary transvascular fluid and protein exchange after thrombin-induced microembolism: differential effects of cyclooxygenase inhibitors. *Am. Rev. Resp. Dis. 132*:70-76.

Johnson, A., Tahamont, M. V., Kaplan, J. E., and Malik, A. B. (1982). Lung fluid balance after pulmonary embolization: effects of thrombin vs. fibrin micro-aggregates. *J. Appl. Physiol. 52*:1565-1570.

Johnson, A., Tahamont, M. V., and Malik, A. B. (1983). Thrombin-induced lung vascular injury: role of fibrinogen and fibrinolysis. *Am. Rev. Resp. Dis. 128*:38-44.

Johnson, A., Blumenstock, F. A., Hussain, M., and Malik, A. B. (1984). Differential effects of complement activation induced by cobra venom factor on pulmonary transvascular fluid and protein exchange. *Am. J. Pathol. 114*: 410-417.

Johnson, A., Perlman, M. B., Blumenstock, F. A., and Malik, A. B. (1986). Superoxide dismutase prevents the thrombin-induced increase in lung vascular permeability: role of superoxide in mediating the alterations in lung fluid balance. *Circ. Res. 59*:405-415.

Jones, R., Reid, L., Zapol, W. M., Tomashefski, J. F., Kirton, O. C., and Kobayashi, K. (1985). Pulmonary vascular pathology: human and experimental studies. In *Acute Respiratory Failure*. Edited by W. M. Zapol and K. J. Falke. Marcel Dekker, New York, pp. 23-160.

Julien, M., Hoeffel, J. M., and Flick, M. R. (1986). Oleic acid lung injury in sheep. *J. Appl. Physiol. 60*:433-440.

Kenzora, J. L., Perez, J. E., Bergmann, S. R., and Lange, L. G. (1984). Effects of acetyl glyceryl ether of phosphorycholine (platelet activating factor) on ventricular preload, afterload, and contractility in dogs. *J. Clin. Invest. 74*:1193-1203.

Kubo, K., and Kobayashi, T. (1985). Effects of OKY-046, a selective thromboxane synthetase inhibitor, on endotoxin-induced lung injury in unanesthetized sheep. *Am. Rev. Resp. Dis. 132*:494-499.

Lamy, M., Fallat, R. J., Koeniger, E., Dietrich, H.-P., Ratcliff, J. L., Eberhart, R. C., Tucker, H. J., and Hill, J. D. (1976). Pathologic features and mechanisms of hypoxemia in adult respiratory distress syndrome. *Am. Rev. Resp. Dis. 114*:267-284.

Lewis, R. A., and Austen, K. F. (1984). The biologically active leukotrienes: biosynthesis, metabolism, and pharmacology. *J. Clin. Invest. 73*:889-897.

Lichey, J., Friedrich, T., Franke, J., Nigam, S., Priesnitz, M., and Oeff, K. (1984). Pressure effects and uptake of platelet-activating factor in isolated rat lung. *J. Appl. Physiol. 57*:1039-1044.

Light, R. B., Mink, S. N., and Wood, L. D. H. (1981). Pathophysiology of gas exchange and pulmonary perfusion in pneumococcal lobar pneumonia in dogs. *J. Appl. Physiol. 50*:524-530.

Loyd, J. E., Newman, J. H., English, D., Ogeltree, M. L., Meyrick, B. O., and Brigham, K. L. (1983). Lung vascular effects of phorbal myristate acetate in awake sheep. *J. Appl. Physiol. 54*:267-276.

Lupi-Herrera, E., Sandoval, J., Bialostozky, D., Seoane, M., Martinez, M. L., Bonetti, P. F., Reyes, P., and Barrios, R. (1981). Extrinsic allergic alveolitis caused by pigeon breeding at a high altitude (2,240 meters). *Am. Rev. Resp. Dis. 124*:602-607.

McDonald, J. W. D., Ali, A., Townsend, E. R., and Cooper, J. D. (1983). Thromboxane synthesis by sources other than platelets in association with complement-induced pulmonary leukostasis and pulmonary hypertension in sheep. *Circ. Res. 52*:1-6.

McMurtry, I. F., and Morris, K. G. (1986). Platelet-activating factor causes pulmonary vasodilation in the rat. *Am. Rev. Resp. Dis. 134*:757-762.

Martin, B. A., Dahlby, R., Nichols, I., and Hogg, J. C. (1981). Platelet sequestration in lung with hemorrhagic shock and reinfusion in dogs. *J. Appl. Physiol. 50*:1306-1312.

Meyrick, B., and Brigham, K. L. (1983). Effects of *Escherichia coli* endotoxin on the pulmonary microcirculation of anesthetized sheep. Structure: function relationships. *Lab. Invest. 48*:458-470.

Meyrick, B. O., and Brigham, K. L. (1984). The effect of a single infusion of zymosan-activated plasma on the pulmonary microcirculation of sheep. *Am. J.Pathol. 114*:32-45.

Meyrick, B., and Brigham, K. L. (1986). Repeated *Escherichia coli* endotoxin-induced pulmonary inflammation causes chronic pulmonary hypertension in sheep: structural and functional changes. *Lab. Invest. 55*:164-176.

Meyrick, B., Miller, J., and Reid, L. (1972). Pulmonary oedema induced by ANTU, or by high or low oxygen concentrations in rat—an electron microscopic study. *Brit. J. Exp. Pathol. 53*:347-358.

Meyrick, B., Gamble, W., and Reid, L. (1980). Development of Crotolaria hypertension: hemodynamic and structural study. *Am. J. Physiol. 239*:H692-H702.

Meyrick, B., Niedermeyer, M. E., Ogletree, M. L., and Brigham, K.L. (1985). Pulmonary hypertension and increased vasoreactivity caused by repeated indomethacin in sheep. *J. Appl. Physiol. 59*:443-452.

Miller, W. C., Rice, D. L., Kreusel, R. G., and Bedrossian, W. M. (1978). Monocrotoline model of noncardiogenic pulmonary edema in dogs. *J. Appl. Physiol. 45*:962-965.

Milligan, S. A., Hoeffel, J. M., and Flick, M. R. (1985). Endotoxin-induced acute lung injury in unanesthetized sheep is prevented by catalase. *Am. Rev. Resp. Dis. 131*:A422.

Mitzner, W., and Sylvester, J. T. (1981). Hypoxic vasoconstriction and fluid filtration in pig lungs. *J. Appl. Physiol. 51*:1065-1071.

Mizus, I., Summer, W., Farrukh, I., Michael, J. R., and Gurtner, G. H. (1985). Isoproterenol or aminophylline attenuate pulmonary edema after acid lung injury. *Am. Rev. Resp. Dis. 131*:256-259.

Mlczoch, J., Tucker, A., Weir, E. K., Reeves, J. T., and Grover, R. F. (1978). Platelet-mediated pulmonary hypertension and hypoxia during pulmonary microembolism. *Chest 74*:648-653.

Montgomery, A. B., Stager, M. A., Carrico, C. J., and Hudson, L.D. (1985). Causes of mortality in patients with the adult respiratory distress syndrome. *Am. Rev. Resp. Dis. 132*:485-489.

Nagasaka, Y., Bhattacharya, J., Nanjo, S., Gropper, M. A., and Staub, N. C. (1984). Micropuncture measurement of lung microvascular pressure profile during hypoxia in cats. *Circ. Res. 54*:90-95.

Newman, J. H., McMurtry, I. F., and Reeves, J. T. (1981). Blunted pulmonary pressor responses to hypoxia in blood perfused, ventilated lungs isolated from oxygen toxic rats: possible role of prostaglandins. *Prostaglandins 22*: 11-20.

Newman, J. H., Loyd, J. E., English, D. K., Ogletree, M. L., Fulkerson, W. J., and Brigham, K. L. (1983). Effects of 100% oxygen on lung vascular function in awake sheep. *J. Appl. Physiol. 54*:1379-1386.

Ngeow, Y. K., and Mitzner, W. (1983). Pulmonary hemodynamics and gas exchange properties during progressive edema. *J. Appl. Physiol. 55*:1154-1159.

O'Brien, R. F., Makarski, J. S., and Rounds, S. (1985). Studies on the mechanism of decreased angiotensin I conversion in rat lungs injured with alpha-naphthylthiourea. *Exp. Lung Res. 8*:243-259.

O'Brien, R. F., Robbins, R. J., and McMurtry, I. F. (1987). Endothelial cells in cullure produce a vasoconstrictor substance. *J. Cell Physiol. 132*:263-270.

O'Brodovich, H., Andrew, M., Silver, R., and Coates, G. (1983). Assessment of coagulation cascade during air microembolization ofthe lung. *J. Appl. Physiol. 55*:1743-1747.

Ogletree, M. L., Oates, J. A., Brigham, K. L., and Hubbard, W. C. (1982). Evidence for pulmonary release of 5-hydroxyeicosatetraenoic acid (5-HETE) during endotoxemia in unanesthetized sheep. *Prostaglandins 23*:459-468.

Ogletree, M. L., Begley, C. J., King, G. A., and Brigham, K. L. (1986). Influence of steroidal and nonsteroidal anti-inflammatory agents on the accumulation of arachidonic acid metabolites in plasma and lung lymph after endotoxemia in awake sheep. *Am. Rev. Resp. Dis. 133*:55-61.

Ohkuda, K., Nakahara, K., Binder, A., and Staub, N. C. (1981). Venous air emboli in sheep: reversible increase in lung microvascular permeability. *J. Appl. Physiol. 51*:887-894.

Olanoff, L. S., Reines, H. D., Spicer, K. M., and Halushka, P. V. (1984). Effects of oleic acid on pulmonary capillary leak and thromboxanes. *J. Surg. Res. 36*:597-605.

Olson, N. C., Brown, T. T., and Anderson, D. L. (1985). Dexamethasone and indomethacin modify endotoxin-induced respiratory failure in pigs. *J. Appl. Physiol. 58*:274-284.

Pace, J. B. (1978). Pulmonary vascular response to sodium nitroprusside in anesthetized dogs. *Anesth. Analg. 57*:551-557.

Perkett, E. A., Brigham, K. L., and Meyrick, B. (1986). Increased vasoreactivity and chronic pulmonary hypertension following thoracic irradiation in sheep. *J. Appl. Physiol. 61*:1875-1881.

Perkowski, S. Z., Havill, A. M., Flynn, J. T., and Gee, M. H. (1983). Role of intrapulmonary release of eicosanoids and superoxide anion as mediators of pulmonary dysfunction and endothelial injury in sheep with intermittent complement activation. *Circ. Res. 53*:574-583.

Perlman, M. B., Lo, S. K., and Malik, A. B. (1986). Effect of prostacyclin on pulmonary vascular resonse to thrombin in awake sheep. *J. Appl. Physiol. 60*:546-553.

Permutt, S. (1985). The role of pulmonary arterial pressure in experimentally induced acute lung injury. In *Acute Respiratory Failure*. Edited by W. M. Zapol and K. J. Falke. Marcel Dekker, New York, pp. 227-239.

Pilati, C. F., and Maron, M. B. (1985). Pulmonary hemodynamics and lung water content during splanchnic ischemic shock. *J. Appl. Physiol. 58*: 1577-1584.

Piper, P. J., and Galton, S. A. (1984). Generation of leukotriene B4 and leukotriene E4 from porcine pulmonary artery. *Prostaglandins 28*:905-914.

Prewitt, R. M., and Wood, L. D. H. (1981). Effect of sodium nitroprusside on cardiovascular function and pulmonary shunt in canine oleic acid pulmonary edema. *Anesthesiology 55*:537-541.

Raj, J. U., Hazinski, T. A., and Bland, R. D. (1985). Oxygen-induced lung microvascular injury in neutropenic rabbits and lambs. *J. Appl. Physiol. 58*:921-927.

Reeves, J. T., and Grover, R. F. (1974). Blockade of acute hypoxic pulmonary hypertension by endotoxin. *J. Appl. Physiol. 36*:328-332.

Reeves, J. T., Groves, B. M., and Turkevich, D. (1986). Controversies in medicine: the case for treatment of selected patients with primary pulmonary hypertension. *Am. Rev. Resp. Dis. 134*:342-346.

Rubanyi, G. M., and Vanhoutte, P. M. (1985). Hypoxia releases a vasoconstrictor substance from the canine vascular endothelium. *J. Physiol. 364*: 45-56.

Rutili, G., Kvietys, P., Martin, D., Parker, J. C., and Taylor, A. E. (1982). Increased pulmonary microvascular permeability induced by naphthylthiourea. *J. Appl. Physiol.* *52*:1316-1323.

Saldeen, T. (1976). Trends in microvascular research: the microembolism syndrome. *Microvasc. Res.* *11*:227-259.

Schneider, R. C., Zapol, W. M., and Carvalho, A. C. (1980). Platelet consumption and sequestration in severe acute respiratory failure. *Am. Rev. Resp. Dis.* *122*:445-451.

Shasby, D. M., Vanbenthuysen, K. M., Tate, R. M., Shasby, S. S., McMurtry, I. F., and Repine, J. E. (1982). Granulocytes mediate acute edematous lung injury in rabbits and in isolated rabbit lungs perfused with phorbal myristate acetate: role of oxygen radicals. *Am. Rev. Resp. Dis.* *125*:443-447.

Sibbald, W. J., Paterson, N. A. M., Holliday, R. J., Anderson, R. A., Lobb, T. R., and Duff, J. H. (1978). Pulmonary hypertension in sepsis: measurement by the pulmonary arterial diastolic-pulmonary wedge pressure gradient and the influence of passive and active factors. *Chest* *73*:583-591.

Sibbald, W. J., Anderson, R. R., Reid, B., Holliday, R. L., and Driedger, A. A. (1981). Alveolo-capillary permeability in human septic ARDS: effect of high-dose corticosteroid therapy. *Chest* *79*:133-142.

Snapper, J. R., Bernard, G. R., Hinson, J. M., Hutchison, A. A., Loyd, J. E., Ogletree, M. L., and Brigham, K. L. (1983a). Endotoxemia-induced leukopenia in sheep. Correlation with lung vascular permeability and hypoxemia but not with pulmonary hypertension. *Am. Rev. Resp. Dis.* *127*:306-309.

Snapper, J., Hutchison, A., Ogletree, M., and Brigham, K. L. (1983b). Effects of cyclooxygenase inhibitors on the alterations in lung mechanics caused by endotoxemia in the unanesthetized sheep. *J. Clin. Invest.* *72*:63-76.

Snapper, J. R., Hinson, J. M., Hutchison, A. A., Lefferts, P. L., Ogletree, M.L., and Brigham, K. L. (1984). Effects of platelet depletion on the unanesthetized sheep's pulmonary response to endotoxemia. *J. Clin. Invest.* *74*:1782-1791.

Snow, R. L., Davies, P., Pontoppidan, H., Zapol, W. M., and Reid, L. (1982). Pulmonary vascular remodeling in adult respiratory distress syndrome. *Am. Rev. Resp. Dis.* *126*:887-892.

Spragg, R. G., Abraham, J. L., and Loomis, W. H. (1982). Pulmonary platelet deposition accompanying acute oleic acid-induced pulmonary injury. *Am. Rev. Resp. Dis.* *126*:553-557.

Sugita, T., Hyers, T. M., Dauber, I. M., Wagner, W. W., McMurtry, I. F., and Reeves, J. T. (1983). Lung vessel leak precedes right ventricular hypertrophy in nomoncrotoline-treated rats. *J. Appl. Physiol.* *54*:371-374.

Tahamont, M. V., and Malik, A. B. (1983). Granulocytes mediate the increase in pulmonary vascular permeability after thrombin embolism. *J. Appl. Physiol.* *54*:1489-1495.

Tate, R. M., and Repine, J. E. (1983). State of the art: neutrophils and the adult respiratory distress syndrome. *Am. Rev. Resp. Dis. 128*:552-559.

Tate, R. M., Morris, H. G., Schroeder, W. R., and Repine, J. E. (1984). Oxygen metabolites stimulate thromboxane production and vasoconstriction in isolated saline-perfused rabbit lungs. *J. Clin. Invest. 74*:608-613.

Tate, R. M., Vanbenthuysen, K. M., Shasby, D. M., McMurtry, I. F., and Repine, J. E. (1982). Oxygen-radical-mediated permeability edema and vasoconstriction in isolated perfused rabbit lungs. *Am. Rev. Resp. Dis. 126*:802-806.

Teague, W. G., Berner, M. E., Scheerer, R. A., Clyman, R. I., and Bland, R. D. (1987). Lung microvascular injury inhibits pulmonary vasoconstriction in lambs. (Abstr.) *Clin. Res. 35*:244A.

Tomashefski, J. F., Davies, P., Boggis, C., Greene, R., Zapol, W. M., and Reid, L. M. (1983). The pulmonary vascular lesions of the adult respiratory distress syndrome. *Am. J. Pathol. 112*:112-126.

Toung, T. J. K., Bordos, D., Benson, D. W., Carter, D., Zuidema, G. D., Permutt, S., and Cameron, J. L. (1976). Aspiration pneumonia: experimental evaluation of albumin and steroid therapy. *Ann. Surg. 183*:179-184.

Traber, D. L., Adams, T., Sziebert, L., Stein, M., and Traber, L. (1985). Potentiation of lung vascular response to endotoxin by superoxide dismutase. *J. Appl. Physiol. 58*:1005-1009.

Utsunomiya, T., Krauz, M. M., Shepro, D., and Hechtman, H. B. (1981). Prostaglandin control of plasma and platelet 5-hydroxytryptamine in normal and embolized animals. *Am. J. Physiol. 241*:H766-H771.

Utsunomiya, T., Krausz, M. M., Dunham, B., Valeri, C. R., Levine, L., Shepro, D., and Hechtman, H. B. (1982a). Modification of inflammatory response to aspiration with ibuprofen. *Am. J. Physiol. 243*:H903-H910.

Utsunomiya, T., Krausz, M. M., Levine, L., Shepro, D., and Hechtman, H. B. (1982b). Thromboxane mediation of cardiopulmonary effects of embolism. *J. Clin. Invest. 70*:361-368.

Vanhoutte, P. M., Rubanyi, G. M., Miller, V. M., and Houston, D. S. (1986). Modulation of vascular smooth muscle contraction by the endothelium. *Ann. Rev. Physiol. 48*:307-320.

Vito, L., Dennis, R. C., Weisel, R. D., and Hechtman, H. B. (1974). Sepsis presenting as acute respiratory insufficiency. *Surgery, Gynecol. Obstet. 138*:896-900.

Voelkel, N. F., Worthen, S., Reeves, J. T., Henson, P. M., and Murphy, R. C. (1982). Nonimmunological production of leukotrienes induced by platelet-activatng factor. *Science 218*:286-288.

Voelkel, N. F., Stenmark, K. R., Reeves, J. T., Mathias, M. M., and Murphy, R. C. (1984). Actions of lipoxygenase metabolites in isolated rat lungs. *J. Appl. Physiol. 57*:860-867.

Wagenvoort, C. A. (1980). Lung biopsy specimens in the evaluation of pulmonary vascular disease. *Chest 77*:614-625.

Watkins, W. D., Huttemeier, P. C., Kong, D., and Peterson, M. B. (1982). Thromboxane and pulmonary hypertension following *E. coli* endotoxin infusion in sheep: effect of an imidazole derivative. *Prostaglandins 23*:273-285.

Weigelt, J. A., Gewertz, B. L., Aurbakken, C. M., and Synder, W. H. (1982). Pharmacologic alterations in pulmonary artery pressure in the adult respiratory distress syndrome. *J. Surg. Res. 32*:243-248.

Weir, E. K., Mlzcoch, J., Reeves, J. T., and Grover, R. F. (1976). Endotoxin and prevention of hypoxic pulmonary vasoconstriction. *J. Lab. Clin. Med. 88*: 975-983.

Weitzenblum, E., Ehrhart, M., Rasoholinjanahary, J., and Hirth, C. (1983). Pulmonary hemodynamics in idiopathic pulmonary fibrosis and other interstitial pulmonary diseases. *Respiration 44*:118-127.

Westcott, R. N., Fowler, N. O., Scott, R. C., Hauenstein, V. D., and McGuire, J. (1951). Anoxia and human pulmonary vascular resistance. *J. Clin. Invest. 30*:957-970.

Wilkerson, R. D. (1977). Possible role for prostaglandins in the production of alterations in pulmonary function during splanchnic arterial occlusion shock. *J. Pharmacol. Exp. Ther. 201*:753-761.

Winn, R., Harlan, J., Nadir, B., Harker, L., and Hildebrandt, J. (1983). Thromboxane A2 mediates lung vasoconstriction but not permeability after endotoxin. *J. Clin. Invest. 72*:911-918.

Zapol, W. M., and Snider, M. T. (1977). Pulmonary hypertension in severe acute respiratory failure. *New Engl. J. Med. 296*:476-480.

Zapol, W. M., Rie, M. A., Frikker, M., Snider, M. T., and Quinn, D. A. (1985). Pulmonary circulation during adult respiratory distress syndrome. In *Acute Respiratory Failure*. Edited by W. M. Zapol and K. J. Falke. Marcel Dekker, New York, pp. 241-271.

13

Role of Humoral Mediators in the Pulmonary Vascular Response to Pulmonary Embolism

ASRAR B. MALIK and ARNOLD JOHNSON*

Albany Medical College
Albany, New York

I. Introduction

Pulmonary embolism is a common clinical event that accounts for approximately 500,000 deaths per year. Pulmonary embolism results in alteration in pulmonary function such as an increase in the $\dot{V}/\dot{Q}$ due to an increased alveolar dead space in the obstructed lung segments (Moser, 1979). The clinical manifestation of the altered $\dot{V}/\dot{Q}$ state is the arterial hypoxemia that occurs secondary to increased alveolar dead space and increased blood flow to nonobstructed areas [even though there may be an attempt to increase ventilation to those areas in order to maintain normal $\dot{V}/\dot{Q}$ (Moser, 1979)].

Pulmonary embolism can result from migration of deep venous thrombosis (Moser, 1979) and other particulates such as fat embolism, tumor emboli, amniotic fluid, and a variety of foreign bodies (Moser, 1979). The emboli may be considered macroemboli of varying size that lodge in extraalveolar pulmonary vessels or microemboli that obstruct the pulmonary microcirculation. The purpose of this review is to describe the pulmonary vascular responses (i.e., pulmon-

---

*Present affiliation: Veterans Administration Medical Center, Albany, New York

ary hemodynamic alteration and pulmonary edema) to embolism and the mechanisms that are currently hypothesized to mediate the response.

II. Determinants of Pulmonary Vascular Resistance After Acute Pulmonary Embolism

A. Mechanical Factors

Pulmonary embolism can increase pulmonary vascular resistance (PVR) by the obstruction of pulmonary blood vessels. However, vascular obstruction of 50-60% of the pulmonary vascular cross-sectional area is required to increase PVR (Okhuda et al., 1978). The decrease in cross-sectional area depends on the size of the emboli, which affects their distribution, that is, whether obstruction occurs in small or large pulmonary arteries. Macroemboli obstructing lobar or segmental pulmonary arteries result in a greater reduction in the cross-sectional area than microemboli obstructing pulmonary arterioles and capillaries (Malik, 1983). Thus, a greater number of microemboli are required to decrease the same amount of cross-sectional area and increase PVR compared to macroemboli (Malik, 1983).

The reason PVR does not increase until at least 60% of the pulmonary vascular bed is obstructed is in part related to the increase in pulmonary arterial pressure following embolism. Increased pressure recruits vessels in underperfused lung regions [i.e., zones I and II defined by West (1964)], which increases the perfused portions of the pulmonary vasculature. In addition, the increase in pulmonary arterial pressure dilates the already perfused vessels, which increases the vascular cross-sectional area and thus dampens the rise in PVR.

B. Humoral Factors

Pulmonary embolization is associated with the release of humoral agents that contribute to the magnitude of the rise in PVR (Malik, 1983). These substances are released frrom blood-formed elements [e.g., leukocytes (Harlan, 1985) and platelets (Vaage, 1982)], the plasma phase during clot formation (Saldeen, 1979), and the lung parenchymal cells (e.g., endothelium, macrophages, and mast cells) (Harlan, 1985; Peters et al., 1987). Most studies have concentrated on platelets and neutrophils as the primary sources of these pulmonary vasoactive mediators.

Platelets

Platelets release substances from three intracellular sources (Vaage, 1982): (1) dense granules, (2) alpha granules, and (3) the phospholipid membrane. The dense granules contain and release upon stimulation serotonin and adenosine diphosphate (ADP), both of which are pulmonary vasoconstrictor agents (Brigham and Owen, 1975; Minnear et al., 1982; Demling et al., 1985). Alpha granules release platelet-derived growth factor (PDGF), which may have a direct pulmonary vasoconstrictor effect and may also activate the release of other pulmonary vasoactive mediators (Deuel and Huang, 1984). The platelet lipid membranes generate metabolites of arachidonic acid including TxA_2, PGH_2, and 12-HETE (Vaage, 1982; Piper, 1984). TxA_2 and PGH_2, which may share similar receptors (Munoz et al., 1986), constrict vascular smooth muscle and increase the resistance in isolated perfused lungs (Hyman et al., 1978; Farrukh et al., 1985; Johnson, unpublished observation). The inhibition of thromboxane synthetase attenuates the initial rise in PVR but not the secondary and sustained increase after endotoxin (Kubo and Kobayashi, 1985), complement activation (Gee et al., 1986), bone marrow (Winn et al., 1981), phorbol myristate acetate (PMA) (Allison et al., 1986), and thrombin (Garcia-Szabo et al., 1984); therefore, TxA_2 is partially responsible for the alterations in pulmonary hemodynamics in a variety of lung injury models.

The 12-lipoxygenase metabolite (12-HETE), which is released by platelets and neutrophils (depending on species involved), does not induce pulmonary vasoconstriction directly (Burhop et al., 1988) but enhances neutrophil migration and activation (Piper, 1984); therefore, 12-HETE may mediate its effect via release of neutrophil-derived products. Platelet activating factor (PAF) is also released by platelets (Vaage, 1982) and can activate neutrophils (Lin et al., 1982; Valone and Goetze, 1983; Gay et al., 1984; Gimbrone et al., 1985), which in turn may result in the generation of vasoactive substances. PAF has been shown to contract pulmonary vascular smooth muscle and increase PVR in the isolated perfused lung preparation (Hamasaki et al., 1984) and in awake animals (Burhop et al., 1986). In low concentration, however, PAF appears to be a pulmonary vasodilator in the rat (McMurtry and Morris, 1986). The role of PAF following pulmonary embolism remains to be determined, since specific PAF receptor antagonists have been only recently developed. The platelet-derived 12-HETE and PAF may be a primary mechanism by which platelets interact with neutrophils. The concept of platelet-neutrophil interaction is important, since platelet-induced responses (e.g., the rise in PVR) may be amplified by the secondary activation of neutrophils.

Neutrophils

Neutrophils contain enzymes that generate PAF (Lynch et al., 1979) and pulmonary vasoconstrictor products of arachidonic acid metabolism such as TxA_2, LTB_4, and the peptidoleukotrienes (LTC_4, LTD_4, and LTE_4) (Toldstein et al., 1978; Piper, 1984). The infusion of LTB_4 or peptidoleukotrienes in experimental animals resulted in increases in PVR (Kadowitz and Hyman, 1984; Ahmed et al., 1985; Noonan et al., 1985; Albert et al., 1987). The role of peptidoleukotrienes in mediating the postembolism rise in PVR is unclear, although these agents have been implicated in contributing to a rise in PVR during alveolar hypoxia (Morganroth et al., 1984, 1985). The action of the peptidoleukotrienes is partially mediated by the release of TxA_2 (Noonan and Malik, 1986), and in some species there is a direct vasoconstrictor effect of these leukotrienes (Piper, 1984).

Activated neutrophils also release oxygen-derived free radicals ($O_2^{\cdot}$, OH-H_2O_2), which may cause vasodilation (Burke and Wolin, 1987) or vasoconstriction (Tate et al., 1984; Rubanyi and Vanhoutte, 1986; McDonald et al., 1987) via the release of TxA_2 (Tate et al., 1984). The infusion of superoxide dismutase into sheep following thrombin-induced pulmonary microembolism attentuated the rise in PVR (Johnson et al., 1986). This effect was independent of TxA_2 generation and may be attributed to inhibition of generation of endothelium-derived relaxing factor (EDRF) induced by the superoxide anion (Vanhoutte et al., 1986).

The mechanism of neutrophil activation after pulmonary microembolism is an area of intense investigation. The generation of putative mediators after complement activation (e.g., C5a) (Muller-Eberhard, 1975) and the clotting cascade (e.g., thrombin) (Zimmerman et al., 1985; Bizios et al., 1986) may contribute to neutrophil activation. As previously mentioned, the release of PAF or 12-HETE from platelets after embolism may also be involved since these mediators may be particularly crucial in amplification of neutrophil activation.

Plasma Factors

Generation of clotting factors such as thrombin in the plasma phase has been shown to constrict smooth muscle (Haver and Namm, 1983, 1984), which can mediate pulmonary vasoconstriction. Thrombin infusion increased the PVR in isolated perfused lungs independent of blood-formed elements (Horgan et al., 1987b). Thrombin also induces platelet aggregation, which may in turn release pulmonary vasoactive products from platelets (Vaage, 1982).

The vascular response to pulmonary embolism may also be influenced by nonclotting humoral factors generated in the plasma. The peptide bradykinin does not induce a significant degree of pulmonary vasoconstriction (Minnear et al., 1983). Evidence also indicates that bradykinin does not contribute to the pulmonary vasoconstrictor effect of embolism (Kivlen et al., 1982). The activation of complement and fibrinolytic cascades generates vasoactive peptides, C3a and C5a, and fragment D, all of which are thought to increase PVR (Saldeen, 1974; Johnson et al., 1986a) in animal studies. However, the role of these peptides in pulmonary embolism response remains unclear.

C. Endothelium

The endothelium releases substances that antagonize as well as promote the pulmonary vasoconstriction induced by embolization. For example, the endothelium generates PGI_2 (Grondelle et al., 1984; McIntyre et al., 1985; Clark et al., 1986), which dampens the pulmonary vasoconstriction induced by pulmonary embolism (Perlman et al., 1986) or hypoxia (Hales et al., 1978). Thus, the data support a role of PGI_2 in modulating the PVR rise during pulmonary embolism. In addition, PGI_2 is an antiaggregatory agent for platelets and neutrophils and may prevent the generation of pulmonary vasoactive factors from platelets (Vaage, 1982) and neutrophils (Camuss et al., 1983).

Thrombin generation after pulmonary intravascular coagulation directly stimulates the release of PGI_2 from the endothelium (Hong et al., 1978). Platelet interactions with the endothelium may provide the substrates PGG_2 and PGH_2 for the PGI_2 synthetase located in the endothelium (Moncada and Vane, 1979), i.e., via the "endoperoxide steal" hypothesis.

In addition to PGI_2, the endothelium releases endothelium-derived relaxant factor (EDRF) (Vanhoutte et al., 1986; Greenberg et al., 1987), which may modulate the rise in PVR. Platelet vasoconstrictor substances that are generated during thrombosis (Vaage, 1982) such as thrombin (Horgan et al., 1987b) and serotonin (Brigham and Owen, 1975) can release EDRF (Furchgott, 1983), but whether EDRF is generated after pulmonary embolism has not been examined. Anoxia inhibits EDRF release (Furchgott, 1983), and it is possible that tissue ischemia induced by embolism may promote an increase in PVR by inhibition of EDRF release. EDRF generation is inhibited by superoxide anion production (Rubanyi and Vanhoutte, 1986): therefore, neutrophil activation after pulmonary microembolism may lead to inhibition of release of EDRF and the enhanced pulmonary vasoconstrictor response.

D. Neural Factors

Sympathetic and parasympathetic efferents innervate the pre- and postcapillary pulmonary vessels (Harris and Heath, 1977); however, the extent of the innervation is highly species dependent (Harris and Heath, 1977). Activation of α-adrenergic receptor subtype with norepinephrine or stellate ganglion stimulation results in an increase in PVR (Hakim et al., 1979, 1981). Blockade of autonomic activity by treatment with the ganglionic receptor antagnoist hexamethonium attenuated the pulmonary vasoconstrictor response to pulmonary embolism in dogs (Malik, 1983). Infusion of β-adrenergic agonists also prevented the rise in PVR following pulmonary embolization (Minnear et al., 1986), whereas the blockade of β-adrenergic receptors with propranolol enhanced the response (Minnear et al., 1986), suggesting that β-adrenergic receptor activation modulates the pulmonary vasomotor tone. Whether sympathetic activation is involved in mediating pulmonary vasomotor tone changes is a matter of conjecture, since the results with pharmacological blockers may reflect the nonspecific nature of these drugs.

The role of the parasympathetic system in the pulmonary vasomotor alteration is equally unclear. Activation of muscarinic receptors in pulmonary vessels by vagal stimulation or with acetylcholine elicits either vasodilation or vasoconstriction, depending on the mode of muscarinic activation, the experimental species, and the vessel under study (Harris and Heath, 1977). It is generally accepted that muscarinic activation decreases PVR (Harris and Heath, 1977), yet direct application of acetylcholine to vessel strips without endothelial lining contracts vascular smooth muscle (Furchgott, 1983), suggesting that muscarinic activation of vessel preparations releases EDRF, which thereby reduces the degree of vasoconstriction. The role of acetylcholine is further confounded by acetylcholine-induced inhibition of norepinephrine release due to prejunctional inhibition of sympathetic nerve terminals (Bevan and Brayden, 1987).

Nonsympathetic-parasympathetic nerves also innervate pulmonary vessels, and their stimulation releases peptidergic transmitters (Said et al., 1980; Bevan and Brayden, 1987). Two widely studied neuropeptides are vasoactive intestinal peptide (VIP) and substance P. VIP relaxes pulmonary vascular smooth muscle and is a weak pulmonary vasodilator in situ (Nanoliwada et al., 1985), and substance P is a potent pulmonary vasoconstrictor both in isolated smooth muscle and in the isolated perfused lung (Tanaka and Grimstein, 1985; Worthen et al., 1985). Substance P-induced increase in vasomotor tone is partly dependent on the generation of thromboxane (Selig et al., 1988). Another recently discovered vasoactive peptide released by endothelial cells in response to thrombin and other factors (Yanagisawa et al. 1988; Horgan et al., 1988) may also be important. The role of these peptides in the pulmonary vascular responses to embolism and other challenges such as alveolar hypoxia needs to be explored.

III. Increase in Lung Vascular Permeability After Pulmonary Embolism

A. Vascular Endothelial Injury

Pulmonary vascular injury and pulmonary edema are common pathological findings after embolism (Saldeen, 1979; Schnells et al., 1980; Malik, 1983). The vascular injury is dependent on the site of embolism, since large emboli do not result in vascular injury (i.e., increased lung vascular permeability to protein) (Johnson and Malik, 1981) unless the macroemboli produce marked increases in pulmonary arterial pressure (>55 mmHg) (Rippe et al., 1984), whereas emboli in smaller vessels of the lung are usually associated with vascular injury and smaller increases in pulmonary arterial pressures (Malik, 1983). Pulmonary microemboli are commonly observed with vascular injury in adult respiratory distress syndrome (ARDS) (Saldeen, 1979; Schnells et al., 1984).

The microemboli consist of fibrin "plugs" with platelets and neutrophils entrapped in the fibrin network (Saldeen, 1979). The vascular endothelium is the primary site of injury, but the alveolar epithelium is also affected in the more lethal cases (Malik, 1983). Focal endothelial gaps, endothelial cell swelling, and in increase in intracellular vacuolization may be present in pre- and post-capillary vessels as well as capillaries. The effect of endothelial injury is an increase in vascular permeability to protein and in the extravascular water content (Malik, 1983).

B. Mechanisms of Vascular Injury

Mechanical Factors

The large increase in pulmonary arterial pressure induced by pulmonary embolism deserves attention as a factor in the development of vascular injury (Rippe et al., 1984). Studies have shown that pulmonary vascular pressures greater than 55 mmHg rupture the endothelial barrier and increase capillary filtration rate in the isolated perfused lung (Rippe et al., 1984). Vessel barotrauma is more likely to occur if there is a concomitant decrease in pulmonary vascular compliance (e.g., with restriction of the pulmonary vascular bed following embolism) associated with a rise in pulmonary arterial pressure (Malik, 1985). Thus, an excessive pressure rise may be an important pathogenic event in the mediation of lung vascular injury. Pressure-induced injury would be expected to occur primarily in the precapillary vessels, where the pressure would be the highest. Whether this occurs is not clear. Pulmonary edema is present in the obstructed as well as the nonobstructed regions after embolism (Lee et al., 1979), suggesting that cellular and humoral mechanisms are more important than mechanical factors in the pathogenesis of vascular injury.

Cellular Mechanisms

The neutrophil has been implicated as the effector cell mediating lung vascular injury (Harlan, 1985) following pulmonary microembolism (Tahamont and Malik, 1983). Neutrophils are found in the pulmonary microcirculation in ARDS patients (Schnells et al., 1980; Powe et al., 1982) and in models of acute lung injury in experimental animals (Brigham and Meyrick, 1984). Depletion of circulating neutrophils prevents lung vascular injury following pulmonary microembolism induced with glass beads (Johnson and Malik, 1980; Johnson and Malik, 1982), air (Flick et al., 1981), and thrombin (Tahamont and Malik, 1983). However, not all models of lung injury (e.g., PMA-induced lung injury) seem to be dependent on neutrophils (Dyer and Snapper, 1986). Also, the neutrophil depletion studies remain inconclusive, since a causal relationship has not been established; that is, the repletion of neutrophils during the lung challenge with the injury-inducing agents has not been done to determine whether the protective effect can be reversed.

Although the exact basis of neutrophil activation after pulmonary embolism remains unclear, the activation process may be explained by several mechanisms. Generation of complement system-derived peptides C3a and C5a occurs during coagulation (Muller-Eberhard, 1975; Zimmerman et al., 1977). These peptides are potent neutrophil chemotactic and aggregating agents and are also capable of stimulating neutrophils to release toxic oxidants and proteases (Muller-Eberhard, 1975). PAF (McIntyre et al., 1986), leukotriene B_4 (Gay et al., 1984; Gimbrone et al., 1985), tumor necrosis factor (TNF) and interleukin-1 (Bevilacqua et al., 1985; Goldblum et al., 1987) may participate in regulating neutrophil function following pulmonary embolism by promoting neutrophil adherence to vascular endothelium, neutrophil aggregation, and the release of neutrophil-derived toxic oxidants and proteases.

Macrophage activation results in the generation of LTB_4 (Bonney et al., 1985) and monokines such as interleukin-1 TNF (Le et al., 1987). Macrophages obtained from sheep after thrombin-induced pulmonary embolism resulted in endothelial injury after the application of macrophages to an endothelial monolayer (Ferro et al., 1987). Macrophage-neutrophil interactions need to be studied further, since they may hold the key to how lung vascular injury is mediated by neutrophils (Pennington et al., 1985; Schwartz and Monroe, 1986).

The activated neutrophil may injure the endothelium by release of oxygen-derived free radicals (i.e., O_2^-, H_2O_2, $OHCl^\cdot$, and OH^-) and proteases (i.e., elastase, collagenases, cathepsins). These oxidants alter the cell membrane viscosity (Block et al., 1986), cytoskeletal components (Hinshaw et al., 1986; Snyder et al., 1985), the molecular structure of interstitial components (Weiss and Regiani, 1984), and perturb membrane lipid homeostasis, all of which lead to cell injury (Demling et al., 1986; Dise et al., 1987). The infusion of superoxide dismutase (the enzyme that induces catalysis of $O_2^\cdot$ to H_2O_2 and O_2) prevented the embolism-induced lung vascular injury (Johnson et al., 1986), supporting an important role for $O_2^\cdot$ in the pathogenesis of lung vascular injury. The role of neutrophil proteases in lung vascular injury is less clear, although elastase and collagenase are generated during pulmonary injury (Lee et al., 1981; Christner et al., 1985). Neutrophil elastase injures pulmonary cells in vitro and in vivo (Janoff, 1983; Peterson et al., 1987) and is released during blood coagulation (Plow, 1982); thus its role in pulmonary embolism may be important. Oxidants also inhibit anti-protease activity (especially a_1 anti-trypsin, which inhibits elastase activity) (Bieth, 1985; Ossanna et al., 1986); thus, there is an intimate relationship between the generation of oxidants and protease activity.

Platelets

Platelets do not appear to play a role in the induction of lung vascular injury following pulmonary microembolism. Platelet depletion did not prevent the microembolism-induced lung vascular injury after glass bead (Binder et al., 1980), endotoxin (Snapper et al., 1984), or thrombin (Tahamont and Malik, 1983) embolism. Platelet release products, however, are involved in mediating the rise in PVR, since twice the number of glass emboli were required to increase the

PVR in platelet-depleted animals as in control animals (Binder et al., 1980). Platelet adherence and activation after embolism may occur secondary to generation of thrombin (Nemerson and Nossel, 1982) and neutrophil-derived products such as PAF (Chesney et al., 1982).

Although platelets do not appear to be involved in mediating vascular injury, they may in fact serve to maintain endothelial integrity (Gimbrone et al., 1969; Tranzer and Baumgartner, 1967). Adding platelets to platelet-depleted sheep (in which lung vascular permeability was increased) restored normal pulmonary transvascular fluid and protein fluxes (Lo et al., 1988). This function of platelets may be a nutritive one [i.e., humorally mediated effect of platelet-derived factors or platelet-derived growth factor (PDGF) (Deuel and Haung, 1984)] on the endothelium or the result of adherence of platelets to endothelial "gaps" (Tranzer and Baumgartner, 1967) that limit transvascular fluid and protein exchange.

IV. Metabolic Response of Vascular Endothelium to Pulmonary Embolism

A. Metabolism of Mediators by Pulmonary Endothelium

The vascular endothelium participates actively in regulating the circulating concentrations of substances that affect pulmonary vasomotor tone. These humoral factors are also capable of modifying or mediating vessel wall injury. Since vascular obstruction after embolism decreases the vascular surface area and microembolism induces endothelial injury (Schnells et al., 1980), the ability of the vascular endothelium to regulate the local concentrations of mediators may be impaired. This may alter the homeostatic response to embolism.

The vascular endothelium metabolizes PGE_1 (Anderson and Eling, 1976; Gillis et al., 1986), norepinephrine (Flink et al., 1982), bradykinin (O'Brodovich et al., 1985), and serotonin (Gillis et al., 1986), resulting in inactive by-products of these factors (Said, 1982). The concentrations of these mediators in the pulmonary effluent decreases to barely detectable levels on first passage through the lung. Interestingly, these factors are generated in the lung after embolization, and thus a disruption in the lung's ability to degrade these factors may effect their circulating concentrations. The activity of enzymes responsible for uptake and degradation of norepinephrine and serotonin does not appear to be affected after embolization (Flink et al., 1982) or lung injury (Dawson et al., 1985), but redistribution of blood flow after uneven vascular obstruction decreases the transit time through the nonobstructed lung segments and vascular surface area, resulting in decreased removal of these vasoactive mediators. The activity of angiotensin-converting enzymes (ACE) (which is responsible for the conversion of angiotensin I to the vasoactive angiotensin II and for the inactivation of bradykinin) is not decreased during hypoxia, but there is a decrease in the transit time, resulting in decreased total removal of substrate (O'Brodovich et al., 1985); however, the effect of embolism and lung injury on ACE activity needs to be resolved (Dobuler et al., 1982). In contrast, PGE_1 is degraded by the prostaglandin dehydrogenase, and its K_m may be decreased by embolism (Gillis et al., 1986).

Increased concentration of vasoactive substances such as norepinephrine, serotonin, and PGE_1 in the lung effluent following embolism may lead to alterations in pulmonary vasomotor tone and fluid exchange in the downstream vessels. Since endothelial injury is a feature of pulmonary microembolism (Malik, 1983), its effect on how the endothelium handles the circulating mediators needs to be better characterized.

B. Release of Mediators by Endothelium

Prostaglandins

Pulmonary embolism results in the release of PGI_2 in reponse to a variety of substances that are generated as a result of pulmonary embolism such as thrombin (Garcia-Szabo et al., 1984), arachidonic acid (Selig et al., 1986), and H_2O_2 (Harlan, 1985). PGI_2 serves to counter the pulmonary vasoconstriction induced by embolism, since it dilates pulmonary vessels (Perlman et al., 1986) and antagonizes platelet aggregation and activation (Vaage, 1982). The effect of PGI_2 occurs through the intracellular elevation of cAMP in smooth muscle, since increased cAMP concentration induced by dibutyryl AMP (Farrukh et al., 1987) and phosphodiesterase inhibitors results in lowering of PVR (Mizus et al., 1985). PGI_2 decreases the transvascular fluid filtration associated with thrombin-induced pulmonary embolism (Perlman et al., 1986), although this is the result of a decrease in the capillary hydrostatic pressure rather than the prevention of the vascular injury (Perlman et al., 1986).

The disruption of the endothelial lining results in decreased PGI_2 release (Zmuda et al., 1977), which may enhance the effect of embolism; for example by producing a greater increase in PVR and increased platelet and neutrophil adherence to the subendothelial matrix.

Endothelium-Derived Relaxing Factor (EDRF)

The pulmonary vascular response to embolism may be influence by the release of EDRF from the vascular endothelium (Furchgott, 1983). EDRF is known to be generated following addition of vasoconstrictor substances such as bradykinin, PAF, and thrombin to vessel wall strips containing the endothelial lining (Furchgott, 1983; Vanhoutte et al., 1986); however, the release of EDRF from the pulmonary circulation may be quite different, since the pulmonary vascular bed constricts in response to humoral mediators such as histamine and bradykinin (Harris and Heath, 1977), which are systemic vasodilators. This difference is not confined to these mediators, since it is well known that alveolar hypoxia constricts pulmonary vessels but dilates peripheral vessels (Hales et al., 1978). EDRF is inactivated by the generation of $O_2\cdot$ (Rubanyi and Vanhoutte, 1986), and therefore the enhancement of the pulmonary vasoactive response after neutrophil activation may be the result of inhibition of generation of EDRF.

Antithrombotic Actions of Endothelium

Vascular endothelium also regulates the degree and duration of thrombosis after pulmonary embolism. For example, the release of PGI_2 antagonizes platelet aggregation (Vaage, 1982) and thus modulates the degree of thrombosis. In addition, the binding of thrombin to thrombomodulin receptors (Marayama et al., 1985) on the endothelium activates protein C with the cofactor protein S (Clouse and Comp, 1986) [these enzymes are located on the endothelium (Clouse and Comp, 1986)]. The activated protein C inhibits the activities of factors VIII and V, resulting in the inhibition of thrombosis by interacting with the intrinsic path of coagulation and the inactivation of prothrombin, respectively (Clouse and Comp, 1986). Heparan sulfates lining the subendothelium matrix (Matzner et al., 1985) also antagonize thrombosis. The heparins bind with antithrombin III for the effective inactivation of thrombin (Nemerson and Nossel, 1982). Finally, thrombin and other procoagulants release plasminogen activator [which converts the zymogen plasminogen to plasmin (Mullertz, 1979)] from the endothelium (Nemerson and Nossel, 1982). Plasmin is responsible for inducing fibrinolysis after pulmonary embolism (Saldeen, 1979; Malik, 1983). The importance of fibrinolysis in lung vascular injury after embolism is inferred from studies in patients in which acute lung injury is associated with decreased fibrinolytic activity due to increased antiplasmin activity (Saldeen, 1979).

Reperfusion Injury After Embolism

Pulmonary reperfusion injury after embolization may be an important clinical entity due to the increased use of fibrinolytic agents such as urokinase, streptokinase, and tissue plasminogen activator to reinitiate perfusion to embolized areas (Levinson et al., 1986). Reperfusion lung injury occurs in experimental models in which the vascular bed is obstructed for a period of time (the time of occlusion varied from 2 to 24 hr) followed by a period of reperfusion (Barie, et al., 1981; Barie and Malik, 1982). Pulmonary edema secondary to increased lung vascular permeability ensues during the reperfusion phase, and there is an associated increase in PVR (Horgan et al., 1987a). It has been proposed by McCord (1987) that the enzyme xanthine dehydrogenase is converted during tissue ischemia to xanthine oxidase due to increase in intracellular Ca^{2+}, which activates Ca^{2+}-dependent proteases, converting the dehydrogenase to the active oxidase form of the enzyme. Ischemia also induces the dephosphorylation of

ATP to adenosine with increased purine catabolism to hypoxanthine due to a decrease in oxidative phosphorylation (McCord, 1987). During reperfusion, the increased O_2 and the intracellular hypoxanthine are available to xanthine oxidase for the intracellular generation of superoxide anion (O_2-) and uric acid. Superoxide can dismutate (by the action of superoxide dismutase at physiologic pH) to H_2O_2, which provides the reaction substrates for generation of hydroxyl radical (OH) or the halogenated oxidants (OHC1) formed by neutrophil enzyme myeloperoxidase (Test et al., 1984). Oxidants may contribute to increased vasoreactivity and may also mediate lung vascular injury following the lysis of pulmonary thrombi (McCord, 1987). Reperfusion induced pulmonary edema and lung vascular injury have been demonstrated in isolated perfused lungs (Horgan et al., 1987a) and in whole animals after pulmonary vascular occlusion (Barie et al., 1981; Barie and Malik, 1982).

Endothelium-Derived Mediators of Endothelial Injury

The vessel lining cells release mediators that are potentially destructive to the endothelium itself. These substances may be generated after thrombosis. For example, pulmonary artery cultured endothelial cell releases neutrophil chemoattractants (Farber et al., 1985, 1986), interleukin-1 (Cybulsky et al., 1986; Libby et al., 1986), oxygen radicals (Selvaraj et al., 1987), or leukotrienes (Piper and Galton, 1984) in response to a number of inflammatory agents. These endothelial cell-derived mediators may directly induce endothelial injury and increase vascular permeability; however, their role in amplifying the response is an exciting area of new investigation.

The endothelium is not an innocent bystander that suffers the consequences of mechanical and humoral insults following pulmonary embolism. The endothelium has the capacity to control its environment and to promote homeostasis. The balance of these endothelial factors is a likely determinant of the severity of lung vascular injury and edema.

V. Pulmonary Vascular Response to Chronic Embolism

A. Adaptations to Increased Pulmonary Arterial Pressure

The degree of pulmonary vascular smooth muscle increases in response to chronic pulmonary embolism manifested as both hyperplasia and hypertrophy (Wagenvoort and Wagenvoort, 1979). Whether the remodeling is similar to that observed with chronic hypoxia is unclear (Snow et al., 1982; Jones et al., 1984; Kirton and Jones, 1987). In the normal lung, arteries ranging in diameter from 500-1000 μm to small arteries of 60-70 μm contain varying amounts of smooth muscle, with the smaller arteries having less smooth muscle than the larger vessels (Wagenvoort and Wagenvoort, 1979). In chronic pulmonary hypertension, the arterioles 30-40 μm in diameter contain greater amounts of smooth muscle than normal vessels of this size (Wagenvoort and Wagenvoort, 1979). Increase in PVR in chronic embolism may occur primarily as the result of increased smooth muscle causing a decreased internal luminal diameter. The increase in smooth muscle also results in altered pulmonary vasoreactivity to mediators generated during embolism (Malik, 1983).

The mechanism of smooth muscle growth in chronic embolism is unknown, although processes quite similar to smooth muscle growth occurring in atherosclerosis may be activated. The genetic regulation of smooth muscle growth is an important area of study. Thrombi contain platelets and monocytes that release smooth muscle growth factors such as the platelet-derived growth factors (Deuel and Huang, 1984), which may be important in pulmonary vascular smooth growth after embolism. Recent studies indicate that pulmonary vascular remodeling during hypoxia is dependent on polyamines (Atkinson et al., 1987) and collagen synthesis (Kerr et al., 1987). It has also been observed that coagulation induces release of endothelium-derived PDGF and mitogen activity (Gajdusek et al., 1986), and endothelial cells exposed to hypoxia release mitogens for smooth muscle cells (Vender et al., 1987); supporting the notion that intravascular coagulations and blood stasis initiates the growth process. All these conditions may be present in the circulation following embolism.

B. Recanalization of Vessels

The patency of the vascular lumen is preserved after pulmonary embolism by fibrinolysis of thrombi (Mullertz, 1979). Vascular endothelium releases plasminogen activator, which converts the plasminogen to plasmin (Mullertz, 1979); however, endothelial injury may result in impairment of fibrinolysis (Saldeen, 1979) and thus in prolonged vascular obstruction. The residual thrombi become incorporated within the vessel intima (Wagenvoort and Wagenvoort, 1979), resulting in a decrease in vessel diameter and sustained increase in PVR. This may be an explanation for the persistent pulmonary hypertension in chronic thrombosis that does not respond to vasodilator therapy (Moser, 1979).

VI. Summary

The pulmonary circulation receives the entire cardiac output, rendering the pulmonary circulation especially susceptible to the effects of embolism. The pulmonary vascular bed actively participates in the response to embolism. It does not simply act as a sieve for particulates in the circulation. Important cellular and humoral mechanisms are activated. The pulmonary vascular bed responds in such a manner so as to decrease the effects of emboli and maintain normal $\dot{V}/\dot{Q}$ balance and fluid exchange, e.g., through fibrinolysis activation and PGI_2 release. However, maladaptations can occur. For example, the endothelial cells have the ability to generate and express factors (e.g. endothelin) whose potency is only recently being appreciated. The factors also include neutrophil chemotoxins, adherence-inducing agents, and oxygen-derived free radicals. The balance of these mediators determines the extent of the rise in PVR and the development of lung vascular injury and lung tissue edema.

Acknowledgment

Supported by HL-32418 and a grant from the Veteran's Administration.

References

Ahmed, T., Marchette, B., Wanner, A., and Yerger, L. (1985). Direct and indirect effects of leukotriene D_4 on the pulmonary and systemic circulations. *Am. Rev. Resp. Dis. 131*:554-558.

Albert, R. K., Greenberg, G., Grist, R. J., Luchtel, D., and Henderson, W. R. (1987). Leukotrienes C_4 and D_4 do not increase filtration coefficient of excised perfused guinea pig lungs. *J. Appl. Physiol. 62*:1-9.

Allison, R. C., Marble, K. T., Hernandez, E. M., Townsley, M. I., and Taylor, A. E. (1986). Attenuation of permeability lung injury after phorbal myristate acetate by verapamil and OKY-046. *Am. Rev. Resp. Dis. 134*:93-100.

Anderson, M. W., and Eling, T. E. (1976). Prostaglandin removal and metabolism by isolated perfused rat lung. *Prostaglandins 11*:645-777.

Atkinson, J. E., Olson, J. W., Altiere, R. J., and Gillespie, M. N. (1987). Evidence that chronic pulmonary vascular remodeling in rats is polyamine dependent. *J. Appl. Physiol. 62*:1562-1568.

Barie, P. S., and Malik, A. B. (1982). Effect of pulmonary arterial occlusion on lung fluid exchange. *J. Appl. Physiol. 53*:543-548.

Barie, P. S., Hakim, T. S., and Malik, A. B. (1981). Effects of pulmonary artery occlusion on extravascular fluid accumulation. *J. Appl. Physiol. 50*:102-106.

Bevan, J. A., and Brayden, J. E. (1987). Non-adrenergic neural vasodilator mechanisms. *Circ. Res. 60*:309-326.

Bevilacqua, M. P., Pober, J. S., Wheeler, M. E., Cotran, R. S., and Gimbrone, M. A. (1985). Interleukin-1 acts on cultured vascular endothelium to increase the adhesion of polymorphonuclear leukocytes, monocytes and related cell lines. *J. Clin. Invest. 76*:2003-2111.

Bieth, J. G. (1985). The antielastase screen of the lower respiratory tract. *Eur. J. Resp. Dis. 139*:57-61.

Binder, A. S., Kageler, W., Perel, A., Flick, M. R., and Staub, N. C. (1980). Effect of platelet depletion on lung microemboli in sheep. *J. Appl. Physiol. 48*:414-420.

Bizios, R., Lai, L., Fenton, J. W., and Malik, A. B. (1986). Thrombin induced chemotaxis and aggregation of neutrophils. *J. Cell Physiol. 128*:483-490.

Block, E. R., Patel, J. M., Angelides, K. J., Sheridan, N. P., and Garg, L. C. (1986). Hyperoxia reduces plasma membrane fluidity: a mechanism for endothelial cell dysfunction. *J. Appl. Physiol. 60*:826-835.

Bonney, R. J., Opas, E. E., and Humes, J. L. (1985) Lipoxygenase pathways of macrophage. *Fed. Proc. 44*:2933-2936.

Brigham, K. L., and Meyrick, B. (1984). Interactions of granulocytes with the lungs. *Circ. Res. 54*:623-635.

Brigham, K. L., and Owen, P. J. (1975). Mechanism of the serotonin effect on lung transvascular fluid flux and protein movement in awake sheep. *Circ. Res. 36*:761-770.

Burhop, K. E., Zee, H. van der, Bizios, R., Kaplan, J. E., and Malik, A. B. (1986). Pulmonary vascular response to platelet-activating factor in awake sheep and the role of cyclooxygenase products. *Am. Rev. Resp. Dis. 134*: 548-554.

Burhop, K. E., Selig, W. M., and Malik, A. B. (1988). Monohydroxyeicosatraenoic acids induce pulmonary vasoconstriction and edema. *Circ. Res 62*: 687-698.

Burke, T. M., and Wolin, M. S. (1987). Hydrogen peroxide elicits pulmonary arterial relaxation and guanylate cyclase activation. *Am. J. Physiol. 252*: 721-732.

Camuss, G., Tetta, C., and Bussolino, F. (1983). Inhibitory effect of prostacyclin on neutropenia induced by intravenous injection of platelet-activating factor (PAF) in the rabbit. *Prostaglandins 25*:343-351.

Chesney, C., Pifer, C. D., Byers, L. W., and Murihead, E. E. (1982). Effect of platelet-activating factor (PAF) on human platelets. *Blood 59*:582-585.

Christner, P., Fein, A., Goldberg, S., Lippmann, M., Abrams, W., and Weinbaum, G. (1985). Collagenase in the lower respiratory tract of patients with adult respiratory distress syndrome. *Am. Rev. Resp. Dis. 131*:690-695.

Clark, M. A., Littlejohn, D., Mong, S., and Crooke, S. T. (1986). Effect of leukotrienes, bradykinin, and calcium ionophore (A23187) on bovine endothelial cells: release of prostacyclin. *Prostaglandins 31*:157-166.

Clouse, L. H., and Comp, P. C. (1986). The regulation of hemostasis: the protein C system. *New Engl. J. Med. 314*:1288-1304.

Cybulsky, M. I., Colditz, I. G., and Moviat, H. Z. (1986). The role of interleukin-1 in neutrophil leukocyte emigration induced by endotoxin. *Am. J. Pathol. 124*:367-372.

Dawson, C. A., Christensen, C. W., Rickaby, D. A., Linehan, J. H., and Johnston, M. R. (1985). Lung damage and pulmonary uptake of serotonin in intact dogs. *J. Appl. Physiol. 58*:1761-1766.

Demling, R. H., Wong, C., Fox, R., Hechtman, H. and Huval, W. (1985). Relationship of increased lung serotonin levels to endotoxin induced pulmonary hypertension in sheep: effects of a serotonin antagonist. *Am. Rev. Resp. Dis. 132*:1257-1261.

Demling, R. H., LaLonde, C., Li-Juan, J., Ryan, P., and Fox, R. (1986). Endotoxemia causes increased lung tissue lipid peroxidation in unanesthetized sheep. *J. Appl. Physiol. 60*:2094-2100.

Deuel, T. F., and Huang, J. S. (1984). Platelet-derived growth factor. *J. Clin. Invest. 74*:669-676.

Dise, C. A., Clark, J. M., Lambertsen, C. J., and Goodman, D. B. P. (1987). Hyperbaric hyperoxia reversibly inhibits erythrocyte phospholipid fatty acid turnover. *J. Appl. Physiol. 62*:533-538.

Dobuler, K. J., Catravas, J. D., and Gillis, C. N. (1982). Early detection of oxygen induced lung injury in conscious rabbits. *Am. Rev. Resp. Dis. 126*: 534-539.

Dyer, E. L., and Snapper, J. R. (1986). Role of circulating granulocytes in sheep lung injury produced by phorbol myristate acetate. *J. Appl. Physiol. 60*: 576-589.

Farber, H. W., Center, D. M., and Rounds, S. (1985). Bovine and human endothelial cell production of neutrophil chemoattractant activity in response to components of the angiotensin system. *Circ. Res. 57*:889-902.

Farber, H. W., Weller, P. F., Rounds, S., Beer, D. J., and Center, D. M. (1986). Generation of lipid neutrophil chemoattractant activity by histamine stimulated cultured endothelial cells. *J. Immunol. 137*:2918-2924.

Farrukh, I. S., Michael, J. R., Summer, W. R., Adkinson, N. F., and Gurtner, G. H. (1985). Thromboxane induced pulmonary vasoconstriction: involvement of calcium. *J. Appl. Physiol. 58*:34-44.

Farrukh, I. S., Gurtner, G. H., and Michael, J. R. (1987). Pharmacological modification of pulmonary vascular injury: possible role of cAMP. *J. Appl. Physiol. 62*:47-54.

Ferro, T. J., Moore, C. C., and Malik, A. B. (1987). Increased endothelial cell monolayer permeability induced by bronchoalveolar cells. *Am. Rev. Resp. Dis. 135*:A189.

Flick, M. R., Perel, A., and Staub, N. C. (1981). Leukocytes are required for increased lung vascular permeability after microembolization in sheep. *Circ. Res. 48*:344-351.

Flink, J. R., Pitt, B. R., Hammond, G. L., and Gillis, N. C. (1982). Selective effect of microembolization of pulmonary removal of biogenic animals. *J. Appl. Physiol. 52*:421-427.

Furchgott, R. F. (1983). Role of endothelium in responses of vascular smooth muscle. *Circ. Res. 53*:558-573.

Gajdusek, C., Carbon, S., Ross, R., Nawroth, P., and Stein, D. (1986). Activation of coagulation release endothelial cell mitogens. *J. Cell Biol. 103*:418-428.

Garcia-Szabo, R. R., Kern, D. F., and Malik, A. B. (1984). Effects of OKY-046 and OKY-1581 on pulmonary vascular response to thrombin. *Prostaglandins 28*:851-866.

Gay, J. C., Beckman, J. K., Brash, A. R., Oates, J. A., and Lukens, J. N. (1984). Enhancement of chemotactic factor stimulated neutrophil oxidative metabolism by leukotriene B_4. *Blood 64*:780-785.

Gee, M. H., Perkowski, S. Z., Tahamont, M. V., Flynn, J. T., and Wasserman, M. A. (1986). Thromboxane as a mediator of pulmonary dysfunction during intravascular complement activation. *Am. Rev. Resp. Dis. 133*:264-273.

Gillis, C. N., Pitt, B. R., Wiedmann, H. P., and Hammond, G. L. (1986). Depressed prostaglandin E_1 and 5-hydroxytryptamine removal in patients with adult respiratory distress syndrome. *Am. Rev. Resp. Dis. 134*:739-744.

Gimbrone, M. A., Aster, R. H., Cotrane, R. S., Corkery, I., Jandl, U. H., and Folkman, J. (1969). Preservation of vascular integrity in organs perfused in vitro with a platelet rich medium. *Nature (Lond.) 222*:33-36.

Gimbrone, M. A., Brock, A. F., and Schafer, A. I. (1985). Leukotriene B_4 stimulates polymorphonuclear leukocyte adhesion to cultured vascular endothelial cell. *J. Clin. Invest. 74*:1552-1555.

Goldblum, S. E., Cohen, D. A., Gillespie, M. N., and McClain, C. J. (1987). Interleukin-1 induced granulocytopenia and pulmonary leukostasis in rabbits. *J. Appl. Physiol. 62*:122-128.

Goldstein, I. M., Malmsten, C. L., Kindahl, H., Kaplan, H. B., Radmark, O., Samuelsson, B., and Weissman, G. (1978). Thromboxane generation by human peripheral blood poolymorphonuclear leukocytes. *J. Exp. Med. 148*:787-791.

Greenberg, B., Rhoden, K., and Barnes, P. J. (1987). Endothelium-dependent relaxation of human pulmonary arteries. *Am. J. Physiol. 252*:H434-H438.

Grondelle, A. V., Worthen, G. S., Ellis, D., Mathias, M. M., Murphy, R. C., Strife, R. J., Reeves, J. T., and Voelkel, N. F. (1984). Altering hydroxydynamic variables influences PGI_2 production by isolated lungs and endothelial cells. *J. Appl. Physiol. 57*:388-395.

Hakim, T. S., Zee, H. van der, and Malik, A. B. (1979). Effect of sympathetic serve stimulation on pulmonary transvascular fluid and protein exchange. *J. Appl. Physiol. 47*:1025-1030.

Hakim, T. S., Zee, H. van der, and Malik, A. B. (1981). Adrenoceptor control of lung fluid balance. *J. Appl. Physiol. 51*:68-72.

Hales, C. A., Rouce, E. T., and Slate, J. L. (1978). Influence of aspirin and indomethacin on variability of alveolar hypoxic vasoconstriction. *J. Appl. Physiol. 45*:33-39.

Hamasaki, Y., Mojarad, M., Saga, T., Tai, H. H., and Said, S. I. (1984). Platelet activating factor raises airway and vascular pressures and induces edema in lungs perfused with platelet-free solution. *Am. Rev. Resp. Dis. 129*:742-746.

Harlan, J. M. (1985). Leukocyte-endothelial cell interactions. *Blood 65*:513-525.

Harris, P., and Heath, D. (1977). Pharmacology of the pulmonary circulation. In *The Human Pulmonary Circulation*, Churchill Livingstone, New York, pp. 182-210.

Haver, V. M., and Namm, D. H. (1983). Generation of a vasoactive substance in human plasma during coagulation. *Blood Vessels 20*:92-98.

Haver, V. M., and Namm, D. H. (1984). Characterization of the thrombin induced contraction of vascular smooth muscle. *Blood Vessels 21*:53-63.

Hinshaw, D. B., Sklar, L. A., Bohl, B., Schraufstatter, I. U., Hyslop, P. A., Rossi, M. W., Spragg, R. G., and Cochrane, C. G. (1986). Cytoskeletal and morphologic impact of cellular oxidant injury. *Am. J. Pathol. 123*:454-464.

Hong, S. L., McLaughlin, N. J., Tzeng, C., and Patton, G. (1985). Prostacyclin synthesis and deacylation of phospholipids in human endothelial cells; comparison of thrombin, histamine and ionophore A23187. *Thromb. Res. 38*:1-10.

Horgan, M. J., Everitt, J., and Malik, A. B. (1987a). Reperfusion lung injury: protective effect of allopurinol. *Am. Rev. Resp. Dis. 135*:260.

Horgan, M. J., Fenton, J. W., III, and Malik, A. B. (1987b). α-Thrombin induced pulmonary vasoconstriction. *J. Appl. Physiol. 63*:1993-2000.

Horgan, M. J., Moon, D. G., Blumenstock, F. A., and Malik, A. B. (1988). Release of a lipid pulmonary vasoconstrictor by thrombin: distinct from cyclooxygenase and lipoxygenase metabolites. *FASEB J. 2*:A1506 (#7023).

Hyman, A. L., Spannhake, E. W., and Kadowitz, P. J. (1978). Prostaglandins and the lung. *Am. Rev. Resp. Dis. 117*:111-136.

Janoff, A. (1983). Proteases and lung injury. *Chest 83*:545-585.

Johnson, A., and Malik, A. B. (1980). Effect of granulocytopenia on lung extravascular fluid accumulation after microembolism. *Am. Rev. Resp Dis. 122*: 561-566.

Johnson, A., and Malik, A. B. (1981). Effect of different sized microemboli on lung fluid exchange. *J. Appl. Physiol. 57*:461-464.

Johnson, A., and Malik, A. B. (1982). Pulmonary edema after glass bead microembolization: protective effect of granulocytopenia. *J. Appl. Physiol. 52*: 155-161.

Johnson, A., Cooper, J., and Malik, A. B. (1986a). Pulmonary leukostasis after complement activation: effect on lung vascular permeability in unanesthetized sheep. *J. Appl. Physiol. 61*:2202-2209.

Johnson, A., Perlman, M. B., Blumenstock, F. A., and Malik, A. B. (1986). Superoxide dismutase prevents the thrombin induced increase in lung vascular permeability: role of superoxide in mediating the alterations in lung fluid balance. *Circ. Res. 54*:405-415.

Jones, R., Zapol, W. M., and Reid, L. (1984). Pulmonary artery remodeling and pulmonary hypertension after exposure to hyperoxia for 7 days. *Am. J. Pathol. 117*:273-285.

Kadowitz, P. J., and Hyman, A. L. (1984). Analysis of responses to leukotriene D_4 in the pulmonary vascular bed. *Circ. Res. 55*:707-717.

Kerr, J. S., Ruppert, C. L., Tozzi, C. A., Neubauer, J. A., Frankel, H. M., Yu, S. Y., and Riley, D. J. (1987). Reduction of chronic hypoxic pulmonary hypertension in the rat by an inhibitor of collagen production. *Am. Rev. Resp. Dis. 135*:300-306.

Kirton, O. C., and Jones, R. (1987). Rat pulmonary artery restructuring and pulmonary hypertension induced by continuous *Escherichia coli* endotoxin infusion. *Lab. Invest. 56*:198-210.

Kivlen, C. M., Johnson, A., Pittman, T., Guile, A. E., and Malik, A. B. (1982). Effect of converting enzyme inhibition on pulmonary edema after microembolization. *J. Appl. Physiol. 53*:1546-1550.

Kubo, K., and Kobayashi, T. (1985). Effects of OKY-046, a selective thromboxane synthetase inhibitor on endotoxin induced lung injury in unanesthetized sheep. *Am. Rev. Resp. Dis. 132*:493-499.

Le, J., and Vilcek, J. (1987). Tumor necrosis factor and interleukin 1: cytokines with multiple overlapping biological activities. *Lab. Invest. 56*:234-248.

Lee, B. C., Zee, H. van der, and Malik, A. B. (1979). Site of pulmonary edema after regional pulmonary embolization. *J. Appl. Physiol. 47*:556-560.

Lee, C. T., Fein, A. M., Lippman, M., Holtzman, H., Kimbel, P., and Weinbaum, G. (1981). Elastolytic activity in pulmonary lavage fluid from patients with adult respiratory distress syndrome. *New Engl. J. Med. 304*:192-196.

Levinson, R. M., Shure, D., and Moser, K. M. (1986). Reperfusion pulmonary edema after pulmonary artery thromboendarterectomy. *Am. Rev. Resp. Dis. 134*:1241-1243.

Libby, P., Ordovas, J. M., Auger, K. R., Robbins, A. H., Biring, L. K., and Dinarello, C. A. (1986). Endotoxin and tumor necrosis factor induce interleukin-1 gene expression in adult human vascular endothelial cell. *Am. J. Pathol. 124*:179-185.

Lin, A. H., Morton, D. R., and Gorman, R. R. (1982). Acetyl glyceryl ether phosphorylcholine stimulates leukotriene B_4 synthesis in human polymorphonuclear leukocytes. *J. Clin. Invest. 70*:1058-1065.

Lo, S. K., Burhop, K. E., Kaplan, J. E., and Malik, A. B. (1988). Role of platelets in maintenance of pulmonary vascular permeability to protein. *Am. J. Physiol. (Heart and Circulation)*:254:H763-H771.

Lynch, J. M., Lotner, G. Z., Betz, S. J., and Henson, P. M. (1979). The release of a platelet activating factor by stimulated rabbit neutrophils. *J. Immunol. 123*:1219-1226.

McCord, J. (1987). Oxygen derived free radicals: a link between reperfusion injury and inflammation. *Fed. Proc. 46*:2402-2406.

McDonald, R. J., Berger, E. M., and Repine, J. E. (1987). Neutrophil derived oxygen metabolites stimulate thromboxane release, pulmonary artery pressure increases and weight gain in isolated perfused rat lungs. *Am. Rev. Resp. Dis. 135*:957-959.

McIntyre, T. M., Zimmerman, G. A., Satoh, K., and Prescott, S. M. (1985). Cultured endothelial cells synthesize both platelet-activating factor and prostacyclin in response to histamine, bradykinin and adenosine triphosphate. *J. Clin. Invest. 76*:271-280.

McIntyre, T., Zimmerman, G. A., and Prescott, S. M. (1986). Leukotrienes C_4 and D_4 stimulate human endothelial cells to synthesize platelet-activating factor and bind neutrophils. *Proc. Natl. Acad. Sci. USA 83*:2204-2208.

McMurtry, I. F., and Morris, K. G. (1986). Platelet activating factor causes pulmonary vasodilation in the rat. *Am. Rev. Resp. Dis. 134*:757-762.

Malik, A. B. (1983). Pulmonary microembolism. *Physiol. Rev. 63*:1114-1207.

Malik, A. B. (1985). Mechanisms of neurogenic pulmonary edema. *Circ. Res. 57*:1-18.

Marayama, I., Bell, E., and Majerus, P. W. (1985). Thombomodulin is found on endothelium of arteries, veins, capillaries, and lymphatics and on syntrophoblast of human placenta. *J. Cell. Biol. 101*:363-371.

Matzner, Y., Bar-Ner, M., Yahalom, J., Ishai-Michaeli, R., Fuks, Z., and Vlodavsky, I. (1985). Degradation of heparan sulfate in the subendothelial extracellular matrix by a readily released heparanase from human neutrophils. *J. Clin. Invest. 76*:1306-1313.

Minnear, F. L., Moon, D. G., Kaplan, J. E., and Malik, A. B. (1982). Effect of ADP induced platelet aggregation on lung fluid balance. *Am. J. Physiol. 11*:645-561.

Minnear, F. L., Johnson, A., and Malik, A. B. (1986). B-Adrenoreceptor modulation of pulmonary transvascular fluid and protein exchange. *J. Appl. Physiol. 60*:266-274.

Minnear, F. L., Kivlen, C. M., and Malik, A. B. (1983). The effect of bradykinin on lung vascular permeability in sheep. *J. Appl. Physiol. 55*:1078-1084.

Mizus, I., Summer, W., Farrukh, I., Michael, J. R., and Gurtner, G. H. (1985). Isoproterenol or aminophylline attenuate pulmonary edema after acid lung injury. *Am. Rev. Resp. Dis. 131*:256-259.

Moncada, S., and Vane, J. R. (1979). Pharmacology and endogenous role of prostaglandins, endoperoxides, thromboxane A_2 and prostacyclin. *Pharmacol. Rev. 30*:293-331.

Morganroth, M. L., Reeves, J. T., Murphy, R. C., and Voelkel, N. F. (1984). Leukotriene synthesis and receptor blockers block hypoxic pulmonary vasoconstriction. *J. Appl. Physiol. 56*:1340-1346.

Morganroth, M. L., Stenmark, K. R., Norris, K. G., Murphy, R. C., Mathias, M., Reeves, J. T., and Voelkel, N. F. (1985). Diethylcarbamazine inhibits acute and chronic hypoxic pulmonary hypertension in awake rats. *Am. Rev. Resp. Dis. 131*:488-492.

Moser, K. M. (1979). Pulmonary vascular obstruction due to embolism and thrombosis. In *Pulmonary Vascular Diseases*. Edited by K. M. Moser. Marcel Dekker, New York, pp. 341-386.

Muller-Eberhard, H. J. (1975). Complement. *Ann. Rev. Biochem. 44*:697-724.

Mullertz, S. (1979). The fibrinolytic system. *Scand. J. Haem. (Suppl.) 34*:15-23.

Munoz, N. M., Shioya, T., Murphy, T. M., Primack, S., Dame, C., Sands, M. F., and Leff, A. R. (1986). Potentiation of vagal contractile response by thromboxane mimetic U-46619. *J. Appl. Physiol. 61*:1173-1179.

Nandiwada, P. A., Kadowitz, P. J., Said, S. I., Mojarad, M., and Hyman, A. L., (1985). Pulmonary vasodilation responses to vasoactive intestinal peptide in the cat. *J. Appl. Physiol. 58*:1723-1728.

Nemerson, Y., and Nossel, H. L. (1982). The biology of thrombosis. *Ann. Rev. Med. 33*:479-488.

Noonan, T., Kern, D. F., and Malik, A. B. (1985). Pulmonary microcirculatory responses to leukotriene B_4, C_4, and D_4 in sheep. *Prostaglandins 30*:419-439.

Noonan, T. C., and Malik, A. B. (1986). Pulmonary vascular response to leukotriene D_4 in unanesthetized sheep: role of thromboxane. *J. Appl. Physiol. 60*:765-768.

O'Brodovich, H., Kay, J., and Coates, G. (1985). Bradykinin is degraded in hypoxic lungs and does not affect epithelial permeability. *J. Appl. Physiol. 59*:1185-1190.

Okhuda, K., Nakahara, K., Weidner, J., Binder, A., and Staub, N. C. (1978). Lung fluid exchange after uneven pulmonary artery obstruction in sheep. *Circ. Res. 43*:152-161.

Ossanna, P. J., Test, S. T., Matheson, N. R., Regiani, S., and Weiss, S. J. (1986). Oxidative regulation of neutrophil elastase-alpha-1-proteinase inhibitor interactions. *J. Clin. Invest. 77*:1939-1951.

Pennington, J. E., Rossing, T. H., Boerth, L. W., and Lee, T. H. (1985). Isolation and partial characterization of a human alveolar macrophage derived neutrophil activating factor. *J. Clin. Invest. 75*:1230-1237.

Perlman, M. B., Lo, S. K., and Malik, A. B. (1986). Effect of prostacyclin on pulmonary transvascular fluid and protein exchange after thrombin in awake sheep. *J. Appl. Physiol. 60*:546-553.

Peters, S. P., Schleimer, R. P., Naclerio, R. M., Macglashan, D. W., Togias, A. G., Proud, D., Freeland, H. S., Fox, C., Adkinson, N. F., and Lichtenstein, L.

M., (1987). The pathophysiology of human mast cells. *Am. Rev. Resp. Dis. 135*:1146-1200.

Peterson, M. W., Stone, P., and Shasby, D. M. (1987). Cationic neutrophil proteins increase transendothelial albumin movement. *J. Appl. Physiol. 62*:1521-1530.

Piper, P. J. (1984). Formation and actions of leukotrienes. *Physiol. Rev. 64*: 744-761.

Piper, P. J., and Galton, S. A. (1984). Generation of leukotriene B_4 and leukotriene E_4 from porcine pulmonary artery. *Prostaglandins 28*:905-913.

Plow, E. F. (1982). Leukocyte elastase release during blood coagulation. *J. Clin. Invest. 69*:564-572.

Powe, J. E., Short, A., Sibbald, W. J., and Driedger, A. A. (1982). Pulmonary accumulation of polymorphonuclear leukocytes in the adult respiratory distress syndrome. *Crit. Care Med. 10*:712-718.

Rippe, B., Townsley, M., Thigpen, J., Parker, J. C., Korthuis, R. J., and Taylor, A. E. (1984). Effects of vascular pressures on the pulmonary microvasculature in isolated dog lungs. *J. Appl. Physiol. 57*:233-239.

Rubanyi, G. M., and Vanhoutte, P. M. (1986). Oxygen derived free radicals endothelium and responsiveness of vascular smooth muscle. *Am. J. Physiol. 250*:815-821.

Said, S. I.(1982). Metabolic functions of the pulmonary circulation. *Circ. Res. 50*:325-333.

Said, S. I., Mutt, V., and Erdos, E. G. (1980). The lung in relation to vasoactive polypeptides. *CIBA Found. Symp. 78*:217-237.

Saldeen, T. (1979). The microembolism syndrome: a review. In *The Microembolization Syndrome*. Edited by T. Saldeen. Almqvist and Wiksell, Stockholm, pp. 7-44.

Schnells, G., Voigt, W. H., Redl, H., Schlag, G., and Glatzl, A. (1980). Electronmicroscopic investigation of lung biopsies in patients with post-traumatic respiratory insufficiency. *Acta Chir. Scand. (Suppl.) 499*:9-20.

Schwartz, B. S., and Monroe, M. C. (1986). Human platelet aggregation is initiated by peripheral blood mononuclear cells exposed to bacterial lipopolysaccharide in vitro. *J. Clin. Invest. 78*:1136-1141.

Selig, W. M., Noonan, T. C., Kern, D. F., and Malik, A. B. (1986). Pulmonary microvascular responses to arachidonic acid in isolated perfused guinea pig lungs. *J. Appl. Physiol. 60*:1972-1979.

Selig, W. M., Burhop, K. E., Garcia, J. G. N., and Malik, A. B. (1988). Substance P induced pulmonary vasoreactivity in the guinea pig lung: mechanism of the response. *Circ. Res. 62*:196-203.

Selvaraj, P. M., Goodwin, J. D., and Ryan, U. S. (1987). Superoxide anion release by pulmonary endothelium: response to phorbol ester and Ca ionophore. *Fed. Proc. 46*:1401.

Snapper, J. R., Hinson, J. M., Hutchinson, A. A., Lefferts, P. L., Ogletree, M. L., and Brighton, K. L. (1984). Effects of platelet depletion on the unanesthetized sheep's pulmonary response to endotoxemia. *J. Clin. Invest. 74*: 1782-1791.

Snow, R. L., Davies, P., Pontoppidan, H., Zapol, W. M., and Reid, L. M. (1982). Pulmonary vascular remodeling in adult respiratory distress syndrome. *Am. Rev. Resp. Dis. 126*:887-892.

Snyder, L. M., Foster, N. L., Trainor, J., Jacobs, J., Leb, L., Lubin, B., Chiu, D., Shoket, S., and Mohandas, N. (1985). Effect of hydrogen peroxide exposure on normal human erythrocyte deformability, morphology, surface characteristics and spectrin-hemoglobin cross linking. *J. Clin. Invest. 76*: 1971-1977.

Tahamont, M. V., and Malik, A. B. (1983). Granulocytes mediate the increase in pulmonary vascular permeability after thromboembolism. *J. Appl. Physiol. 54*:1489-1495.

Tanaka, D. T., and Grimstein, M. M. (1985). Vasoactive effects of substance P on isolated rabbit pulmonary artery. *J. Appl. Physiol. 58*:1291-1297.

Tate, R. M., Morris, H. G., Schroeder, W. R., and Repine, J. E. (1984). Oxygen metabolites stimulate thromboxane production and vasoconstriction in isolated saline-perfused rabbit lungs *J. Clin. Invest. 74*:608-613.

Test, S. T., Lampert, M. B., Ossanna, P. J., Thoene, J. G., and Weiss, S. J. (1984). Generation of nitrogen-chlorine oxidants by human phagocytes. *J. Clin. Invest. 74*:1341-1349.

Tranzer, J. P., and Baumgartner, H. R. (1967). Filling gaps in the vascular endothelium with blood platelets. *Nature 216*:1126-1128.

Vaage, J. (1982). Intravascular platelet aggregation and pulmonary injury. *Ann. NY Acad. Sci. 384*:301-318.

Valone, F. H., and Goetze, E. J. (1983). Enhancement of human polymorphonuclear leukocyte adherence by the phospholipid mediators 1-O-hexadecyl-2=acetyl-*SN*-glycero-3-phosphorylcholine (AGEPC). *Am. J. Pathol. 113*:85-89.

Vanhoutte, P. M., Rubanyi, G. M., Miller, V. M., and Houston, D. S. (1986). Modulation of vascular smooth muscle contraction by the endothelium. *Ann. Rev. Physiol. 48*:307-320.

Vender, R. L., Clemmons, D. R., Kwock, L., and Friedman, M. (1987). Reduced oxygen tension induces pulmonary endothelium to release a smooth muscle cell mitogen(s). *Am. Rev. Resp. Dis. 135*:622-627.

Wagenvoort, C. A., and Wagenvoort, N. (1979). Pulmonary vascular bed: normal anatomy and response to decrease. In *Pulmonary Vascular Disease*. Edited by K. M. Moser. Marcel Dekker, New York, pp. 1-109.

Weiss, S. J., and Regiani, S. (1984). Neutrophils degrade subendothelial matrices in the presence of alpha-1-proteinase inhibitor. *J. Clin. Invest. 73*:1297-1303.

West, J. B., Dollery, C. T., and Nainmark, A. (1964). Distribution of blood flow in isolated lung; relation to vascular and alveolar pressures. *J. Appl. Physiol. 19*:713-724.

Winn, R., Maunder, R., and Harlan, J. (1987). Lung lymph flow after bone marrow injection into goats was reduced by indomethacin. *J. Appl. Physiol. 62*:762-767.

Worthen, G. S., Gumbay, R. S., Tanaka, D. T., and Grunstein, M. M. (1985). Opposing hemodynamic effects of substance P on pulmonary vasculature in rabbits. *J. Appl. Physiol. 50*:1098-1103.

Yanagisawa, M., Kurihara, H., Kimura, S., Tomobe, Y., Kobaayashi, M., Miksui, Y., Yazaki, Y., Goto, K., and Masaki, T. (1988). A novel potent vasoconstrictor peptideproduced by vascular endothelial cells. *Nature 392*:411-415.

Zimmerman, G. A., McIntyre, T. M., and Prescott, S. M. (1985). Thrombin stimulates the adherence of neutrophils to human endothelial cells in vitro. *J. Clin. Invest. 76*:2235-2246.

Zimmerman, T. S., Fierer, J., and Rothberger, H. (1977). Blood coagulation and the inflammatory response. *Semin. Haematol. 14*:391-404.

Zmuda, A., Dembinska-Kiec, A., Chytkowski, A., and Gryglewski, R. J. (1977). Experimental atherosclerosis in rabbits. Platelet aggregation, thromboxane A_2 generation, and anti-aggregatory potency. *Prostaglandins 14*:1035 1042.

14

Mechanisms of Pulmonary Hypertension in Chronic High Flow States

MARLENE RABINOVITCH

University of Toronto and
The Hospital for Sick Children
Toronto, Ontario, Canada

I. Introduction

The congenital cardiac defect with a left-to-right shunt best typifies the "chronic high flow state" associated with pulmonary hypertension. The development of structural changes in the pulmonary arteries in this condition leads to elevation in vascular resistance, the single most important impediment to a successful surgical outcome (DuShane et al., 1976). This chapter will describe the determinants of pulmonary hypertension in high flow states and will address the nature of the vascular changes and new concepts related to their mechanism of development. The latter, based on an explosion of new information about the cell biology of the vessel wall, will ultimately lead to improved understanding and treatment of this condition.

II. Determinants of Pulmonary Hypertension in Chronic High Flow States

The first description of severe pulmonary hypertension related to a high flow state was a case report of a 32-year-old man with progressive exercise intolerance and cyanosis, who died in congestive heart failure after an episode of hemoptysis (Eisenmenger, 1897). Postmortem examination revealed a large ventricular septal defect with overriding of the aorta. Many years later it was observed that the symptoms this man had also occurred in patients with a variety of congenital cardiac defects such as patent ductus arteriosus, atrial septal defect, or atrioventricular septal defect (Bing et al., 1947; Besterman, 1961; Reid et al., 1964; Newfeld et al., 1977). In these lesions there is initially left-to-right shunting, but later, in some patients, a progressive elevation in pulmonary vascular resistance develops, causing reversal of the shunt and cyanosis. The pathologic basis for this clinical entity, which came to be known as the Eisenmenger syndrome (Wood, 1959), was the development of structural changes in the peripheral pulmonary arteries, originally described as "endarteritis obliterans" (Civin and Edwards, 1950). Thus the term "pulmonary vascular obstructive disease" was commonly applied to describe the functional state.

Natural history studies revealed that among the different congenital cardiac defects with left-to-right shunts, and even among patients with the same abnormality, the incidence of this complication and the rate of its progression varied considerably (Nadas and Fyler, 1972) (Table 1). For example, approximately 15% of infants with a large unrestrictive ventricular septal defect develop progressive elevation in pulmonary vascular resistance associated with vascular disease, and this will usually occur either in late infancy or in early childhood (Hoffman and Rudolph, 1965). If surgical repair is carried out in the first two years of life, especially in the first 8 months, then increased pulmonary vascular resistance rarely persists (Rabinovitch et al., 1984), but if it is delayed beyond 2 years, then persistent elevation is inevitable and progressive disease likely (DuShane et al., 1976). Even those patients who manifest only a mild degree of elevation in pulmonary vascular resistance at rest will usually exhibit a more severe increase with exercise (Friedli et al., 1974; Hallidie-Smith et al., 1977). Infants with a large patent ductus arteriosus have the same incidence and rate of development of pulmonary vascular disease as those with an unrestrictive ventricular septal defect (Rudolph and Nadas, 1962; Reid et al., 1964). Patients with a secundum atrial septal defect in which high flow is unaccompanied by high pressure, however, usually do not develop elevated pulmonary vascular resistance until after the third decade (Besterman, 1961). Even then, the pulmonary vascular disease is more slowly progressive. It is for this reason and also because of the relative technical ease of the operation that some centers including our own have opted to repair secundum atrial septal defects in adult patients if there is still a substantial net left-to-right shunt despite severe elevation in pulmonary vascular resistance and advanced vascular changes (DiSesa et al., 1983). The initial results, in particular, relief of symptomatology, are encouraging, but it remains to be seen whether long-term outcome will be affected. Rarely, infants with a secundum atrial septal defect will have rapidly progressive pulmonary vascular disease

Table 1 Factors Determining the Development of Pulmonary Vascular Disease in Patients with Common Varieties of Congenital Heart Disease[a]

	Major Factors					Minor Factors	
	P_{pa}	P_{pv}	QPA	PO_{2PA}	PO_{2SA}	Hematocrit	PVD
ASD, secundum	–	–	+	+	–	–	Unlikely
ASD, primum	–	±	+	+	–	–	Possible
TAVC	+	+	+	+	±	±	Highly probable
Large VSD	+	±	+	+	–	–	Probable
with mitral disease	+	+	+	+	–	–	Virtually certain
TF	–	–	–	–	+	+	Unlikely till late
with Potts	+	±	+	+	–	±	Probable
TGA	±	±	+	+	±	+	Virtually certain
with VSD	+	+	+	+	±	+	Certain

[a]The abbreviations used are: PVD, pulmonary vascular disease; P, pressure; PV, pulmonary vein; Q, flow; PA, pulmonary artery; SA, systemic artery; P_{pa} mean pulmonary artery pressure; P_{pv}, mean pulmonary venous pressure; PO_{2PA}, oxygen pressure in pulmonary artery; PO_{2SA}, oxygen pressure in systemic artery; QPA, flow pulmonary artery.

Source: Adapted from Nadas and Fyler: (1972), p. 684.

in the first year of life (Haworth, 1983). In some of these cases we have observed associated pulmonary vein stenosis, a condition that is frequently difficult to detect clinically.

Virtually all patients with common atrioventricular canal develop severe and irreversible increased pulmonary vascular resistance in childhood. The majority do so by 2 years of age, but in some this has been observed as early as the first year and rarely it occurs by 6 months (Newfeld et al., 1977). The combination of an unrestrictive ventricular and atrial septal defect and frequently associated mitral regurgitation seems to increase the risk over that expected with a simple ventricular septal defect. Moreover, the fact that many of these patients with Downs syndrome with chronic upper airway obstruction and pulmonary congestion seems to add to the risk of operation, although these variables have not been satisfactorily sorted out.

The combination of a ventricular septal defect with coarctation of the aorta also seems to increase the risk of rapidly progressive pulmonary vascular changes either because the left atrial pressure is frequently elevated or because the ventricular pressures may be higher. The combination of an unrestrictive ventricular septal defect with d-transposition of the great arteries increases the risk of severe elevation in pulmonary vascular resistance in the first year of life from 8 to 40% (Newfeld et al., 1974) as does a large patent ductus arteriosus (Waldman et al., 1977). This probably reflects the additional contribution of cyanosis and polycythemia to the combined determinants of high pulmonary flow and pressure and high left atrial pressure (Table 1). There have even been reports of patients with simple d-transposition who develop progressive elevation in pulmonary vascular resistance after surgical repair even though they had normal values preoperatively (Rosengart et al., 1975; Berman et al., 1978; Edwards and Edwards, 1978). In some of these cases, microthrombi have been identified in peripheral arteries, and it has been assumed that severe polycythemia had been a predisposing influence. The combination of high flow, high pressure, and cyanosis as seen in truncus arteriosus also increases the risk of early permanent elevation in pulmonary vascular resistance even after 6 months (Marcelletti et al., 1976).

The fact that a given patient with a specific cardiac abnormality develops rapidly progressive elevation in pulmonary vascular resistance whereas another does not probably reflects an as yet unknown genetic predisposition. The latter will be better understood only when progress is made in defining the specific cellular mechanisms governing the development of the vascular changes.

III. Assessment of Pulmonary Hypertension in Chronic High Flow States

Detecting the patient with a given congenital cardiac defect who will develop pulmonary vascular disease at all or who will do so particularly rapidly is difficult. Clinical and radiologic manifestations are those of advanced disease (Weidman et al., 1963). Electrocardiography (Johnson et al., 1950), vectorcardiography (Chou et al., 1973), conventional echocardiography (Mills et al., 1980), and radionuclide studies (Rabinovitch et al., 1981b) are relatively nonspecific. Doppler two-dimensional echocardiography may prove more reliable (Marx et al., 1985). Early cardiac catheterization is, however, to date the most definitive way to assess the level of pulmonary vascular resistance and the risk of rapidly progressive pulmonary vascular disease. Criteria have been established to distinguish patients in whom, even after repair, persistent elevation in pulmonary resistance is likely (Mair et al., 1971): a difference in oxygen saturation between pulmonary arteries and veins of greater than 2.5 vol % or an absolute level of pulmonary vascular resistance of greater than 10 $\mu \cdot m^2$. Values in the range between 8 and 10 $\mu \cdot m^2$ are considered borderline but very promising that a decrease to 6$\mu \cdot m^2$ or less can be achieved with the administration of oxygen, tolazoline, or prostacyclin. While the estimate of pulmonary vascular resistance by the Fick principle is most precise when oxygen consumption is measured, the value obtained reflects the functional state at only one point in time and the measurement is influenced by a variety of factors: the level of sedation under which the patient is examined or the presence of pulmonary disease causing hypoxic vasoconstriction (Vogel et al., 1967), the level of hematocrit (Rosenthal et al., 1970), and the amount of flow through systemic collateral vessels (Keane et al., 1973). Thus, in certain cases, in addition to the hemodynamic assessment, an evaluation of the structural state of the pulmonary vascular bed can provide useful information.

Techniques of wedge angiography have been developed to assess preoperatively the structural state of the pulmonary vascular bed. Changes that can be evaluated qualitatively – sparsity of aborization of the pulmonary tree, abrupt termination, tortuosity and narrowing of small arteries, and reduced background capillary filling – generally reflect advanced vascular changes and indicate already severe elevation in pulmonary vascular resistance (Nihill and McNamara, 1978). We described a quantitive pulmonary wedge angiographic technique that predicts a broad range of vascular abnormalities (Rabinovitch et al., 1981c) (Fig. 1). A balloon catheter is first directed to the origin of the axial artery of the posterior basal segment of the lower lobe (the right lung is usually chosen). Contrast material is injected, and the injection is filmed on biplane cine. The rate of tapering of the arteries is evaluated by measuring the length of segment between 2.5 and 1.5 mm lumen diameter. The abruptness of tapering correlates in severity with the degree of abnormality in the peripheral arteries and hence the potential for persistent elevation in pulmonary vascular resistance after surgical repair (Rabinovitch et al., 1984). Decreased background filling with contrast material (assessed qualitatively) and increased pulmonary circulation time, a feature that can be measured quantitively from the cineangiogram, generally re-

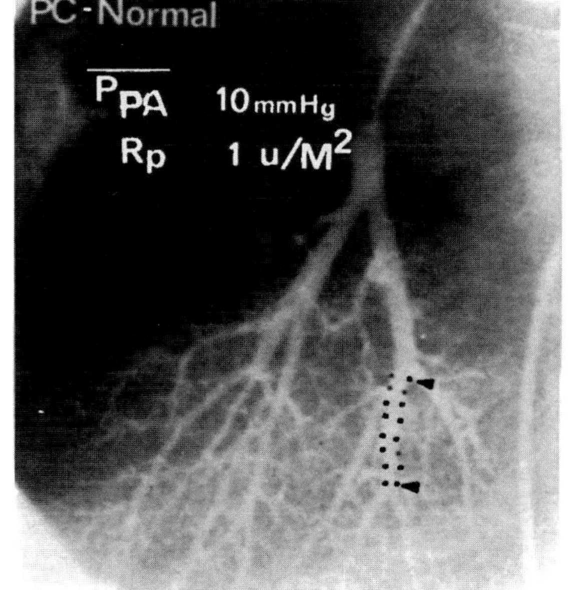

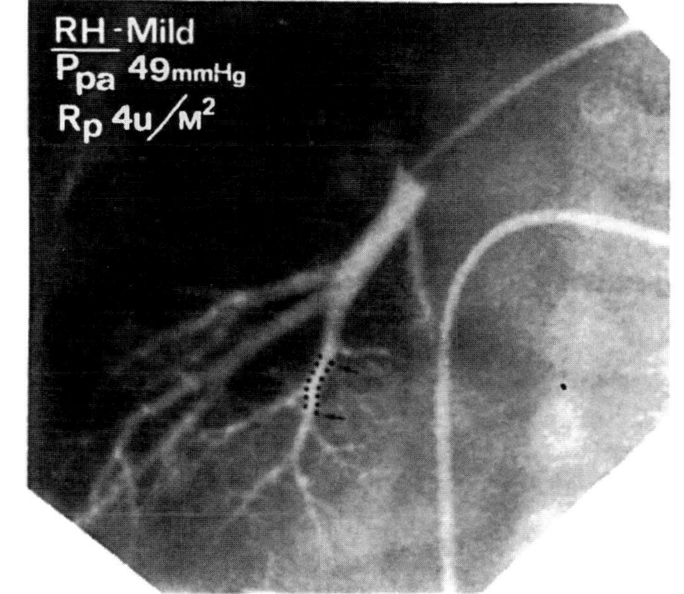

(A)

Figure 1 (A) Left: A wedge angiogram shows gradual tapering of the axial artery in a child with d-transposition of the great arteries (TGA) and normal pulmonary arterial pressure (P_{PA}) and resistance (R_p). Approximate segment length between 2.5 and 1.5 mm internal diameter is marked off (arrows). Right: A wedge angiogram in a child with a VSD shows rapid tapering of the artery and a decrease in "background haze" when there is increased pulmonary artery pressure and resistance. An approximate segment length between 2.5 and 1.5 mm internal diameter is marked off (arrows). (B) Left: A wedge angiogram with a more abrupt taper and decrease in "background haze." Right: In a child with more severe pulmonary hemodynamic impairment and irreversible vascular changes, there is very abrupt tapering and absent background filling of small vessels. (Reproduced with permission from Rabinovitch et al., 1981c).

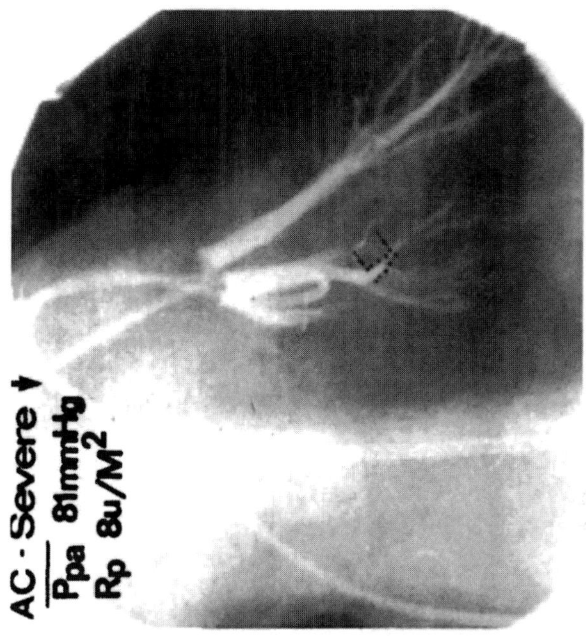

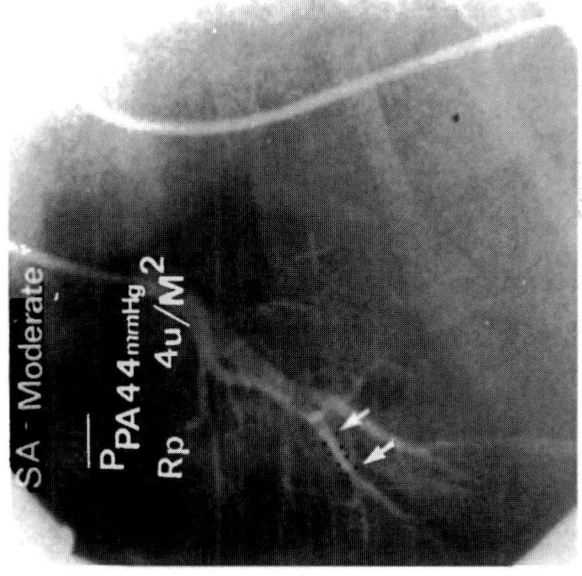

(B)

flect advanced disease. There are, however, some pitfalls in the interpretation of the wedge angiogram. An incomplete injection will give the false impression of decreased background filling, and incomplete occlusion of the vessel by the balloon will make the circulation time falsely rapid. Previous placement of a pulmonary artery band will result in abrupt tapering owing to poststenotic dilatation. Moreover, some patients with advanced vascular disease will not have abrupt tapering because the intimal hyperplasia has extended into larger preacinar arteries, narrowing the lumen uniformly. The same will be true of patients who have had severe vasoconstriction from birth and develop progressive vascular changes and severe elevation of pulmonary resistance without ever having had much of a left-to-right shunt. Both groups will, however, have markedly decreased background filling and a prolongation of the pulmonary circulation time.

When the hemodynamic measurement of pulmonary vascular resistance and findings on the wedge angiogram are in agreement that the disease is severe and irreversible, then further assessment of the structural state of the pulmonary vascular bed by evaluating a lung biopsy is usually just confirmatory. However, when data appear discrepant or are difficult to interpret, or in borderline cases, we have analyzed lung biopsy tissue to predict potential for reversibility of disease and risk of operation (Rabinovitch et al., 1981a).

IV. Nature of Pulmonary Vascular Changes in Chronic High Flow States

As early as 1935, from study of autopsy material, the different types of pulmonary vascular lesions occurring in patients with congenital heart defects were recorded (Brenner, 1935). In 1958, it was suggested that there was a progression of structural changes, grades I through VI (Heath and Edwards, 1958a) (Fig. 2). Grades I and II, medial hypertrophy and cellular intimal hyperplasia, respectively, were considered mild and probably reversible. Grade III, lumen occlusion from intimal hyperplasia, is characterized by little cellularity and by fibroelastosis, the so-called onionskinning pattern. Grade IV represents the formation of dilatation complexes and plexiform lesions. The latter results from medial thin-

Figure 2 Heath-Edwards classification of pulmonary vascular changes. (Top Left) Grade I: medial hypertrophy; elastin Van Gieson stain (EVG), X150. (Top Right) Grade II: cellular intimal proliferation in an abnormally muscular artery. EVG, X250, (Middle Left) Grade III: occlusive changes. Media is thickened due to fasciculi of longitudinal muscle, and vessel is all but occluded by fibroelastic tissue. EVG, X150. (Middle Right) Grade IV: dilatation. Vessel is dilated, and media is abnormally thin (arrow). Lumen is occluded by fibrous tissue. (Lower Left) Plexiform lesion. (Lower Right) Fibrinoid necrosis. EVG, X150. (Reproduced with permission from Wagenvoort et al., 1964.)

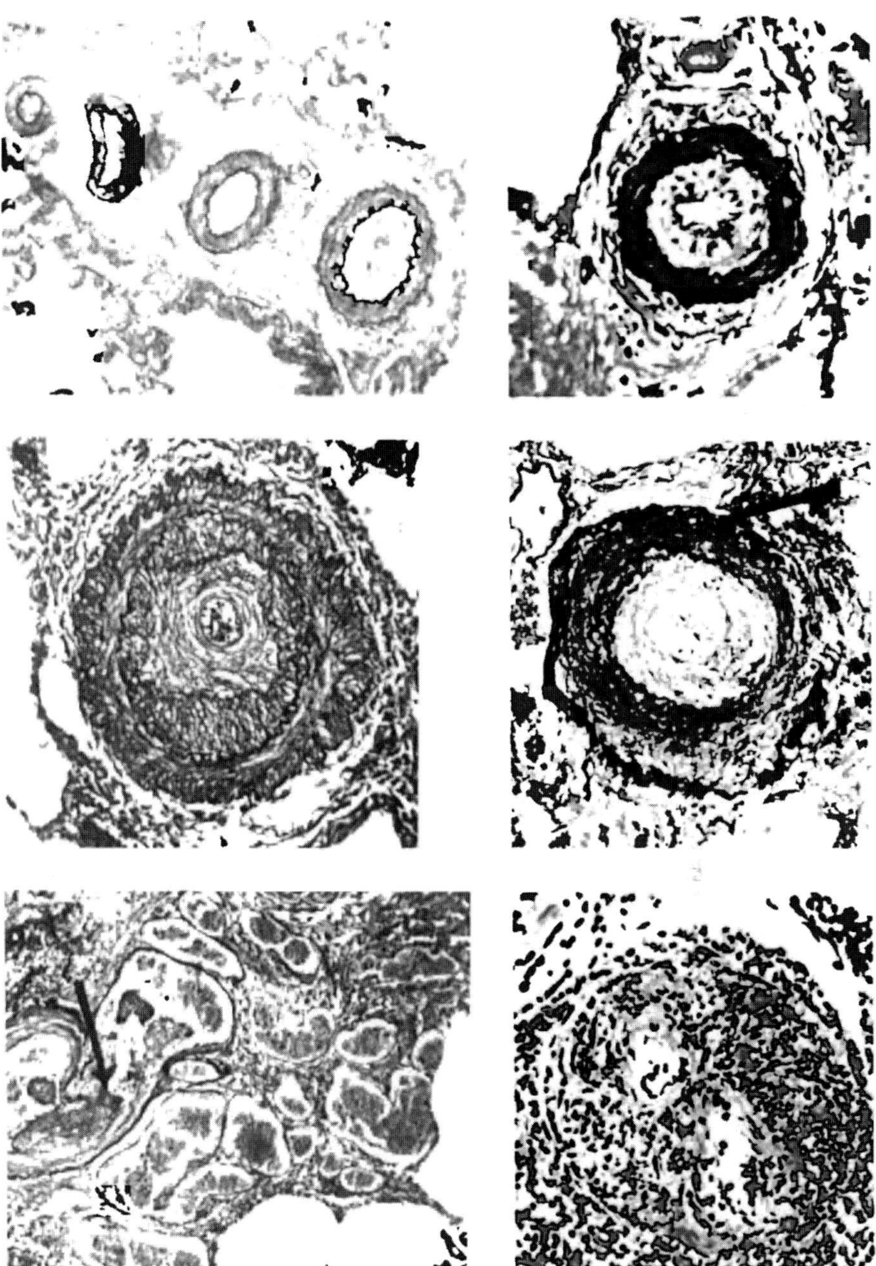

ning and atrophy and the development of small bypass channels around occluded vessels. Grade III is thought to be partially reversible at best in that some degree of elevated pulmonary vascular resistance will probably persist. Grade IV reflects structural changes associated with a progressive increase in pulmonary vascular resistance. Grades V and VI are terminal changes, V being angiomatoid formation and VI fibrinoid necrosis. The more advanced vascular changes indicating irreversible disease seem to take time to develop and have been most frequently identified in older children (Heath and Edwards, 1958b). It was, therefore, more difficult to establish in infants and young children, structural changes that predicted severe and fixed elevation in pulmonary vascular resistance. Several investigators tried to quantitate the degree of medial hypertrophy, but their measurements did not correlate closely with the preoperative level of pulmonary vascular resistance or with its change postoperatively (Naeye, 1966).

In the 1970s a new approach was developed to study pulmonary vascular changes in infants with congenital heart defects, the premise being that in a young lung it was likely that the features related to growth and development would be perturbed. Thus, reintroducing a technique of injecting lungs at postmortem, both the normal features of postnatal pulmonary vascular growth and development and the abnormalities that are associated with chronic high flow states were quantitatively assessed (Hislop and Reid, 1973; Hislop et al., 1975). After injecting the pulmonary vascular bed, arteriograms were generated that revealed that at birth all the preacinar generations were present, but small peripheral arteries could not be delineated and so the background was dark. With increasing age, the preacinar arteries grew in size, and also the background gradually filled in with a "haze" of small vessels that could not be resolved as single lines owing to their size and density.

On microscopic examination of the lung, it was observed that in the neonate the normally muscular arteries are most thickwalled, but at birth, with the fall in pulmonary vascular resistance, they begin to dilate. This occurs in the smallest vessels, those $<250\,\mu m$, in the first few days of life, and in the larger proximal arteries, up to the hilum, within the next few months. The peripheral intraacinar arteries are nonmuscular at birth, but gradually over months to years as they grow in size they become more muscular. Thus respiratory bronchiolus arteries become muscular by the first year of life, and alveolar duct arteries, in early childhood. The ratio of alveoli to arteries at birth is approximately 20:1, but alveoli proliferate rapidly, particularly in the first 2 years of life and so do arteries; in fact, the ratio of alveoli to arteries actually decreases, being 16:1 at the end of the first year, 12:1 at the end of the second, and 10:1 thereafter. It was observed that these normal features of pulmonary vascular growth and development are altered in the presence of a chronic high flow, high pressure state such as that produced by a ventricular septal defect (Fig. 3). The wall

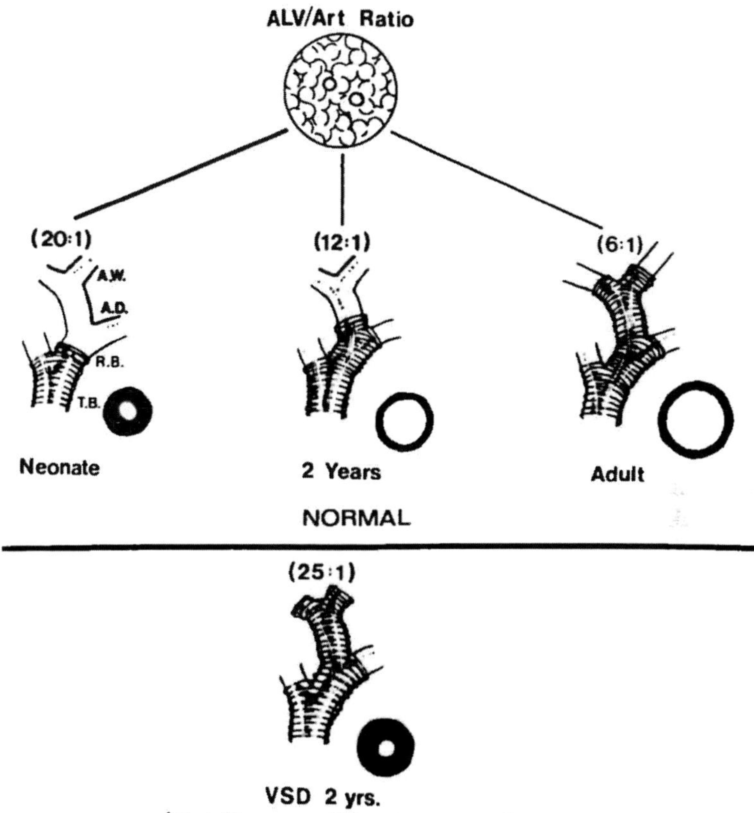

Figure 3 Schema of normal peripheral pulmonary arterial development and abnormal development in a child with a ventricular septal defect and high pulmonary arterial pressure and resistance at 2 years. Normally, muscle extends with age into arteries more peripheral within the acinus; the wall thickness of the normally muscular arteries decreases, and there is a decreasing ratio of alveoli to arteries, indicating an increase in the number of arteries. In a child with a ventricular septal defect, abnormalities in all three features of normal growth and remodeling may be seen, that is, "precocious" extension of muscle into peripheral arteries, medial hypertrophy of muscular arteries, and a reduced concentration of arteries, i.e., increased alveolar arterial ratio. T.B., artery accompanying a terminal bronchiolus; R.B., artery accompany a respiratory bronchiolus; A.D., artery accompanying an alveolar duct; A.W., artery accompanying an alveolar wall; ALV-Art, alveolar arterial ratio. (Reproduced with permission from Rabinovitch et al., 1978.)

thickness of the normally muscular arteries fails to regress from birth, and there is additional medial hypertrophy; muscle "extends" precociously into arteries that are located peripherally and are normally nonmuscular. The peripheral arteries do not grown normally in that they are small and decreased in number. The latter is reflected by an increased ratio of alveoli to arteries. Alveolar multiplication and differentiation is, however, normal. Since there is no regional variation in the severity of these structural abnormalities assessed quantitatively (Haworth and Reid, 1978), application of the morphometric technique of analysis of lung biopsy tissue is feasible.

From lung biopsy studies, we observed that the severity of altered growth and development of the pulmonary vascular bed is correlated with the hemodynamic state. Three progressively severe stages are seen (Rabinovitch et al., 1978) (Fig. 4).

Grade A There is abnormal extension of muscle into small peripheral arteries that are normally nonmuscular only or, in addition, a mild increase in medial wall thickness of the normally muscular arteries is present (less than 1.5X normal). These patients have increased pulmonary blood flow but, generally, normal mean pulmonary artery pressure. Meyrick and Reid (1980) have shown from ultrastructural studies of lung biopsy tissue that the basis for this change is a differentiation to smooth muscle of the precursor cells, the pericyte in the normally nonmuscular region of the artery and the intermediate cell in the partially muscular region. Since arteries become more muscular as they increase in size, it is tempting to speculate that in the setting of the altered hemodynamics of a chronic high flow, high pressure state, it is the mechanical stretch of the cells that initiates the structural change. This mechanism is being addressed in our experimental studies, which will be discussed.

Figure 4 Morphometric features on lung biopsy tissue. (Left) A 2-year-old child with a ventricular septal defect and normal pulmonary arterial pressure. (Right) A 2-year-old with a defect of the atrioventricular canal and increased pulmonary artery pressure and resistance. (Top) Alveolar wall arteries, nonmuscularized on left and surrounded by a complete muscular coat on right, x175. (Middle) Artery accompanying respiratory bronchiolus (RB), (left) with wall thickness only slightly increased, (right) with wall thickness greatly increased x70. Arrows denote external diameter and medial width. (Bottom) An abundance of small arteries (arrows) relative to alveoli (left) and only one small artery in a similar microscopic field (right). Elastic Van Gieson stain. (Reproduced with permission from Rabinovitch et al., 1978.)

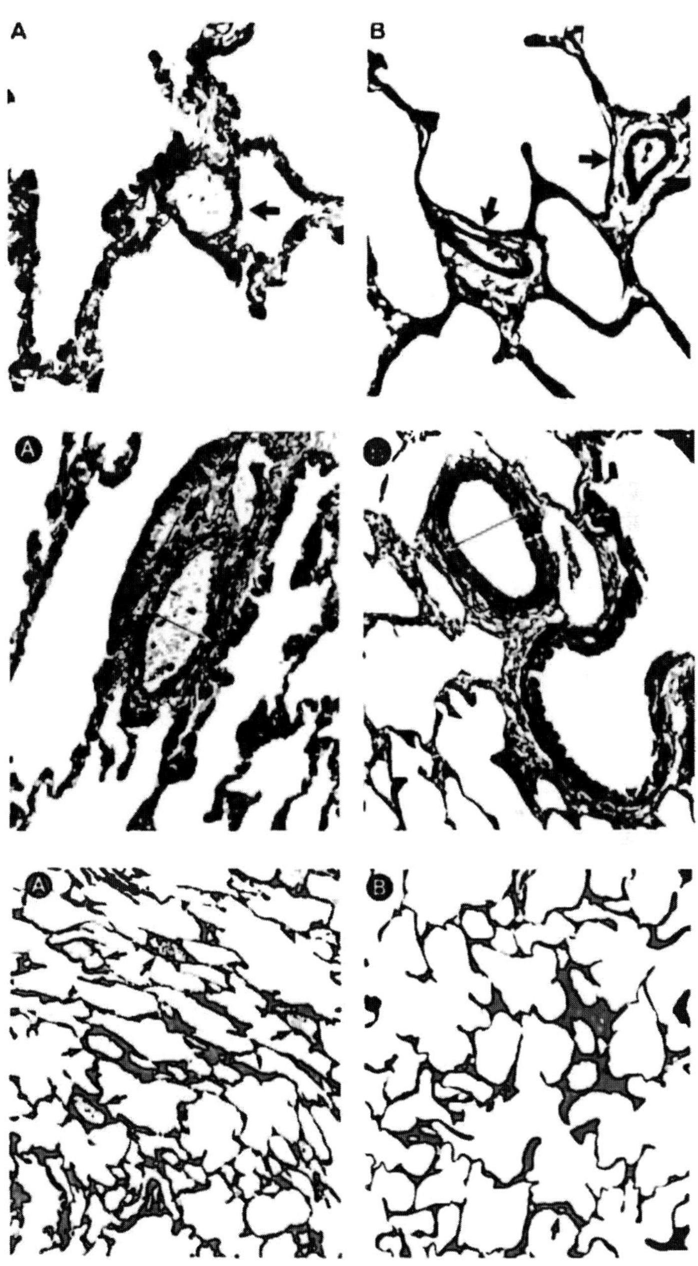
A
B
A
B
A
B

Grade B As in grade A, there is increased extension of muscle, but in addition there is more severe medial hypertrophy of normally muscular arteries. When medial wall thickness is greater than 1.5 times but less than 2 times normal (grade B mild), mild pulmonary hypertension is usually present. When medial wall thickness is more than twice normal (grade B severe), pulmonary hypertension is always present and often with pressure values greater than half the systemic level. The medial wall thickness is due to hypertrophy as well as hyperplasia of preexisting smooth muscle cells and an increase in the intercellular connective tissue proteins (Meyrick and Reid, 1980).

Grade C In addition to the findings of late grade B, arterial concentration is reduced, and usually arterial size also. Patients with these changes have elevation in pulmonary vascular resistance of greater than 3.5 $\mu \cdot m^2$. When arterial number is greater than half normal (grade C mild), pulmonary vascular resistance is often less than 6 $\mu \cdot m^2$, whereas if arterial number is less than half normal it is generally higher. The basis for grade C is likely the failure of new vessels to grow normally, although some loss of arteries may also occur (Meyrick et al., 1974).

Whether and to what extent abnormal growth and structural remodeling of the pulmonary vascular bed are permanent and result in functional impairment has been determined by correlating these features with postoperative hemodynamic studies. We correlated both the quantitative features of abnormal growth and remodeling of the pulmonary arteries and the qualitative changes described by Heath and Edwards with the hemodynamic behavior of the pulmonary circulation in the immediate postoperative period in the intensive care unit and one year later at the time of routine cardiac catheter study (Rabinovitch et al., 1984). Patients with grade A or grade B mild changes have normal pulmonary arterial pressures in the early postoperative period or only a minimal degree of elevation. Those with more severe medial hypertrophy, i.e., grade B severe and Heath-Edwards I, usually have elevated values. The pulmonary hypertension observed is frequently labile and usually can be controlled with a combination of hyperventilation and vasodilators (Jones et al., 1981). The nature of this increased pulmonary vascular reactivity resulting in "pulmonary hypertensive crises" will be addressed. Both the presence and the severity of pulmonary hypertension in the early postoperative period are increasingly predictable when there are more advanced changes on lung biopsy, i.e., reduced artery number (grade C) and intimal hyperplasia (Heath-Edwards II) (Fig. 5A).

One year after repair, however, patients operated on within the first 8 months of life tend to have normal pulmonary hemodynamics regardless of the severity of vascular change on lung biopsy, as do all patients with abnormalities of grade B severe (Heath-Edwards I) regardless of their age at repair. Patients

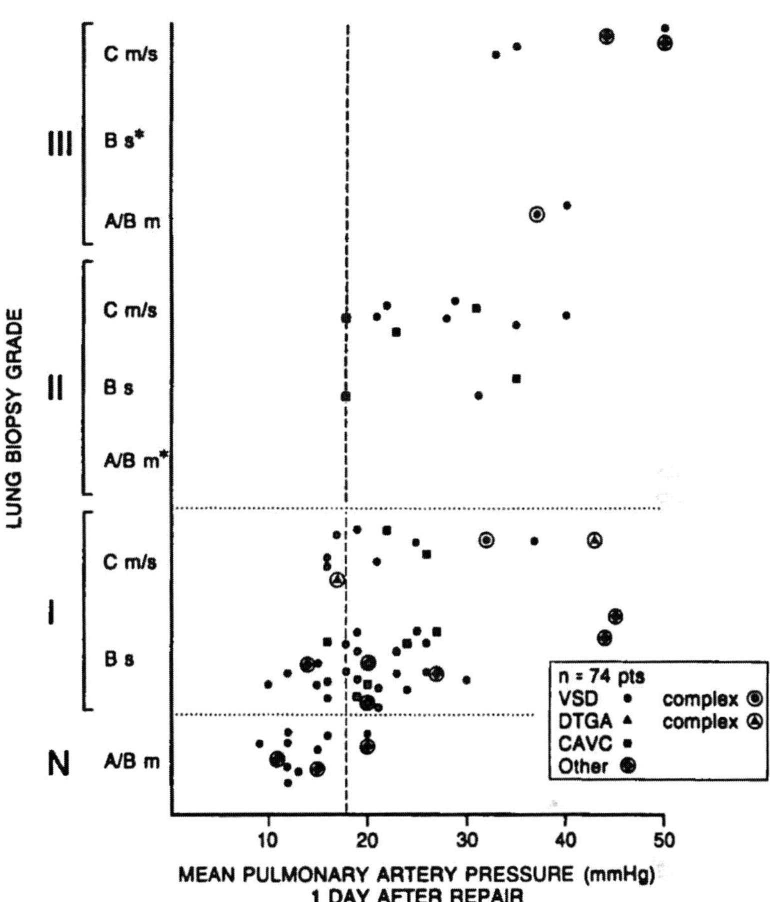

Figure 5A Lung biopsy grade is correlated with mean pulmonary arterial pressure recorded the day after surgical repair. The dashed vertical lines separate the normal from the abnormally elevated pressure values, and the dotted horizontal lines separate the biopsy grades. Note that with the more severe Heath-Edwards changes on lung biopsy tissue there is a trend toward a greater proportion of patients with elevated pulmonary arterial pressures and higher values. A, B, C, are morphometric grades; m, mild; s, severe. N, I, II, III are Heath-Edwards grades. N, normal, *, no patients in this group; VSC, ventricular septal defect; DTGA, d-transposition of the great arteries; CAVC, complete atrioventricular canal; complex, associated abnormality. (Reproduced with permission from Rabinovitch et al., 1984.)

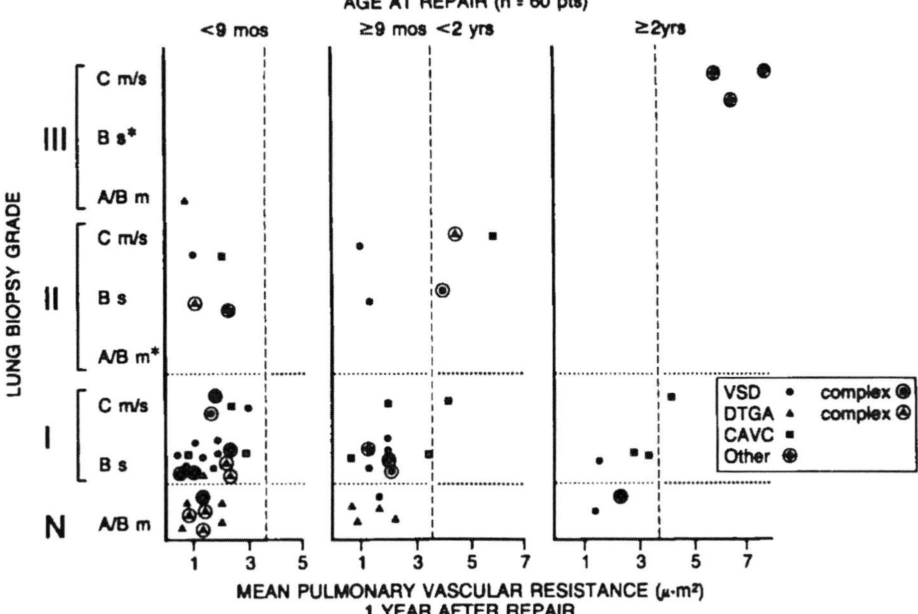

Figure 5B Graph correlating lung biopsy grade with pulmonary vascular resistance 1 year after cardiac repair. Patients who underwent repair within the first 8 months of life, but not those operated upon later, had normal pulmonary vascular resistance regardless of the severity of their structural changes. (Reproduced with permission from Rabinovitch et al., 1984.)

operated on between 9 months and 2 years of life with grade C and Heath-Edwards II or more severe structural changes may have persistent elevation in pulmonary vascular resistance, and this appears inevitable in those operated on after 2 years of life (Fig. 5B).

V. Control of the Reactive Pulmonary Circulation

A major challenge in pediatric cardiology is to understand and control the reactive pulmonary circulation, which can be particularly problematic in the early postoperative period after repair of a congenital heart defect. The "pulmonary hypertensive crisis," as it has been called, is thought to result from interaction of vascular endothelium with platelets and leukocytes which, following cardiopulmonary bypass and hypothermia may more easily degranulate (Biggar et al., 1984) and release potent vasoconstrictor agents, in particular thromboxanes (Addonizio et al., 1980) and leukotrienes (Yokochi et al., 1982). In recent studies, an increased density of neuroepithelial bodies (Cutz et al., 1984) has been observed in the airways of patients at risk of this complication (Cutz et al., 1986). These neuroendocrine cells contain bombesin and serotonin, also known to be potent vasoconstrictors. Since most of the pulmonary hypertensive crises occur upon weaning from the ventilator, it is tempting to speculate that swings in airway pressure might lead to degranulation of the neuroepithelial cells and release of the vasoconstrictor substances. It is also conceivable that the hypertensive pulmonary arteries lack or are unresponsive to the endothelial dependent relaxing factor (Furchgott, 1983; Vanhoutte et al., 1986), as has been demonstrated in atherosclerotic systemic arteries (Jayakody et al., 1987).

Various methods of managing postoperative increased pulmonary vascular reactivity have been proprosed, including prolonged anesthesia with fentanyl (Hickey et al., 1985) and vasodilators such as tolazoline (Jones et al., 1981). In our own unit, we have benefited from continuous monitoring of pulmonary arterial and left atrial pressure. To maintain the pulmonary arterial pressure at less than or equal to half systemic level, we institute hyperventilation (pCO_2 25-30 mmHg) and if necessary continue for several postoperative days. Thereafter, weaning from the ventilator can usually be accomplished slowly and with the help of intravenous vasodilators: specifically, we give alpha antagonists such as nitroglycerin followed by phenoxybenzamine if there is evidence that left ventricular dysfunction may be aggravating the problem: beta agonists, salbutamol or isoproterenol, are helpful if there is a component of pulmonary congestion. Almost all patients can be weaned from this therapy after one week.

There are, however, a few patients who maintain a high level of pulmonary vascular resistance and are refractory to vasodilator therapy despite what appear to be mild vascular changes on light microscopy (medial hypertrophy) and others who develop rapidly progressive pulmonary vascular disease despite early diagnosis and timely intervention. In our most recent lung biopsy studies on patients with congenital heart defects and pulmonary hypertension, we are trying to learn more about the nature of altered endothelial platelet, leukocyte, and endothelial smooth muscle interactions that may be relevant to the mechanism of heightened pulmonary vascular reactivity and to the development of progressive pulmonary vascular disease (Rabinovitch et al., 1986, 1987; Turner-Gomes and Rabinovitch, 1988).

Using scanning and transmission electron microsopy, we have identified structural changes in pulmonary vascular endothelial cells that suggest altered function and the potential for abnormal interaction with circulating blood elements, platelets and leukocytes (Rabinovitch et al., 1986). On scanning electron microscopy, the endothelial surface of normal thin-walled pulmonary

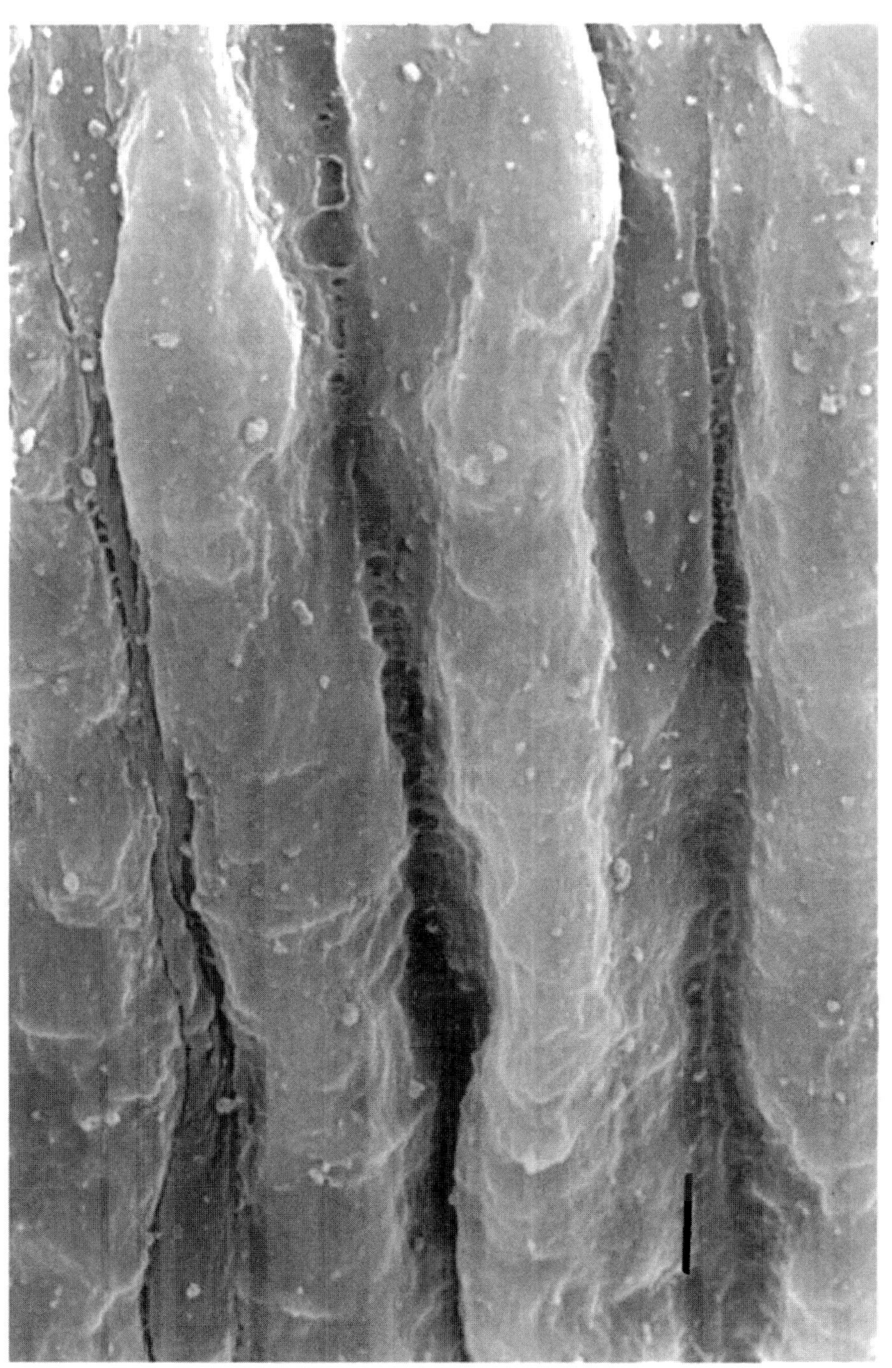

(a)

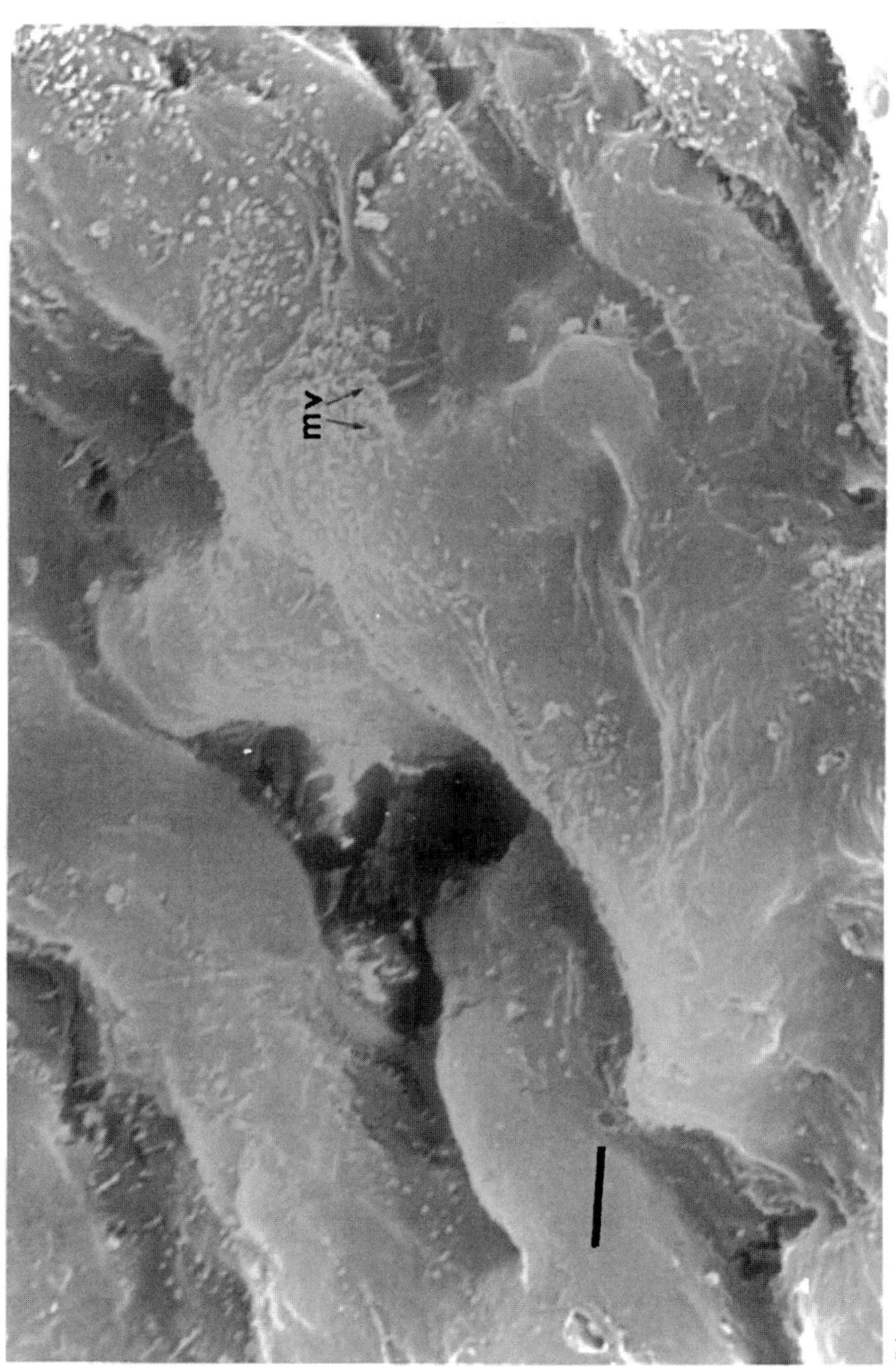
mv
(b)

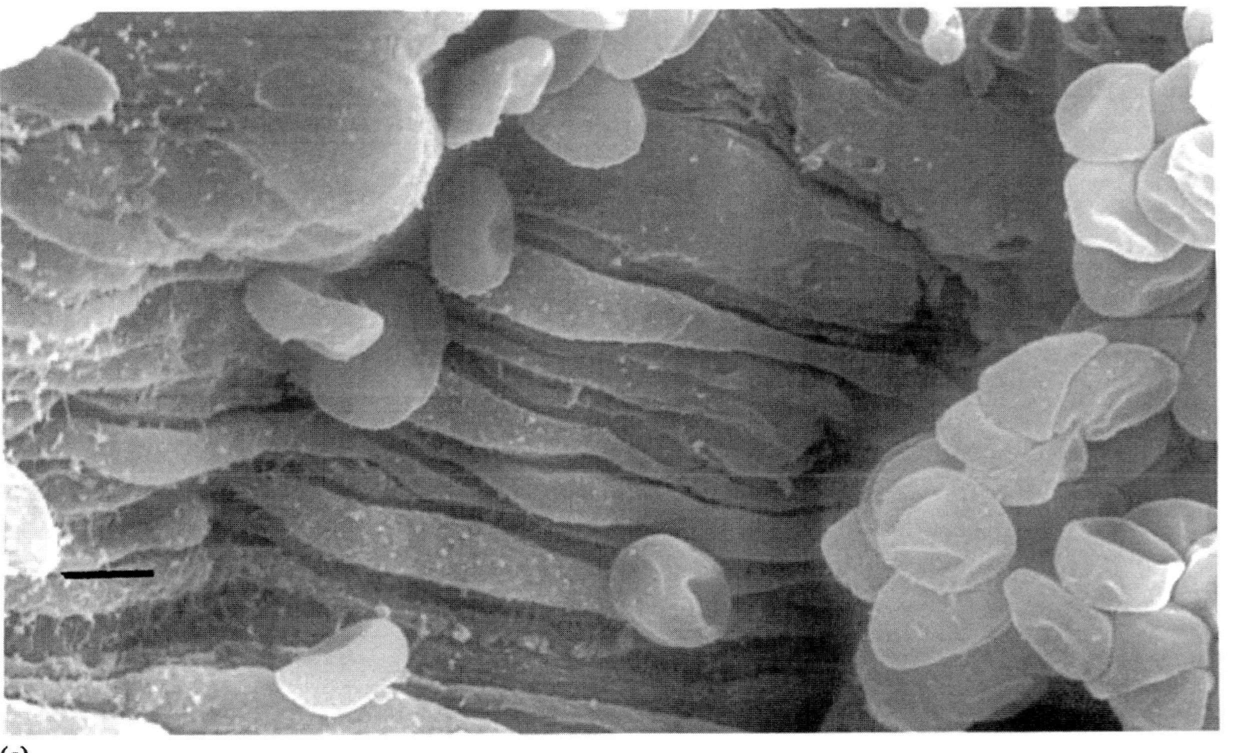

(c)

Figure 6 Scanning electron photomicrographs of pulmonary artery endothelial surfaces. (a) Normal pulmonary artery shows "corduroy pattern," neat, closed aligned ridges. (b) Hypertensive pulmonary artery shows "cable" pattern, deep knotted ridges, and numerous microvilli (MV). (c) Hypertensive pulmonary artery from a patient with advanced structural changes shows chenille pattern with misshapen endothelial cells. Magnification X 810. (Re-

arteries has a "corduroy-like" appearance in that the cells form narrow even ridges (Fig. 6). In contrast, the endothelial surface of hypertensive thick-walled pulmonary arteries has a "cable-like" texture in that the cells form deep, twisted ridges (Fig. 6). In patients with advanced pulmonary vascular changes, the endothelial surface exhibits a chenille pattern in which high ridges alternate with narrow, twisted misshapen ones (Fig. 6). The hypertensive endothelium is therefore coarse relative to the normotensive and may be predisposed to interact abnormally roughly with marginating blood elements such as platelets and leukocytes. This might result in the release of pulmonary vasoconstrictor substances and smooth muscle mitogens. In very preliminary studies, we have identified platelet activating factor, a phospholipid produced by endothelial cells (Zimmerman et al., 1985) and known to be a pulmonary vasoconstrictor (Stimler and O'Flaherty, 1983) and platelet aggregator, in the plasma of patients with increased pulmonary arterial pressure and heightened postoperative pulmonary vascular reactivity (Turner-Gomes and Rabinovitch, 1988).

On transmission electron microscopy, it is evident that the altered endothelial surface of hypertensive pulmonary arteries is associated with abnormalities in the concentration of the intracytoplasmic components. There is an increased density of microfilament bundles and rough endoplasmic reticulum (Fig. 7). The former suggests an altered cytoskeleton that may serve to keep the endothelium well anchored to the subendothelium, whereas the latter indicates increased protein synthesis and metabolic activity. The subendothelium of the muscular arteries is also abnormal in that there appear to be degradation and neosynthesis of the internal elastic lamina (Fig. 8).

Further studies were designed to try to identify what the products of increased endothelial metabolism might be. We hypothesized that since endothelial cells produce factor VIII (Von Willebrand), an increase in this protein may cause platelet adhesion, and this may also result in release of pulmonary vasoconstrictor substances and smooth muscle mitogens (Rabinovitch et al., 1987). Using an immunoperoxidase stain for factor VIII, we observed that hypertensive pulmonary arteries stain densely whereas nonhypertensive vessels do not (Fig. 9). We then measured the circulating levels of the factor VIII molecule, both the antigenic component VIII:Ag) and the biologic, measured as ristocetin-induced platelet agglutination (VIII:rist). While VIII:Ag levels were significantly higher in patients with congenital heart defects and elevated pulmonary arterial pressure than in those with normal pressure, in only a few was there a concomitant elevation in VIII:rist. This indicated that the molecule being synthesized was lacking in biologic activity (Fig. 10), and indeed, further multimeric analysis of the factor VIII being produced revealed lack of the high molecular weight components (Fig. 11). Thus it appeared that the endothelium in most patients with congenital heart defects and pulmonary hypertension might actually be less conducive to platelet adhesion and the formation of platelet fibrin microthrombi.

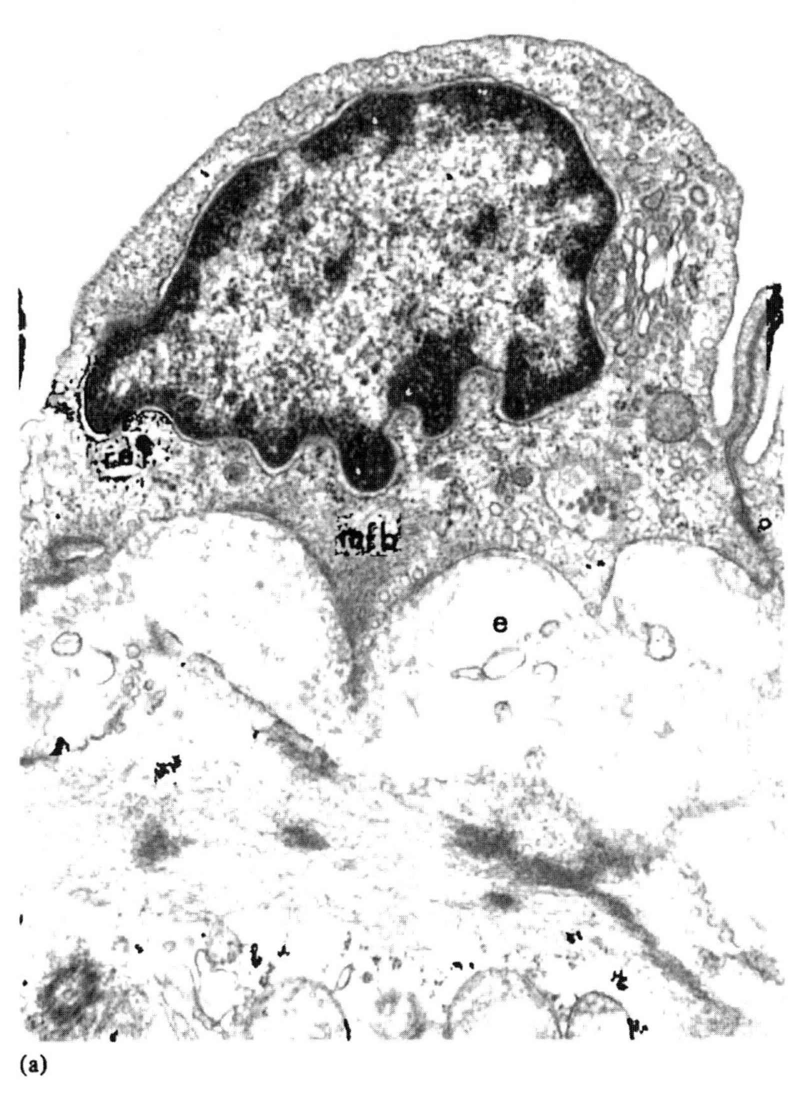

(a)

Figure 7 Transmission electron photomicrographs of pulmonary artery endothelial cells. Compared to normal endothelial cell in (a), endothelial cell in (b), from hypertensive pulmonary artery, shows increased rough endoplasmic reticulum (rer) and microfilament bundles (mfb) X 34,000. (Reproduced with permission from Rabinovitch et al., 1986.)

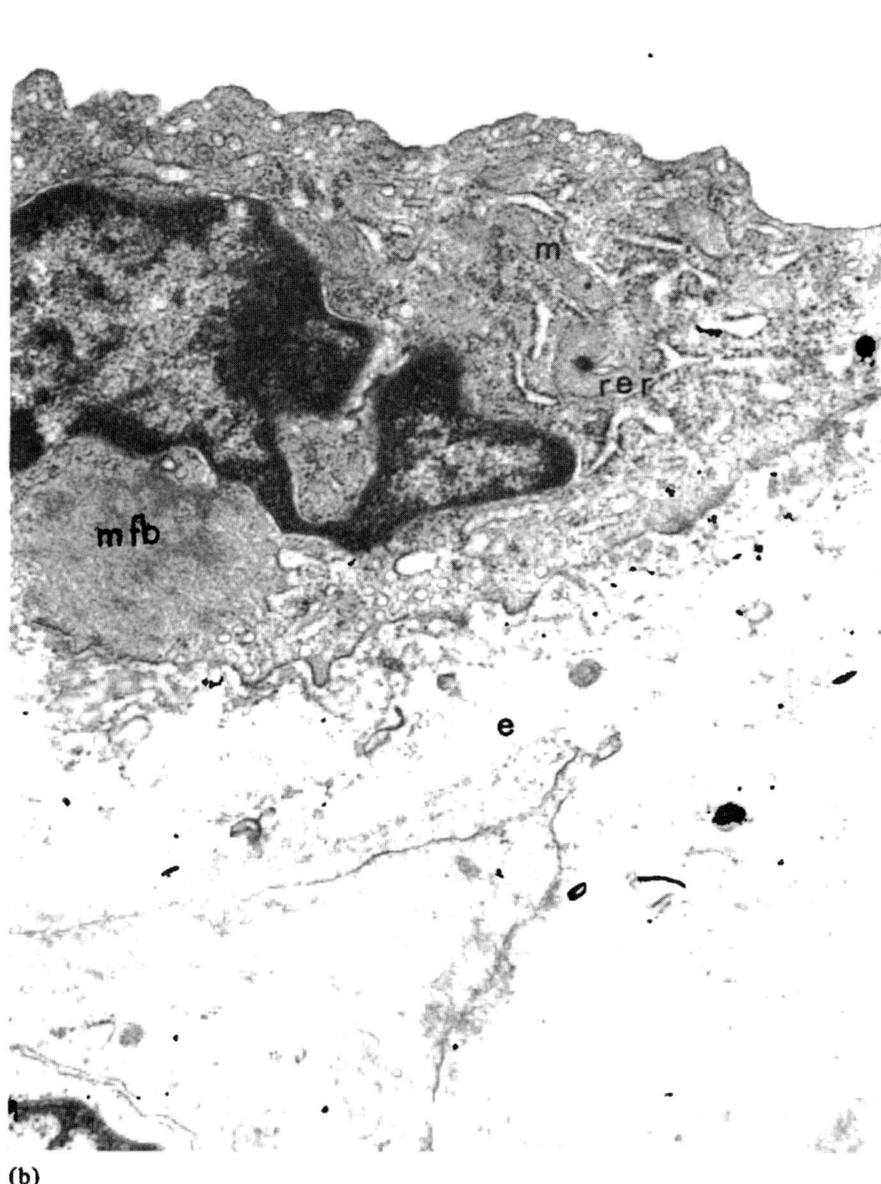

(b)

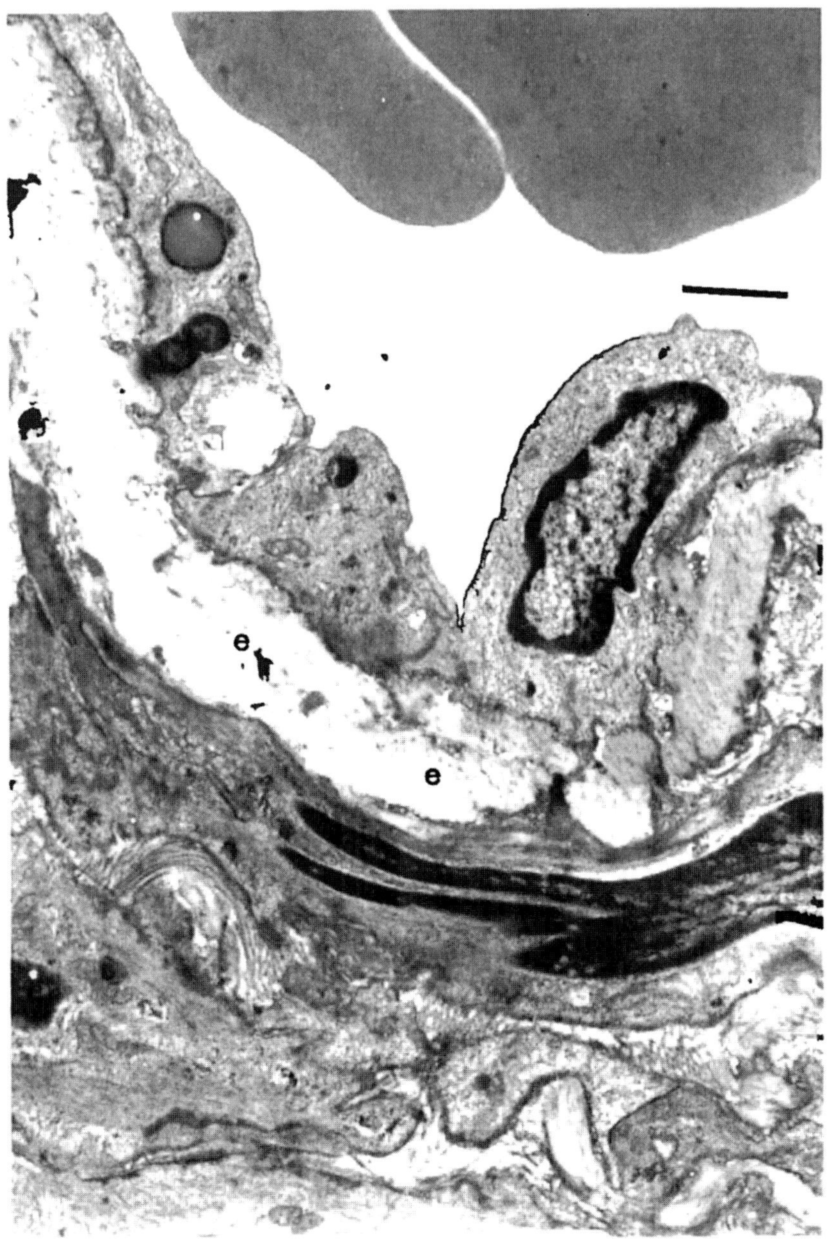

(a)

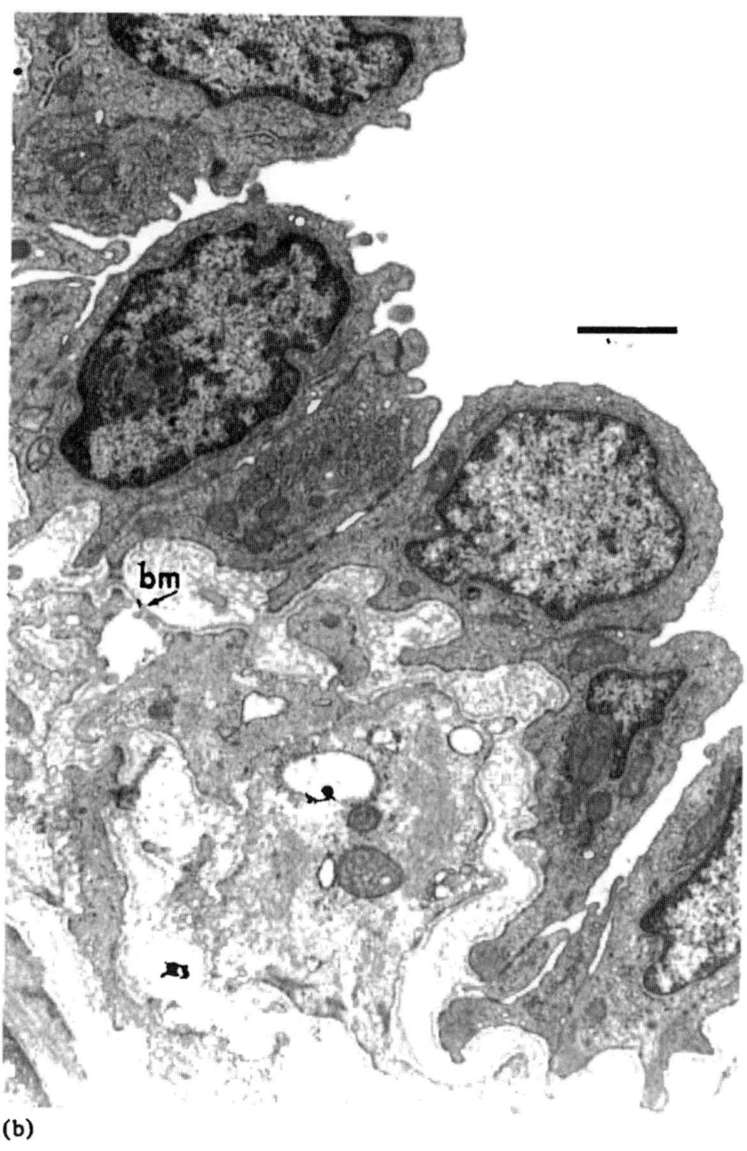

(b)

Figure 8 (a) A section of a pulmonary artery 92 μm in diameter in a patient with normal pulmonary arterial pressure shows an intact elastic lamina. (b) In a section from a pulmonary artery 108 μm in diameter in a patient with increased pulmonary blood flow and pressure, microfibrillar material is present in the subendothelium but no true internal elastic lamina. The endothelial and smooth muscle cells are separated by only a thick basement membrane (bm). A myoendothelial contact is seen (e). Bar = 1μm in both. (Reproduced with permission from Rabinovitch et al., 1986.)

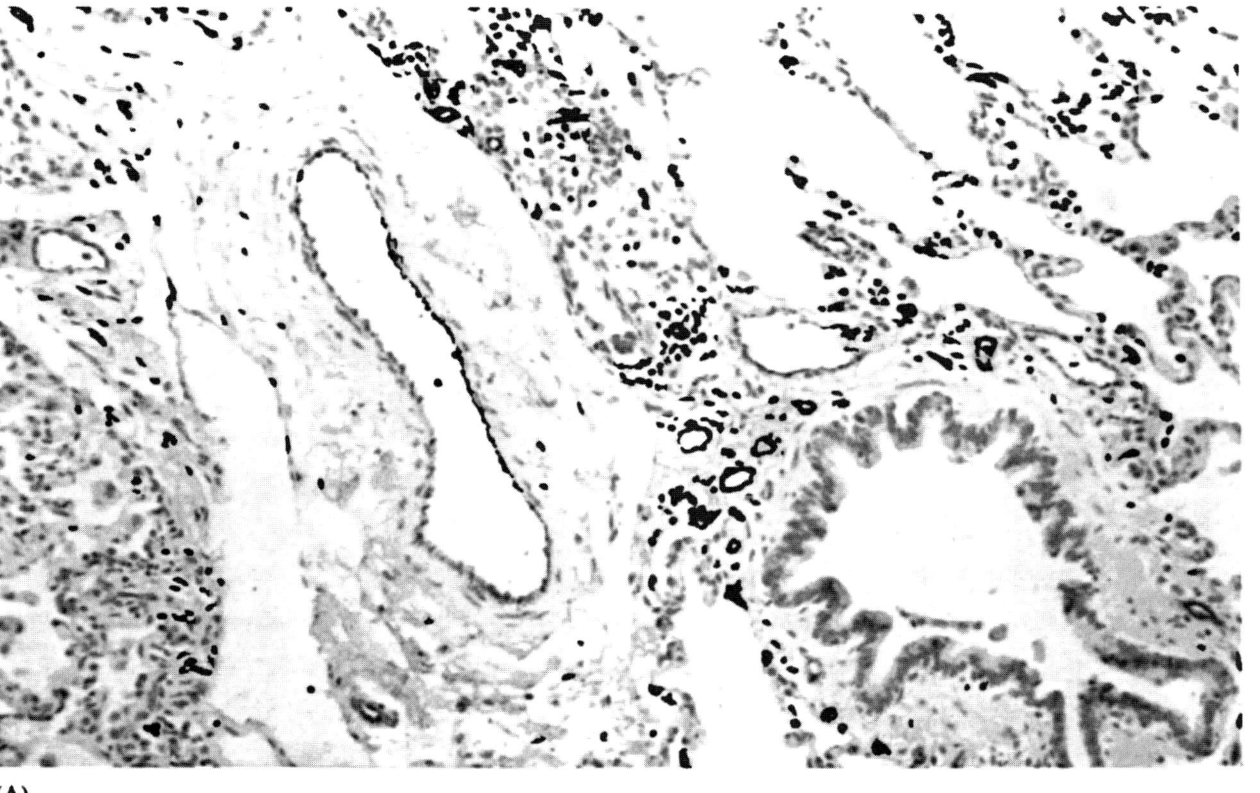

(A)

Figure 9 Lung biopsy section from a patient with normal pulmonary artery pressure (A) and with pulmonary hypertension in (B). Note thin-walled pulmonary artery in (A) with light rim of endothelial immunoperoxidase stain for factor VIII and thick-walled pulmonary artery in (B) with deeply positive endothelial stain. Magnification X16O. (Reproduced with permission from Rabinovitch et al., 1987.)

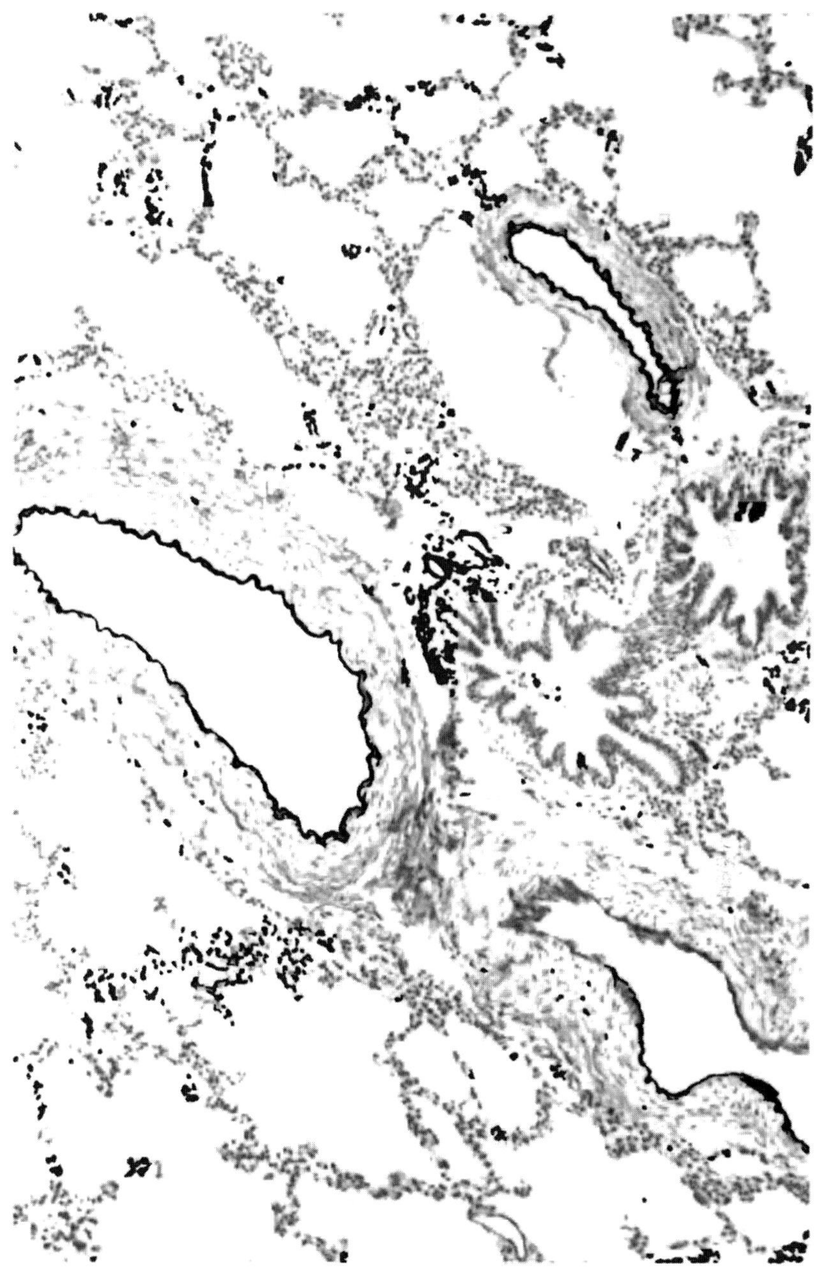

(B)

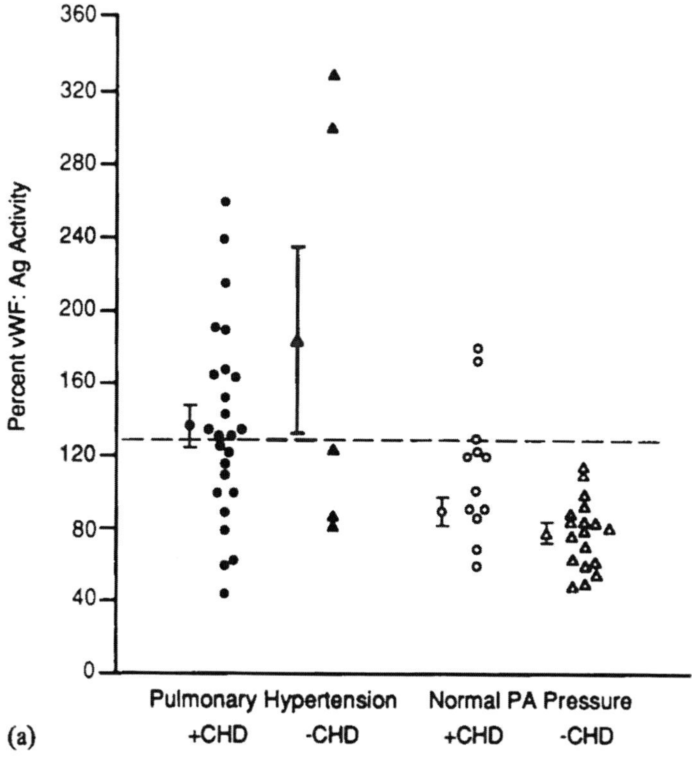

Figure 10 (a) Graph of percent of von Willebrand factor antigenic activity (vWF:Ag) in individual patients in the following four groups (●) pulmonary hypertension (PH) with (+) congenital heart disease (CHD); (▲) PH without (−) /CHD; (○) normal pulmonary artery pressure (nl P_{pa}) + CHD; (△) nl P_{pa} − CHD. Upper limits of normal vWG:Ag activity in our laboratory. Next to individual values is mean ± standard error for the group. Patients with PH and CHD have significantly higher values than those with nl P_{ps} without CHD, $p<0.05$. (b) Few patients with PH and increased vWF:Ag have increased vWF:rist.

The factor VIII abnormality did not correlate with the severity of vascular change, suggesting that this feature may occur early in the course of the disease. While the mechanism causing the multimeric abnormality is not known, it is conceivable that the endothelial cells are producing a protease that is cleaving the factor VIII molecule. Further and most recent observations in lung biopsy tissue and in experimental studies suggest that a process of ongoing proteolysis and

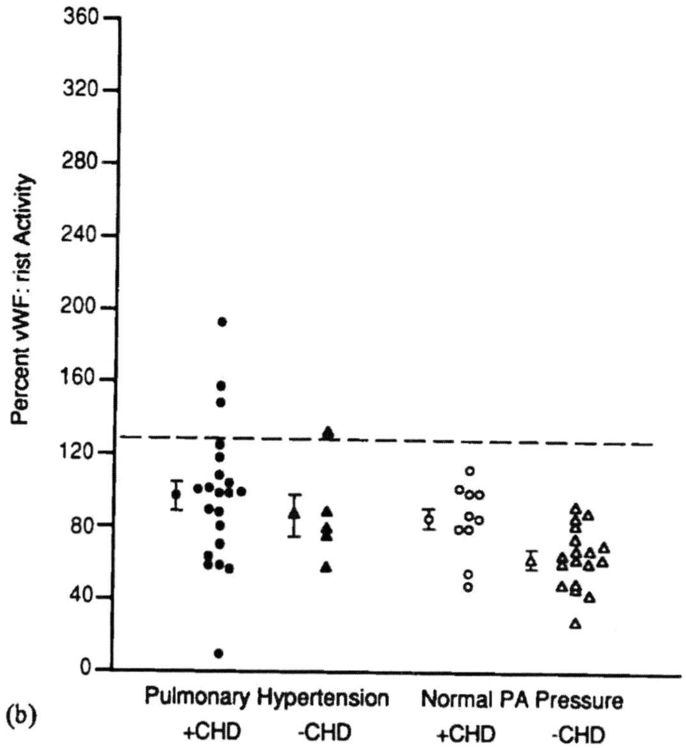

(b)

increased synthesis of connective tissue proteins in the subendothelium and media may be important in the pathogenesis of progressive pulmonary vascular disease (Rabinovitch et al., 1986; Boucek et al., 1987; Todorovitch-Hunter and Rabinovitch, 1988).

VI. Mechanism of Development of Pulmonary Vascular Changes

Experimental studies have been undertaken to determine the effects of high flow and high pressure on the pulmonary vascular bed. High pulmonary flow alone via pneumonectomy or pulmonary artery banding or ligation results in minimal if any elevation in pulmonary arterial pressure and structural changes in the vessels (Rudolph et al., 1961; Friedli et al., 1975; Kato et al., 1971; Davies et al., 1982; Haworth et al., 1981; Rabinovitch et al., 1983). Slight elevation in pul-

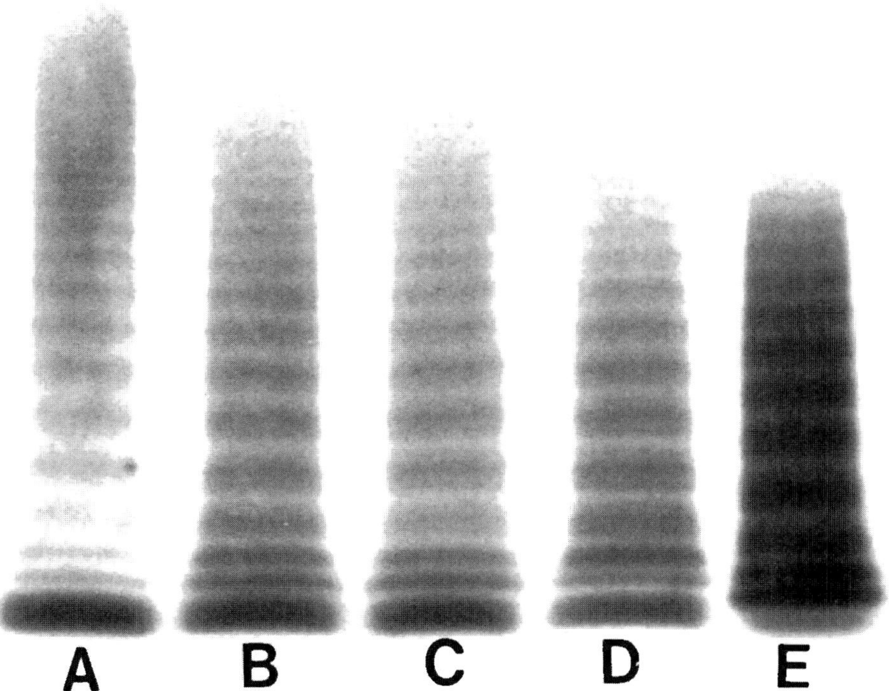

Figure 11 Multimeric patterns for vWF:Ag:Lane A, normal pooled plasma; lanes B, C, and D, patients with pulmonary hypertension and loss of high molecular weight forms; lane E, hemophil concentrate (low molecular weight forms only).

monary arterial pressure is accompanied by extension of muscle into peripheral arteries. Aortopulmonary shunts surgically created in growing piglets (Rendas et al., 1979) are associated with a progressive increase in pulmonary arterial pressure associated with the development of structural changes, specifically extension of muscle into peripheral arteries, medial hypertrophy of muscular arteries, and reduced arterial number. Takedown of the shunts during the period of rapid lung growth results in regression of the structural changes and pulmonary hypertension (Rendas and Reid, 1983). Creation of large aortopulmonary shunts, particularly into a single pulmonary artery, in dogs results in rapidly progressive pulmonary vascular changes (Ferguson and Varco, 1955; Blank et al., 1961). These studies document the development of pulmonary vascular changes

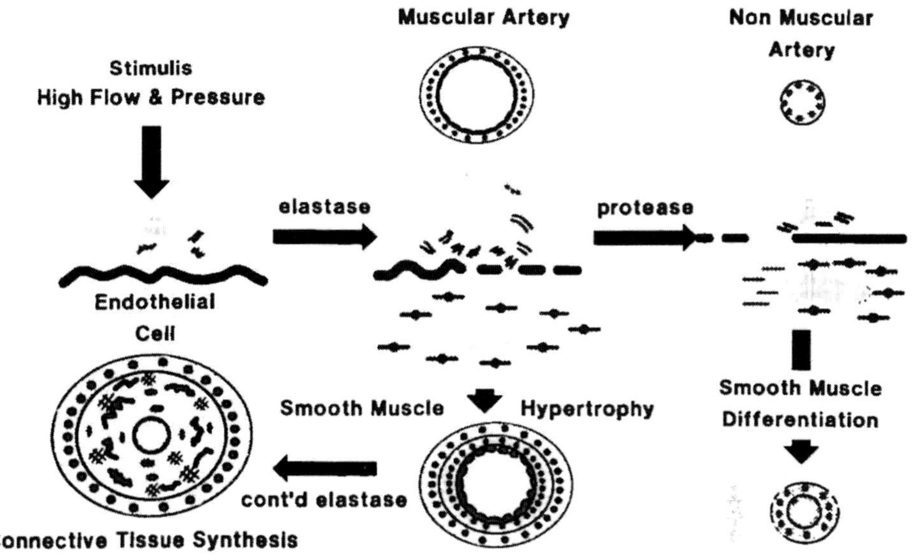

Figure 12 Schema of hypothesis concerning mechanism of development of pulmonary vascular changes with high flow, high pressure states as outlined in the test.

in the setting of high pulmonary flow and pressure. Based on lung biopsy studies and experimental observations in animal models, we have developed a hypothesis of the pathogenesis of pulmonary vascular disease in response to high flow states that we are currently exploring in cell culture systems (Fig. 12).

A stimulus – in this case, the high pulse pressore of a congenital heart defect with a left-to-right shunt – alters endothelial cells both structurally and functionally, and this affects their interactions with marginating blood elements. Because of endothelial dysfunction or in association with neutrophil degranulation, there is abnormal release of proteases in the subendothelium. In the peripheral, normally nonmuscular arteries we speculate that this leads to degradation of some of the basement membrane or other extracellular matrix proteins (Mainardi et al., 1980), encouraging the differentiation of precursor cells to mature smooth muscle cells, a phenomenon described in other cell systems (Mecham and Senior, 1985). The end result is abnormal muscularization of small vessels. In the normally muscular arteries, we speculate that increased elastase activity leads to breakdown of elastin and perhaps other extracellular matrix proteins as well. This, we hypothesize, has two possible effects. It may facilitate transfer of growth factors and mitogens, leading to smooth muscle hyperplasia (Ross et al., 1974; Gajdusek et al., 1980). In addition, breakdown of elastin may stimulate neosynthesis (Faris et al., 1986) via smooth muscle hypertrophy, and this may result in increased production of collagen as well. Continuous elastase activity results in altered distribution of these connective tissue proteins with increasing encroachment on the lumen and stiffening of the vessel wall.

In the newborn lamb with a ventricular septal defect experimentally created (Boucek et al., 1985), there is evidence of increased elastin synthesis in the large central and hilar pulmonary arteries. Stress-strain relationships in the isolated vessels, however, suggest little elastin, and morphometric analysis of ultrastructure reveals a decreased proportion of mature amorphous elastin and an altered distribution as islands rather than as laminae (Boucek et al., 1987). These changes in the large arteries precede evidence of abnormal muscularization of the peripheral vessels, suggesting that the increased distensibility of the central and hilar vessels may absorb some of the hemodynamic effect of the high flow and pressure. The same type of abnormality is observed in our studies of rats in which pulmonary vascular disease was induced by an injection of the toxin monocrotaline (Todorovich-Hunters et al., 1988).

Based on the hypothesis that regardless of the etiology, the mechanism of development of pulmonary vascular changes is remarkably similar, we have investigated rats injected with the toxin monocrotaline in which pulmonary vascular endothelial injury is associated with the subsequent development of muscularization of peripheral arteries, medial hypertrophy of muscular arteries, and decreased artery number. Specifically we assessed whether the elastase inhibitor SC39026 (Searle) might counteract the increased protease activity in the subendothelium and thereby prevent abnormal muscularization of peripheral arteries and medial hypertrophy of muscular arteries (Ilkiw et al., 1987). This agent is a serine protease inhibitor that specifically inhibits neutrophil serine protease. Neutrophils have been implicated early in the course of the monocrotaline injury, and neutrophil serine protease degrades type IV collagen, a basement membrane protein, as well as elastin (Mainardi et al., 1980). We observed that SC39026 does in fact significantly decrease muscularization of peripheral artieries, and this correlates with lower levels of pulmonary arterial pressure. There is, however, only a trend toward increased preservation of medial elastin and decreased medial wall thickness of normally muscular arteries.

VII. Cell Culture Systems

To begin to effectively answer questions related to cellular functions and interactions it is advantageous to study cells in culture. Various techniques have been used to evalute shear stress in vitro (vanGrondelle et al., 1984). Since, in the compliant pulmonary vascular bed, features of pressure as well as stretch are probably important, we devised a technique that would allow us to pulsate

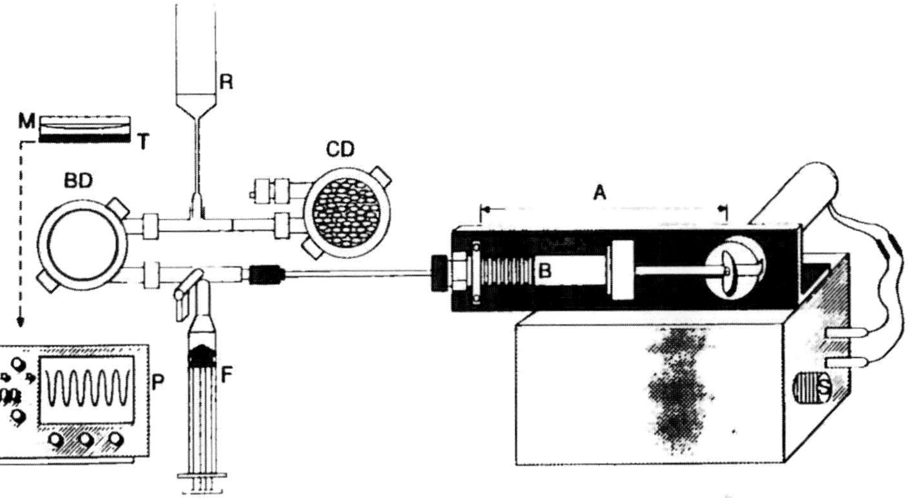

Figure 13 A drawing of the cell pulsation apparatus described in text. CD, cell dome; BD, blank dome; A, amplitude of excursion; T, transducer; S, speed control; P, pressure tracing.

endothelial or smooth muscle cells from large central or small microvessels (Ryan et al., 1978, 1982) at a given pulse pressure and frequency (Rabinovitch et al., 1988) (Fig. 13). Essentially, we grow the cells to confluence on the flexible polyvinyl chloride membrane of a pressure dome (Hewlett-Packard). Then the dome is attached to a reciprocating generator pump. The pump consists of a piston that drives fluid back and forth and a reservoir. By varying the amplitude of excursion of the piston, a given pulse pressure can be set, and by adding fluid from the reservoir to the closed system the mean pressure is established. In our first series of experiments, we pulsated endothelial cells from both large central and small microvessels at 100/60 or 20/10 mmHg pressure for 48 hr at 60 times per minute and have compared the ultrastructural features to those of cells grown on the transducer domes but not pulsated (Rabinovitch et al., 1988). On morphometric analysis, there were no significant differences in the qualitative or quantitative assessment of endothelial intracytoplasmic components (Fig. 14).

Having been assured, in this way, that the endothelial cells had not been damaged by the pulsation, we proceeded with experiments to try to identify whether a mitogen was being released by pulsated endothelial cells that would stimulate the hypertrophy and hyperplasia of smooth muscle cells. Rather than

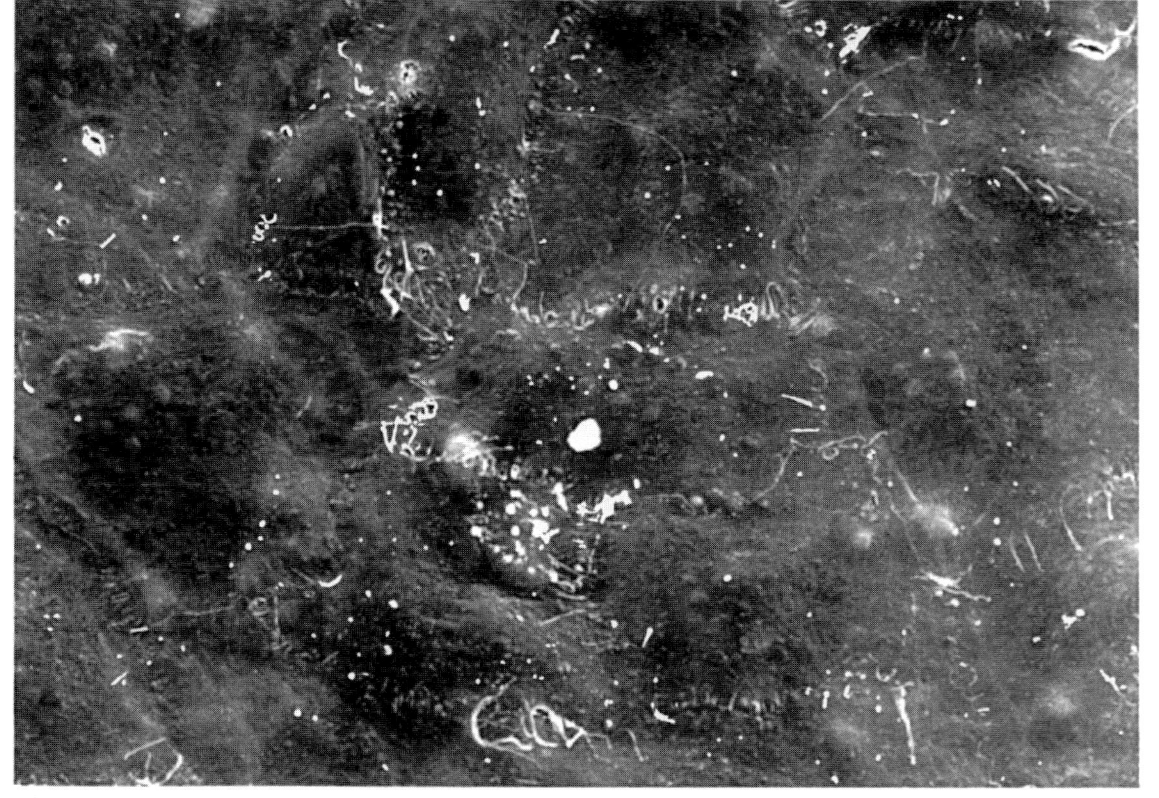

(a)

Figure 14 (a) SEM and (b) TEM of endothelial cells on flexible polyvinyl chloride membrane after 48-hr pulsation at high pressure 100/60 mmHg, 60 times per minutes. Note intact monolayer in SEM with filopodia and junctions and healthy ultrastructural appearance in (b) with microfilament bundles (f), mitochondria (m), and rough endoplasmic reticulum (rer). Magnification (a) X200, (B) X35,000.

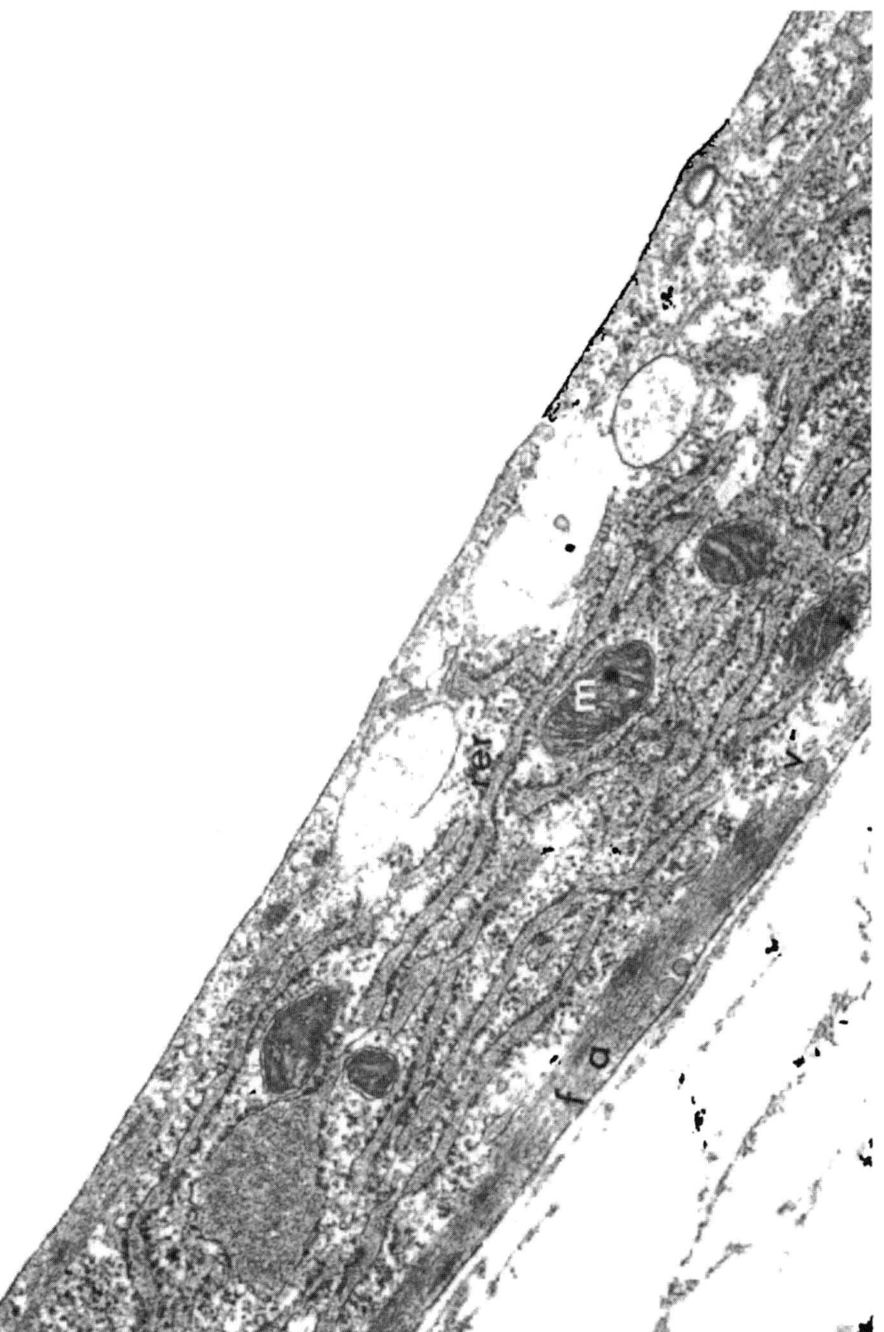

(b)

identify a mitogen, we found evidence that pulsated pulmonary endothelial cells, especially those from microvessels, appear to release an inibitor of smooth muscle hypertrophy and hyperplasia (Rabinovitch and Bothwell, 1987; Bothwell and Rabinovitch, 1988). When we pulsate smooth muscle cells directly, those from microvessels appear to release an "autoinhibitor," but pulsated large vessel smooth muscle cells do not have this property. Thus it appears that the smooth muscle hypertrophy and hyperplasia that is associated with the development of pulmonary vascular changes in response to high flow states is the result of a mitogen our system is not designed to identify, perhaps because it comes from circulating blood elements such as platelets (Ross et al., 1974). The endothelial and microvessel smooth muscle inhibitor that is apparent in our system probably serves to limit the magnitude of the response. Future studies will be directed at trying to identify what this growth inhibitor might be so that in the future its action might be enhanced. Release of prostaglandins has been observed in endothelial cells under conditions of high shear (van Grandelle et al., 1984) and prostaglandins I_2 and E_2 as well as metabolites of D_2 are potent inhibitors of smooth muscle cell DNA synthesis (Owen, 1985). Growth factors such as platelet-derived growth factor (PDGF) are known to release prostaglandins by activating protein kinase C and the phosphoinositol pathway, and this could be part of the mechanism of inhibition (Coughlin et al., 1985). Alternatively, other agents such as transforming growth factor β may be involved. The latter can stimulate or inhibit cell growth depending upon protease activity, (Lyons et al., 1988) other growth factors in the environment, and perhaps the cell type (Roberts et al., 1985). Direct measurement of protease activity in cultured cells (Leake et al., 1983) is possible using a variety of assays.

VIII. Conclusions

A great deal of new knowledge is currently available to better explore the mechanism of development of pulmonary vascular changes in chronic high flow states. Future studies could then be directed at uncovering the genetic regulation of these structural changes. This will ultimately lead to better therapeutic avenues aimed at retarding progression or inducing regression of pulmonary vascular disease.

References

Addonizio, V. P., Jr., Smith, J. B., Strauss, J. F., III, Colman, R. W., and Edmunds, L. H., Jr. (1980). Thromboxane synthesis and platelet secretion during cardiopulmonary bypass with bubble oxygenation. *J. Thorac. Cardiovasc. Surg.* *79*:91-96.

Berman, W., Jr., Whitman, V., Pierce, W. S., and Waldhausen, J. A. (1978). The development of pulmonary vascular obstructive disease after successful Mustard operation in early infancy. *Circulation 58*:181-185.

Besterman, E. (1961). Atrial septal defect with pulmonary hypertension. *Brit. Heart. J. 23*:587-598.

Biggar, W. D., Bohn, D. J., Kent, G., and Hamilton, G. (1984). Neutrophil migration in vitro and in vivo during hypothermia. *Infect Immunol. 46*: 857-859.

Bing, R. J., Vandam, L. D., and Gray, F. D. (1947). Physiological studies in congenital heart disease. *Bull. Johns Hopkins Hosp. 80*:323-347.

Blank, R. H., Muller, W. H., and Damman, J. F. (1961). Experimental pulmonary hypertension. *Am. J. Surg. 101*:143-153.

Bothwell, T., and Rabinovitch, M. (1988). A pulmonary artery smooth muscle growth inhibitor released from endothelial cells stretched at high pulsatile pressure. *FASEB J. 2*:A1577.

Boucek, M. M., Chang, R., and Synhorst, D. P. (1985). Hemodynamic consequences of inotropic support with digoxin and amrinone in lambs with ventricular septal defect. *Pediatr. Res. 19*:887-891.

Boucek, M. M., Roos, P. J., Minto, A., Moss, S., and Rabinovitch, M. (1987). Alteration of pulmonary artery connective tissue properties following ventricular septal defect in lambs. *Pediatr. Res. 21*:382A.

Brenner, O. (1935). Pathology of hypertensive pulmonary vascular disease. *Circulation 18*:533-547.

Chou, T., Masangkay, M. P., Young, R., Conway, G. F., and Helm, R. A. (1973). Simple quantitative vectorcardiographic criteria for the diagnosis of right ventricular hypertrophy. *Circulation 48*:1262-1267.

Civin, W. H., and Edwards, J. E. (1950). Pathology of the pulmonary vascular tree. *Circulation 2*:545-552.

Coughlin, S. R., Lee, W. M. F., Williams, P. W., Giels, G. M., and Williams, L. T. (1985). c-myc gene expression is stimulated by agents that activate protein kinase C and does not account for the mitogenic activity of PDGF. *Cell 43*:243-251.

Cutz, E., Gillan, J. E., and Track, N. S. (1984). Pulmonary endocrine cells in the developing human lung and during neonatal adaptation. In *Endocrine lung in Health and Disease*. Edited by K. L. Becker and L. Gazdar. Saunders, Philadelphia, pp. 210-231.

Cutz, E., Chan, W., Wong, V., Bienkowski, E., and Rabinovitch, M. (1986). Pulmonary neuroendocrine cells in normal human lung and in pulmonary hypertension. *Lab. Invest. 54*:14A.

Davies, P., McBride, P., Murray, G. F., Wilcox, B. R., Shallal, J. A., and Reid, L. (1982). Structural changes in the canine lung and pulmonary arteries after pneumonectomy. *J. Appl. Physiol. 53*:859-864.

DiSesa, V. J., Cohn, L. H., and Grossman, W. (1983). Management of adults with congenital bidirectional cardiac shunt, cyanosis and pulmonary vascular obstruction: successful operative repair in 3 patients. *Am. J. Cardiol.* *51*:1495-1497.

DuShane, J. W., Kongrad, E., Ritter, D. G., and McGoon, D. C. (1976). The fate of raised pulmonary vascular resistance after surgery in ventricular septal defect in the child after congenital heart surgery. In *The Child with Congenital Heart Disease After Surgery*. Edited by B. S. Langford Kidd and R. D. Rowe. Futura, Mount Disco, NY, pp. 299-312.

Edwards, W., and Edwards, J. E. (1978). Hypertensive pulmonary vascular disease in D- transposition of the great arteries. *Am. J. Cardiol.* *41*:921-924.

Eisenmenger, V. (1988). Die angeborenen Defecte der Kammerscheidewand des Herzen. *Z. Klin. Med. Suppl.* *132*:1.

Faris, B., Toselli, P., Kispert, J., Wolfe, B. L., Pratt, C. A., Mogayzel, P. J., Jr., and Franzblau, C. (1986). Elastase effect on the extracellular matrix of rat aortic smooth muscle cells in culture. *Exp. Mol. Pathol.* *45*:105-117.

Ferguson, D. J., and Varco, R. L. (1955). The relation of blood pressure and flow to the development and regression of experimentally induced pulmonary arteriosclerosis. *Circ. Res.* *3*:152-158.

Friedli, B., Kidd, B. S., Mustard, W. T., and Keith, J. D. (1974). Ventricular septal defect with increased pulmonary vascular resistance. *Am. J. Cardiol.* *33*:403-409.

Friedli, B., Kent, G., and Kidd, L. (1975). The effect of increased pulmonary blood flow on the pulmonary vascular bed in pigs. *Pediatr. Res.* *9*:547-553.

Furchgott, R. F. (1983). Role of endothelium in responses of vascular smooth muscle. *Circ. Res.* *53*:557-573.

Gajdusek, C., DiCorleto, P., Ross, R., and Schwartz, S. M. (1980). An endothelial cell-derived growth factor. *J. Cell Biol.* *15*:467-470.

Grondelle, A. van, Worthen, G. S., Ellis, D., Mathias, M. M., Murphy, R. C., Strife, R. J., Reeves, J. T., and Voelkel, N. F. (1984). Altering hydrodynamic variables influences PGI_2 production by isolated.

Hallidie-Smith, K. A., Wilson, R. S. E., Hart, A., and Ziedgard, E. (1977). Functional status of patients with large ventricular septal defect and pulmonary vascular disease 6 to 16 years after surgical closure of their defect in childhood. *Brit. Heart J.* *39*:1093-1101.

Haworth, S. G. (1983). Pulmonary vascular disease in secondum atrial septal defect in childhood. *Am. J. Cardiol.* *51*:265-272.

Haworth, S. G., and Reid, L. (1978). A morphometric study of regional variation in lung structure in infants with pulmonary hypertension and congenital heart defect. A justification of lung biopsy. *Brit. Heart J.* *40*:825-831.

Haworth, S. G., deLeval, M., and McCartney, F. J. (1981). Hypo and hyperperfusion in the immature lung: pulmonary arterial development following ligation of the left pulmonary artery in the newborn pig. *J. Thorac. Cardiovasc. Surg. 82*:281-292.

Heath, D., and Edwards, J. E. (1958a). The pathology of hypertensive pulmonary vascular disease. *Circulation 18*:533-547.

Heath, D., and Edwards, J. E. (1958b). The relation of medial thickness of small muscular pulmonary arteries to survival in patients with ventricular septal defect and patent ductus arteriosus. *Thorax 13*:267-271.

Hickey, P. R., Hansen, D. D., Wessel, D. L., Lang, P., Jonas, R. A., and Elixson, E. M. (1985). Blunting of stressing responses of the pulmonary circulation of infants by Fentanyl. *Anaesth. Anala. 64*:1137-1142.

Hislop, A., and Reid, L. M. (1973). Pulmonary arterial development during childhood: branching pattern and structure. *Thorax 28*:129-135.

Hislop, A. Haworth, S. G., and Reid, L. M. (1975). Quantitative structural analysis of pulmonary vessels in isolated ventricular septal defects in infancy. *Brit. Heart J. 37*:1014-1021.

Hoffman, J. I. E., and Rudolph, A. M. (1965). The natural history of ventricular septal defect in infancy. *Am. J. Cardiol. 16*:634-653.

Iikiw, R., Todorovich, L., Shin, J., and Rabinovitch, M. (1987). An elastase inhibitor may prevent monocrotaline induced pulmonary hypertension. (Abstr.). *Fed. Proc. 46*:730.

Jayakody, L., Senaratne, M., Thompson, A., and Kappagoda, T. (1987). Endothelium-dependent relaxation in experimental atherosclerosis in the rabbit. *Circ. Res. 60*:251-264.

Johnson, J. B., Felter, M. L., West, J. R., and Cournand, A. (1950). The relation between electrocardiographic existence of right ventricular hypertrophy and pulmonary arterial pressure in patients with chronic pulmonary disease. *Circulation 1*:536-550.

Jones, O. D. H., Shore, D. F., Rigby, M. L., Leijala, M., Scallan, J. Shineborne, E. A., and Lincoln, J. C. R. (1981). The use of tolazoline hydrochloride as a pulmonary vasodilator in potentially fatal episodes of pulmonary vasoconstriction after cardiac surgery in children. *Circulation 64*: Supp. 11: 134-139.

Kato, H., Kidd, L., and Olley, P. M. (1971). Effects of hypoxia on pulmonary vascular reactivity in pneumonectomized puppies and mini-pigs. *Circ. Res. 28*:397-402.

Keane, J. F., Ellison, R. C., Rudd, M., and Nadas, A. S. (1973). Pulmonary blood flow and left ventricular volumes with transposition of the great arteries and intact ventricular septum. *Brit. Heart J. 35*:521-526.

Leake, D. S., Hornebeck, W., Brechemier, D., Robert, L., and Peters, T. J. (1983) *Biochim. Biophy. Acta 761*:41-47.

Lyons, R. M., Keski-Oja, J., and Moses, H. L. (1988). Proteolytic activation of latent transforming growth factor B from fibroblast conditioned medium. *J. Cell. Biol. 106*:1659-1665.

Mainardi, C. L., Dixit, S. N., and Kang, A. H. (1980). Degradation of type IV collagen by a proteinase isolated from human polymorphonuclear leukocyte granules *J. Biol. Chem. 255*:5435-5441.

Mair, D. D., Ritter, D. G., Ongley, P. A., and Helmholz, M. F., Jr. (1971). Hemodynamics and evaluation for surgery of patients with complete transposition of the great arteries and ventricular septal defect. *Am. J. Cardiol. 28*:632-640.

Marcelletti, C., McGoon, D. C., and Mair, D. D. (1976). The natural history of truncus arteriosus. *Circulation 54*:108-111.

Marx, G. R., Allan, H. D., and Goldberg, S. J. (1985). Doppler echocardiographic estimation of systolic pulmonary artery pressure patients with interventricular communications. *J. Am. Coll. Cardiol. 6*:1132-1137.

Mecham, R. P. and Senior, R. M. (1985). Extracellular matrix promotes elastogenic differentiation in ligament fibroblasts in *Extracellular Matrix Structure and Function*. Alan R. Liss, New York, pp. 383-392.

Meyrick, B., and Reid, L. M. (1980). Ultrastructural findings in lung material from children with congenital heart defects *Am. J. Pathol. 101*:527-537.

Meyrick, B., Clarke, S. W., Symons, C., Woodgate, D., and Reid, L. (1974). Primary pulmonary hypertension. A case report including electronmicroscopic study. *Brit. J. Dis. Chest 68*:11-20.

Mills, P., Amara, I., McLaurin, L. P., and Graige, B. (1980). Noninvasive assessment of pulmonary hypertension from right ventricular isovolumic contraction time. *Am. J. Cardiol. 46*:272-276.

Nadas, A. S., and Fyler, D. F. (1972). *Pediatric Cardiology*. W. B. Saunders, Philadelphia.

Naeye, R. L. (1966). Pulmonary arterial bed in ventricular septal defect: a quantiative study of anatomic features in early childhood. *Circulation 34*: 962-970.

Newfeld, E. A., Paul, M. H., Muster, A. J., and Idriss, F. S. (1974). Pulmonary vascular disease in complete transposition of the great arteries. A study of 200 patients. *Am. J. Cardiol. 34*:75-82.

Newfeld, E. A., Sher, M., Paul, M. H., and Higashi, N. (1977). Pulmonary vascular disease in complete atrioventricular canal defect. *Am. J. Cardiol. 39*: 721-726.

Nihill, M. R., and McNamara, D. G. (1978). Magnification pulmonary heart disease and pulmonary hypertension. *Circulation 58*:1094-1106.

Owen, N. E. (1985). Prostacyclin can inhibit DNA synthesis in vascular smooth muscle cells. In *Prostaglandins, Leukotrienes and Lipoxins*. Edited by M. Bailey, Plenum Press, New York, pp. 193-204.

Rabinovitch, M., and Bothwell, T. (1987). An inhibitor of smooth muscle growth is released by cells pulsated at high pressure. *Fed. Proc. 46*:730.

Rabinovitch, M., Haworth, S. G., Castaneda, A. R., Nadas, A. S., and Reid, L. (1978). Lung biopsy in congenital heart disease: a morphometric approach to pulmonary vascular disease. *Circulation 58*:1107-1122.

Rabinovitch, M., Castaneda, A. R., and Reid, L. (1981a). Lung biopsy with frozen section as a diagnostic aid in patients with congenital heart defects. *Am. J. Cardiol. 47*:77-84.

Rabinovitch, M., Fischer, K. C., and Treves, S. (1981b). Quantitative thallium-201 myocardial imaging in assessing right ventricular pressure in patients with congenital heart defects. *Brit. Heart J. 45*:198-205.

Rabinovitch, M., Keane, J. F., Fellows, K. E., Castaneda, A. R., and Reid, L. (1981c). Quantitative analysis of the pulmonary wedge angiogram in congenital heart defects. Correlation with hemodynamic data and morphometric findings in lung biopsy tissue. *Circulation 63*:152-164.

Rabinovitch, M., Konstam, M. A., Gamble, W. J., Papanicolaou, N., Aronovitz, A. J. Treves, S., and Reid, L. (1983). Changes in pulmonary blood flow affect vascular response to chornic hypoxia in rats. *Circ. Res. 52*:432-441.

Rabinovitch, M., Keane, J. F., Norwood, W. I., Castaneda, A. R., and Reid, L. (1984). Vascular structure in lung biopsy tissue correlated with pulmonary hemodynamic findings after repair of congenital heart defects. *Circulation 69*:655-667.

Rabinovitch, M., Bothwell, T., Mullen, M., and Hayakawa, B. N. (1988). High-pressure pulsation of central and microvessel pulmonary artery endothelial cells. *Am. J. Physiol. 254*:C338-C343.

Rabinovitch, M., Bothwell, T., Hayakawa, B. N., Williams, W. G., Trusler, G. A., Rowe, R. D., Olley, P. M. and Cutz, E. (1986). Pulmonary artery endothelial abnormalities in patients with congenital heart defects and pulmonary hypertension. A correlation of light with scanning electron microscopy and transmission electron microscopy. *Lab. Invest. 55*:632-653.

Rabinovitch, M., Andrew, M., Thom, H., Trusler, G. A., Williams, W. G., Rowe, R. D., and Olley, P. M. (1987). Abnormal endothelial factor VIII associated with pulmonary hypertension and congenital heart defects. *Circulation 76*:1043-1052.

Reid, J. M., Stevenson, J. G., Coleman, E. N., Barclay, R. S., Welsh, T. M., Fyfe, W. M., and Inal, J. A. (1964). Moderate to severe pulmonary hypertension accompanying patent ductus arteriosus. *Brit. Heart J. 26*:600-605.

Rendas, A., Lennox, S. and Reid, L. (1979). Aortopulmonary shunts in growing pigs. *J. Thorac Cardiovasc Surg. 77*:109-118.

Rendas, A. and Reid, L. (1983). Pulmonary vasculative after connection of autopulmonary shunts. *J. Thorac. Cardiovasc. Surg. 85*:911-916, 1983.

Roberts, A. B., Anzano, M. A., Wakefield, L. M., Roche, N. S., Stern, and Sporn, M. B. (1985). Type β transforming growth factor: a bifunctional regulator of cellular growth. *Proc. Natl. Acad. Sci. USA 82*:119-123.

Rosengart, R., Rishbein, M., and Emmanoulides, G. C. (1975). Progressive pulmonary vascular disease after surgical correction (Mustard procedure) of transposition of the great arteries with intact ventricular septum. *Am. J. Cardiol. 35*:107-111.

Rosenthal, A., Nathan, D. G., Marty, A. T., Button, L. N., Miettinen, O. S., and Nadas, A. S. (1970). Acute hemodynamic effects of red cell volume reduction in polycythemia of cyanotic congenital heart disease. *Circulation 42*:297-307.

Ross, R., Glomset, J., Kariya, B., and Harker, L. (1974). A platelet derived serum factor that stimulates the proliferation of arterial smooth muscle cells in vitro. *Proc. Natl. Acad. Sci. USA 71*:1207-1210.

Rudolph, A. M., and Nadas, A. S. (1962). The pulmonary circulation and congenital heart disease. Consideration of the role of the pulmonary circulation in certain systemic-pulmonary communications. *New Engl. J. Med. 267*:968-974, 1022-1028.

Rudolph, A. M., Neuhauser, E. B. D., Golinko, R. J., and Auld, P. A. M. (1961). Effects of pneumonectomy on pulmonary circulation in adult and young animals. *Circ. Res. 9*:856-861.

Ryan, U., Clements, E., Habliston, D., and Ryan, J. W. (1978). Isolation and culture of pulmonary artery endothelial cells. *Tissue Cell 10*:535-554.

Ryan, U. S., White, L. A., Lopez, M., and Ryan, J. W. (1982). Use of microcarriers to isolate and culture pulmonary microvascular endothelium. *Tissue Cell 14*:597-606.

Stimler, N. P., and O'Flaherty, J. T. (1983). Spasmogenic properties to platelet activating factor. Evidence for a direct mechanism in the contractile response of pulmonary tissues. *Am. J. Pathol. 113*:75-84.

Todorovich-Hunter, L., Johnson, D., Ranger, P., Keeley, F., and Rabinovitch, M. (1988). Altered elastin and collagen synthesis associated with progressive pulmonary hypertension induced by monocrotaline: a biochemical and ultrastructural study. *Lab. Invest.* 58:184-195.

Todorovich-Hunter and Rabinovitch, M. (1988) Non serine elastase-like activity in the pulmonary artery of rats with monocrotaline-induced pulmonary hypertension. *Am. Rev. Resp. Dis. 137*:209 (abstract).

Turner-Gomes, S., Andrew, M. and Rabinovitch, M. (1988). Altered factor VIII and coagulation abnormalities in congenital heart disease: perioperative predisposition to platelet microthrombin. *Pediatr. Res. 23*:226A (abstract)

Turner-Gomes, S., and Rabinovitch, M. (1988). Platelet activating factor - its role in the genesis and propagation of pulmonary vascular reactivity in patients with congenital heart disease and pulmonary hypertension. *Am. Rev. Resp Dis. 137*:533 (abstract).

Vanhoutte, P. M., Rubanyi, G. M., Miller, V. M., and Hurston, D. S. (1986). Modulation of vascular smooth muscle contraction by the endothelium. *Ann. Rev. Physiol. 48*:962-968.

Vogel, J. H. K., McNamara, D. C., and Blount, S. G., Jr. (1967). Role of hypoxia in determining pulmonary vascular resistance in infants with ventricular septal defect. *Am. J. Cardiol. 20*:346-349.

Wagenvoort, C. A., Heath, D. A., and Edwards, J. E. (1964). *The Pathology of the Human Vasculature*. Charles C. Thomas, Springfield, Il.

Waldman, J. D., Paul, M. H., Newfeld, E. A., Muster, A. J., and Idriss, F. S. (1977). Transposition of the greater arteries with intact ventricular septum and patent ductus arteriosus. *Am. J. Cardiol. 39*:232-238.

Weidman, W. H., DuShane, J. W., and Kincaid, O. W. (1963). Observations concerning progressive pulmonary vascular obstruction in children with venricular septal defects. *Am. Heart J. 65*:148-154.

Wood, P. (1959). The Eisenmenger syndrome of pulmonary hypertension with reversed central shunting. *Brit. Med. J. 2*:701-755.

VanGroudelle, A., Worthen, G. S., Ellis, D., Mathias, M. M., Murphy, R. C., Strife, R. J., Reeves, J. T., and Voelkel, N. F. (1984). Altering hydrodynamic variables influences PGI_2 production by isolated lungs and endothelial cells. *J. Appl. Physiol. 57*:388-395.

Yokochill, K., Olley, P. M., Sideris, E., Hamilton, F. Hutrtanen, D., and Coceani, F. (1982). Leukotriene D_4; a potent vasoconstrictor of the pulmonary and systemic circulations in the newborn lamb. In *Leukotrienes and other Lipoxygenase Products*. Edited by B. Samuelsson. Raven Press, New York, pp. 221-214.

Zimmerman, G. A., McIntyre, T. M., and Prescott, S. M. (1985). Production of PAF by human vascular endothelial cells: evidence for a requirement for specific agonists and modulation by prostacyclin. *Circulation 72*:718-727.

15

Etiologic Mechanisms in Primary Pulmonary Hypertension

NORBERT F. VOELKEL

University of Colorado Health Sciences Center
and Webb-Waring Lung Institute
Denver, Colorado

E. KENNETH WEIR

VA Medical Center and University
of Minnesota School of Medicine
Minneapolis, Minnesota

I. Introduction

"Primary pulmonary hypertension" is a clinical term used to describe patients who have pulmonary hypertension in the absence of a detectable cause, such as congenital intracardiac shunts; pulmonary emboli involving the proximal pulmonary arteries; collagen-vascular disease; or lung disease involving the airways or parenchyma. Other causes to be ruled out include an elevated left heart filling pressure (>12 mmHg), whatever the underlying reason; hypoventilation syndromes; residence at high altitude; parasitic disease, such as schistosomiasis; peripheral pulmonary artery stenoses; sickle cell disease; choriocarcinoma; and the intravenous injection of pulverized pills, leading to talc emboli and granulomas. When these possible etiologies have been excluded, patients with a mean resting pulmonary arterial pressure in excess of 25 mmHg are considered to have primary pulmonary hypertension (Rich et al., 1987).

II. Pathologic Classification

It might be thought that the relatively small number of patients isolated by this rigorous diagnostic screen would be fairly homogeneous. However, while the patients appear similar clinically, several "distinct pathologic entities" have been described when the lung vessels are examined histologically at autopsy or biopsy. A World Health Organization meeting in Geneva in 1973 concluded that the clinical picture of primary pulmonary hypertension could be the result of plexogenic pulmonary arteriopathy, recurrent pulmonary thromboembolism, or pulmonary veno-occlusive disease (Hatano and Strasser, 1975). The data in Table 1 indicate the relative frequency of these three pathologic subsets in three large series.

Recently it has been suggested that a fourth pathologic appearance, that of pulmonary capillary hemangiomatosis, should be included as a possible cause of primary pulmonary hypertension (Kay and Heath, 1985). In this condition the lung parenchyma, the pleura, and the walls of bronchi, pulmonary arteries, and veins are invaded by sheets of capillaries or small venules. In some cases a secondary intimal fibrosis of the pulmonary veins may occur, making the distinction from pulmonary veno-occlusive disease difficult. To say that this is a disorder of angiogenesis does not bring us closer to the etiology, except to focus attention on the mechanisms which normally stimulate and control vessel growth (D'Amore and Thompson, 1987).

Pulmonary veno-occlusive disease can easily be distinguished histologically from the plexogenic and microthromboembolic forms of primary pulmonary hypertension. The predominant lesions in the pulmonary veins are intimal proliferation and fibrosis, which may be eccentric, suggesting prior thrombosis. Muscularization of the small pulmonary veins can also occur. The intimal proliferation affects both large and small veins (Heath et al., 1971). Demographically, pulmonary veno-occlusive disease is different from other forms of primary pulmonary hypertension in that the incidence is about the same in both sexes. It has been suggested that several factors, such as viral infections (McDonnell et al., 1981), chemotherapeutic agents (Lombard et al., 1987), or immune reactions (Corrin et al., 1974), might cause pulmonary veno-occlusive disease. If this is correct, then the histologic appearance of pulmonary veno-occlusive disease may be a nonspecific response to a variety of injuries (Wagenvoort, 1976). Fifteen years ago, it was suggested that toxic or infective agents might attack pulmonary venous endothelial cells, inhibit lysis, encourage thrombosis and cause intimal proliferation (Editorial, 1972). It is important to consider that plexogenic and microthromboembolic arteriopathies may similarly be parts of the spectrum of late nonspecific pulmonary arterial responses to a number of injurious stimuli.

III. Plexogenic and Microthromboembolic Arteriopathies: Discrete Pathologic Entities or Late, Nonspecific, Histologic Changes?

Plexogenic lesions are seen not only in primary pulmonary hypertension but also in pulmonary hypertension occurring in association with left to right

Table 1 Histologic Characteristics of Primary Pulmonary Hypertension

	Wagenvoort and Wagenvoort, 1970	Wagenvoort, 1980	Bjornsson and Edwards, 1985
Number of Cases	156	40	80
Thromboembolic	20%	30%	56%
Plexogenic	71	35	28
Veno-occlusive	3	5	6
Other	6	30	10

intracardiac shunts, portal hypertension, schistosomiasis, and aminorex ingestion. It follows that the lesions themselves are not specific for one form of primary pulmonary hypertension. Similarly thrombotic lesions may be observed in the small pulmonary arteries of patients with pulmonary hypertension secondary to scleroderma (Wagenvoort and Wagenvoort, 1977) or systemic lupus erythematosus (Fayemi, 1976), as well as in patients with plexogenic arteriopathy. Consequently, they cannot be considered specific for one form of primary pulmonary hypertension. It is usually not possible to determine from the histologic appearance whether the thrombi are the result of thrombosis in situ or embolism. In the case of embolism the initial pathology clearly lies in the systemic veins, not in the muscular pulmonary arteries. However, in many cases of primary pulmonary hypertension a site of systemic venous thrombosis cannot be identified (Bjornsson and Edwards, 1985).

Although plexogenic lesions and thrombotic lesions may not be limited to specific forms of primary pulmonary hypertension, there are other features of plexogenic and thrombotic arteriopathy. Plexogenic arteriopathy will characteristically have marked medial hypertrophy and concentric, laminar, "onion-skin" intimal fibrosis, in addition to plexiform lesions. The most clear cut cases of thrombotic arteriopathy have eccentric intimal fibrosis, modest medial hypertrophy and evidence of recanalization of thrombi (Wagenvoort, 1980). When such classic features are compared from two different cases of primary pulmonary hypertension, it may seem obvious that they are "distinct pathological entities" (Hatano and Strasser, 1975). However, in some subjects the histopathologic lesions of plexogenic and thromboembolic pulmonary hypertension coexist in similar proportions (Bjornsson and Edwards, 1985). These instances could be explained as plexogenic arteriopathy complicated by secondary thrombosis or embolism, or it could be considered that the initial pathologic mechanism gave rise to features of both plexogenic and thrombotic arteriopathies as late, nonspecific reactions to damage or dysfunction of the vessel wall. The second, "nonspecific" explanation would be strengthened if a single etiologic stimulus could be shown to give rise in one individual to the pattern of plexogenic arteriopathy, and in an other individual to the pattern of thrombotic arteriopathy. This observation has been made by three groups of workers studying the pulmonary vascular pathology associated with aminorex ingestion, portal hypertension, and familial primary pulmonary hypertension.

A review of the pathology of 17 cases of primary pulmonary hypertension associated with aminorex ingestion, classified 15 as plexogenic, one as thromboembolic, and one as being either thromboembolic or plexogenic with thromboembolism (Heath and Kay, 1978). A study of 12 patients with primary pulmonary hypertension associated with portal hypertension, found three to have plexogenic arteriopathy, seven to have both plexogenic arteriopathy and thromboembolism, one to have only thromboembolic lesions, and one to have only medial hypertrophy (Edwards et al., 1987). The third report described three families with familial primary pulmonary hypertension. In each family one individual had predominantly plexogenic arteriopathy, while another had predominantly thromboembolic arteriopathy (Lloyd et al., 1987).

Thus, a single stimulus or circumstance can give rise to a spectrum of histologic responses, depending presumably on the genetic and environmental factors influencing the individual. It is easy to see how endothelial dysfunction could lead to the production of a growth factor, causing medial proliferation and migration into the intima, and also to abnormalities of coagulation, platelet adherence, and fibrinolysis. This concept has recently been discussed in more detail (Weir et al., 1988).

IV. Vasoconstriction and Vasoproliferation

Paul Wood (1956) proposed a "vasoconstrictive factor" in primary pulmonary hypertension, having found in some of the patients that pulmonary vasodilators acutely decreased pulmonary arterial pressure. Subsequently, arguments for (Fowler, 1950; Dresdale, 1954; Yu, 1958, Farrar, 1963; Sedziwy, 1966), and against (Blount, 1967) increased vascular tone initiating the vascular lesions have been raised. The structural evidence for vasoconstriction began with Staemmler, whose studies in 1937 suggested that spasm of arterioles led to vascular muscle hypertrophy. In 1957, Short found "arterial contracture" in postmortem arteriograms of patients with primary pulmonary hypertension. The finding that arterial medial hypertrophy is the dominant lesion in the lungs of infants and young children dying of primary pulmonary hypertension, has recently been reviewed (Haworth, 1988). It is of interest that Chapman et al., (1957) attributed the increased medial thickening to a proliferation of connective tissue rather than to the muscular component. Physiological evidence for the presence of vasoconstriction in primary pulmonary hypertension since the early publications (Wood, 1956; Dresdale et al., 1951) has largely consisted of the acute, and more recently also chronic, pulmonary vasodilatation in certain patients. Reeves et al. (1986) made a case for the individualized treatment of selected patients with primary pulmonary hypertension with vasodilators. This group documented by careful review of the recent literature, several cases with successful long-term reduction of pulmonary vascular resistance on chronic vasodilator therapy. Of 53 patients with an initial acute lowering of pulmonary vascular resistance, 33 went on to show continued improvement. Thus, vasoconstriction is at least one component in the pathogenesis of pulmonary hypertension in many patients with primary pulmonary hypertension. It is, however, doubtful that it is the only important component. Wagenvoort (1973) argued that if vasoconstriction was indeed responsible for the plexiform lesions then the vasoconstriction must be far more severe than usually seen in humans, because hypoxia is considered a potent vasoconstricting mechanism and yet leads only to medial hypertrophy without progression to more advanced lesions. Anderson et al. (1973) suggested that the primary abnormality may reside in the endothelium which may synthesize vasoactive agents. Alternatively, the injured endothelium may either produce growth factors and proliferate to ultimately accomplish total or near total lumen obliteration, or it may respond to factors like platelet-derived growth factor (PDGF) or even angiogenesis factors like the recently identified tumor-derived angiogenic factor isolated from the Walker 256 carcinoma (Kull et al., 1987).

Because the angioproliferative aspects of primary pulmonary hypertension cannot be overlooked, future work must focus on the role of the pulmonary vascular muscle cell and its crosstalk with endothelial cells and fibroblasts. Voelkel et al. (1977) described increased ^{3}H thymidine incorporation into lung parenchyma of hypoxic rats. The peak increase was observed after three days of high altitude exposure. Autoradiographic studies indicated that the lung vascular smooth muscle cells incorporated the DNA synthesis marker (Niedenzu et al., 1981). Adrenalectomy increased the hypoxia-induced thymidine incorporation suggesting perhaps that the lung proliferative events were under steroid hormone control. Recent work (Mecham et al., 1987; Tozzi et al., 1988; Rabinovitch, 1988) begins to examine the role of matrix proteins in the development of pulmonary hypertensive vascular diseases. Increased collagen and elastin synthesis occurs, orchestrated by the phenotypically altered smooth muscle cell as shown in the bovine neonatal high altitude pulmonary hyptertension model (see Stenmark this volume). The schematic (Fig. 1) attempts to integrate our current thinking regarding the angioproliferative events in primary pulmonary hypertension.

High pressure or noxious stimuli may act as expression factors which cause endothelial injury. In a susceptible individual the "incubation" of subintimal cell layers with serum factors, platelet factors, and possibly proliferation-promoting principles from other organs may start an exuberant activity of cell growth and synthesis of matrix proteins. This then leads to the typical vascular morphology with its occlusive (onion skin intimal proliferation) and restrictive (adventitia cuff made of collagen and elastin) elements.

Fairly early histologic findings have been reported in two cases (Rao et al., 1969; Heath et al., 1987). The first patient died when a catheter perforated the right ventricle. Hemodynamically he had severe pulmonary hypertension, which was very responsive to vasodilator agents. Histological examination of the small muscular pulmonary arteries showed predominantly medial hypertrophy but also "prominent endothelial cells." The second patient had a lung biopsy in 1981 and further histologic studies in 1986 at the time of heart-lung transplantation. In 1981, there was pronounced medial hypertrophy in the small

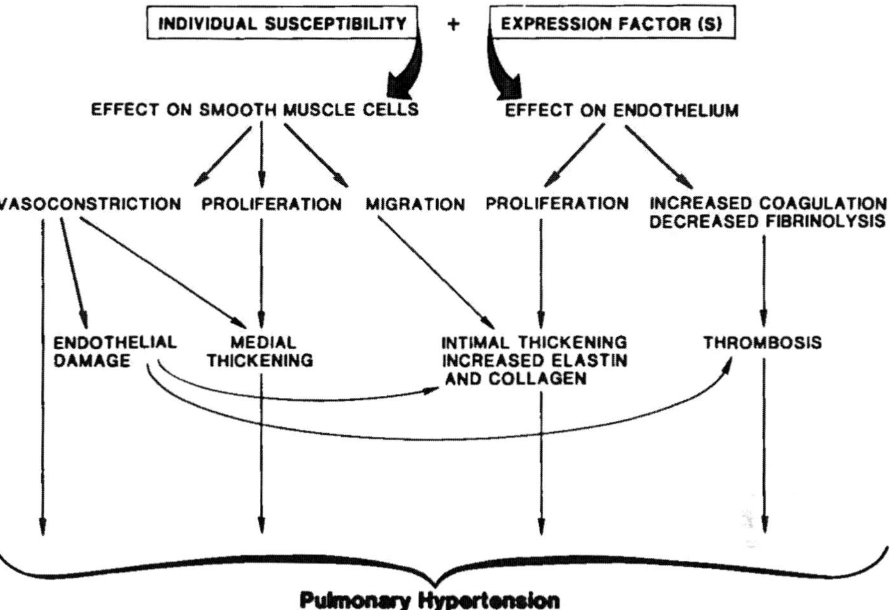

Figure 1 Potential pathways in the pathogenesis of chronic pulmonary hypertension.

pulmonary arteries and proliferation of "myofibroblasts," which could be seen crossing the internal elastic lumina and encroaching on the lumen. By 1986, plexiform lesions and concentric laminar intimal proliferation were evident (Heath et al., 1987). Previous electron microscopic studies have identified such proliferating cells as myofibroblasts (Smith and Heath, 1979). Similar proliferation and migration has been observed in the systemic vessels of rats with spontaneous systemic hypertension (Haudenschild et al., 1980).

These observations raise several questions. Does the endothelium send a signal which causes the proliferation of pulmonary arterial smooth muscle cells, some of which cross into the intima, or does the signal for proliferation arise in the media itself, with only secondary involvement of the endothelium? In each case, what induces the signal? The control of cell proliferation is considered in detail in Chapter 16, but it is clear that there is intense interaction between vascular endothelial and smooth muscle cells. Endothelial cells can stimulate (Zerwes and Risau, 1987) or inhibit (Benitz et al., 1987) smooth muscle growth. Smooth muscle cells can stimulate (Winkles et al., 1987) or inhibit (Orlidge and D'Amore, 1987) endothelial cell growth. Regulation can also be imposed by other substances, such as transforming growth factor-beta (Sporn et al., 1986), insulin-like growth factor 1 (Pfeifle et al., 1987), or thrombospondin (Majack et al., 1988). It is easy to see how a virus or other etiologic stimulus could induce production of a growth factor, or prevent production of a growth inhibitor. Transformation of some cells by a virus, such as the simian sarcoma virus (SSV), can result in the production of a molecule-like platelet-derived growth factor (PDGF). Similarly, endotoxin and alpha-thrombin both can cause cultured vascular endothelial cells to synthesize and secrete a molecule like PDGF (Fox and DiCorleto, 1984; Harlan et al., 1986). PDGF could easily be responsible for the proliferation and migration of medial smooth muscle cells observed in primary pulmonary hypertension (Heath et al., 1987). Once initiated, the production of PDGF by smooth muscle cells might become autonomous (Nilsson et al., 1985; Sjolund et al., 1988). When the normal systems of checks and balances are disturbed, cellular proliferation and structural remodeling may result.

V. Interaction of Endothelial and Smooth Muscle Cell Dysfunction to Cause Pulmonary Hypertension

From the preceding discussion, it is apparent that we do not know whether the initial lesion in primary pulmonary hypertension occurs in the endothelium or the smooth muscle, or indeed in some other system involving perhaps the production of alpha-thrombin, or the secretion of growth factors by macrophages (Nathan, 1987). As the vascular changes are confined to the pulmonary circulation, it might seem more likely that the problem arises in the pulmonary vascular endothelium or smooth muscle rather than in circulating leukocytes or in changes of coagulation or fibrinolysis.

Some insight may be gained from other forms of pulmonary hypertension. In the case of intracardiac shunts, high flow presumably initiates pulmonary hypertension through the effects of increased shear stress on the endothelium or through reactive vasoconstriction. This etiology produces a histologic picture very similar to that of primary pulmonary hypertension. In this instance, once endothelial injury or dysfunction is present, platelets and other blood elements are almost certainly involved, but the search for the first derangement of function should focus on the endothelium or possibly the smooth muscle. In the case of portal hypertension, caused perhaps by cirrhosis, the stimulus for pulmonary vascular changes could be repeated exposure to endotoxin which is not metabolized in the liver (Meyrick et al., 1986), or could be secondary to the action of thrombin on the endothelium, which will be discussed later. In these patients, the pulmonary vascular pathology is the same as that in primary plexogenic pulmonary hypertension. On one hand, the initiating stimulus comes from outside the lungs but on the other, the fact that only a very small percentage of those who have portal hypertension also develop pulmonary hypertension implies individual susceptibility, perhaps involving endothelial dysfunction.

Figure 1 illustrates the concept that factors acting on the smooth muscle or the endothelium, or both, can produce the histologic features of intimal proliferation, intimal fibrosis, and medial hypertrophy, as well as thrombosis. Interaction between the endothelium and smooth muscle is also important, as mentioned earlier. The endothelium forms both relaxing and constricting substances as discussed in Chapter 18. A decrease in the former, or an increase in the latter, could promote vasoconstriction. Conversely, vasoconstriction could cause endothelial damage. Endothelial dysfunction can result in the release of PDGF on the abluminal surface of the endothelial cell, which might cause smooth muscle proliferation and migration in primary pulmonary hypertension (Zerwes and Risau, 1987).

It has been noted that the half-life of fibrinogen is decreased in primary pulmonary hypertension (Langleben et al., 1985) and the possibility that endothelial dysfunction might have a procoagulant effect is intriguing. The complexity of the interactions can be illustrated by the opposing effects that a single substance, such as thrombin, can have on the wall of a vessel. Thrombin can work against thrombosis by stimulating prostacyclin production (Jaffe et al., 1987), by activating protein C (Esmon, 1987), by causing the secretion of tissue plasminogen activator (Erickson et al., 1985), and by stimulating production of endothelium-dependent relaxing factor (DeMay and Vanhoutte, 1982). It can also be a procoagulant, by cleaving fibrin and fibrinogen, by platelet activation, by stimulating PDGF production (Harlan et al., 1986), and by inducing the secretion of platelet-activating factor (Prescott et al., 1986), interleukin 1 (Nawroth et al., 1986), or factor VIII antigen (Levin et al., 1982) from endothelial cells. It is easy to see how an increased procoagulant activity or decreased antithrombotic activity could lead to fibrin deposition orr platelet aggregation. A preliminary report suggests that some primary pulmonary hypertension patients may have a decreased fibrinolytic capacity (Fuchs et al., 1981) and a similar observation was made in seven members of a primary pulmonary hypertension family (Inglesby and Singer, 1973). Another study found no evidence of a defect in fibrinolysis in a different primary pulmonary hypertension family (Tubbs et al., 1979).

The likelihood of endothelial dysfunction is indicated by a recent report on von Willebrand factor (vWF) abnormalities in primary pulmonary hypertension (Geggel et al., 1987). Four of six patients had an increase in the lower molecular weight multimers of vWF and all six showed an increase in the ratio of vWF function (Ristocetin-cofactor activity) to vWF concentration (vWF-related antigen). Too much emphasis should not be placed on measurements of ristocetin-cofactor activity as it may not accurately reflect the physiological function of vWF (Giddings, 1986). However, as the endothelial cells synthesize and secrete vWF, the observed abnormalities could be either a marker of endothelial dysfunction or possibly a pointer to a pathophysiologic mechanism. Abnormalities of von Willebrand factor have been noted in several other conditions such as thrombotic thrombocytopenic purpura and disseminated intravascular coagulation, as well as in patients with pulmonary hypertension secondary to congenital heart disease (Rabinovitch et al., 1987). In the latter patients the endothelium of the pulmonary arteries showed a markedly increased intensity of immunostaining for vWF antigen. They also had fewer high molecular weight multimers of vWF but, in contrast to the primary pulmonary hypertension patients (Geggel et al., 1987), had high plasma levels of vWF antigen.

The fact that abnormalities of the vWF system have been observed in other conditions, as well as in primary pulmonary hypertension, does not indicate whether these abnormalities are a nonspecific secondary response to injury or an essential part of the etiologic mechanism. Von Willebrand factor is present, not only in the Weibel-Palade bodies of endothelial cells, but also in the alpha granules of platelets. It plays an important part in the adherence of platelets to the subendothelium (Giddings, 1986). As the alpha granules also contain platelet-derived growth factor, it is interesting to speculate that these two factors may have a synergistic role in the development of pulmonary hypertension. The potential involvement of platelets in the pathogenesis of several forms of pulmonary hypertension has been reviewed recently (Mlczoch, 1985; Reeves and Herget, 1986).

The etiologic factors which will be considered in the following are: congenital factors, inherited susceptibility and familial pulmonary hypertension, "factors associated with female maturation," thromboembolism, autoimmune mechanisms, dietary pulmonary hypertension, drugs, and severe pulmonary hypertension in patients with hepatic dysfunction.

VI. Congenital Factors

Primary pulmonary hypertension has been described in infancy. The recently described syndrome of persistence of the fetal pulmonary circulation (see Stenmark et al., Chap. 11) may bridge the pathogenetic gap between failure of the lung to adapt to normal extrauterine life and childhood cases of severe pulmonary hypertension. Lichtenstern-Peters and co-workers (1982), described a 18-month-old infant, who was normal in the perinatal period, but developed cyanosis at 1 year of age and signs of pulmonary hypertension (Pap at catheterization was 70/30 mmHg), and died of right heart failure. At autopsy lung histology showed severe vascular lesions including plexogenic lesions. Juaneda and co-workers (1985) reported on a 7-year-old girl who died 6 months after onset of symptoms (general malaise). Antimitochondrial antibodies and antibodies against smooth muscle were present. Intimal thickening and medial hypertrophy of the pulmonary arteries were observed at autopsy. Knauf et al. (1982) described a 4 ½-year-old boy with severe pulmonary hypertension whose lungs demonstrated plexogenic lesions.

The interim report of the NIH registry of patients with primary pulmonary hypertension (Rich et al., 1987) documents 5 patients, of a total of 187, in the age group from 1-10 years with primary pulmonary hypertension and Knight and Wilson (1985) reported on primary pulmonary hypertension in two infant brothers. Thus it appears that a congenital abnormality in the pulmonary circulation, perhaps an inborn susceptibility to vasoconstriction, may be present. Such susceptibility may or may not be grafted onto morphological changes which have been suggested to be present in the syndrome of persistence of the fetal pulmonary circulation, namely: (1) insufficient number of pulmonary arterioles, (2) failure of appropriate growth of new arterioles, or (3) incomplete regression of fetal pulmonary medial hypertrophy (Voelkel and Reeves, 1979). Since the syndrome of persistence of the fetal lung circulation has features in common with adult forms of unexplained pulmonary hypertension, the possibility that the two disorders may be related should be considered. The recent description of a bovine neonatal model of supersystemic pulmonary hypertension and striking alterations of the lung vascular morphology (Stenmark et al., 1987), may mark the beginning of new insights into the important mechanisms involved in the development of severe pulmonary hypertensive disorders.

The combination of two factors appears to contribute to the development of the severe pulmonary hypertension in this bovine model. First, the bovine species is equipped with a strong hypoxic vasoconstriction response (Tucker et al., 1975) and breeding experiments provide cattle with heritable greater susceptibility to hypoxia and high altitude edema formation (Weir et al., 1974; Cruz et al., 1980). These studies set the precedent for a genetic factor or condition involved in the control of pulmonary vascular tone. The second factor of importance may be the pluripotent cellular makeup of the newborn and its cellular growth potential.

The issue of susceptibility to hypoxia was also addressed in a recent study by Fasules et al. (1985) who examined the hypoxic pressor response at heart catheterization of seven children from high altitude, after recovery from high altitude edema. The mean pulmonary artery pressure of the susceptible children after a challenge with 16% inspired oxygen was 56 ±24 but 19±4 mmHg in a group of age-matched nonsusceptible children.

VII. Familial Pulmonary Hypertension

A familial form of pulmonary hypertension was first described by Clarke and co-workers (1927). Since then, numerous reports from many parts of the world have appeared (Lang, 1946; Hood 1968; Kingdon et al., 1966; Tubbs et al., 1977; Asmervik, 1982). Thompson and McRae (1970) suggested an autosomal dominant inheritance. Lloyd and co-workers (1984) recently reviewed 13 families with familial disease in the North American literature and described a family with 6 deaths from primary hypertension in two generations. They also concluded that the transmission was autosomal dominant and excluded an x-linkage of the gene. Knight and Wilson (1985) reviewed cases of familial childhood primary pulmonary hypertension and listed 6 families with sibling involvement. Among those, one of their own patients and the family described by Massound et al. (1970), were four siblings (3 sisters and their brother) who had primary pulmonary hypertension. A possible association between primary pulmonary hypertension and autoimmune diseases does exist (see below) and the observation that the family of one patient with primary pulmonary hypertension may include others with Raynaud's disease may strengthen this link. In the NIH primary pulmonary hypertension study (Rich et al., 1987) only 6.4% of the patients had a familial history. The conclusion must be that primary pulmonary hypertension is only rarely a heritable disease (Newman and Lloyd, 1986), indicating perhaps the importance of expression factors, required for the development of the disease. The early detection of pulmonary hypertension in family members at risk to develop this devastating disease is a clinical challenge, particularly in the absence of early symptoms. Yet, early detection of pulmonary hypertension in members of primary pulmonary hypertension families would permit a description of the natural history of the disease, and further the assessment of the role of vasoconstriction in the pathogenesis of this disorder. A failure to achieve a decrease in pulmonary artery pressure with infusion of a potent pulmonary vasodilator like prostacyclin in patients with early mild to moderate pulmonary hypertension would lead one to doubt the principal pathogenetic importance of vasoconstriction.

VIII. Factors Related to Female Maturation and Pregnancy

Whereas the female to male incidence ratio for primary pulmonary hypertension is 1:1 before puberty and in the infantile cases of familial primary pulmonary hypertension (Knight and Wilson), there is a higher incidence of primary pulmonary hypertension in females in the third decade. The NIH registry with 187 patients, had an overall female to male distribution of 1.7:1 and a female to male ratio of 2.8:1 in the third decade. A Japanese survey of 134 patients with primary pulmonary hypertension (Watanabe and Ogata, 1976) had an overall female to male ratio of 2:1 and a female to male ratio of 3.5:1 in the fourth decade. Further, the disorder was associated with pregnancy in 8 of the

56 women of childbearing age of Wagenvoort's report (1970). There are several reports documenting onset of primary pulmonary hypertension during pregnancy (Feijen et al., 1983), in some cases, in the first trimester. Dawkins and associates (1986) report on 6 pregnant women with primary pulmonary hypertension, two of whom had taken oral contraceptives prior to their pregnancy. Kleiger et al. (1976) reported on 6 women with primary pulmonary hypertension who had taken progestational agents for varying periods of time varying from six months to five years. Notably absent in these cases was evidence for thromboembolic disease. Whereas these associations point toward a female hormonal factor in the pathogenesis of primary pulmonary hypertension, the recent NIH registry data do not support this notion, since there was no particularly strong association with either pregnancy or oral contraceptive use. Thus, at present it is not clear whether earlier reports associating pregnancy and progestational agent use were anecdotal clusters or whether the NIH registry presents a somewhat select group of patients.

Most clinicians agree that pregnancy tends to aggravate pulmonary vascular disease in general, regardless of the etiology (Gatewood and Yu, 1979). Nelson and associates (1985) provide hemodynamic data from a woman with primary pulmonary hypertension obtained before, during, and after delivery, demonstrating progression of the disease (Pap 59/35 - 92/40 mmHg). Feijen and associates discuss the course of a 20-year-old woman, whose brother had primary pulmonary hypertension who developed primary pulmonary hypertension during pregnancy and died 35 days after cesarean delivery of her child.

The reason for the increase in incidence of primary pulmonary hypertension in women of childbearing age is not known. No specific hormone or endocrine modality has yet been identified. Regarding the pulmonary vascular response in the setting of chronic hypoxia, data from animal experiments indicate a greater degree of right ventricular hypertrophy and higher pulmonary artery pressures in male than female (McMurtry et al., 1973; Rabinovitch et al., 1981). Wetzel et al. recently suggested that estradiol could attenuate the acute hypoxic vasoconstriction in sheep. Catecholamines have been proposed to influence vascular tone during menstruation, possibly including that of the lung circulation (Winters et al., 1964). Aminorex fumarate (Menocil), the appetite depressant which had caused a predominantly female epidemic of primary pulmonary hypertension in Europe, can release catecholamines from endogenous stores and may have altered pulmonary vascular tone by such a mechanism. Many investigators share the notion that hormonal influences on the pulmonary circulation are important, however, the important findings have yet to come. Folkman and Ingber point out that "physiological angiogenesis" seems to be a uniquely female affair," occurring during ovulation, repair of the menstruating uterus, and placentation." The authors describe angiostatic steroids like the naturally occurring tetrahydrocortisol, and speculate that low levels of circulating angiostatic steroids may, synergistically with heparinlike molecules, suppress endothelial cell growth. To carry this thought further, one might speculate that a relative decrease of such endothelial cell growth-restraining factors during pregnancy or in the female reproductive life could be an important element in the pathogenetic pattern required to produce primary pulmonary hypertension. Alternatively an overproduction of growth factors- "overpowering" the prevailing angiostatic principles- could act preferentially during the female reproductive period. Estrogens might have a direct effect on endothelial cells, increasing vascular permeability as suggested by Almen and co-workers (1975).

IX. Thromboembolism

The notion that primary pulmonary hypertension was simply a microthrombotic or microembolic disease was prevalent in the 1950s and 1960s. Wagenvoort and Wagenvoort (1970) differentiated primary pulmonary hypertension from recurrent micropulmonary embolism on the basis of (1) bands or webs in the muscular pulmonary arteries, suggesting that thromboembolism had occurred (2) signs of recanalization (multiple channels or eccentric intimal cushions), and (3) less prevalence of medial hypertrophy in the thromboembolic group.

Fuster and co-workers (1984) examined retrospectively the Mayo Clinic's experience with anticoagulant therapy. In their evaluation they found that patients with primary pulmonary hypertension survived longer on anticoagulation therapy (n=78) than those not treated with anticoagulation (n=37). The interpretation of this data is difficult because of the unequal group sizes, the retrospective nature of the analysis and the fact that more than 50% of the patients had thromboembolic disease. Platelet function disturbance and endothelial cell damage have been suggested to be key elements in primary pulmonary hypertension (Mlczoch, 1986). Altered endothelial cell function, possibly represented by a reduction in fibrolytic properties and an imbalance in platelet thromboxane-endothelial cell prostacyclin synthesis (Das, 1981) could well be predisposing factors for in situ thrombosis. Whether or not platelet activation and endothelial dysfunction are primary events, or are frequently encountered but pathophysiologically less important epiphenomena is presently not clear.

X. Autoimmune Disorders

There is a strong association between collagen vascular diseases, in particular systemic sclerosis (Young and Mark, 1978) and systemic lupus erythematosus (Nair et al., 1983; Hovels-Gurich et al., 1986; Schwartzberg et al., 1984; Pines et al., 1982), and "primary" pulmonary hypertension. The table below gives an overview of the various autoimmune diseases, that have been reported in association with primary pulmonary hypertension.

Autoimmune Disorders Associated With PPH
Systemic sclerosis
Mixed connective tissue disease
Systemic lupus
Rheumatoid arthritis
Dermatomyositis
Polymyositis
Polyarteritis nodosa
Chronic active hepatitis
Graves disease
Hashimoto disease

These are all diseases which occur primarily in women. Raynaud's syndrome has been reported in 7-30% of patients with PPH and also to often precede the appearance of symptoms of PPH. In the familial occurrences, family members not afflicted with PPH had Raynaud's syndrome.

In rheumatoid arthritis, lung involvement can occasionally be restricted to a necrotizing angiitis, which then is the substrate of severe pulmonary hypertension. In two cases described by Kay and Banik (1977) and one case by Baydur et al. (1979), the lung vessels were infiltrated with polymorphonuclear neutrophils. Hovels-Gurich et al. (1986) reported the case of a 15-year-old girl with lupus erythematosus and PH whose lung biopsy histology showed plexogenic lesions, with lymphocytes and plasma cells present in periarterial infiltrates, whereas such perivascular infiltrates were absent in the case of a 35-year-old woman described by Nair and associates (1980). Pines and associates (1982) discuss the successful treatment of pulmonary hypertension complicating SLE with corticosteroids in a 49-year-old female patient. Her pulmonary artery pressure decreased from 100/40 to 60/30 mmHg on 60 mg/day of flucortolone. A recent report by Carreras and co-workers (1981) suggested that the so-called lupus anticoagulant may interfere with the vascular production of prostacyclin, which in turn might predispose to thrombosis or vasoconstriction. However, Petri et al. (1987) are of the opinion that lupus-anticoagulant-induced thrombosis was not a major etiologic factor leading to pulmonary hypertension in patients with lupus erythematosus.

Brundage et al. (1984) found a 40% incidence of positive ANA titers (antinuclear antibodies) in 30 patients with PPH and it has been suggested, based on these data, that some patients might have collagen vascular disease confined to the lung. It is not clear at the present time whether the relatively low ANA levels reported are a nonspecific marker of vascular damage or whether follow-up data in these patients would, with passage of time, provide higher titers. A particularly malignant form of pulmonary hypertension appears to be associated with scleroderma (Young and Mark, 1978).

Stuhlinger and co-workers (1978) demonstrated granular deposits of IgG and C_{19} in the lung of a 73-year-old female patient with pulmonary veno-occlusive disease. The deposits were found along the alveolar basal membranes similar to those described by Corrin et al. (1974). Both groups interpreted their findings as deposits of circulating immune complexes. Stuhlinger et al. also identified peripheral lymphocytes sensitized against Type I and Type II collagen. The importance of these results for the pathogenesis of venoocclusive disease is not entirely clear and confirmation by other laboratories is desirable.

XI. Dietary "Primary" Pulmonary Hypertension

From 1967 to 1970 in Switzerland, Austria, and West Germany, a 20-fold increase in unexplained pulmonary hypertension was reported. The clinical, angiographic, and histologic findings resemble the "classic" findings in primary pulmonary hypertension. The epidemic followed the introduction of an appetite depressant agent aminorex (2-amino-5phenyl-2-oxazoline, Menocil) in December 1965 and disappeared soon after the drug had been banned from the market. Approximately 2% of the patients that had taken Menocil developed pulmonary hypertension (Gurtner, 1970). The risk of developing the disease was correlated with the dose, with up to 10% of those taking 320 or more tablets (4.4 g) developing the disease (Greiser, 1973). However, there was no correlation between the severity of the disease and the number of tablets the individual patient had taken (Gurtner, 1970).

The chemical structure of aminorex resembles epinephrine and amphetamine (Kraupp, 1969). A release of catecholamines from endogenous stores by this drug (Kraupp, 1969) has been suggested, as well as a mechanism involving lung serotonin release (Lullmann, 1972; Mielke, 1972). Whereas it was shown that acute administration of aminorex increased the pulmonary vascular resistance in a dose-dependent fashion in anesthetized dogs (Kraupp, 1969), so far all the experimental work to demonstrate the effect of chronic administration on pulmonary hemodynamics and morphology has failed to produce significant alterations (Byrne-Quinn, 1972, Kay, 1971, Kay, 1970, Mielke, 1972). This failure to produce chronic pulmonary hypertension with aminorex in any species investigated usually is explained by the low incidence of pulmonary hypertension, that might be even lower in test animals. A further prerequisite is probably a genetic susceptibility of the pulmonary circulation to constrict or to proliferate when exposed to the offending agent. The aminorex episode suggests that a substance taken orally in humans may induce, by an as yet unknown mechanism, a fatal pulmonary hypertension which resembles primary pulmonary hypertension.

Fahlen et al. (1973) reported two patients who developed pulmonary hypertension during treatment with the antihyperglycemic biguanide phenformin. The pulmonary hypertension subsided on withdrawal of the drug.

In Spain in 1982, several months after ingestion of a rapeseed oil denatured with aniline which had been sold as a cheap cooking oil, an epidemic of more than several thousand cases occurred of what later would be called "toxic oil syndrome." As described by Kay (1985), in the vast majority of the cases, there was an initial ill-defined lung illness with cough, fever, and dyspnea usually associated with the radiographic findings of an interstitial pneumonia. Interestingly, eosinophilia and elevated levels of IgE appeared to be early markers of the disease. Later the patients developed thromboembolic complications, neuropathy, myositis, and Raynaud's abnormalities. Some patients, mostly women, developed pulmonary hypertension, with histological findings of increased pulmonary artery medial thickening, a particular foamy intimal proliferation, and polymorphonuclear neutrophils infiltrating the pulmonary blood vessels. Plexogenic lesions have not yet been described.

Kay suggested that toluidines and analides might have produced free radicals responsible for membrane damage. Alterations in platelet functions in these patients with the "toxic oil" syndrome have been reported. Yet, it is unclear whether a chemical had caused primary endothelial cell damage or caused activation of the immune defense system which accounted for the "graft versus host"-like picture observed in several of these patients.

XII. Primary Pulmonary Hypertension in Patients with Hepatic Cirrhosis and Portal Hypertension

Mantz and Craige (1951) described the first patient with the association of portal hypertension and pulmonary hypertension. The prevalence of primary pulmonary hypertension in a group of 2,459 patients with biopsy-proven hepatic cirrhosis was .61%, – significantly higher than that in an unselected autopsy series (.13%) and also higher than in Ruttner's series (.26%) Both cirrhosis (McDonnell et al., 1983) (alcoholic cirrhosis and postnecrotic cirrhosis) and chronic hepatitis and portal hypertension due to portal vein obstruction, have been described as liver disorders associated with idiopathic pulmonary hypertension. The association between portal hypertension and primary pulmonary hypertension has also been described in young children (Rosenberg et al., 1979)

Naeije et al. (1985) examined 100 patients with liver cirrhosis and measured pulmonary artery pressures. Ten patients had a mean pulmonary artery pressure greater than 20 mmHg; one patient had a mean pulmonary artery pressure of 44 mmHg. In the series of nine patients with liver cirrhosis and primary pulmonary hypertension reporrted by McDonnell et al., 6 were female and 3 were male. All had plexogenic lung vascular lesions and thromboembolism was absent. By what mechanism portal hypertension facilitates development of primary pulmonary hypertension remains obscure.

Attempts to create pulmonary hypertension by surgical production of portal hypertension in rats have so far failed (Chang et al., 1987). Fishman reviewed certain possible mechanisms whereby liver disease could affect the lung circulation. It is of interest that the monocrotaline-induced pulmonary hypertension in rats is always preceded by liver injury.

XIII. Infections

It has been postulated that viral infections might be the origin of primary pulmonary hypertension. A nonspecific infection had been noted particularly in the patients with veno-occlusive disease and an infectious etiology had been postulated to explain the findings of interstitial fibrosis and bronchial mucous gland hyperplasia. As mentioned earlier, others suggested that a virus might selectively attack the pulmonary venous endothelium.

XIV. Conclusion

The pathogenesis of primary pulmonary hypertension remains a fascinating enigma. As discussed above, it is not clear whether plexogenic and microthromboembolic pulmonary arteriopathies are entirely discrete pathologic entities, which happen to have some similar histologic features, or are part of a spectrum of morphologic responses to one or more stimuli, in which the nonspecific histologic appearances are determined by genetic factors, age at onset, etc. The fact that features of both arteriopathies can be seen in association with aminorex administration and portal hypertension, and within families suffering from familial primary pulmonary hypertension, makes it likely that the histologic findings are nonspecific. Attention should be paid to the cellular and molecular mechanisms responsible for smooth muscle migration, intimal proliferation, and thrombosis in situ. The observations regarding the increased incidence in young women, the familial occurrence of the disease, the association with autoimmune disorders, portal hypertension, and the ingestion of certain drugs, should be used as clues to the initial stimulus and the necessary, predisposing substrate for the expression of primary pulmonary hypertension.

References

Almen, T., Hartel, M., Nylander, G., and Olivecrona, H. (1975). The effect of estrogen on the vascular endothelium and its possible relation to thrombosis. *Surg. Gynecol. Obstet. 140*:938.

Anderson, E. G., Simon, G., and Reid, L. (1973). Primary and thrombo-embolic pulmonary hypertension: a quantitative pathological study. *J. Pathol. 110*: 273-293.

Asmervik, J. (1985). Familiaer primaer pulmonal hypertension. *Tidsskr Nor Loegeforen nr. 105*:673-674.

Avasthey, P., and Roy, S. B. (1968). Primary pulmonary hypertension, cerebrovascular malformation, and lymphoedema feet in a family. *Br. Heart J. 30*:769.

Baydur, A., Mongan, E. S., Slager, U. T. (1979). Acute respiratory failure and pulmonary arteritis without parenchymal involvement: demonstration in a patient with rheumatoid arthritis. *Chest 75*:518-520.

Benitz, W. E., Kelley, R. T., and Bernfield, M. (1987). An endothelial cell-derived inhibitor of smooth muscle cell growth has the characteristics of a basement membrane heparan sulfate proteoglycan. *J. Cell. Biol. 105*:220a.

Berliner, S., Shoenfeld, Y., Dean, H., Avisar, R., David, M., and Pinkhas, J. (1982). Primary pulmonary hypertension: a facet of a diffuse angiopathic process. *Respiration 43*:76-79.

Bjornsson, J., and Edwards, W. D. (1985). Primary pulmonary hypertension: a histopathologic study of 80 cases. *Mayo Clin. Proc. 60*:16-25.

Blount, S. G. (1967) Primary pulmonary hypertension. *Mod. Conc. Cardiovasc. Dis. 36*(12):67-72.

Brundage, B. H., Rich, S., and Groves, B. M. (1984). Positive antinuclear antibody tests in primary pulmonary hypertension. *J. Am. Coll. Cardiol. 3*: 596.

Byrne-Quinn, E., and Grover, R. F. (1972) Aminorex (Menocil) and amphetamine: acute and chronic effects on pulmonary and systemic hemodynamics in the calf. *Thorax 27*:127.

Carreras, L. O., Machin, S. J., Deman, R., Defreyn, G., Vermylen, J., Spitz, B., and Van Assche, A. (1981). Arterial thrombosis, intrauterine death and "lupus" anticoagulant: detection of immunoglobulin interfering with prostacyclin formation. *Lancet* 244.

Chang, S. W., Ohara, N., and Voelkel, N. F. (1987). Pulmonary hemodynamic changes in awake, cirrhotic rats: role of platelet activating factor (PAF). APS (Submitted).

Chapman, D. W., Abbott, J. P., and Latsor, J. (1957). Primary pulmonary hypertension: Review of literature and results of cardiac catheterization in 10 patients. *Circulation 15*:35.

Clarke, R. C., Coombs, C. F., Hadfield, G., and Todd, A. T. (1927). On certain abnormalities, congenital and acquired, of the pulmonary artery. *O. J. Med. 21*:51-69.

Corrin, B., Spencer, H., Turner-Warwick, M., and Hamblin, J. J. (1974). Pulmonary veno-occlusion: an immune complex disease? *Virchows Arch. Path Anat. Histol. 364*:81-91.

Cruz, J. C., Reeves, J. T., Russel, B. E., Alexander, A. F., and Will, D. H. (1980). Embryo transplanted calves: the pulmonary hypertensive trait is genetically transmitted (40837).

D'Amore, P., and Thompson, R. W. (1987). Mechanisms of angiogenesis. *Ann. Rev. Physiol. 49*:453-464.

Das, U. N. (1981). Prostaglandins and pulmonary hypertension-further evidence. *Med. Hypotheses 7*:621-624.

Dawkins, K. D., Burke, C. M., Billingham, M. E., and Jamieson, S. W. (1986). Primary pulmonary hypertension and pregnancy. *Chest 89*(3):383-388.

DeMey, J. G., and Vanhoutee, P. M. (1982). Heterogeneous behavior of the canine arterial and venous wall. *Circ. Res. 51*:439-447.

Dresdale, D. T., Michtom, R. F., and Schultz, M. (1954) Recent studies in primary pulmonary hypertension including pharmacodynamic observations on pulmonary vascular resistance. *Bull. N.Y. Acad. Med. 30*:195.

Dresdale, D. T., Schultz, M., and Michtom, R. J. (1951). Primary pulmonary hypertension. I. Clinical and haemodynamic study. *Am. J. Med. 11*:686.

Editorial (1972). Pulmonary veno-occlusive disease. *Br. Med. J. 3*:369.

Edwards, B. S., Weir, E. K., Wedards, W. D., Ludwig, J., Dykoski, R. K., and Edwards, J. E. (1987). Coexistent pulmonary and portal hypertension: morphologic and clinical features. *J. Am. Coll. Cardiol. 10*:1233-1238.

Erickson, L. A., Schleef, R. R., Ny, T., and Loskutoff, D. J. (1985). The fibrinolytic system of the vascular wall. *Clin. Haematol. 14*:513-530.

Esmon, C. T. (1987). The regulation of natural anticoagulant pathways. *Science 235*:1348-1352.

Fahlen, M., Bergman, H., and Helder, G. (1973) Phenformin and pulmonary hypertension. *Br. Heart J. 35*:824-828.

Farrar, J. R. (1963) Idiopathic pulmonary hypertension. *Am. Heart J. 66*:128.

Fasules, J. W., Wiggins, J. W., and Wolfe, R. R. (1985). Increased lung vasoreactivity in children from Leadville, Colorado, after recovery from high-altitude pulmonary edema. *Circulation 72*(5):957-962.

Fayemi, A. O. (1976). Pulmonary vascular disease in systemic lupus erythematosus. *Am. J. Clin. Pathol. 65*:284-290.

Feijen, H. W. H., Hein, P. R., van Lakwijk-Vondrovicova, E. L., and Nijhuis, G. M. M. (1983). Primary pulmonary hypertension and pregnancy. *Eur. J. Obstet. Gynecol. 15*:159-164.

Fowler, N. O., Westcott, R. N., Hanenstein, V. D., Scott, R. G., and McGuire, J. (1950) Observations on autonomic participation in pulmonary arteriolar resistance in man. *J. Clin. Invest. 29*:1387.

Fox, P. L., and DiCorleto, P. E. (1984). Regulation of production of a platelet-derived growth factor-like protein by cultured bovine aortic endothelial cells. *J. Cell. Physiol. 121*:298-308.

Fuchs, J., Mlczoch, J., Niessner, H., and Lechner, K. (1981). Abnormal fibrinolysis in primary pulmonary hypertension. *Eur. Heart J. 2*:168.

Fuster, V., Steele, P. M., Edwards, W. D., Gersh, B. J., Phil, D., McGoon, M. D., and Frye, R. L. 91984). Primary pulmonary hypertension: natural history and the importance of thrombosis. *Circulation 70*(4):580-587.

Gatewood, R. P., Jr., and Yu, P. N. (1979) Primary pulmonary hypertension. In *Progress in Cardiology*. Edited by P. N. Yu and J. F. Goodwin, Lea and Febiger, Philadelphia, 305-349.

Geggel, R. L., Carvalho, A. C. A., Hover, L. W., and Reid, L. M. (1987). Von Willebrand factor abnormalities in primary pulmonary hypertension. *Am. Rev. Resp. Dis. 135*:294-299.

Giddings, J. C. (1986). Von Willebrand factor-physiology. In *Vascular Endothelium in Hemostasis and Thrombosis*. Edited by M. A. Gimbrone. New York, Churchill Livingstone Inc.

Greiser, E. (1973). Epidemiologische Untersuchungen zum Zusammenhang zwischen Appetitzuglereinnahme und Primar vascularen Hypertonie. *Internist 14*:437.

Gurtner, H. P. (1970) *Schweiz. Med. Wochenschr. 100*:2158.

Harlan, J. M., Thompson, P. J., Ross, R. R., and Bowen-Pope, D. F. (1986). Alpha-thrombin induces release of platelet-derived growth factor-like molecule(s) by cultured human endothelial cells. *J. Cell. Biol. 103*:1129-1133.

Hatano, S., and Strasser, T. (1975). Primary pulmonary hypertension. Report on a World Health Organization Meeting. Geneva, Switzerland. pp. 7-45.

Haudenschild, C. C., Prescott, M. F., and Chobanian, A. V. (1980). Effects of hypertension and its reversal on aortic intimal lesions of the rat. *Hypertension 2*:33-44.

Haworth, S. G. (1988). Pulmonary vascular remodeling in neonatal pulmonary hypertension. State of the art. *Chest 93*(3):133S-138S.

Heath, D., and Kay, J. M. (1978). Diet, drugs, and pulmonary hypertension. *Progr. Cardiovasc. 7*:125-140.

Heath, D., Scott, O., and Lynch, J. (1971). Pulmonary veno-occlusive disease. *Thorax 26*:663-674.

Heath, D., Smith, P., Gosney, J., Mulcahy, D., Fox, K., Yacoub, M., and Harris, P. (1987). The pathology of the early and late stages of primary pulmonary hypertension. *Br. Heart J. 58*:204-213.

Hermus, A., Claessens, R. J. J., and Klijn, L. D. (1983). Chronische hepatitis en primaire pulmonale hypertensie. *Ned. Tijdschr Geneeskd 127*(24):1041.

Hood, H. B., Jr. (1968). Primary pulmonary hypertension: Familial occurrence. *Br. Heart J. 30*:336.

Hovels-Gurich, G., Bocking, A., and von Bernuth, G. (1986). Primare pulmonale Hypertension und systemischer lupus erythematodes im Jugendalter. *Klin. Padiatr. 198*:126-128.

Inglesby, T. V., and Singer, J. W. (1973). Abnormal fibrinolysis in familial pulmonary hypertension. *Am. J. Med. 55*:5-14.

Jaffe, E. A. (1985). Physiologic functions of normal endothelial cells. *Ann. N.Y. Acad. Sci. 454*:279-291.

Jones, M. B., Osterhold, R. K., Wilson, R. B., Martin, F. H., Commers, J. R., and Bachmayer, J. D. (1978). Fatal pulmonary hypertension and resolving immune-complex glomerulonephritis in mixed connective tissue disease. *Am. J. Med. 855.*

Juaneda, E., Watson, H., and Haworth, S. G. (1985). An unusual case of rapidly progressive primary pulmonary hypertension in childhood. *Intl. J. Cardiol.* 7:306-309.

Kay, J. M. (1970). Crotalaria pulmonary hypertension. *Prog. Respir. Res. 5*:30.

Kay, J. M., and Banik, S. (1977). Unexplained pulmonary hypertension with pulmonary arteritis in rheumatoid disease. *Br. J. Dis. Chest 71*:53-59.

Kay, J. M., and Heath, D. (1985). Pathologic study of unexplained pulmonary hypertension. *Sem. Resp. Med.* 7:180-192.

Kay, J. M., Smith, P., and Heath, D. (1971) Aminorex and the pulmonary circulation. *Thorax 26*:262-270.

Kingdon, H. S., et al. (1966). Familial occurrence of primary pulmonary hypertension. *Arch. Intern. Med. 118*:422.

Kleiger, R. E., Boxer, M., Ingham, R. E., and Harrison, D. C. (1976). Pulmonary hypertension in patients using oral contraceptives. *Chest 69*(2):143-147.

Knaue, M., Huffman, W., and Uhl, J. (1982). Primary pulmonary hypertension in childhood. *Medizinische Welt 33*(36):1238-1241.

Knight, J. A., and Wilson, J. F. (1985). Primary pulmonary hypertension in childhood; a report on two brothers. *Pediatr. Pathol. 4*:13-23.

Kobayashi, H., Sano, T., Ii, K., Hizawa, K., Yamanoi, A., and Otsuka, T. (1981). Mixed connective tissue disease with fatal pulmonary hypertension. *Acta Pathol. Japan 32*(6):1121-1129.

Kraupp, O. (1969). Studies on the etiology of primary pulmonary hypertension in animal experiments. *Wien Z. Inn. Med. 50*(10):493-496.

Kull, F. C., Brent, D. A., Parikh, I., and Cuatrecasas, P. (1987) Chemical identification of a tumor-derived angiogenic factor. *Science 236*:843-845.

Lang, F. (1948). Die essentielle Hypertonie der Lungenstrombahn und ihr familares Vorkommen. *Deutsch Med. Wschr. 72*:322.

Langleben, D., Moroz, L. A., McGregor, M., and Lisbona, R. (1985). Decreased half-life of fibrinogen in primary pulmonary hypertension. *Thrombosis Res. 40*:577-580.

Levine, J. D., Harlan, J. M., Harker, L. A., Joseph, M. L., and Counts, R. B. (1982). Thrombin mediated release of factor VIII antigen from human umbilical vein endothelial cells in culture. *Blood 60*:531-534.

Lichtenstern-Peters, E., Bein, G., Lange, L., Jimenez, E., Schachinger, H., Schartl, S., and Stoltenburg-Didinger, S. S. G. (1982). Primare pulmonale Hypertonie im Kindesalter. Primary pulmonary hypertension in childhood. *Z. Kardiol. 71*:779-783.

Loyd, J. E., Primm, R. K., and Newman, J. H. Familial primary pulmonary hypertension: clinical patterns. *Am. Rev. Resp. Dis. 129*:194-197, 1984.

Loyd, J. E., Atkinson, J. B., Virmani, R., Pietra, G. G., and Newman, J. H. (1987). Concentric and eccentric intimal fibrosis occur together in families with primary pulmonary hypertension. *Am. Rev. Resp. Dis. 135*:A350.

Lombard, C. M., Churg, A., and Winokur, S. (1987). Pulmonary veno-occlusive disease following therapy for malignant neoplasms. *Chest 92*:871-876.

Lullmann, H., Parwaresch, M. R., Sattler, M., Seiler, K. U., and Siegfriedt, A. (1972). The effects of anorectic agents on the pulmonary pressure and morphology of rat lungs after chronic administration. *Arzneimittelforsch 22*:2096.

Majack, R. A., Goodman, L. V., and Dixit, V. M. (1988). Cell surface thrombospondin is functionally essential for vascular smooth muscle cell proliferation. *J. Cell. Biol. 106*:415-422.

Mantz, F. A., and Craige, E. (1951). Portal axis thrombosis with spontaneous portacaval shunt and resulting cor pulmonale. *Arch. Pathol. 52*:91-97.

Massoud, H., Puckett, W., and Auerbach, S. H. (1970). Primary pulmonary hypertension. A study of the disease in four young siblings. *J. Tenn. Med. Assoc. 63*:299-305.

Mecham, R. P., Whitehouse, L. A., Wrenn, D. S., Parks, W. C., Griffin, G. L., Senior, R. M., Crouch, E. C., Stenmark, K. R., and Voelkel, N. F. (1987). Smooth muscle-mediated connective tissue remodeling in pulmonary hypertension. *Science 237*:423-426.

McDonnell, P. J., Summer, W. R., and Hutchins, G. M. (1981). Pulmonary veno-occlusive disease: morphological changes suggesting a viral cause. *JAMA 246*:667-671.

McMurtry, I. F., Frith, C. H., and Will, D. H. (1973). Cardiopulmonary responses of male and female swine to simulated high altitude. *J. Appl. Physiol. 35*:459-462.

Melmon, K. L., and Braunwald, E. (1963). Familial pulmonary hypertension. *N. Engl. J. Med. 269*:770.

Meyrick, B., and Brigham, K. L. (1986). Repeated *Escherichia coli* endotoxin-induced pulmonary inflammation causes chronic pulmonary hypertension in sheep. Structural and functional changes. *Lab Invest. 55*:164-176.

Mielke, H., Seiler, K. U., Stumpf, U., and Wassermann, O. (1972). Influence of aminorex (menocil) on pulmonary pressure and on the content of biogenic amines in the lungs of rats. *Naunyn Schmiedeberg's Arch. Pharmacol. 274*(s):R79.

Mlczoch, J. (1985). Potential role of platelets in the pulmonary circulation. *Cor Vasa 27*:153-159.

Mlczoch, J. (1986). Cor pulmonale infolge Erkrankungen vorwiegend des Lung-engefaBsystems. *Herz 11*(4):191-196.

Naije, R., Melot, C., Hallemans, R., Mols, P., and Lejeune, P. (1985). Pulmonary hemodynamics in liver cirrhosis. *Sem. Resp. Med. 7*:164-170.

Nair, S. S., Askari, A. D., popelka, C. G., and Kleinerman, J. F. (1980). Pulmonary hypertension and systemic lupus erythematosus. *Arch. Intern. Med. 140*:109.

Nathan, C. F. (1987). Secretory products of macrophages. *J. Clin. Invest. 79*: 319-326.

Nawroth, P. P., Handley, D. A., Esmon, C. T., and Stern, D. M. (1986). Interleukin 1 induces endothelial cell procoagulant while suppressing cell surface anticoagulant activity. *Proc. Natl. Acad. Sci. 83*:3460-3464.

Nelson, D. M., Main, E., Crafford, W., and Ahumada, G. G. (1983). Peripartum heart failure due to primary pulmonary hypertension. *Obstet. Gynecol. 62*(3):58S-63S.

Newman, J. H., and Loyd, J. E. (1986). Genetic basis of pulmonary hypertension. *Sem. Resp. Med. 7*(4):343.

Niedenzu, C., Grasedyck, K., Voelkel, N. F., Bittmann, S., and Lindner, J. (1981). Proliferation of lung cells in chronically hypoxic rats. An autoradiographic and radiochemical study. *Int. Arch. Occup. Environ. Health 48*(2):185-193.

Nilsson, J., Sjolund, M., Palmberg, L., Thyberg, J., and Heldin, C. H. (1985). Arterial smooth muscle cells in primary culture produce a platelet derived growth factor like protein. *Proc. Natl. Acad. Sci. 82*:4418-4422.

Orlidge, A., and D'Amore, P. A. (1987). Inhibition of capillary endothelial cell growth by pericytes and smooth muscle cells. *J. Cell. Biol. 105*:1455-1462.

Petri, M., Rheinschmidt, M., Whiting-O'Keefe, Q., Hellmann, D., and Corash, L. (1987). The frequency of lupus anticoagulant in systemic lupus erythematosus. *Ann. Intern. Med. 106*:524-531.

Pfeifle, B., Boeder, H., and Ditschuneit, H. (1987). Interaction of receptors for insulin-like growth factor I, platelet-derived growth factor, and fibroblast growth factor in rat aortic cells. *Endocrinology 120*:2251-2258.

Pines, A., Kaplinsky, N., Goldhammer, E., Olchovsky, D., and Frankl, O. (1982). Corticosteroid responsive pulmonary hypertension in systemic lupus erthematosus. *Clin. Rheumatol. 1*(4):301-304.

Prescott, S. M., Zimmerman, G. A., and McIntyre, T. M. (1984). Human endothelial cells in culture produce platelet-activating factor (1-alkyl-2-acetyl-sn-glycero-3-phosphocholine) when stimulated with thrombin. *Proc. Natl. Acad. Sci. 81*:3534-3538;

Rabinovitch, M., Gamble, W. J., Miettinen, O. S., and Reid, L. (1981). Age and sex influence on pulmonary hypertension of chronic hypoxia and on recovery. *Am. J. Physiol. 240 (Heart Circ. Physiol. 9)*:H62-H72.

Rabinovitch, M. (1988). Problems of pulmonary hypertension in children with congenital cardiac defects. *Chest 93*(3):119S-126S.

Rabinovitch, M., Andrew, M., Thom, H., Trusler, G. A., Williams, W. G., Rowe, R. D., and Olley, P. M. (1987). Abnormal endothelial factor VIII associated with pulmonary hypertension and congenital heart defects. *Circulation 766*:1043-1052.

Rao, B. N.S., Moller, J. H., and Edwards, J. E. (1969). Primary pulmonary hypertension in a child. *Circulation 40*:583-587.

Reeves, J. T., Groves, B. M., and Turkevich, D. (1986). The case for treatment of selected patients with primary pulmonary hypertension. *Am. Rev. Respir. Dis. 134*:342-346.

Reeves, J. T., and Herget, J. (1984). Experimental models of pulmonary hypertension. In *Pulmonary Hypertension.* Edited by E. K. Weir and J. T. Reeves. New York, Futura Publishing Company, Inc.

Rich, S., Dantzker, D. R., Ayres, S. M., Bergofsky, E. H., Brundage, B. H., Detre, K. H., Fishman, A. P., Goldring, R. M., Groves, B. M., Koerner, S. K., Levy, P. S., Reid, L. M., Vreim, C. E., and Williams, G. W. (1987). Primary pulmonary hypertension, A national prospective study. *Ann. Intern. Med. 107*:216-223.

Rosenberg, L., Silverman, A., and Strain, J. E. (1979). The pediatric corner. *Am. J. Gastroenterol. 71*:427-431.

Ruttner, J. R., Bartschi, J. P., Niedermann, R., and Schneider, J. (1980). Plexogenic pulmonary arteriopathy and liver cirrhosis. *Thorax 35*:133-136.

Samet, P., Bernstein, W. H., and Widrich, J. (1960). Intracardiac infusion of acetylcholine in primary pulmonary hypertension. *Am. Heart J. 60*:433-439.

Schwartzberg, L., Lieberman, D. H., Gertzoff, B., and Ehrlich, G. E. (1984). Systemic lupus erythematosus and pulmonary vascular hypertension. *Arch. Intern. Med. 144*:605-607.

Sedziwy, L., and Kalczynski, J. (1966). Primary pulmonary hypertension in three brothers. *Acta Med. Pol. 7*:401.

Short, D. S. (1957). The arterial bed of the lung in pulmonary hypertension. *Lancet 2*:12-16.

Sjolund, M., Hedin, U., Sejersen, T., Heldin, C., and Thyberg, J. (1988). Arterial smooth muscle cells express platelet-derived growth factor (PDGF) a chain mRNA, secrete a PDGF-like mitogen, and bind exogenous PDGF in a phenotype- and growth state-dependent manner. *J. Cell Biol. 106*:403-413.

Smith, P., and Heath, D. (1979). Electron microscopy of the plexiform lesion. *Thorax 34*:177-186.

Sporn, M. B., Roberts, A. B., Wakefield, L. M., and Assoian, R. K. (1986). Transforming growth factor-beta: biological function and chemical structure. *Science 233*:532-534.

Staemmler, M. (1937). Die thromboendarteritis obliterans der lungenartenrien. *Klin. Wochenschr. 16*:1669.

Stenmark, K., Fasules, J., Voelkel, N. F., Henson, J., Tucker, A., Hyde, D. M., Wilson, H., and Reeves, J. T. (1987). Severe pulmonary hypertension and arterial adventitial changes in newborn calves at 4300m. *J. Appl. Physiol. 62*(2):821-830.

Stuhlinger, W., Michlmayr, G., Mikuz, G., and Braunsteiner, H. (1978). Humarale und zellulare Immunmechanismen bei veno-okklusiver Erkrankung der Lung. *Schweiz Med. Wschr. 108*(22):822.

Thompson, P., and McRae, C. (1970) Familial pulmonary hypertension. Evidence of autosomal dominant inheritance. *Br. Heart J. 32*:758-760.

Tozzi, C. A., Poiani, G. J., Harangozo, A. M., Boyd, C. J., and Riley, D. J. (1988). Pulmonary vascular endothelial cells modulate stretch-induced DNA and connective tissue synthesis in rat pulmonary artery segments. *Chest 93*(3):169S-170S.

Tubbs, R. R., Levin, R. D., Shirley, E. K., and Hoffman, G. C. (1979). Fibrinolysis in familial pulmonary hypertension. *Am. J. Clin. Pathol. 71*:384-387.

Tucker, A., McMurtry, I. F., Reeves, J. T., Alexander, A. F., Will, A. H., and Grover, R. F. (1975). Lung vascular smooth muscle as a determinant of pulmonary hypertension at high altitude. *Am. J. Physiol. 228*:762-767.

Voelkel, N. F., and Reeves, J. T. (1979). Primary pulmonary hypertension. In *Pulmonary Vascular Diseases*. Edited by K. Moser. Marcel Dekker, New York.

Voelkel, N. F., Wiegers, U., Sill, V., and Trautmann, J. (1977). Kinetic study on the lung DNA-synthesis stimulated by chronic high altitude hypoxia. *Thorax 32*:578.

Wagenvoort, C. A. (1976). Pulmonary veno-occlusive disease entity or syndrome? *Chest 69*:82-86.

Wagenvoort, C. A. (1980). Lung biopsies in the differential diagnosis of thromboembolic versus primary pulmonary hypertension. *Prog. Resp. Res. 13*: 16-21.

Wagenvoort, C. A., and Wagenvoort, N. (1970). Primary pulmonary hypertension, a pathologic study of the lung vessels in 156 clinically diagnosed cases. *Circulation 42*:1163-1184.

Wagenvoort, C. A., and Wagenvoort, N. (1977). *Pathology of Pulmonary Hypertension.* J. Wiley &Sons, New York.

Watanabe, S., and Ogata, T. (1976). Clinical and experimental study upon primary pulmonary hypertension. *Jap. Circ. J. 40*(6):603-610.

Weir, E. K., Archer, S. L., and Edwards, J. E. (1988). Chronic primary and secondary thromboembolic pulmonary hypertension. *Chest 93*:149-154.

Weir, E. K., Will, D., Reeves, J. T., Tucker, A., and Grover, R. F. (1974). The genetic factor influencing pulmonary hypertension in cattle at high altitude. *Cardiovasc. Res. 8*:745-749.

Wetzel, R. C., Zacur, H. A., and Sylvester, J. T. (1984). Effect of puberty and estradiol on hypoxic vasomotor response in isolated sheep lungs. *J. Appl. Physiol. 56*(5):1199-1203.

Winkles, J. A., Friesel, R., and Maciag, T. (1987). Smooth muscle cells are a potential vessel wall source for the angiogenic protein HBGF-I. *J. Cell. Biol. 105*:274a.

Winters, W. L., Joseph, R. R., and Learner, N. (1964). Primary pulmonary hypertension and Raynaud's phenomenon. *Arch. Int. Med. 114*:821-830.

Wood, P. (1956). *Diseases of the Heart and Circulation.* Philadelphia, J. Lippincott Co., p. 839.

Wood, P. (1959). Pulmonary hypertension with special reference to the vasoconstrictive factor. *Br. Heart J. 21*:557.

Young, R. H., and Mark, G. J. (1978). Pulmonary vascular changes in scleroderma. *Am. J. Med. 64*:998.

Yu, P. N. (1958). Primary pulmonary hypertension: Resport of 6 cases and review of literature. *Ann. Intern. Med. 49*:1138.

Zerwes, H., and Risau, W. (1987). Polarized secretion of a platelet-derived growth factor-like chemotactic factor by endothelial cells in vitro. *J. Cell. Biol. 105*:2037-2041.

16

Control of Cell Proliferation in Pulmonary Hypertension

LYNNE M. REID and PAUL DAVIES

Harvard Medical School and The Children's Hospital
Boston, Massachusetts

I. Introduction

Proliferation of vascular and migratory cells is an important feature of virtually all types of pulmonary hypertension. While the hypertension points to the significant functional derangement, this diagnosis includes many and varied diseases that differ in their cause, pathogenesis, and pathophysiology. And yet it is useful to consider them together, since the cellular and tissue events characteristic of each focus on injury, repair and adaptation by the vascular bed.

To understand pulmonary hypertension we must understand the structural remodeling caused by the original injury, by adaptation to this injury, and to established pulmonary hypertension. Clinical pulmonary hypertension always is caused by structural change. Constriction represents a reversible component and so can respond to treatment but it is not always present. The basic changes are caused by restriction rather than constriction, restriction based either on the obliteration of arteries or on narrowing of those that are patent. Some of the structural changes are secondary to the pulmonary hypertension per se, but it is becoming increasingly apparent that even this adaptation is modified by the nature of the original injury. For example, the reactivity of the central hypertrophied axial pulmonary arteries is different in the hypertensions caused by hypoxia, hyperoxia, and monocrotaline.

Proliferation of vascular cells is a feature of all types of pulmonary hypertension. Proliferation can occur as part of the original injury – that is, mitogens are released as part of acute damage – it may be part of the repair process or of the adaptation that occurs when pulmonary hypertension (PH) is established. In the idiopathic variety it could even be part of the unexplained intrinsic abnormality of endothelial cells that causes the obliterative vasculitis. The mechanisms by which a stimulus is transduced to proliferation are likely to be different in each case. Each of the four vascular cell types – endothelial cell, smooth muscle cell, pericyte, and fibroblast – is affected, but in types of PH caused by an acute injury the proliferative activity of the various cell types and its timing are very different.

While proliferation is a readily identified end point, it is only one of several cell responses seen in PH. Injury to a cell can result in necrosis, hypertrophy or change in metabolic activity, even in change in phenotype; proliferation is not always part of the reaction. In some situations, as in replacing injured cells, proliferation can only be considered beneficial. A localized constrictor response to localized hypoxia seems beneficial, but the proliferative, restrictive lesion that develops in the precapillary segment that causes hypoxic pulmonary hypertension does not. As part of the process responsible for structural remodeling inflammatory cells often migrate and multiply as do the neighboring cells of the epithelial alveolar lining and the fibroblasts of the interstitium.

In PH the site of primary resistance can be at any level in the lung's vascular loop from the large arteries to the extrapulmonary veins. A given vascular segment can be upstream or downstream from the site of main obstruction so that sometimes it may be adapting to high flow and raised transmural pressure, sometimes it is to the opposite. In this chapter we focus mainly on the types of PH where the early and critical injury is in the microcirculation where the special pre- and postcapillary segments in the alveolar wall bear the brunt of injury and adaptation.

II. Pathophysiology

Pulmonary hypertension, then, is a structural, not a functional, disease. Vasoconstriction is not necessarily a component of PH, although in a given patient it can occur at any time in the story. Typically a reversible constrictive component is a feature even of chronic hypoxic PH, yet not all human subjects or patients show a constrictor response to hypoxic challenge, nor do all experimental animals. In hyperoxic injury, pulmonary vasoconstriction is not a feature. In some patients with established PH, the pressure level shows spontaneous lability; in some, dilators reveal a reversible component; in others, resistance remains fixed. This means that ultimately prevention of PH and restoration of the lung's vascular bed to normal structure and compliance calls for knowledge of the pathogenesis of injury and of the pathophysiology of vasoactive agents that goes beyond simple dilation.

Restriction of an otherwise intact vascular bed is caused by vessel wall remodeling that narrows the lumen (Fig. 1). This is seen in hypoxia and in increased blood flow to the lung, at least in its early stages. At this stage of remodeling, improvement, even reversal, is possible. Disturbances of vascular growth can lead to a hypoplastic vascular bed with vessels too small and/or too few – another way restriction of the lung's vascular volume is produced. Obliteration of vessels, arteries or veins, is an irreversible cause of restriction. The residual bed may dilate to compensate, but all too often the diversion of blood to the persisting bed ultimately represents a high flow injury, leading to vessel wall restructuring and lumen narrowing of the patent vessels.

This adaptation by the patent bed represents a vicious circle of injury that operates in all types of established PH. If cardiac output is normal, the first effect may be to increase velocity of blood flow through the restricted segment to a level no greater than occurs during exercise. In the diseased circulation, however, this increase is maintained; cyclical recruitment of the lung's vessels is reduced or lost. In cases of high flow (as in systemic arteriovenous shunts or in certain congenital heart lesions), cardiac output is increased. In this case there is increased total flow as well as increased velocity. These changes evoke a structural remodeling that restricts cross-sectional area.

Whereas hypoxia typically gives a hypertrophic response with an intact vascular bed, hyperoxia, certainly in its early stages, typically causes an obliterative injury. Then the residual patent bed has to adapt to high flow, and so hypertension per se amplifies the already restrictive injury, In at least some cases of primary pulmonary artery hypertension the acute lesion is obliterative, notably of vessels below 40 μm.

Whether the main block is in large elastic or in muscular arteries as in large artery thromboembolism, the arteries less than 40 μm in diameter as in primary pulmonary artery hypertension, the small veins as in primary pulmonary venous hypertension, or the large veins as in idiopathic perivenous fibrosis, the vessels upstream have to adapt to changed hemodynamic conditions. These include a rise in pressure, an increase in transmural pressure, and a different pulse wave and velocity profile of blood flow. In PH the blood volume distribution in the various vascular segments during the cardiac cycle is important. The distribution of vascular pressures through the lung changes: the apex-to-base gradients typical of zones, I, II, and III are no longer apparent. The impedance of the vascular bed increases. Hypertrophy of each coat of the vascular wall occurs; this involves cell proliferation and an increase in extracellular matrix constituents.

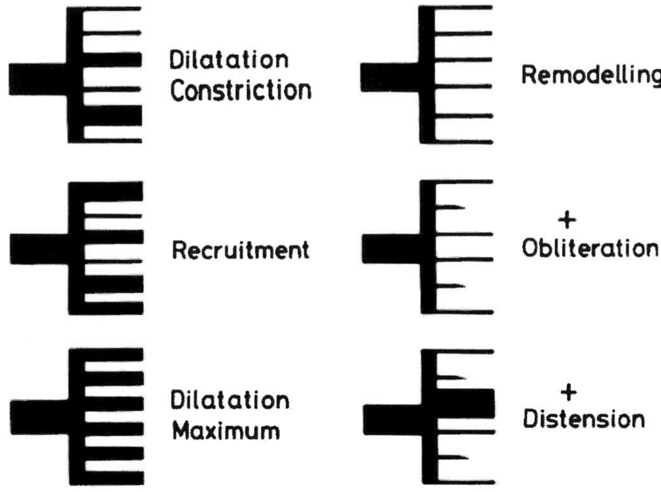

Figure 1 Diagrammatic representation, at left, of variation in diameter in normal bed that expands by dilatation and recruitment of new arteries. In pulmonary hypertension the vascular bed is restricted by structural narrowing of the lumen or by obliteration; to adapt to this, blood flows at increased velocity and residual arteries dilate and then remodel.

Downstream from the site of blockage, adaptation also occurs. This may be an adaptation to virtually no flow or to a change in blood volume distribution and reduced flow rates. Adaptation to "no flow" illustrates the degree of structural remodeling that can occur: contracture of the vessel wall and intimal thickening by cellular and serum products also produces restriction. This can be important in patients with large artery thromboembolism when surgical treatment by excision of clots calls for reflow through these now structurally restricted channels.

A. Smooth Muscle Cells – Proliferation and Differentiation

There is a reciprocal relationship between smooth muscle cell proliferation and differentiation. In the growing vasculature, when smooth muscle cells proliferate they express a "synthetic" phenotype typical of nonmuscle cells, with a predominance of nonmuscle β-actin (Owens and Thompson, 1986; Barja et al., 1986). By contrast, in adult vessels where cells are in the differentiated "contractile" phase, α-actin is its major form. When injury to the adult vessel triggers smooth muscle cell division, this process is reversed and the cells switch their expression of actin to the β and γ isomers (Gabbiani et al., 1984). A change also occurs in intermediate filament proteins so that the ratio of desmin to vimentin is decreased (Gabbiani et al., 1982).

As normal smooth muscle cells become established in culture, similar changes occur in cytoskeletal proteins (Barja et al., 1986) and in cellular metabolism, including induction of ornithine decarboxylase and polyamine synthesis (Thyberg and Fredholm, 1987). In vivo, the switch from "contractile" to "synthetic" is reversible; smooth muscle cells of the injured vessel ultimately stop proliferating and return to a contractile phenotype (Campbell and Campbell, 1985). In culture this can be achieved by manipulating conditions, as by maintaining density, or less effectively, by serum deprivation (Owens et al., 1986).

B. Contracture

Each cell layer can contribute to restriction. The intimal and medial hypertrophy encroach on the lumen. Adventitial hypertrophy is often associated with contracture – that is, narrowing of the external diameter that is not reversible by dilatation or distension of the artery wall. It implies that structure has changed. This could occur in several ways. If constriction and fibrosis both occur the fibrosis perhaps "sets" the artery in its constricted state. Whether the media can change its cellular and intracellular structure to cause contracture without a primary change in the adventitia is not clear: the adventitia would then have to adapt to the smaller artery. Adventitial change alone could lead to contracture if collagen can narrow the lumen even against a normal or raised P_{pa}.

III. Vascular Segments and Their Cells: Targets for Injury, Repair, and Adaptation in Pulmonary Hypertension

Only three types of cells constitute the normal vascular wall – the endothelial cell, the smooth muscle cell or its precursors, and the fibroblast – and yet by their arrangement, their products, and their behavior they produce the variety of channels that characterize the vascular bed. Each of these cell types regularly makes elastin and collagen and the endothelium and muscle cell basement membrane. Even within the lung, strikingly different segments can be distinguished by variation in the arrangement and structure of a given cell type, and extracellular matrix, as well as by sensitivity and reactivity to a variety of physiological and pharmacological stimuli (Reid and Meyrick, 1982). The story continues as one of "threes." Each cell is responsible for one of the three layers of a vessel wall: the endothelial cell for the intima, the smooth muscle cell and the precursor muscle cells, the intermediate cell and pericyte, for the medial or muscular coat, the vascular fibroblast for the adventitia. Within the alveolar wall interstitium, a fibroblast and myofibroblast can also be identified.

In large arteries the adventitial coat is well demarcated and its fibroblasts easily identified. A case can also be made for identifying the vascular fibroblasts in small vessels and capillaries. Here the vascular fibroblast is a single cell running parallel to the transverse plane of section and applied closely to the elastic lamina. It can still be considered distinct from the fibroblast of the interstitium that bridges the space between epithelium and capillary.

In injury this putative advential cell layer often thickens and is distinct from the interstitial fibroblast and fibrosis. Migrant cells move through the vessel wall from either the lumen or the adventitia. The blood is the source of the first; lymphatics, interstitial space, or, in the case of large arteries, vaso vasorum, of the second.

A. Vascular Segments

In considering PH we are mainly concerned with the loop–pulmonary artery to pulmonary vein. There is, in addition, another loop–bronchial artery to true bronchial vein. As described below it is overlap between these loops that suggests a functional significance.

In addition to the triad artery, capillary, and vein the pulmonary vascular loop includes a well defined precapillary and postcapillary segment (Fig. 2) (Reid, 1968). Traversing this pathway within each of these five regions an additional eight segments or levels can be identified by a characteristic structure. For example, the largest central arteries are described as elastic: in addition to the internal and external elastic laminae that define the medial or muscular coat, this layer contains more than five elastic laminae (Fig. 3a, b) that subdivide the thick muscle coat; those with fewer elastic laminae are muscular. Peripherally the central elastic laminae become fragmented and disappear. Although an artery increases in size from birth to adulthood, this change in structure in preacinar arteries is at the same level of branching in fetus and adult (Reid, 1968, 1979). The level of branching in the pulmonary artery can most conveniently be described by reference to the type and generation of the airway that the artery accompanies. These large arteries may be blocked by emboli: invariably they are involved in the adaptation to raised arterial pressure downstream. In the adult, arteries above about 100 μm are elastic and those as small as about 150 μm are muscular. Between this size and the capillary an artery passes through several additional structural changes. Along any arterial pathway from hilum to periphery, whether the loop is short and supplies the central region of the lung or long and passes to the distal pleural surface, a level is reached at which the circumferentially complete medial muscle coat of the artery gives way to a spiral of muscle so that, in cross-section, muscle is identified (at least by light microscopy) in only part of the arterial circumference – this is called a partially muscular artery. This medial muscle disappears from arteries larger than capillaries; these are nonmuscular arteries. We apply the word *artery* to all precapillary ves-

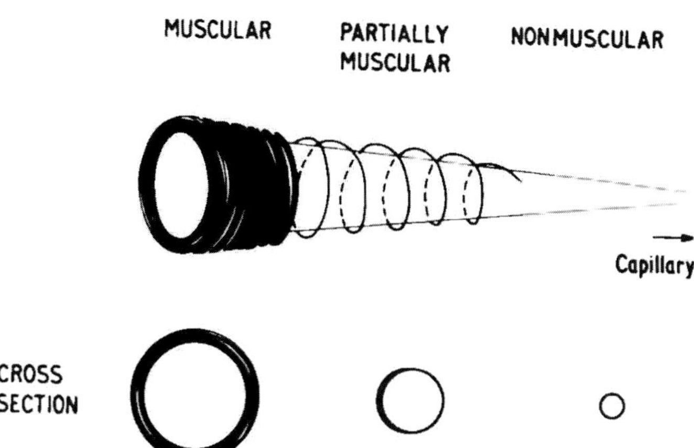

Figure 2 Illustration of pulmonary artery wall showing the arrangement of muscle. Along the pathway of any artery, from hilum to periphery, structure changes as muscle coat diminishes. In cross section the medial muscle coat is either complete (a muscular artery), incomplete (a partially muscular artery), or absent (a nonmuscular artery). (From Reid, 1968, with permission.)

sels to avoid the word *arteriole* since this is used with several different meanings. The transition from one of these structures to another does not always occur at the same size; even in the normal lung the structure of a small artery cannot be predicted from the size. And yet in the normal lung, a given structural type is seen over a set size range, and for any size range the proportion of arteries with a given structure can be predicted. These distributions are similar in the fetus and adult, but during childhood the distribution shifts so that larger vessels are partially muscular or nonmuscular (Davies and Reid, 1970). In many diseases, notably many types of PH, the shift is in the other direction, more precapillary arteries become muscularized.

One feels intuitively that the external diameter of an artery and its wall thickness depend on whether it is constricted or relaxed. A constricted artery has a smaller diameter and a thicker wall (and, of course, its wall thickness as a percentage of external diameter is higher) than the same artery when relaxed. And so to analyze a vascular bed it is necessary to distend (at uniform pressure) the circulation before quantitative analysis of size and wall thickness. Even this may not give the whole story. It is often necessary to know whether the size of an artery is appropriate to its position in the vascular tree and, at this position, appropriate for the age of the subject. This additional information is obtained by considering an artery in its pattern of branching. The pulmonary artery runs with the airway in the same bronchovascular bundle. The artery branches three

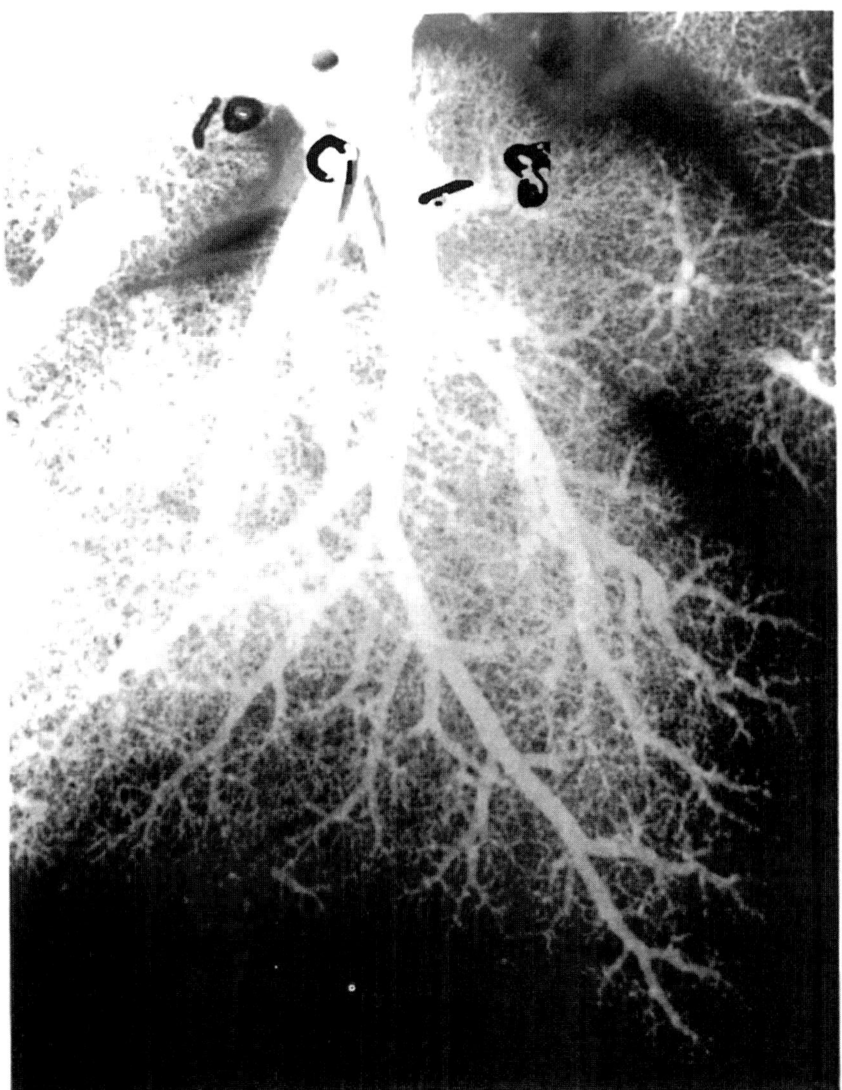

Figure 3 (a) Specimen pulmonary arteriogram. Anterior basal segment (segmental artery 8) in slice of lung 1 cm thick.

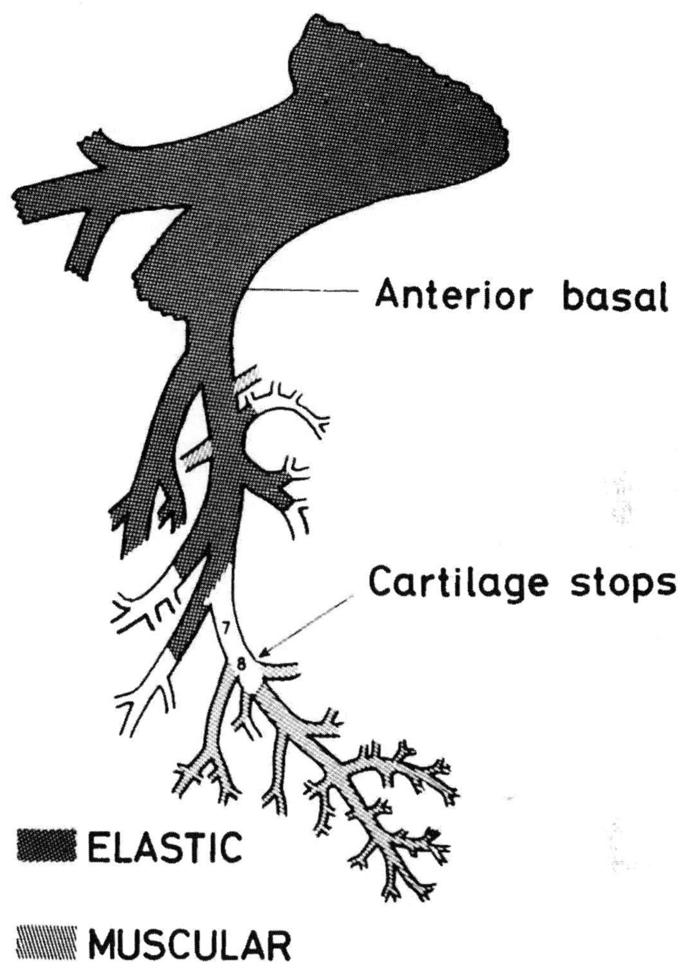

(b) Diagrammatic representation of structure of arterial pathway in (a). This pattern of structure is established in utero. (From Reid, 1979, with permission.)

or four times as often as the airway. It is more convenient to "landmark" the artery by the airway it accompanies since the functional regions of the lung are defined by reference to the airways.

The question of size of an artery is clearly important in the growing lung, in diseases that impair growth, but also in most acquired vascular diseases since the structural changes associated with PH are often associated with contracture (Geggel and Reid, 1984; Haworth et al., 1977; Hislop and Reid, 1981).

B. Double Vascular Supply

The lung has a double arterial supply and a double venous drainage that do not correspond precisely. The pulmonary artery supplies the capillary bed within the alveolar region–that is within the acinus–and also most of the pleura. The bronchial artery supplies the capillary bed in the wall of the airways as far as the respiratory unit and a small region around the hilum of the lung.

The acinus is the respiratory unit of the lung; it is supplied by a terminal bronchiolus – the last generation along any air pathway that has a complete wall. A respiratory bronchiolus has alveoli opening into its lumen: the rest of its wall is lined by respiratory epithelium and includes connective tissue and a muscle layer. The terminal bronchiolus is the airway just proximal to the first respiratory bronchiolus along any pathway. The acinus includes several generations of respiratory bronchioli and of alveolar ducts as well as alveolar sacs and alveoli.

The bronchial and pulmonary arteries with the airway all run within the same bronchovascular connective tissue sheath.

The two venous systems do not correspond to the arterial. Virtually all blood from intrapulmonary structures drains to the pulmonary veins. These receive the bronchial artery blood from bronchial and bronchoalveolar walls as well as from the alveoli and pleura. The true bronchial veins drain to the azygos system, a conventional route for blood starting from the aorta.

The blood draining from airways to the pulmonary veins represents a degree of venous admixture. The blood that circulates from central airways to the azygos system goes directly to the lung's microvessels without "detoxification" systemically (as by the liver).

The blood that drains to pulmonary veins (as from distal airways) will be the source of blood supplying the vaso vasorum of large pulmonary arteries. For example, it is sometimes suggested that hypoxia is sensed in small airways, certainly in the alveolar region. Does the blood from here carry a mediator signal to the adventitial fibroblasts of large pulmonary arteries?

In quantifying arterial structure we use a barium-gelatin suspension that distends arteries as small as 16 μm in diameter, does not pass through the capillary bed, and still permits microscopy and measurement. In the normal bed, arteries are recognized by the injectate in their lumen: the veins are empty. If the vascular bed is diseased, interpretation may be more complex. Much of the data for the structural remodeling in various types of PH is based on quantitative analysis of specimens prepared in this way. The main features that we identify or calculate for each vessel are: external diameter, wall thickness (wall thickness as percent external diameter), structure (elastic, muscular, partially muscular, or nonmuscular), and accompanying airway. The density of filled arteries (or veins) is related to the number of alveoli within the same area and to unit area of a section. Veins run at the edge of any unit whether acinus, lobule, or segment and so cannot be landmarked in the same way. At any level veins receive drainage from several adjacent units.

The veins show a mirror image of the precapillary segment: through the nonmuscular to partially and then to fully muscular vein. In an uninjected system the alveolar vessels of these pre- and postcapillary units are very similar. And yet some lesions are specific to one or the other, e.g., the remodeling in hypoxia affects the precapillary unit. A rise in venous pressure affects both pre- and postcapillary segments.

C. Ultrastructural Features

Electron microscopy has filled in the "gaps" – the details in wall structure in vessels where a medial muscle layer cannot be resolved by light microscopy (Meyrick and Reid, 1982). In the nonmuscular artery, pericytes are found scattered as solitary cells immediately beneath the endothelial cell (Fig. 4). The pericyte lies within the single elastic lamina and parts of it are even within the basement membrane of the endothelial cell. In the muscle-free region of the partially muscular artery an intermediate cell is identified. We used this term because it is intermediate in structure and position between the pericyte and the smooth muscle cell. It has its own basement membrane but still is internal to a single elastic lamina. It has organized microfilaments but no dense bodies. More recently we have combined microdissection with electron microscopy to establish in more detail the structural transition from a fully muscular artery to a capillary, within an acinar segment about half a millimeter long, that proximally would suggest a "resistance artery" to the physiologist, while distally it runs within the alveolar wall (Davies et al., 1986a).

Clinically and experimentally the precapillary unit (and in some forms of disease the postcapillary also) undergoes rapid and striking remodeling so that the cells underlying the endothelium hypertrophy and, in some cases, proliferate and differentiate to form a continuous muscle layer. These cells can be appropriately called precursor smooth muscle cells (Davies et al., 1986a, b).

In the restructuring of many forms of PH these cells have a leading role. Their behavior can be followed in vivo so many of the biological problems and questions considered later can be furnished by reference to tissue changes. It is also desirable that these be explored in vitro as has been done widely for systemic vessels (see Sec. IV). We can culture the cells of the lung's peripheral circulation (Davies et al., 1987c; Jones, 1987b), but in developing this we have learned that the cells of the microvessels are fragile or perhaps coy. This also underlines the difference between the cells from various sites in the circulation – between even large and small pulmonary arteries.

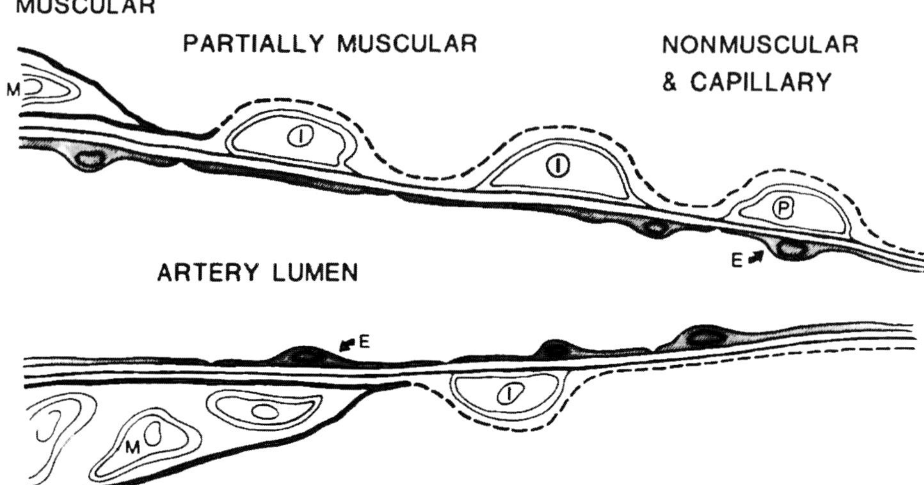

Figure 4 Diagrammatic representation of end of arterial pathway as shown in Figure 2. Electron microscopy reveals additional features of the wall. In the muscle-free region, a pericyte (P) is found in the nonmuscular artery, and an intermediate cell (I) in the nonmuscular part of the partially muscular artery. These are precursor smooth muscle cells. E, endothelial cell, M, muscle cell. (From Davies et al., 1987, with permission).

IV. Factors Stimulating and Inhibiting Vascular Cell Growth

A. Introduction

Growth factors were first identified some decades ago. Currently their investigation is active and exciting in that many new factors and new facts are being reported (Tables 1-3). Since most studies are concerned with the systemic circulation, the relevance to the pulmonary vessels of most of the new knowledge is not yet apparent. Even for the systemic circulation, proof of an in vitro effect is no guarantee of the same effect in vivo. Because an agent can produce an effect does not necessarily mean that it does so biologically.

In PH, proliferation affects all cells of the vessel wall. The causes include injury, repair, and adaptation and the various segments of the vascular bed respond differently. As will be seen in the next section, the biological questions posed by the structural changes in PH do not match those being pursued for systemic vascular disease.

Table 1 Factors Stimulating Vascular Cell Growth[a]

	Target Cell[b]			
	EC	SMC	PC	FIB
EGF	+	+		+
bFGF	+	+		+
Histamine	+			
IGF–I	+	+	+	+
IGF–II	+	+	+	+
IL–1	±			
MDGF (non-PDGFc)	+			
PDGF		+	+P	+
PDGFc		+	+	+P
Platelet factor(s)	+			
Serotonin		+		
TGF–α	+			+
TGF–β	±	±		±
TNF				+
Factor (Vender et al., 1987)		+P1		
Factor(s) (Jones et al., 1987)				+P1
Bloodborne				
aFGF	+			+
Insulin	+	+	+	+

[a]EC, endothelial cell; SMC, smooth muscle cell; PC, pericyte; FIB, fibroblast; EGF, epidermal growth factor; FGF, fibroblast growth factor; (a, acidic; b, basic); IGF, insulin-like growth factor; IL, interleukin; MDGF, macrophage-derived growth factor; PDGF, platelet-derived growth factor; PDGFc, platelet-derived growth factor from cells other than platelets; TGF, transforming growth factor; TNF, tissue necrosis factor.
[b]+P, demonstrated on pulmonary as well as systemic cells; +P1, demonstrated on pulmonary cells only.

Table 2 Factors Stimulating Vascular Cell Growth[a]

	Cell of Origin						
	EC	SMC	PC	FIB	Mast Cell	MON	Platelet
EGF				+			+
bFGF	+					+	
Histamine					+		
IGF–I				+P			
IGF–II				+P			
IL–I	+					+	
MDGF						+	
PDGF							+
PDGFc	+	+				+P	
Platelet factors							+
Serotonin					+		
TGF–α							+
TGF–β						+P	+
TNF				+		+	
Factor (Vender et al., 1987)	+P1						
Factor(s) (Jones et al., 1987)				+P1			

[a]MON, mononuclear cell. For other symbols, see Table 1.

Interest in atherosclerosis has directed much of the investigation in systemic arteries (Schwartz et al., 1986; Ross et al., 1986). For this, migration of smooth muscle cells from media to intima, their multiplication, and interaction with macrophage and lipid are the major cellular events (Davies, 1986). These are changes of large arteries. In the pulmonary artery, atheroma develops only when PH is present (Hayes et al., 1979).

Another major focus of systemic studies is angiogenesis, particularly by tumors and in granulation tissue (Folkman and Klagsbrun, 1987; Fett et al., 1985). This concerns endothelial cell multiplication that provides a vascular network. The role of these in normal growth is not yet clear even in systemic ves-

Table 3 Factors Inhibiting Vascular Cell Growth[a]

	Cell of origin	Target Cell			
		EC	SMC	PC	FIB
Contact-inhibiting membrane molecule(s)	EC	+			
Heparin-like molecule	EC		+P		
EPIF	EC			+P1	
Heparin-like molecule	SMC		+		
Contact-dependent factor	PC	+			
Interferon	MON	+			
Prostaglandins	MON				+P
TGF–β	MON	+	±		
35-40 kD factor	Platelets	+			
Heparin			+P	+P	+
Heparin-binding fragments of fibronectin		+			

[a]For explanation of symbols, see Tables 1 and 2. EPIF endothelial-cell-derived pericyte inhibitory factor.

sels. Tumors in the lung are supplied mainly by bronchial arteries so that systemic artery studies are likely to be relevant to their vascularization.

In lung, angiogenesis is part of the inflammatory process that handles intraalveolar exudate, including cells. These new vessels grow from the pulmonary microcirculation, that is from the capillary and pre- and postcapillary segments. For lung it is not known from what level these new sprouts come: in the systemic circulation, it seems that they are mainly from the postcapillary or venous side. Intraalveolar granulation tissue can result either in effacement of alveolar structure or in absorption of the exudate back into the alveolar wall. Sometimes after an inflammatory process the new vessels as well as the original ones have disappeared.

In the systemic studies much of the focus has been on mitosis by smooth muscle cells. And yet to take one type of PH, that caused by hypoxia, the mitotic activity is later and much less in this cell type than in the adventitial fibroblasts of large arteries or the pericytes of the microcirculation (Meyrick and Reid, 1979a).

The earlier events in PH from either hypoxia or monocrotaline focus attention on the pericyte, although there are differences between the two types (Meyrick and Reid, 1979b). When hypoxia is the cause, the pericyte hypertrophies, proliferates, and then changes phenotype to a smooth muscle cell. It distances itself from the intimal endothelial cell by basement membrane and even by an elastic lamina. To underline differences as well as similarities, after monocrotaline administration the proliferative step seems not to occur although the hypertrophy and differentiation of a muscular media proceed. This occurs more slowly and it seems that the differentiation to smooth muscle cells does not include the development of dense bodies. It appears that the adage still holds that proliferation precedes differentiation.

Most of the studies of systemic arteries have concentrated on growth factors and mitogenesis, but this is only half the story. It is necessary to understand how the homeostasis is maintained, what are the checks as well as the stimuli that maintain normal balance. Growth represents a time of controlled imbalance leading to a new homeostasis.

Once the adult balance is reached, different questions arise, particularly with regard to the way in which vessels adapt to cyclic variation. The heart beat at rest and then the effect of exercise represent an adaptation calling for growth and structural remodeling. Exercise can be considered normal if not necessarily usual. How transduction from work to hypertrophy is carried out is not clear, but the identification of increased metabolism in a fibroblast through change in its ambient electrical field within the normal physiological range provides a clue (McLeod et al., 1987). Injury represents a higher level of activity, where growth factors abound, but inhibitory factors are also critical.

The following sections present something of what is known of the agents that stimulate, and of the fewer that inhibit, the four types of vascular cells. Only a few of these studies have been made on lung cells and/or the exception, the fibroblast, it is the interstitial, not the vascular or adventitial cell that is described. The vascular smooth muscle cell is a candidate for the "most studied." In changes of PH, it is the precursor smooth muscle cell, the pericyte that is more critical than the muscle cell. Since it seems that these cells behave differently in vivo than in vitro, transfer of findings for one to the other must be made with due reserve. The products of inflammatory cells are mentioned, but are not central in the discussion. In various types of PH and at various stages, mediators of injury and factors stimulating and inhibiting growth hypertrophy, mitosis, and differentiation of vascular cells all need to be invoked.

B. Competence and Progression Factors

On the basis of their effect on a mouse fibroblast line (3T3), mitogens have been classified as one of two types – competence or progression. For a quiescent cell of this line, both types of factor must bind to the cell to ensure that it starts to synthesize DNA, it enters the S phase of the cell cycle. The appropriate factor elicits competence by binding to a cell for about 2 hr; this state lasts for a further 13 hr, a period when binding of one or more progression factors is necessary for DNA synthesis (Stiles et al., 1979). In the first experiments, platelet-derived growth factor (PDGF) was used and is still regarded as the classical competence factor; fibroblast growth factor (FGF) is another. Progression factors include epidermal growth factor (EGF), insulin, and somatomedin C (IGF–I) (Leof et al., 1982). While similar behavior is shown by other cells, it does not always strictly apply. Quiescent human fibroblasts pass into S phase in response to either PDGF or EGF (Westermark and Heldin, 1985), while response to PDGF by others include synthesizing their own progression factor (Clemmons and van Wyk, 1985). Since plasma includes progression factors and is included in most culture media, it is not always clear from the literature whether a given cell is capable of making progression factors.

Most work on vascular mitogens has concentrated on systemic cells, especially those involved in atheroma and tumor angiogenesis. While the results are relevant to hypertensive remodeling in the lung, differences in the primary location and morphologic details of change should make us wary of drawing too many parallels.

C. Factors Stimulating Vascular Cell Growth

Endothelial Cell

A large number of factors mitogenic for endothelial cells have been identified, mostly in reference to systemic endothelium. In an appropriate assay system, many of these factors are also angiogenic (D'Amore and Thompson, 1987; Folkman and Klagsburn, 1987). This chapter concentrates mainly on stimulation and inhibition of proliferation; angiogenesis is usually not a feature of pulmonary hypertension.

Systemic

A potentially important example of *autocrine* control of endothelial growth has recently been described for calf aortic and corneal endothelial cells (Vlodavsky et al., 1987a, b). In culture, these cells synthesize basic FGF, a potent, heparin-binding cationic endothelial mitogen. The FGF produced remains bound to the cell and to the subendothelial matrix, possibly to heparan sulfate proteoglycans, and is not found in the medium. Presumably, under normal conditions, it remains bound and inactive as long as the endothelium is confluent and not injured. With loss of confluence, however, the bound FGF could stimulate division of the remaining endothelial cells. This perhaps explains why, in vitro, a lower concentration of FGF is required to produce a given growth rate if endothelial cells are plated at subconfluent density on subendothelial matrix rather than on plastic (Gospodarowicz and Ill, 1980). The binding of FGF by heparin-like molecules in the matrix may be a property similar to that demonstrated for exogenous heparin, which binds both basic and acidic FGFs (Folkman and Klagsbrun, 1987), stabilizes these growth factors and, in the case of aFGF, increases its potency (Schreiber et al., 1985). Thus, when heparin-binding growth factors are also present, exogenous heparin stimulates endothelial proliferation (Thornton et al., 1983; Orlidge and D'Amore, 1986b) though, on capillary endothelial cells its stimulatory effect is not always apparent (Orlidge and D'Amore, 1986a).

Deendothelialization may not be necessary for cell- and matrix-bound FGF to play a role in autocrine growth stimulation. For example, endothelial cell injury could release plasminogen activator that has been shown to degrade the matrix (Bar-Ner et al., 1986) and may free the FGF-heparin-sulfate complex. The FGF itself is freed from the complex if activated platelets release their store of heparinase (Yahalom et al., 1984).

Paracrine stimulation of endothelial cells by resident cells of the vessel wall has not been demonstrated, but some studies suggest this is likely. EGF is a modest endothelial mitogen present in plasma, but until recently a likely local cellular source had not been identified. Human WS-1 fibroblasts have now been shown to produce EGF in culture (Kurobe et al., 1985). Fibroblasts and other cells of the vessel wall are certainly possible sources of this and other mitogens. Insulin-like growth factors I and II (IGF-I and II) are mitogenic for bovine retinal microvascular endothelium, but not for aortic endothelium (King et al., 1985). mRNA for both IGF-I and II is localized in fibroblasts in situ (Han et al., 1987). IGF-I has also been shown by biochemical techniques to be a product of smooth muscle cells (Clemmons, 1984).

Blood-borne mitogens include those normally present such as insulin, which is mitogenic for endothelium from calf retinal capillaries, but not aortic (King et al., 1983) and those resulting from an injury to the vessel wall that promotes thrombosis. Activated platelets release endothelial mitogens, including an EGF-like molecule (Oka and Orth, 1983), and several partially characterized molecules of 45 kD (Miyazono et al., 1987), and 65 and 135kD (King and Buchwald, 1984).

Mast cells also could play a mitogenic role in certain conditions. Rat mast cell granules stimulate proliferation of human newborn foreskin microvascular endothelial cells. The active molecule is histamine, working through the H1 receptor (Marks et al., 1986).

If the initial injury is necrotizing, inflammatory cells are attracted to the site. Of these, mononuclear cells are the major and long-term source of mitogens. They release macrophage derived growth factors (MDGFs). Although a proportion of these is made up of PDGF-like molecules (Shimakado et al., 1985) that fail to stimulate endothelial cells, a remainder has mitogenic activity for endothelium (Polverini and Leibovich, 1984). The extracellular matrix in culture is important in modulating response to growth factors. Laminin, a specific component of the basement membrane, enhances proliferation of microvascular endothelial cells in a full, serum-supplemented medium, whereas type IV collagen, another specific basement membrane component, has less mitogenic effect. When these two matrices are combined, simulating the basement membrane in vivo, proliferation is appreciably less than on laminin alone. During angiogenesis in vivo, laminin is the first to appear around the new capillary sprout. Type IV collagen appears later during morphologic differentiation, when the lumen is formed (Form et al., 1986). The fact that culture conditions critically affect results is demonstrated by the contrasting findings of a more recent study in which bovine adrenal microvascular endothelial cells incorporate less thymidine when grown on laminin than on any of the other matrices tested including type IV collagen (Ingber et al., 1987). In this experiment, cells were tested in a medium with no serum, but with known concentration of specific heparin-binding growth factor.

Over a 7-day period, calf adrenal capillary endothelial cells failed to grow in 40% oxygen; this is in contrast to the fourfold increase in numbers when the cells are cultured under ambient oxygen tension (D'Amore and Sweet, 1987).

Pulmonary

There is no evidence of an *autocrine* mitogenic effect by pulmonary endothelium. One of our experiments suggests that mitogen(s) can be bound by the endothelial matrix (Davies et al., 1987). We have grown rat lung peripheral endothelial cells to postconfluence, and obtained a cell-free substrate by treating a confluent monolayer with nonionic detergent or alkaline solution. When freshly trypsinized endothelial cells are plated onto this substrate in serum-supplemented medium, the substrate promotes their growth, suggesting that growth factor(s) is bound to it (Fig. 5).

In human fetal *pulmonary* tissue a recent in situ hybridization study has localized IGF-I (A and B) and II in fibroblasts of the interlobular septa and within the adventitia of pulmonary vessels (Han et al., 1987). Although insulin binds to main pulmonary artery endothelium more than to vein (Bar et al., 1980), the effects of the IGFs on pulmonary endothelium is unknown.

Smooth Muscle Cells

Systemic

One of the most potent mitogens for smooth muscle cells is platelet-derived growth factor (PDGF). Its discovery was immediately relevant to atheroma because of the involvement of platelets in that lesion. PDGF-like molecules (PDGFc) are now known to be produced by other resident cells of the vessel wall: the endothelial and smooth muscle cells, but not the fibroblast.

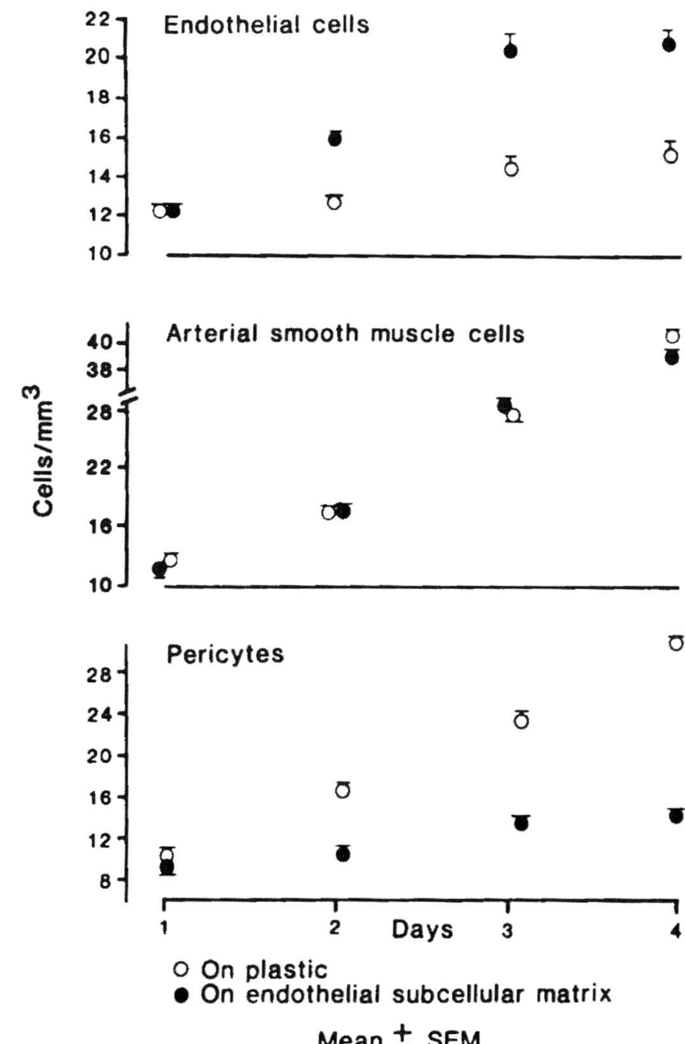

Figure 5 The effect of substrate from rat lung microvascular endothelial cells on culture of pulmonary vascular cells. The endothelial cells were grown to post-confluence and treated with 0.5% aqueous Triton-X. Filled circles indicate cells plated on substrate; open circles are cells placed on plastic. Each point is mean ± SEM. (From Davies et al., 1987c, with permission).

Autocrine stimulation by PDGFc has not been demonstrated directly, but PDGFc is produced in culture by smooth muscle cells obtained from the developing aorta of normal postnatal (13-18 day) rats. Cells from adult (3 month) rats do not secrete the molecule (Seifert et al., 1984).

Paracrine interaction involving PDGF could occur within the vessel wall. Endothelial cells organized into capillary-like tubes in culture do not express c-sis, the protooncogene encoding PDGF B-chain, but actively growing cells do. Confluent endothelial cell monolayers constitutively produce and release molecules homologous with the A (Collins et al., 1987) and B (Collins et al., 1985; Barrett et al., 1985) chains of PDGF, but at low levels. PDGFc release is increased if (1) the cells are injured by endotoxin or phorbol esters (Fox and DiCorleto, 1984); (2) the cells contact activated coagulation Factor X (Gadjusek et al., 1986); or (3) the cells bind α-thrombin (Harlan et al., 1986). Release of PDGFc does not occur when the cells are simply lysed, yet does not require active protein synthesis. It is suggested that a precursor form of the molecule is present within the cell and is activated by the serine protease of thrombin (Harlan et al., 1986). Unlike bFGF, the released PDGFc is not bound by the cell or its matrix (Vlodavsky et al., 1987).

Other molecules that are mitogenic for vascular smooth muscle cells and that could originate in adjacent cells are FGF and EGF (Gospodarowicz et al., 1986). IGF-1 is 10 to 100 times more potent a mitogen for calf aortic smooth muscle cells than IGF-II or insulin (King et al., 1985).

Serotonin is a mitogen (Nemecek et al., 1986) that could be blood borne or released from mast cells – common cells in the vessel wall – or from platelets following activation.

An important consequence of established hypertension is an increase in the transmural pressure load on the wall of vessels proximal to the sites of increased resistance. This pressure load increases stretch in both the longitudinal and circumferential axes. Its cellular effects have been investigated using rat aortic smooth muscle cells growing on an elastic membrane that is subjected to uniaxial stretch (10% increase in length) at a frequency of 52 times/min. After 8 hr, incorporation of thymidine and total DNA are unaffected, but incorporation of proline, presumably into matrix proteins, is increased (Leung et al., 1976, 1977).

Pulmonary artery smooth muscle cells from the near-term fetal calf fail to proliferate in serum deprived of PDGF (Benitz et al., 1986a, b), so presumably, they are not capable of producing their own. In this respect they differ from aortic smooth muscle cells from the young postnatal rat (Siefert et al, 1984). Exposure of the fetal calf pulmonary cells to low oxygen tensions (below 50 mmHg) in a serum-supplemented medium reduces their proliferative rate, but the effect is not selective for pulmonary cells: the growth of cells from the calf aorta is also reduced by this level of hypoxia (Benitz et al., 1986a, b). A paracrine effect by the endothelial cell, specific for pulmonary smooth muscle cells may override this hypoxic growth suppression. Calf pulmonary artery endothelial cells, exposed in culture to *anoxia* for periods up to 24 hr, release a mitogen for pulmonary artery smooth muscle cells (Vender et al., 1987). Unlike PDGFc, a cationic molecule with competence activity only, it is anionic and has both competence and progression activity.

Pericyte

Systemic

Systemic pericytes share some of the characteristics of smooth muscle cells, including expression of α-isoactin (Herman and D'Amore, 1985), smooth muscle myosin (Joyce et al., 1984), and cGMP-dependent protein kinase (Joyce et al., 1985), but because they have not been as intensively investigated, we know much less about them. We do not know, for example, if pericytes release PDGFc normally or after injury. Serum mitogens enhance their growth in culture.

Calf retinal pericytes proliferate in response to IGF-I and II as well as to insulin, but IGF-I has the greatest mitogenic effect (King et al., 1985).

Calf retinal pericytes exposed to 40% oxygen in culture exhibit the same growth rate as cells under ambient oxygen tension (D'Amore & Sweet, 1987). In this respect they differ from the endothelial cells obtained from the same site which fail to grow in high oxygen.

Pulmonary

Rat lung pericytes have a similar morphology in culture to pericytes from systemic sites. At low density, they spread widely on the substratum, are not contact inhibited, and, indeed, readily form multilayered nodules. They are positive for smooth muscle and nonmuscle myosin (Davies et al., 1987c). In serum-supplemented medium they grow more slowly than smooth muscle cells from the rat main pulmonary artery, but, like them, also respond to PDGF (Davies, personal observation).

Fibroblast

Systemic

Autocrine stimulation of systemic fibroblast growth has not been demonstrated. These cells produce EGF and IGF-I and II, all progression factors, so that replication could be stimulated if a competence factor were available. Adjacent smooth muscle cells, in the developing vessel or when injured, are a *paracrine* source of PDGFc, the classical competence factor. Calf aortic endothelial cells release fibroblast mitogens that include PDGFc (DiCorleto, 1984). Endothelium also synthesizes bFGF, another competence factor, and interleukin-1 (IL-1) (Harlan, 1985), a potent mitogen of human neonatal fibroblasts (Libby et al.,

1985). IL-1 is also a product of mononuclear cells. Its mitogenic effect is selective for fibroblasts, but *not* for smooth muscle cells (Libby et al., 1985). In this respect it differs from PDGF, which acts on both. Tumor necrosis factor (TNF), derived from mononuclear cells activated by inflammatory stimuli, is another fibroblast mitogen, but the concentrations required to produce an effect are higher than with IL-1 (Le and Vilcek, 1987). It acts synergistically with insulin and increases the expression of EGF receptors by fibroblasts (Palombella et al., 1987). TNF induces the production of IL-1 in fibroblasts themselves (Le et al., 1987), in mononuclear cells (Dinarello et al., 1986), and stimulates endothelial cells to release IL-1 (Nawroth et al., 1986).

Pulmonary

In the lung, the interstitial fibroblast has been much studied due to its importance in interstitial fibrosis (Goldstein and Fine, 1986). Much less is known of the adventitial fibroblast, the one most pertinent to the remodeling of pulmonary hypertension. Because their response to a given injury differs, these two cells are likely to exhibit behavioral differences. In hypoxia and persistent pulmonary hypertension of the newborn (PPHN), it is the adventitial cell that increases, whereas, in diffuse fibrosis, it is the interstitial fibroblast that proliferates selectively.

Evidence of *autocrine* secretion by pulmonary interstitial fibroblasts has been found. Fibroblasts obtained in culture from full-term (180 days) baboons release into the medium one or more factors mitogenic for fibroblasts from the lungs of normal, 1-year old baboons (Jones et al., 1987). The fact that the stimulation is only seen when there is serum or PDGF present in the test medium indicates that the factor(s) has progression activity. It is produced whether the donor lungs are ventilated or not. Fibroblasts from baboons delivered prematurely at 140 days do not release mitogens, even after ventilating the animals under normal conditions, but after ventilating the animals in 100% oxygen for 6 days, the fibroblasts obtained from the lungs do. Ventilation with 100% oxygen for 24 hr is insufficient to give this effect.

A similar result is obtained in lung fibroblasts from hamsters, but this time in the adult (Jones et al., 1987b). While cells from adult hamsters normally do not release an autocrine factor, cells from hamsters exposed to 100% oxygen for as little as 4 days release one or more factors that once again have progression activity.

Paracrine interactions involving the lung fibroblast are common. Alveolar, and presumably interstitial, macrophages synthesize IL-1, a potent mitogen, and TGF-β, a factor of considerable interest because it stimulates collagen production (Goldstein and Fine, 1986). Its role in proliferation is inconsistent. While it stimulates proliferation of a murine fibroblast line (Shipley et al., 1985), it does not stimulate human embryonic lung fibroblasts (Fine and Goldstein,

1987). Its promotion of collagen production, however, is consistent. Collagen deposition in the adventitia contributes appreciably to vessel restriction and is a particularly notable feature of several forms of pulmonary hypertension, especially PPHN.

D. Factors Inhibiting Vascular Cell Growth

The selectivity of the mitogenic response may be due to the presence of controlling, i.e., inhibitory mechanisms. These are also relevant in defining normal homeostasis and are considered in this section.

Endothelial Cells

Systemic

Endothelial cells from all sites are contact inhibited in culture, reflecting their normal state in situ. Although the control mechanisms have not been completely worked out, an inhibitory molecule is located within the membrane of confluent cells (Heimark and Schwartz, 1985; Teitel, 1986). Loss of confluence results in cell migration and proliferation.

A "*paracrine*" type of inhibitory control on systemic microvascular endothelial cells is exerted in culture by systemic pericytes. The inhibition requires contact between the two cell types (Orlidge and D'Amore, 1987b). Other inhibitors of endothelial growth include TGF-β. Paradoxically, this can exhibit angiogenic activity. Its contrasting effects are also shown on other cells and seem to depend on a variety of conditions. Its ability to promote nonanchorage-dependent proliferation of rat kidney fibroblasts, for example, depends on culture in soft agar and a synergistic action with either EGF or its close homologue TGF-a (Roberts et al., 1981). When the cells are grown in monolayer culture, it antagonizes the stimulatory effects of EGF (Roberts, 1985). TGF-β blocks FGF-stimulated endothelial proliferation (Hotta and Baird, 1986). When added to rat heart endothelial cells, it reduces the number of high-affinity EGF receptors, while EGF-induced expression of specific competence genes, c-myc, JE, KC, is decreased (Takehara et al., 1987). Its growth-suppressive effect in this study is irreversible, whereas in others it acts only temporarily. For example, when added to bovine aortic endothelial cells experimentally "wounded" by introducing a break in the cell monolayer, TGF-β inhibits repleciation and migration, but only for 24 hr (Heimark et al., 1986). TGF-β is a product of mononuclear cells.

Platelets have recently been found to release a factor that inhibits thymidine uptake by porcine aortic endothelial cells. The molecule is heat labile with a size of 35-40 kD (Brown and Clemmons, 1986).

In contrast to the stimulatory effect of some matrix components, those fragments of fibronectin that bind heparin are inhibitory for aortic endothelial cells (Homandberg et al., 1985). This mechanism may serve to confine endothelial growth to the intima, even when the basement membrane is damaged. This may partly explain the inhibitory effect on endothelial growth of tissue extracts.

Pulmonary

Pulmonary endothelial cells display the same kind of contact inhibition of growth as systemic, so that loss of confluence in vivo is likely to result in increased migration and growth. Deendothelialization, however, is a rare occurence in the lung and certainly not a necessary prerequisite for pulmonary hypertensive remodeling. Exposure, for example, to oxygen tensions that cause desquamation of the alveolar epithelium cause subendothelial edema, but little or no frank loss of the intimal lining (see Fig. 8).

No inhibitory mechanisms specific to pulmonary endothelium have been found so far.

Smooth Muscle Cells

Systemic

Autocrine reduction of bovine aortic smooth muscle growth is given by heparan sulfate molecules present on the cells and released into the culture medium. The molecule released by postconfluent cells has eight times the inhibitory potency as that produced by exponentially growing cells (Fritz et al., 1985).

A paracrine type of reduction of smooth muscle cell growth has been much investigated. Bovine aortic endothelial cells release into the medium a heparin-like molecule that reduces the proliferation of aortic smooth muscle cells (Castellot et al., 1981). The effect is most pronounced when the endothelium is confluent and the smooth muscle cells are growth arrested, and can be increased if the endothelial cells have been or the smooth muscle cells are grown on a preparation of subendothelial matrix (Herman and Castellot, 1987).

Exogenous heparin reduces the growth of systemic smooth muscle cell cultures. The anticoagulant properties of heparin are not important for this effect, which is given by fragments as small as pentasaccharides. The 3-*O*-sulfate on the repeated glucosamine residues appears critical to the inhibition (Castellot et al., 1986). Although heparin is endocytosed by the smooth muscle cell by a receptor-mediated mechanism (Castellot et al., 1985), it is not known if this is important to its suppression of growth. Addition of EGF prevents the heparin effect (Reilly et al., 1987), but PDGF, even at concentrations 200 times greater than controls, does not (Reilly et al., 1987). Heparin stimulates the synthesis of a 38 kD protein (Majack and Bornstein, 1985).

TGF-β inhibits serum- or PDGF-mediated proliferation of rat aortic smooth muscle cells plated at subconfluent density (Majack, 1987). On the other hand, at a density high enough to provide maximum cell-cell contact, TGF-β stimulates both proliferation and change in cell morphology such that the cells form multilayered nodules. As with heparin, the inhibition of smooth muscle proliferation caused by TGF-β is accompanied by the synthesis by the muscle cells of a 38 kD protein.

Pulmonary endothelial cells from the main artery of the late gestation calf shows a paracrine effect on smooth muscle cells. They release into the culture medium a factor that is inhibitory for smooth muscle cells from the same site (Benitz, personal communication). The inhibitory molecule resembles heparin and is not produced if the endothelial cells are exposed in culture to hypoxia. This effect differs from that demonstrated by Vender et al. (1987) in which medium conditioned by pulmonary endothelial cells (again from the calf, but postnatal) has a slight mitogenic effect on smooth muscle under ambient culture conditions; this is amplified by exposure of the endothelial cells to anoxia. The difference could be due to the pre- and postnatal ages of the donor animals or to the different effects of hypoxia and anoxia.

Pulmonary

Exogenous heparin reduces the exponential growth of rat pulmonary artery smooth muscle cells in 10% serum-supplemented medium (Davies et al., 1987a) and, at a similar concentration of heparin, of near-term calf-pulmonary artery smooth muscle cells (Benitz et al., 1986b). Dextran sulfate has a similar effect, but dermatan-, chondroitin-4-, and chondroitin-6-sulfates have no effect on proliferation (Benitz et al., 1986a).

Pericytes

Systemic

Heparin (obtained from Hepar) reduces the growth of retinal pericytes, as determined by a maximal reduction of 50% in cell number at the end of a period in which untreated cells underwent three population doublings (Orlidge and D'Amore, 1986a). Chondroitin- and dermatan-sulfate did not have this effect.

Pulmonary

Heparin (also from Hepar, and at the same concentration of 100 μg/ml) reduces the number of rat lung pericytes as early as 3 days after its addition, and the reduction is still apparent after 6 days, but at this stage the doubling time of the cells is unaffected. In contrast, the effect on the number of smooth muscle cells plated at the same density is first seen 7 days after adding heparin and is accompanied by a slower doubling time (Davies et al., 1987a).

Pulmonary endothelial cells inhibit pericyte growth by a contact-dependent effect. A substrate prepared by removing confluent microvascular endothelial cells with either nonionic detergent or alkaline solutions is inhibitory to the growth of lung pericytes plated at low density. Smooth muscle cells from the main pulmonary artery are unaffected, while endothelial cell proliferation is stimulated (Davies et al., 1987a).

Fibroblasts

Systemic

Heparin suppresses the growth of chicken fibroblasts (Balks et al., 1985). Heparan sulfate-containing glycosaminoglycans are produced by vascular smooth muscle cells, and although their primary effect may be autoinhibition, they are also likely to affect the adjacent fibroblasts within the adventitia. As with smooth muscle cells, heparin suppression of fibroblast growth can be reversed specifically by EGF (Balks et al., 1985).

Pulmonary

In considering the factors likely to be inhibitory for the adventitial fibroblast, one is again forced to examine the information on the interstitial fibroblast, recognizing that this is not necessarily a relevant cell type.

Proliferation of the interstitial fibroblast is inhibited by prostaglandins (Goldstein and Polgar, 1982). These could be produced by the fibroblast itself, but in interstitial fibrosis are also a product of infiltrating mononuclear cells (Elias et al., 1985).

That a typical hormone, insulin, and similar molecules, insulin-like growth factors I and II (IGF-I and IGF-II), are included with growth factors illustrates the overlap between the recently discovered factors and hormones as conventionally accepted. The chemical mediator or factor circulating in tissue fluid, whether delivered via the blood or from local cells, modifies cell behavior in a way analogous to a hormone: extending the name to the autocrine/paracrine/endocrine system, it reflects widespread chemical control that serves homeostasis of the organism while allowing for local variation, demand and injury

Increase in the production of a factor is perhaps detected as raised blood or tissue level, but local events determine what the effect will be. Local concentration is one aspect, but availability of the factor and its correct molecular configuration activation are more important for binding to the target cell. It is at this stage that membrane receptors, their number and affinity, are critical. The metabolic state of the cell determines whether a signal is received and transduced. Receptor expression and signal transduction are in turn affected by additional considerations such as cell attachment to particular matrices, and exposure to other growth factors or agents that alter cell metabolism. Each of these can potentiate or antagonize the original response.

Although the signals for vascular cells are likely to be highly conserved, the conditions prevailing in the pulmonary circulation are sufficiently different from the systemic to alter cellular response.

V. Varieties of Pulmonary Hypertension

The story of mediators and growth factors unfolded in the last section has something of the quality of a fairy tale, at least when related to pulmonary hyper-

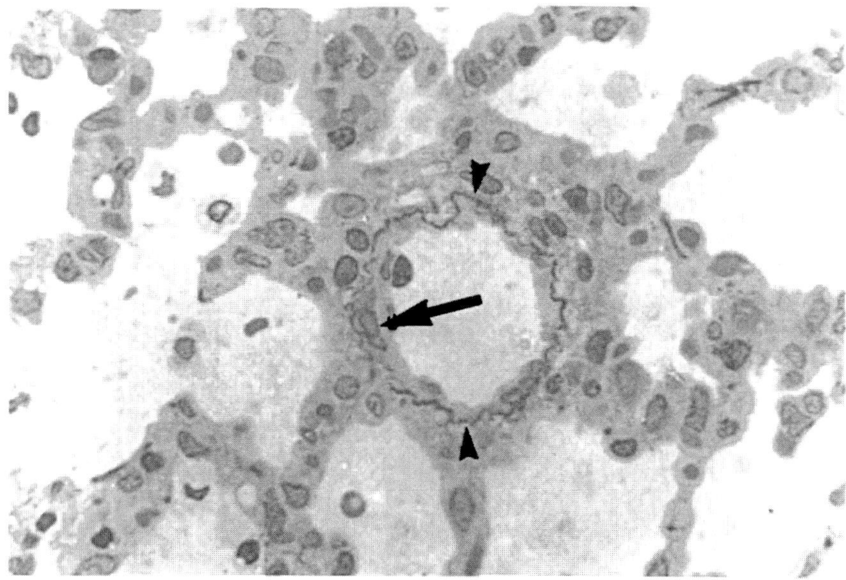

Figure 6 (a) Light micrograph of a nonmuscular artery at alveolar duct level from a rat chronically exposed to hypoxia. The artery shows the earliest stage of structural remodeling with a hypertrophied precursor cell (arrow) apparent between the endothelium and single elastic lamina (arrowheads). 1000X.

tension. Are these actors really the fairies that do the good and bad things in the lung? That is what we must explain. First for several types of PH we will describe some of the key biological facts established. We will then try to transfer the events in the in vitro story of growth and inhibition to explain the findings in PH. This will be highly speculative perhaps even a little fantastic as befits a good fairy tale.

The PH caused by hypoxia, the alkaloid monocrotaline, or hyperoxia are first described and compared. For these three types in addition to morphometric analysis of arterial remodeling in experimental studies, activity of arterial cells has been quantified: for the hyperoxia we are able to draw on limited preliminary data. Each of these types is represented in clinical PH. Monocrotaline is an endothelial toxin, and like hyperoxia, is associated with necrotic injury and major obliterative lesions that cause PH and lead to further adaptation by the residual patent bed. Hypoxia represents a metabolic injury without necrosis that causes PH by structural remodeling, polycythemia, and usually a degree of vasoconstriction (not seen in the other two). Their story is a parable that makes clear the variety of injury and response seen in the pulmonary hypertensions.

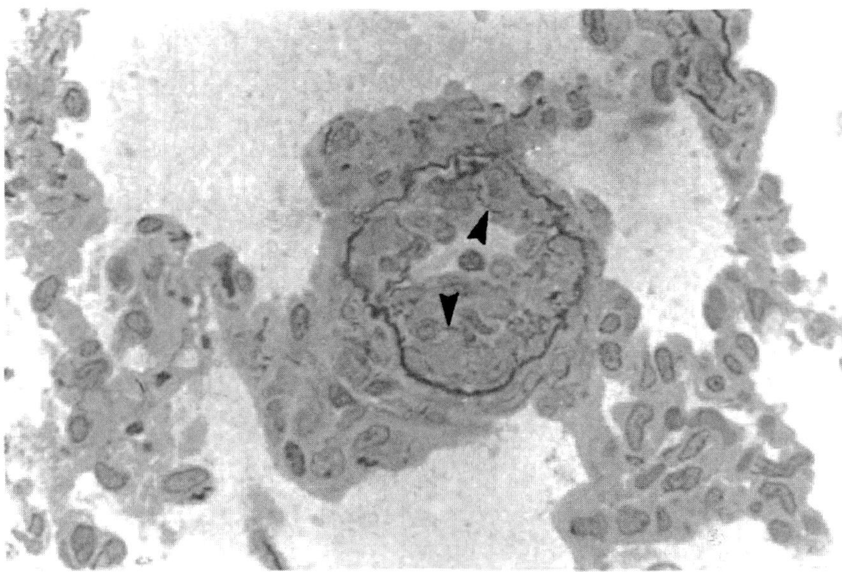

(b) Light micrograph of an artery at alveolar duct level from a rat exposed to hypoxia for 14 days. The precursur cells have proliferated to form a new medial layer. They have also laid down a network of additional elastic fibers (arrowheads). Both micrographs 1000X. (From Davies et al., 1985 with permission.)

A. Hypoxia

The response of the pulmonary vascular bed to hypoxia is associated with restriction of cross-sectional area at all arterial levels from the hilum to the periphery. Proliferation of some cells is a striking feature (Hislop and Reid, 1976). Hypoxia is marked by hypertrophy and hyperplasia – the cells respond in a positive way and yet such a response is injury – it is a significant shift from normal balance (Fig. 6a, b). A striking feature is the rapidity with which adaptation to hypoxia changes vascular structure (Meyrick and Reid, 1978, 1979a, b, c). It is tempting but probably quite erroneous to invoke return to the fetal pattern. All systems were first conditioned, in utero, to hypoxia and so within each cell is the biological memory of its function under relatively hypoxemic conditions. Does hypoxia turn this on or does postnatal adaptation represent a diferent metabolic pattern from the fetal?

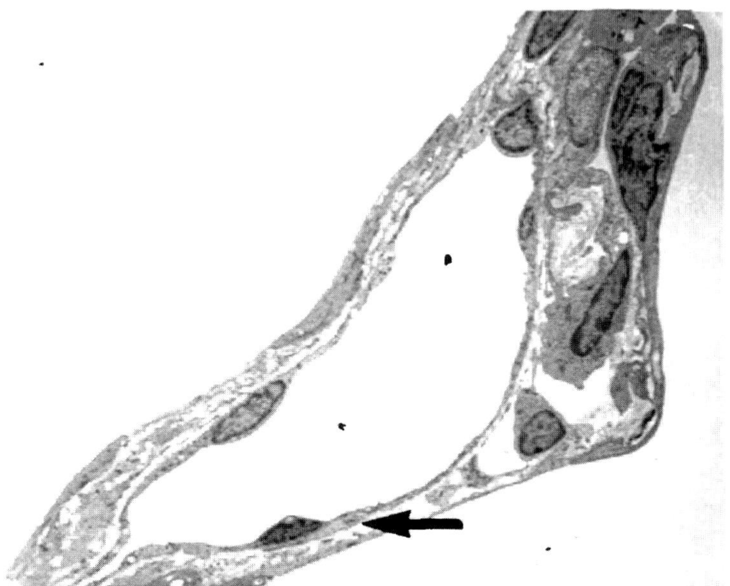

Figure 7 **(a)** Electron micrograph of a nonmuscular artery within the alveolar wall from normal rat. Its wall consists of one layer of endothelial cells; a single pericyte is present (arrow) beneath the endothelium. 2600X. (From Davies et al., 1986, with permission).

Responses to Acute Hypoxia

Acute challenge with hypoxia provides a vasoconstriction that reverses rapidly on return to air. It persists if the animal continues exposure to hypoxia but still reverses rapidly on return to air (Freid and Reid, personal communication).

With continuing hypoxia/hypoxemia, there is a steady rise in pulmonary artery pressure, we commonly use 10 days or more to establish changes (Rabinovitch et al., 1979). This hypertension persists even when the animal is returned to air and the residual pressure is greater than the original vasoconstrictor response. Most, but not all, animals respond to acute hypoxia with acute vasoconstriction. As exposure continues, this increase in absolute terms is greater than the original response, but as a percent rise on baseline it is similar.

We have learned recently that there are still animals that do not respond to acute hypoxia even when structural remodeling has occurred (Hu et al., 1987). There are "nonresponders" among people and among most experimental animals. No dilator has been shown to prevent the PH of chronic hypoxia although the right ventricular hypertrophy (RVH) (taken as a sign of rise in resistance)

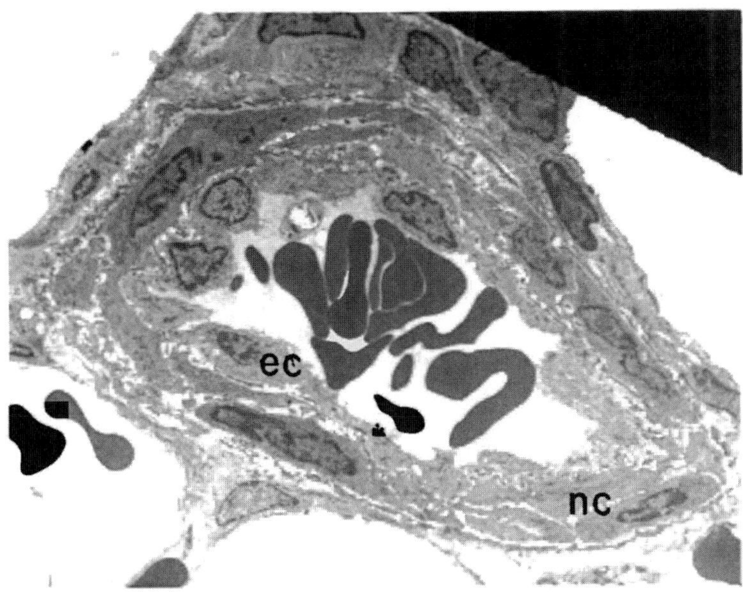

(b) Electron micrograph of an artery at distal alveolar duct level from a rat exposed to hypoxia for 14 days. The artery wall is thick, consisting of proliferated new muscle cells (NC) that are now morphologically similar to smooth muscle cells. The endothelial cells (EC) are hypertrophied. 2800X.

may be reduced. The steady rise in pressure based on structural remodeling is independent of the acute constrictor response.

The acute constrictor response is given by the normal and remodeled vascular bed. In the restructured bed it shows a different sensitivity to antagonists that point to a difference in mediator or receptor responsible for the hypoxic constrictor response or in the metabolism of the muscle cell (McMurtry et al., 1976). In the normal bed and intact rat, nifedipine blunts the acute hypoxic pressor response (Geggel and Reid, personal communication). It does not modify the response by the chronically remodeled bed.

Response to Chronic Hypoxia

The chronic PH of hypoxia is based on three features: acute vasoconstriction, polycythemia (Fried et al., 1983), and structural remodeling. Structural changes reflecting changed cell activity are apparent in large and small arteries within hours of starting hypoxic exposure (the veins seem relatively spared) (Fig. 7a, b). The following account is based on exposure of rats to hypoxia during 10-14 days (Meyrick and Reid, 1979a-c, 1980a, b; Rabinovitch et al., 1979).

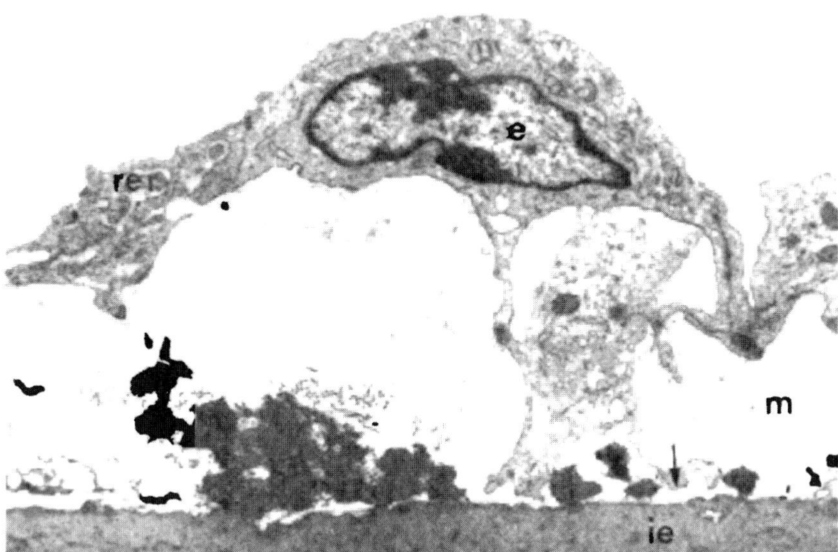

Figure 8 Electron micrograph of the wall of the hilar pulmonary artery from a rat after 3 days in normoxia following 10 days exposure to hypoxia. Extensive edema is present in the subendothelial space without loss of endothelium. Elastin is deposited as an extra layer on the luminal surface of the internal lamina (ie). 9000X. (From Meyrick and Reid, 1980b, with permission).

Large Preacinar and Pulmonary Artery

In the large pulmonary artery the media and adventitia both increase in tissue mass and thickness: and there is a reduction in external diameter of the artery (measured from external elastic lamina to external elastic lamina). The adventitia doubles in thickness during the first 3 days. After one week it is more than three times thicker than normal. The media lags behind a little. This increase in adventitial mass virtually leads the pulmonary circulatory response. The endothelial cells hypertrophy, and their basal surface becomes separated from the elastic almina by edema: at its edge it stays tethered to the lamina. The pocket of tissue fluid seems designed to concentrate locally bioactive factors. Figure 8, taken 3 days after return to the air, illustrates this as well as the rapid production of elastin that the endothelial cell has produced during recovery.

After 24 hr of hypoxia, the labeling index of the adventitial fibroblast shows a sixfold increase, rising further by day 3 to an eightfold increase (Fig. 9). By the end of a week it is three times the normal level and flattens here for the next few days (14 days is the maximum time studied). Because the pressure does

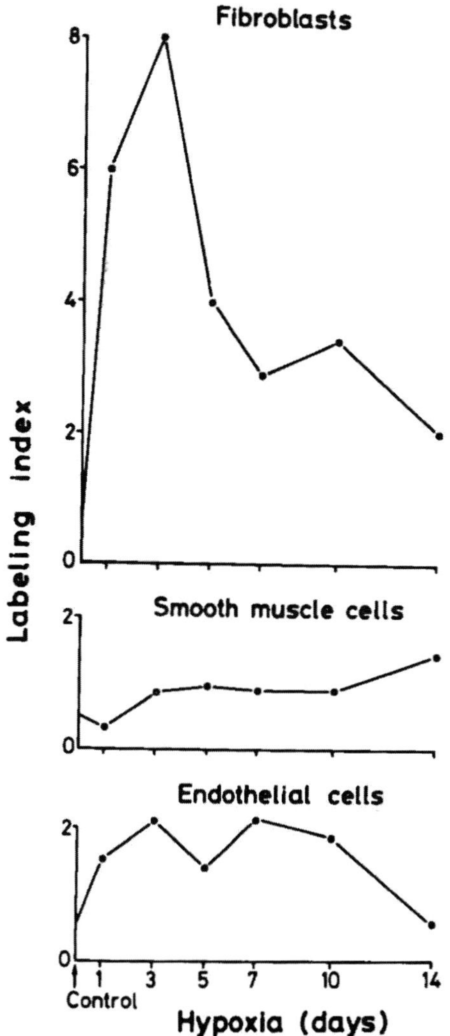

Figure 9 Labeling index of adventitial fibroblasts, medial smooth muscle cells, and endothelial cells of the hilar muscular artery of the rat exposed to hypoxia for up to 14 days. (From Meyrick and Reid, 1979b, with permission).

rise immediately on hypoxic exposure, it could be considered that this increase is pressure driven, which we have previously suggested. The small rise in pressure due to constriction, in the early days, however, seems too small to explain the striking fibroblast activity and the early effect seems more likely to be a meta bolic effect of hypoxia.

Endothelial cell show a slight but sustained increase, somewhat less than a doubling of mitotic activity virtually throughout this period. Pressure, per se, has given a small increase to these cells. The muscle of the media shows only a slight but sustained increase.

The medial thickening owes a lot to increase in extracellular matrix. The organelles that show the greatest relative increase in the smooth muscle cells are those that synthesize protein, not the contractile elements such as myofilaments (see Sec. IIA for consideration of the synthetic and contractile phases of vascular smooth muscle).

Intraacinar Arteries

In the normal rat, the intraacinar arteries are mainly nonmuscular or partially muscular: these with small resistance muscular arteries are the vessels that in the microcirculation show hypertrophy and hyperplasia of their constituent cells. This produces the structural remodeling responsible for the development of PH.

In the partially and nonmuscular arteries, the pericyte and intermediate cell population rapidly hypertrophy, and by light microscopy, are obvious by day 3. By day 5 nearly 20% of these cells are labeled (Fig. 10). This falls off, but at day 14 still about 8% take up thymidine. This cell population shows an early burst of mitosis.

Although the endothelial cell is closely associated with the pericyte and intermediate cell – they are situated within a single elastic lamina and in the case of the pericyte even the same basement membrane – the endothelial cell does not show a peak of mitosis until day 7, which is short-lived and affects only 8% of the population.

What is clear is that the pericyte multiplies, differentiates, produces a basement membrane and an elastic lamina that separates it from the endothelial cell: it continues to hypertrophy and differentiate to a smooth muscle cell Fig. 11a, b).

In the small resistance arteries of the periphery, that is those with a complete medial coat, between two elastic laminae, the smooth muscle cells showed a modest increase in labeling. Here again it was the fibroblast that most increased its labeling, but much less than at the hilum, to twice that seen under baseline conditions.

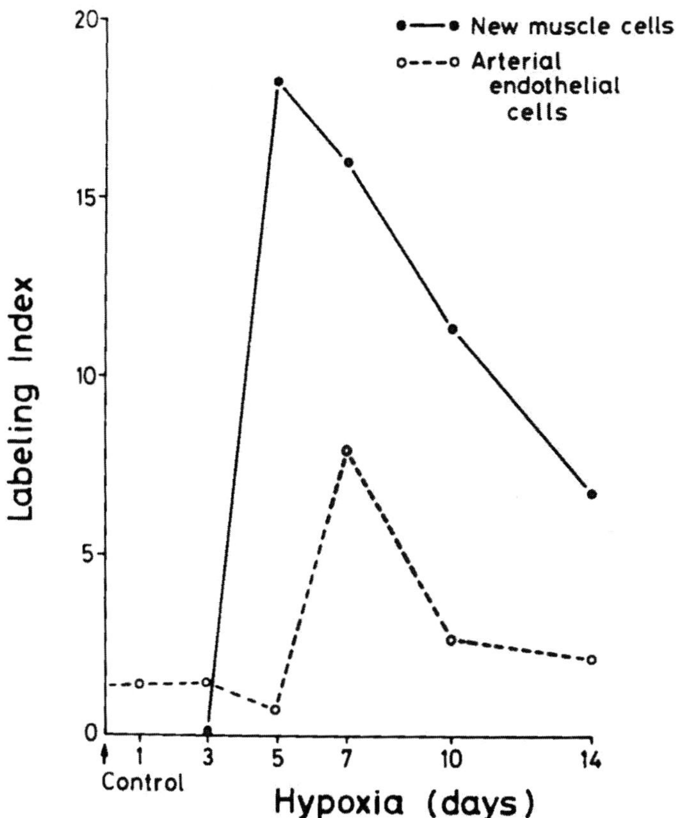

Figure 10 Labeling index of intraacinar new muscle cells (solid circles) and arterial endothelial cells (open circles) in the rat exposed to hypoxia for up to 14 days. (From Meyrick and Reid, 1979b, with permission).

What is the effect on the capillary and blood gas barrier? During the first week, interstitial cells of the alveolar wall and capillary endothelial cells show a modest increase in labeling to about 3% maximum at any time. The epithelial cells show a burst at about day 7. An increase in nuclear number of the alveolar wall is apparent during the first week. It does not seem to be associated with cell death.

At day 1 the alveolar wall is like the control. At day 3 the interstitial cells show about a fourfold increase in labeling: endothelial cells also show an increase, but a smaller one. Some intracapillary monocytes are labeled. Their density decreases during exposure.

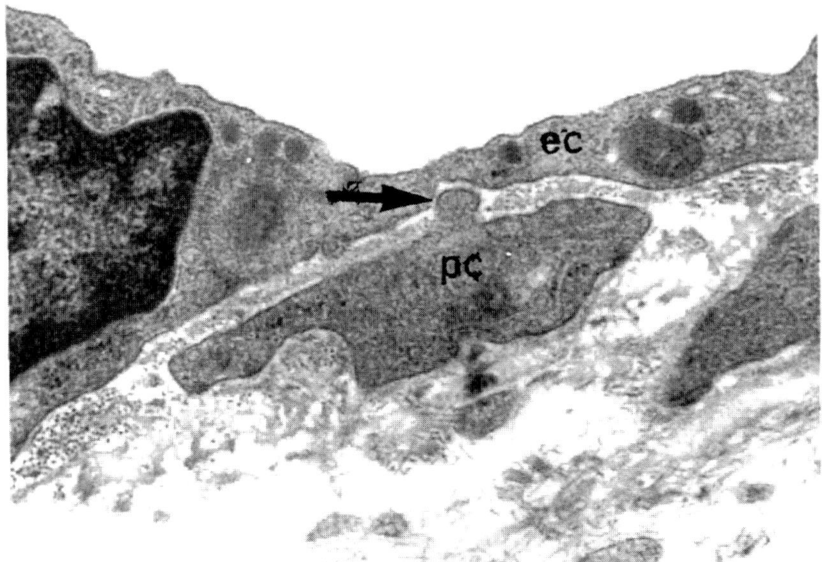

Figure 11 (a) Electron micrograph of the wall of a nonmuscular artery at alveolar wall level, from a normal rat. Beneath the endothelium (ec) is a solitary pericyte (pc). The endothelial basement membrane is interrupted by a process of the pericyte that forms a "peg-and-socket" junction (arrow) with the endothelial cell. 46,000X. (From Davies et al., 1986, with permission).

The large pulmonary arteries are likely to adapt to the pressure rise as hypoxia continues. In a series of experiments we reduced flow to the left lung of the rat by banding the left pulmonary artery (Rabinovitch et al., 1983). This made it possible to separate the effect of hypoxia from the changes due to pressure. In the left lung the muscle extension and muscle hypertrophy were less than in the right but the density of filled arteries was not affected. This points to endothelial swelling as a critical response to hypoxia, the other changes may reflect increased flow and pressure.

Administration of heparin to rats during chronic hypoxic exposure does not reduce the level of P_{pa} but shows a trend to reduce RVH (Hu et al., 1987). Structural remodeling is reduced in two ways: at the periphery it is less, particularly at the alveolar duct level, where fewer arteries have become muscularized. At this level the pericyte is the major precursor smooth muscle cell. Heparin, perhaps, is preventing mitosis of the cell at the stage it is still relatively isolated and solitary. In cell culture we have shown that heparin reduces the number of pericytes from the pulmonary bed when they are still at low density.

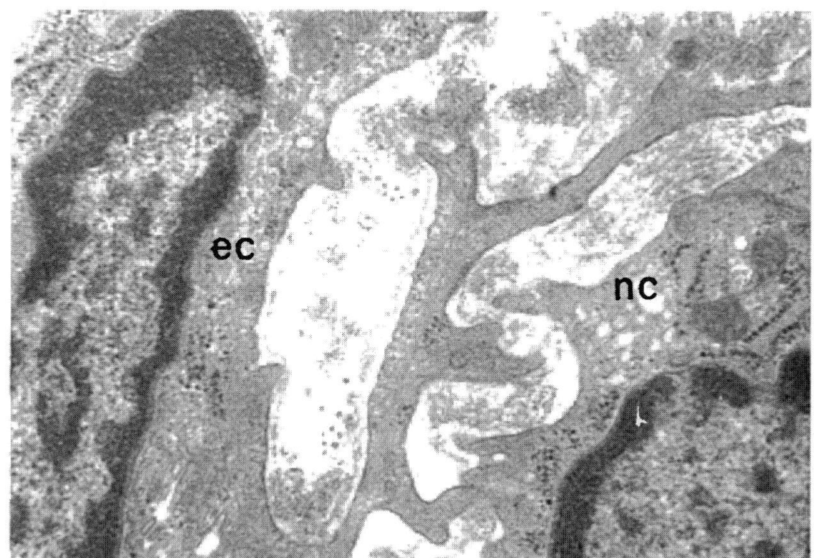

(b) Electron micrograph of the adluminal surface of a "new" muscle cell in a remodeled artery from a rat exposed to hypoxia for 14 days. Unlike the pericyte in the normal nonmuscular artery, the new cell (nc) forms an elaborate, branched process that contracts the endothelial cell (ec). 40,500X. (From Davies et. al., 1987b, with permission).

The second effect shown only at the higher dose was to reduce the narrowing caused in the large arteries by hypoxia. Since lessening of RVH also was only seen with the higher dose, this suggests that the reduced impedence by large arteries contributes. The reduction in peripheral restructuring was similar in both groups. It seems that this is not enough in itself to reduce P_{pa} or the work of the right ventricle. Heparin reduces the growth of chicken fibroblasts. Perhaps in the large arteries heparin reduced fibroblast multiplication: it does not seem to do so in the smaller ones.

Hypoxia itself seems to be the critical stimulus, since with return to air the arteries of the alveolar wall and duct mostly return rapidly, at least by light microsopy, to normal size (Fried and Reid, 1984). The newly muscularized arteries are reduced in number. The arteries with respiratory bronchioli do not seem to revert to normal as quickly; these represent hypertrophy and hyperplasia of the intermediate cell, a precursor smooth muscle cell that is, in its phenotype, closer to a smooth muscle.

Preliminary ultrastructural results show that for the "new" muscle cells the film does not rewind: The cells do not show simple regression but a series of abnormalities, including accumulation of glycogen (Davies, personal communication).

Factors and Mediators of Structural Remodeling in Hypoxic PH

There is no obvious candidate among the growth factors for the pattern of mitotic activity seen in hypoxia. Some cells show a short-lived burst, in others increased activity is maintained longer, while in yet others the effect is minimal but maintained. The absence of inflammatory cells emphasizes that the resident cells of the vascular wall are likely contributors. But other organs, other systems, react to hypoxia so that local factors will act in an environment containing increased levels of circulating hormones from sympathetic nerves and the suprarenal. The mast cell whose degranulation has been invoked as a contributor to hypoxic PH can release serotonin and histamine, shown under other circumstances to promote the replication of smooth muscle and endothelial cells, respectively. The heparin released would also be expected to potentiate endothelial growth, but would reduce smooth muscle proliferation. It is now known that hypoxic (anoxic) endothelial cells from large pulmonary arteries produce a factor that stimulates growth-arrested smooth muscle cells from the large pulmonary artery. Our own studies, however, show that smooth muscle cells from the chronically hypoxic rat grow more slowly than those from normoxic large arteries in the rat. If the growth factor has an effect, it is in somewhat elevated levels of the smooth muscle cell of the media, but at day 14 when pressure is well established the higher count is likely to be caused by pressure.

Hypoxic endothelial cells have been seen in culture to produce a mitogen for smooth muscle. It is of interest, but biologically does not seem to be the key response in PH. The real question is what is the cause of the fibroblast response. This seems to be the more important change.

The remodeled artery has a reduced lumen and external diameter. How has fibrosis produced contracture. In hypoxia constriction occurs in the large pulmonary arteries as well as the microcirculation. Or is it that contraction of fibrous tissue overcome the increased transmural pressure.

That the density of fibroblast in adventitia and smooth muscle in media decreases emphasizes the importance of the extracellular matrix in the media and collagen in adventitia.

The intriguing puzzle is the cause for the adventitial fibroblast's rapid and large response to hypoxia that is maintained over several days. This occurs before a significant pressure rise, suggesting increased transmural pressure is not the trigger. The modest rise seen early in the endothelial cells has also returned to baseline by the time that the pressure rise is well established.

Factors produced by the resident cells principally include PDGFc, known to stimulate fibrobasts and also smooth muscle cells. Hypoxia itself emerges as a candidate, possibly acting through cellular metabolic pathways to stimulate the mitotic response to mitogens that are at normal concentrations. The endothelial cells of the microcirculation produces a substrate that inhibits the pericyte. This is likely to be important in homeostasis.

The proliferation of the pericyte during hypoxia suggests that failure of this inhibiting control occurs. Does the hypoxic endothelial cell no longer produce the appropriate conditions? Or is the pericyte no longer susceptible?

The fact that this inhibitory mechanism is contact dependent, localized in the subendothelium, suggests that loss of contact is the first step. This could be an effect of hypoxia on one or both cell types. Loss of contact could also remove an inhibition, demonstrated in systemic cells, of endothelium by pericytes. Hypoxia-induced disruption of the subendothelial matrix could release matrix-bound bFGF, a possible mitogen for pericytes and a particularly likely one for the endothelial cells. The delay in the mitotic peak – day 5 for pericytes, day 7 for endothelial cells – is difficult to explain. Once again, hypoxia could be the culprit, reducing cell sensitivity to mitogens.

Within 3-4 days of release from the endothelial cell-derived pericyte inhibiting factor (EPIF), most of the pericyte population of the precapillary segment have hypertrophied: then the burst of mitotic activity is apparent. A simple explanation could be that this hypertrophy is premitotic. Hypertrophy per se will not do it as it is not seen in the hyperoxic injury. But it is likely that the metabolic high oxygen damage is very different from low oxygen damage.

The single burst of endothelial mitosis at day 7 also could be easily explained if the inhibition of the endothelium by pericyte is reasserted. An inhibitory effect of pericyte for endothelial cells has been described for systemic cells. If a similar action runs in pulmonary cells it is still strange that the effect is so late and short-lived. This could represent an effect of hypoxia peculiar to the endothelium or an autocrine or paracrine effect from another vascular cell is a possibility.

If hypoxia is sensed in the alveoli and peripheral small airways, the possibility cannot be excluded that a mediator produced here drains with the pulmonary veins and then through the bronchial artery supply to the vaso vasorum of the large pulmonary arteries, specifically stimulating the fibroblasts. Numerous agents stimulate interstitial fibroblasts; there is little reason to choose any of them for stimulation of the adventitial fibroblast.

B. Monocrotaline

Monocrotaline, the alkaloid obtained from the seeds of the ground plant *Crotalaria spectabilis*, is an endothelial cell toxin (Kay and Heath, 1969) that causes pulmonary hypertension associated with obliteration of many small pulmonary arteries (Hislop and Reid, 1974; Meyrick and Reid, 1979a). This obliterative vascular injury places it with hyperoxia and yet we will see there are striking differences between them in the pattern of cell proliferation caused by the original injury, that accompanies subsequent healing or the adaptation to established hypertension.

The monocrotaline injury causes increased endothelial permeability and reduced endothelial clearance of drugs. Platelets and fibrin thrombi form. In the lung's microcirculation, interaction of these humoral and formed cellular vascular constituents with the various cells of the vessel wall occurs. And yet vasoconstriction does not seem to be a part of this injury, although utlimately increased vasoreactivity is demonstrated. If oral administration is used, it is possible to study recovery in the animals.

Pulmonary hypertension ultimately develops – whether after a single injection or daily ingestion in food. In either case it takes about 4 weeks or longer for pulmonary hypertension to become established (Meyrick et al., 1980) (Fig. 12). By this time, in addition to cardiac right ventricular hypertrophy, and an increased medial thickness of elastic and muscular pulmonary arteries, the small precapillary arteries show structural remodeling. The number of small arteries that fill with a barium gelatin injectate is reduced: ghost arteries are seen that represent the stage of obliteration before disappearance. The patent and persisting precapillary arteries show, even by light microscopy, the presence of a coat of smooth muscle in arteries more distal and smaller than normal. RVH is detected and significant at day 21 and like the various vascular changes, continues to increase to day 35.

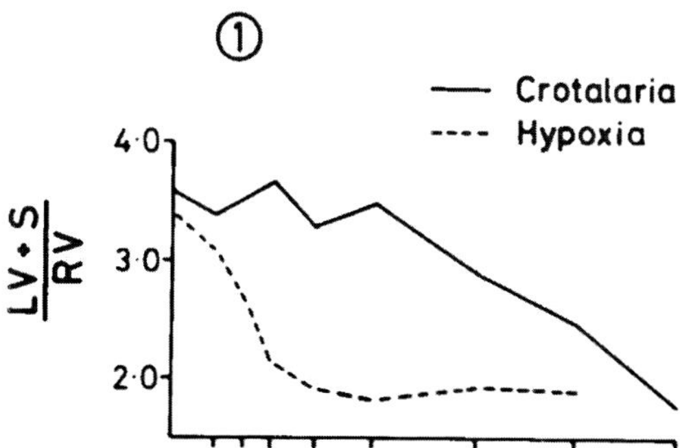

Figure 12 Right ventricular hypertrophy (RVH) follows the development of pulmonary hypertension. Both occur rapidly in hypoxia and much more slowly after monocrotaline, whether ingested or injected. (From Reid et al., 1986, with permission).

Hemodynamic Changes

Hypertension follows the structural changes in this model since neither the vasoconstriction nor polycythemia occur that are confounding and additional factors in hypoxia. By day 3 these new muscle cells are seen in some normally nonmuscular arteries. After monocrotaline, PH is first apparent at day 14 and is doubled by day 28 (Meyrick et al., 1980). Medial thickness of normally muscular arteries is apparent from day 7, reaches significance in small arteries from day 10 and in larger ones from day 14. The reduction in density of filled arteries is apparent by day 14 and is significant by day 21. By days 15 and 20 about a third of the peripheral arteries have been "lost" – that is, they no longer fill with the injectate: this reflects both obliteration and lumen narrowing. By day 30, more than half the arteries are missing. It is between day 15 and 30 that new peripheral muscle is particularly obvious – perhaps ths is better stated as muscle newly apparent. The hypertrophy of the precursor muscle cells could be part of the original injury, but it could reflect the relative increase in flow in the patent vascular bed.

If monocrotaline administration is used and appropriately controlled the rats survive and recovery occurs in that RVH returns to normal. The obliterated arteries do not become patent. The degree of arterial restructuring that persists is evidently not enough to raise baseline resistance, presumably vascular reserve is reduced.

Large and Preacinar Arteries

Proliferation of the pulmonary vascular and alveolar wall cells during these various phases has been followed by uptake of ^{3}H-thymidine (Meyrick and Reid, 1982). There is an increase in vascular wall mass in both hilar (intrapulmonary) and peripheral arteries. It will be seen that the final balance derives from cell hypertrophy, cell necrosis, and cell hyperplasia.

In the hilar arteries the medial thickness did not alter during the first two weeks; during the second two it rose steadily so that it was about three times normal by the end of 5 weeks. An increase in smooth muscle division was slight but significant at 3 days and then rose at 21 days (Fig. 13). (Pressure rise is apparent only after 14 days). This suggests that the early stimulus was from a mediator effect of injury and that the increased transmural pressure is likely to be the second. The fibroblasts of the adventitia show an early rise at day 7, when the endothelial cells do also. These lead the muscle and could also represent the effect of early injury.

The late burst at day 21 (not apparent at day 18) is present in all three cell types, whereas endothelial and muscle cells then fall, the adventitial fibroblast increases further to day 28. By day 35, levels are virtually back to baseline. In endothelial cells the effect is to give an increase in endothelial cell num-

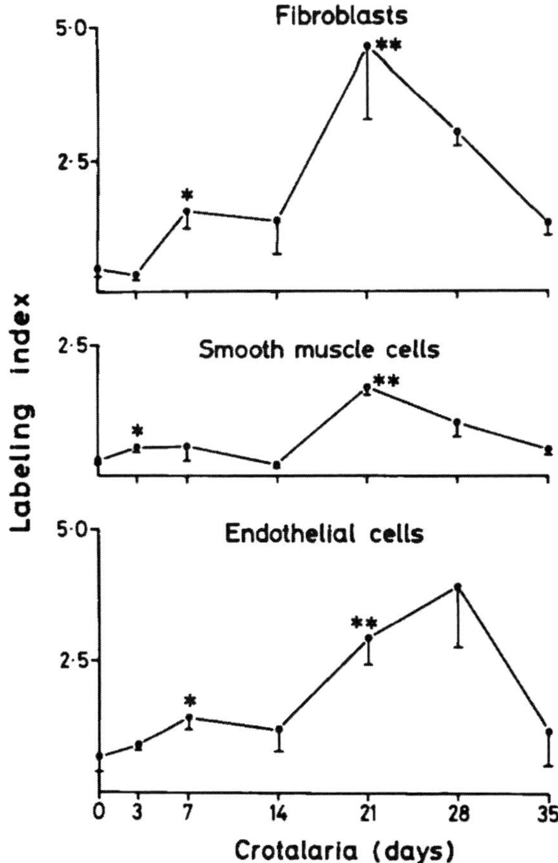

Figure 13 Labeling index of adventitial fibroblasts, medial smooth muscle cells, and endothelial cells of the hilar intrapulmonary artery from rats fed *Crotalaria*. The single asterisks indicate the first significant increase in ^{3}Hthymidine uptake, and the double asterisks the second. (From Meyrick and Reid, 1982, with permission).

ber and in relative density. The concentration of fibroblasts indicates that necrosis of these cells has occurred and that intercellular matrix increases. Smooth muscle cell concentration falls, virtually because of increase in matrix, at least early on.

At day 14, and not before, electron-dense smooth muscle and adventitial cells are seen: this either indicates delayed injury or is a secondary effect mediated by inflammatory cells and mediators. The toxic alkaloid appears to be eliminated from the system.

Intraacinar

Within the acinus the small arteries and veins show a different pattern of adaptation. Obstructive ghost arteries are seen. Density of filled arteries falls and then returns to the control values. It does not seem that obliterated arteries are restored. This suggests rather that the patent bed adapts to increased flow through it. Newly muscularized arteries are not apparent in this model of injury until day 14 (much later than the 3 days of hypoxia). Their number increases steadily until at day 35 they represent about 80% of small filled arteries.

Pressure again follows this remodeling, though whether it is the effect of injury or the result of increased velocity and flow through the residual bed is not clear (Meyrick et al., 1980). It is tempting to accept the latter as being the stimulus. At day 14 PH is present in the large arteries, medial hypertrophy occurs one week later.

Within the microcirculation days 7-21 show an increased level of endothelial multiplication, with a peak at day 14 (Meyrick and Reid, 1982) (Fig. 14). Is this the burst of mitosis to replace the injured cells? The venous endothelial cells show a slight increase at day 7 of the continued feeding. This is slight – less than the arterial – but more persistent. What is of interest is that the pericytes and new smooth muscle cells, so obvious a part of the wall, show no mitotic activity. Hypertrophy, not hyperplasia, is the basis for the newly muscularized arteries. In the alveolar region, in a given area of lung section, the alveolar epithelial cells show a similar density of labeled cells at the peak times to the adventitia: then return to baseline. Fibroblast mitosis is up at day 14 and then also at days 28 and 35. Monocytes show no increase at any time.

The labeling rate of the arterial endothelial cells is 40 times the normal value. In the few normally muscular arteries in the intraacinar region, no increase is seen in the adventitial fibroblasts. These are resistance arteries and do not constrict.

Edema is present at 14 days and more marked at 28. Platelet plugs are seen at 21 days.

The timing of changes within small vein endothelial cells is similar to that of some of the hilar arteries. Pulmonary venous blood circulates to the vaso vasorum of the hilar arteries; a similar agent that stimulates the arterial and venous endothelial of the microcirculation could be the stimulus to fibroblasts and smooth muscle of the hilum.

The late appearance of obviously injured and necrotic cells in the media and adventitia of the hilum suggests that mitogenic products could be released from these cells about day 14.

A striking feature of this model is the failure of any mitotic burst in the "precursor muscle cells" that hypertrophy in the microcirculation. Perhaps earlier the endothelial cell is well able to maintain the inhibitory effect on

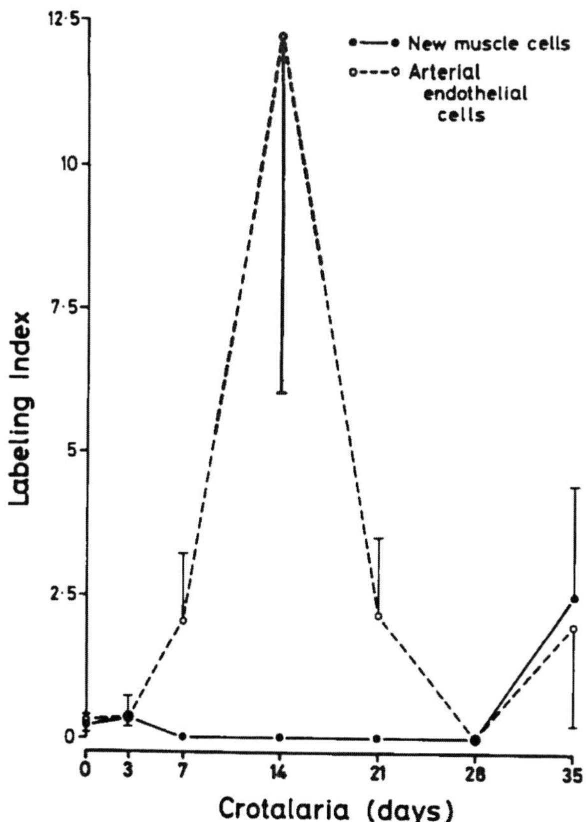

Figure 14 Labeling index of new muscle cells and arterial endothelial cells after feeding *Crotolaria spectabilis*. Endothelial cells are labeled after 3 days, maximally at 14 days; the labeling of new muscle cells is seen only at the end of the experiment. (From Meyrick and Reid, 1982, with permission).

the pericyte that we have postulated, or injury to the pericyte has modified the way the cells respond.

Response to the noxious agent seems to be determined by level of the vascular bed. In a simple way it seems that the endothelium throughout the lung would receive a dose of toxin. And yet the arrangement recently described of a crenated internal elastic lamina even when an artery is distended could well offer a degree of protection to surface endothelium at such a level (Davies et al., 1985).

The platelet and its products in some way contribute to the PH of monocrotaline since their depletion at 1 week after injury reduces (but does not inhibit) RVH (Hilliker et al., 1983). RVH reflects arterial obliteration or vascular remodeling, so it is likely that the final common pathway of this effect is the smooth muscle cell or endothelial cell obliteration. If PDGF is the cause, it seems this effect is not through the release of TXB_2. This statement is based on the study of the effect of dazmegrel a TXB_2 synthetase inhibitor (Langleben and Reid, 1985).

Since PH evolves slowly even after a single injection of Monocrotaline (Mct), it suggests that the Mct effect is modified partly through activation of some biological control system during the early hours of injury, but then becomes self-sustaining. Methylprednisolone given to cover the first 20 hr after injection somewhat reduces RVH and vessel loss. Its effect is even greater if it does not start until 24 hr after injection but then is given daily (Langleben and Reid, 1985) (Fig. 15).

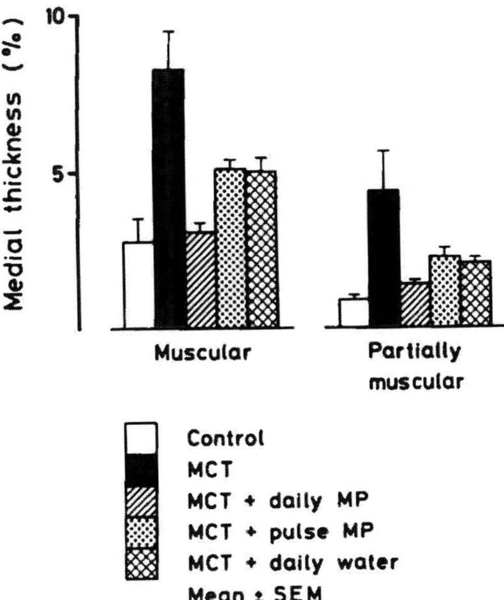

Figure 15 Effect of methylprednisolone (MP) injection on the increased medial thickness that results from a single injection of monocrotaline. A daily intraperitoneal (IP) injection of MP is most protective. A high-dose pulse of MP, given as two injections at the time of MCT, is protective, but less so. A daily IP injection of water for 21 days following MCT offers protection equal to pulse MP, possibly from release of autologous steroid hormone. (From Langleben and Reid, 1985, with permission).

Methylprednisolone reduced RVH and medial thickness, and the percentage of arteries developing completely or partially muscular walls. It is simplest to interpret this effect as being due to reduction of endothelial injury with less obliteration and less stimulus to structural remodeling, since rise in pulmonary vascular resistance is less. It could be that there is also a stabilizing effect on platelets so that if the remodeling is the result of a growth factor, not a flow effect, there would be an additive effect. Methylprednisolone does reduce edema so there is reason to think that this contributes to the PH. Whether it is the mediator release or cellular response after 24 hr that is significant we cannot say.

Monocrotaline is accepted as toxic to endothelial cells and yet at the hilum the peak in endothelial cell mitosis seen at 7 days is mild, no more than that caused by hypoxia. At the periphery, the Mct effect is similar to the hilum (but less here than after hypoxia). Monocrotaline does cause a second burst of mitotic activity between days 21 and 28 (hypoxia does not). In the first 2 weeks the fibroblast and smooth muscle cell show low activity. At day 21 all three show a higher level – a burst of activity through all the cells of the vessel wall. Only the endothelial cell rises higher by day 28. In the other two cells, mitosis falls. Since this rise corresponds with the pressure rise it is possible that this is the stimulus. Mediators of acute injury released by the agent could be responsible for the first activity.

At the periphery also, the difference from hypoxia is striking. After Mct virtually no mitotic activity is seen in the precursor smooth muscle cells. The endothelium, however, shows mitotic activity spread over at least 3 weeks with a peak at day 14. The enothelium of small veins shows a different response from the precapillary. The cells maintain a moderate level of increase through several weeks, with a small peak at day 7. Is damage to the veins less? Normally vein endothelium shows a higher fibrinolytic activity – it is less thrombogenic. This is not satisfactory, since other platelet activity would be expected to be less, not more.

Replacement of injured cells is likely to be a factor. Of known mitogens, and because platelets accumulate in this injury, PDGF can be considered. But the paradox is that there is no response by the pericyte, the precursor muscle cell that in vitro is more responsive to PDGF than is the endothelial cell. Does this reflect a different metabolic effect on the two cell types by the same injury? Or is the endothelial cell more fragile than the contractile cells.

C. Hyperoxia

The potentially toxic nature of oxygen is demonstrated clinically and by experimental studies. Experimentally, tensions greater than $FiO_2$0.8 rapidly produce obvious injury to the normal lung, although clinically tensions as low as 0.6

have been reported to produce injury that leads to edema. This injury differs from that due to hypoxia in that it causes frank necrosis of pulmonary cells including those comprising vessel walls. The severity of lung injury is related to the oxygen tension. In our experimental studies we use $FiO_2 0.87$: the animals survive chronic exposure to this tension, although with progressively severe PH. This is based on obliterative vascular structural injury and structural remodeling by the patent bed (Fig. 16).

Exposure of rats to 85% oxygen causes necrosis of the cells lining the air/blood barrier – particularly of the type I pneumocyte and the pulmonary capil-

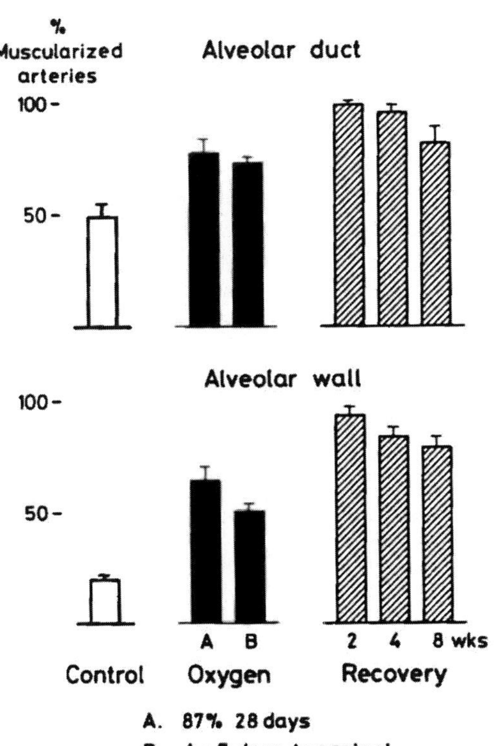

Figure 16 Percentage of muscularized (muscular and partially muscular) alveolar duct and alveolar wall arteries (mean ± SEM) in control rats and in five groups of rats exposed to 87% oxygen for 28 days (hyperoxia). A, hyperoxia alone; B, hyperoxia + weaning to air over 7 days by daily 10% reduction in oxygen concentration; recovery = B + 2, 4, or 8 weeks of breathing air. (From Jones et al., 1983, with permission).

lary endothelial cell (Crapo et al., 1978, 1980). While at an early stage epithelial cells desquamate, leaving large areas of the alveolar wall bare, this rarely happens on the endothelial surface. After several days exposure, endothelial cells in the capillaries are seen to be necrotic.

An early feature of adaptation that occurs in the capillaries as well as in the small segments up- and downstream is hypertrophy of the endothelial cells. This partly reflects stimulated production of antioxidant enzyme systems occurring in the endothelial cell cytoplasm (Crapo and Tierney, 1974). Hypertrophy also occurs in the subendothelial precursor smooth muscle cells, principally the pericyte (Jones et al., 1981). In distal segments this may be a similar metabolic response to oxidant injury. The overall effect is to obliterate some arteries and restrict the lumen of others. This augments the developing PH by increased velocity of blood flow in the patent arteries and also stimulates changes in upstream vessels as the cells adapt to the increased pressure load.

The cellular inflammatory response changes during continuing exposure, depending rather on the degree of initial injury (Barry and Crapo, 1985). In 100% oxygen, for example, platelets are sequestered in the pulmonary vessels followed somewhat later by polymorphonuclear leukocytes. At 87% O_2 a widespread acute inflammatory infiltrate is rarely seen (Jones et al., 1984b, 1985b). By day 7 however, monocytes have accumulated in the vessel wall and alveolar space: they become numerous as exposure continues.

The remodeling of the small arteries at alveolar duct and alveolar wall level is not accompanied by obvious phenotypic changes in the precursor cells. In hypoxia the pericyte develops into a typical of a smooth muscle cell. These features are seen however, if the animals are weaned back to normoxia, which seems to represent a relative hypoxia. In proximal resistance arteries, structural remodeling is manifested as medial thickening and probably represents an adaptation to increased pressure. These vessels are different in their mechanical property from vessels adapted to monocrotaline or hypoxia (Coflesky et al., 1987). So the original injury modifies the way even the large arteries behave in PH.

Recovery from Hyperoxia

Return to air does not immediately produce regression of these lesions (Jones et al., 1985b). It is associated with additional and different injury. Weaning to air and normoxia cause further damage and different adaptation (Fig. 17). Even weaning to air, necessary if the rats are to survive, has the effect of relative hypoxia, and a vasoconstriction occurs. Additional precapillary arteries develop a media-like layer of cells derived from the subendothelial precursor cells. Increased elastin is deposited below the endothelium, separating the precursor muscle cells, and also around each "new" smooth muscle cell. A prominent layer of collagen is laid down in the adventitia.

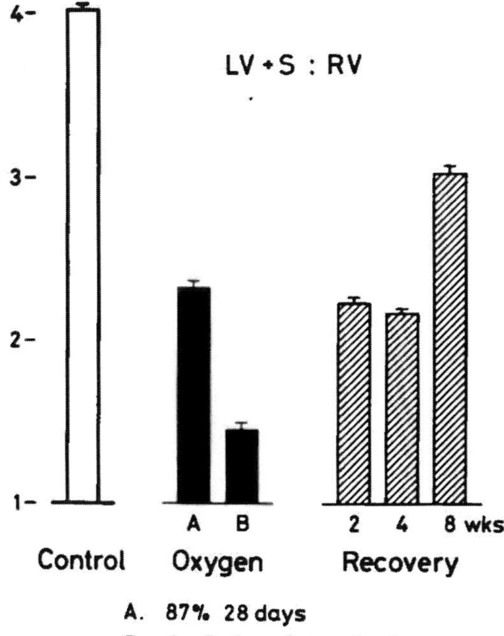

Figure 17 The ratio left ventricle plus septum to right ventricle (LV + S to RV) is a measure of right ventricular hypertrophy. This develops during exposure to 87% oxygen (A) and increases further after weaning to air (over 7 days by 10% daily reduction in oxygen concentration) (B), indicating an injury of weaning. It reverses somewhat during the first 4 weeks of recovery in air but even after 8 weeks is not back to normal. (From Jones et al., 1983, with permission).

Cell Proliferation in Hyperoxia

These studies were carried out on four groups of rats: hyperxia (studied at 1, 4, 7, 10, and 28 days), hyperoxia (28 days) + weaning (1 or 7 days), and hyperoxia (28 days) + weaning (7 days) + air (1, 2 or 4 weeks): untreated controls were examined at 1, 4, 7, 10, and 28 days.

After 3 days, pulmonary artery pressure is still normal but by 7 days it is elevated – from about 17 mm Hg to 26 mmHg – and right ventricular hypertrophy can be detected. Neither vasoconstriction nor polycythemia seem to contribute to this: the obliteration of small arteries reduces the density of patent intraacinar small arteries by as much as one-third to one-half. This obliterative vascular lesion seems to be the most important single cause of the hypertension; the patent arteries are also narrowed by restructuring.

The lumen of the hilar pulmonary arteries is reduced due to reduction in external diameter and medial thickening. Encroachment on the lumen occurs and the adventitial collagen "sets" this narrower artery – an example of contracture (see Sect. IIB). Intimal thickening by hyaline material also adds to lumen narrowing. This is another example of the way intimal thickening develops from nonspecific vascular debris, presumably from cells and serum. Thymidine labeling has not yet been completed for large arteries, but we draw on preliminary analysis of the peripheral ones. High oxygen does not increase thymidine labeling of smooth muscle cells. The endothelial cell and pericyte show their peak at day 4, the adventitial fibroblast at day 7 (Jones et al., 1987a). Its peak is the largest of any of the vascular cells. Considering the effect of hyperoxia on vessels less than 100 μm in diameter, an obviously different pattern of cell division is seen from that produced by hypoxia. Again, no obvious candidate presents to explain the patterns of the hyperoxic injury. Even the injury of weaning, which can be considered relative hypoxia, offers a different pattern from a first hypoxic exposure. Since hyperoxia produces necrosis we can invoke a broad range of mitogens released from migrating cells and yet the smooth muscle cell, the cell type most often suggested to respond to PDGF in systemic arteries, showed no increase in mitosis until day 28 of hyperoxia. The pericyte scarcely responded. The fibroblast responds by day 4 and continues to show a high level of activity. The endothelial cell shows its first peak at day 7. The response of the fibroblast with none by smooth muscle cell suggests that interleukin-1 derived from endothelial cells and/or mononuclear cells could be the effective agent. TGFβ, another product of the mononuclear cell, is likely to promote collagen synthesis. It might even be induced within the fibroblasts by the action of TNF and also released from the mononuclear cells.

During the relative hypoxia of weaning, neither the fibroblast nor pericyte show any measured mitotic activity yet the population of smooth muscle cells maintain a raised level of division. PDGF is not sufficiently selective to explain this. The endothelial cells also increase their mitotic rate. It is now that fibrosis, in the interstitium particularly, becomes obvious. This could simply represent activity from the increased population of fibroblasts produced by hyperoxia or it could be the response of the changed fibroblast to TGFβ released from a relatively hypoxic mononuclear population.

Relative hypoxia per se seems not to be a trigger of fibroblast division. Endothelial cells react to weaning and air with a higher level of mitotic activity. This is maintained, whereas the first hypoxic challenge caused only a peak. The presence of endothelial mitogens released from the mononuclear cells is a possibility. The alveolar epithelial cell, which gave a greater mitotic response to hyperoxia than the endothelial, responds less than the endothelial to the relative hypoxia of weaning to air.

D. Comment

A clear conclusion from the above is that as a tissue adapts to a new environment the phenotype of the constituent cells changes and persists so that a given environment elicits an abnormal response. A relatively simple example of this is seen in vitro. In culture pericytes and smooth muscle cells from chronically hypoxic rats grew more slowly than from control rats, even in a mitogenically rich culture medium and in ambient air. These cells do not rapidly revert to the normal pattern. Pericyte growth is slowed by heparin in the first days, smooth muscle cell, only after 7 days. This pattern is preserved in the hypoxic cells (Davies, personal communication).

The account of these three models makes clear our deficient knowledge in the action of growth factors that are known to cause proliferation of cells within the vascular wall with respect to PH. Better understanding of baseline sensitivity peculiar to the various cell types could be important, but intriguing questions are posed by the time relationships of the bursts of mitotic activity.

A cautionary tale can be told of the angiogenesis – action in vitro that is important and impressive. It is a pharmacological factor, angiogenin (Marx, 1987; Weiner et al., 1987). What is in doubt is whether in vivo it is being made in the right place at the right time to contribute to active angiogensis during growth. The latter is a widespread assumption for its action, although its discoverers disclaim such a hypothesis.

From these studies a plea can be made for greater correlation between in vitro and in vivo results. Our knowledge of the biological changes in PH means that in investigating PH the questions we formulate for in vitro studies should reflect this knowledge and not be a repetition or continuation of the studies using systemic vascular cells.

These three experimental models have been considered in some detail, since patterns and ratios of proliferation have been established. The following are comments on several other types of hypertension considered briefly in their clinical form mainly to emphasize the details of injury and where cell proliferation contributes to the structural changes.

E. Persistent Pulmonary Hypertension in the Newborn

In PPHN abnormal proliferation and differentiation of vascular cells occurs. PH is the normal condition of the pulmonary circulation before birth. At birth, mainly because of air breathing, pressure and resistance fall rapidly, because of two types of adaptation, one functional and one structural. In the arterial bed, particularly the small arteries dilate (Rudolph et al., 1977), and the structure of small mostly muscular arteries, changes so that the wall is more compliant (Fig. 18) (Hislop and Reid, 1981). Presumably, all layers of the wall become more compliant so that the external diameter and lumen increase, and

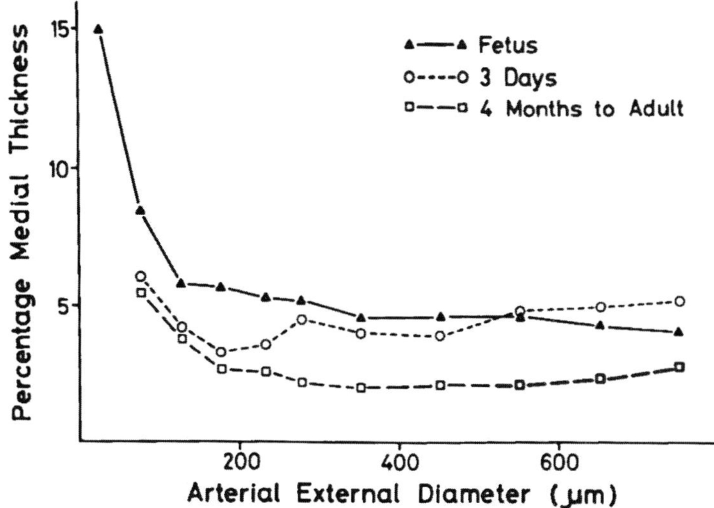

Figure 18 Arterial wall thickness (WT) as percentage of external diameter (ED) calculated by [(2xWT/ED)x100]. Arteries of all sizes are thicker in the fetus than in the adult. Soon after birth, the increase in compliance of small arteries is apparent by a decrease in wall thickness and an increase in external diameter (judged at similar levels in branching pattern). (From Reid, 1979, with permission).

the wall, notably the media, thins. PH can persist in the newborn because these adaptive changes fail (Gersony et al., 1969). When PPHN occurs and is fatal, other structural abnormalities are usually found (Haworth and Reid, 1976; Murphy et al., Reid, 1981, 1984). Normally in the newborn, the alveolar wall arteries are free of muscle: in fatal PPHN they are nearly always fully muscularized arteries with a thick media (Fig. 19). This is several muscle layers thick, and because of the small size of the arteries as a percent of wall thickness, this is in the high fetal range. In fatal cases the wall of these arteries has not shown the reduction in thickness associated with the increase in compliance. The adventitia is well developed and consists of dense collagen. Lymphatics are identified in this sheath (this is a level at which the lymphatics are not usually present in the newborn). The density of the alveoli and alveolar wall arteries is normal and suggests that the lung had developed normally until relatively near term. The well organized artery wall indicates that the changes had developed at least several weeks before birth. Distension by injection shows that these arteries are usually strikingly small.

The proximal normally muscular preacinar arteries typically show increased medial and adventitial thickness. The media is a well-developed

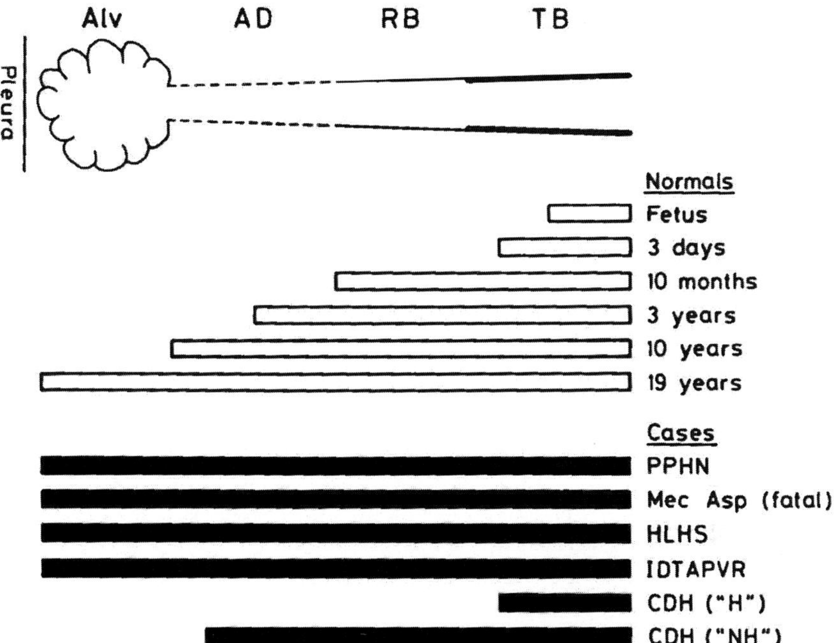

Figure 19 Muscle extension within the acinus in normal children and in newborns with pulmonary hypertension. The acinus is the respiratory unit supplied by a terminal bronchiolus (TB). In the fetus, muscular arteries are not found with the respiratory bronchiolus (RB) or beyond. During childhood, they extend further, until in the adult they reach alveolar ducts (AD) and distal alveoli (Alv).

muscle layer, the adventitia dense collagen. The size is often reduced.

The increased compliance that occurs normally at birth in the adjacent upstream segment has quite often occurred normally. This underlines the different behavior of the resistance arteries upstream from the precapillary segment. The latter is confined to the arterial site of the capillary bed, and therefore represents either a receptor abnormality of the arterial segment or a mediator effect that is peculiar at this site.

It is useful to distinguish the idiopathic or unexplained variety from cases where cause of the prenatal abnormality has been identified. In the latter, we have at least one link in the chain of responsible events, although we do not yet know what signals are produced or how they are transduced to the abnormal cellular events that have taken place.

In the idiopathic variety we start with the vascular restructuring and try to work back to the mediators and cellular dialogue that have produced them.

Experimental studies and clinical investigation have failed to indicate the nature of the disturbance that leads to the characteristic cellular restructuring typical of the idiopathic form. It has been claimed often in the literature that hypoxemia of the infant is a cause of PPHN. There is reason to question this even as a hypothesis, since children born at altitude do not necessarily have PPHN and infants of cyanotic mothers also do not have this condition. Experimental studies in which detailed morphometry has been performed and where hemodynamic studies have been carried out in the newborn have shown in both rat (Geggel et al., 1986a) and guinea pig (Murphy et al., 1986) that neither the hemodynamic findings nor the structural characteristics of the idiopathic variety are present.

Another suggested model is the feeding of indomethacin to the infant – the suggestion being that intermittent closure of the ductus could produce PH (of complete closure, usually results in death of the fetus). In the guinea pig, administration of indomethacin to the mother for several weeks before delivery has not produced the changes of PPHN in the offspring (deMello et al., 1987). The possibility that the guinea pig is relatively resistant to this effect needs to be considered, but although an acute closure of the ductus has been shown to temporarily produce PH its presence in the newborn has not been established (Levin et al., 1978).

In human cases of idiopathic PH the partially and nonmuscular parts of the precapillary arterial segment have developed into an artery which is too small, has the structure of a mature artery, that is an internal and external elastic lamina, and also a collagenous adventitial sheath that is strickingly dense.

Considering the human cases of PPHN where a cause can be identified, it seems that hypoplasia represents one large group of cases and increased flow another (Geggel and Reid, 1984). In these two groups the same message is probably being delivered to the peripheral vascular bed. If a small lung accepts the normal or usual output of the right ventricle that would be appropriate to body weight, then there is not only an increased velocity of flow through those of the vascular channels but also a net increase in flow per unit volume of lung (Goldstein and Reid, 1980). In the cases of diversion of flow or of high cardiac output before birth to a normal lung there is an abnormally high flow to the lung.

Cases of a congenital heart disease (CHD) offer an important and vicarious experiment. For example, total anomalous pulmonary venous drainage (Haworth and Reid, 1977a) and obstructive lesions of the left side of the heart (Haworth and Reid, 1977b) cause structural remodeling of the precapillary vessels similar to the idiopathic form of PPHN. It is of interest that in the latter group the mechanical effect produces a muscularization of the venous, that is the postcapillary, segment as well as of the arterial or precapillary. The pericyte and intermediate cell on the venous side of the capillary are capable of differentiating to a mature muscle cell and of organizing a muscular vessel just as are the precapillary cells.

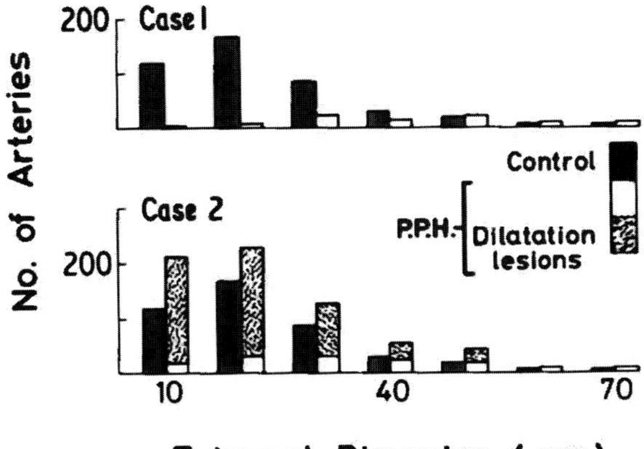

Figure 20 Reduction in the number of nonmuscular arteries less than 40 μm in diameter in primary pulmonary hypertension (PPH). Case 1: The patient with the shortest clinical history had no dilatation lesions. Case 2: A patient with a longer clinical history did have dilatation lesions. (From Anderson et al., 1973, with permission).

F. Primary Pulmonary Hypertension: Arterial or Venous

In PPAH the reason for the microvascular lesion that causes hypertension is unexplained. In patients wtihout clinical or pathological thromboembolism, examined soon after symptoms developed, we have identified an obliterative lesion of arteries less than 40 μm in diameter (Anderson et al., 1973). It seems that this developing stage of obliteration is short-lived, evidence of acute change in the vessel wall and "ghost arteries" during the phase of obliteration and disappearance are rare. In one patient we found that the arteries less than 40 μm were reduced to about 4% of normal (Fig. 20). This stage explains the strickingly low diffusion found in some of these patients. Survival is probably only possible if the residual bed dilates. As this occurs presumably the factor improves. Larger arteries may well be affected also. In most fatal cases it is difficult to determine the original lesion or the level at which most damage has occurred. High pressures upstream and raised velocity through the narrowed peripheral bed produce a restructuring of the small residual arteries. The early lesion of the small arteries suggests endothelial injury or disease. Fenestrated capillary walls have been found ultrastructurally, along with an increase in connective tissue fibrils in the nonmuscular wall (Meyrick et al., 1974). Recently we have demonstrated disturbed endothelial function in the abnormal ratio of von Willebrand antigen to von Willebrand ristocetin cofactor activity (Geggel et al., 1987). Whereas the concentration of the protein is normal or low, the activity is considerably increased. By contrast, nonspecific injury gives both a high concentration of the von Willebrand antigen but also an appropriate activity that maintains this ratio in the normal range of 1. Our more recent analysis of additional cases confirms this abnormality and suggests that this pattern is of the familial as well as sporadic variety (Carvalls et al., personal communication). The veins are relatively normal. Downstream the cross-sectional area is virtually within the normal range and injury from increased rate of flow does not occur.

In the idiopathic form of PVHN the brunt falls on the veins (Davies and Reid, 1982; Geggel et al., 1984). The restriction of the vascular bed at this level follows either an obliterative lumen lesion or the lumen narrows from perivenous fibrosis. The hyperplastic intimal lesion is illustrated in Figure 21. The nature of the cells has not been established, but intimal cells can be expected to contribute, although whether muscle cells also take part has not been established. In the case of intimal lesions, proliferation could be one expression of injury but this must be severe enough to cause obliteration.

In the case of perivenous fibrosis, as in the spontaneous variety that affects vessels or the secondary involvement seen with mediastenitis, fibroblasts seem to play a major part, indicating that the contracting force of the fibroblast or the fibers it produces exceeds that of the transmural pressure. The stimulus to fibroblast proliferation has not been identified.

Whether the primary obliteration and restriction is on the arterial or venous side of the capillary bed, upstream the vessels show hypertrophy and hypoplasia of all coats that is presumed to be in response to the increased transmural pressure. While interesting as a model of interaction between cells of the vascular wall this change would not seem important in causing disability. In fact, it is such a physiological hypertrophic response by right ventricle and large vessel wall that probably determines survival of the patient.

G. High Flow, Low Flow Injury

An artery adapts structurally to reduced (Langille and O'Donnell, 1986) as well as to increased flow. A model of reduced flow is the shut down in flow that occurs in the wall of abscess cavities in the lung, as in a tuberculosis cavity. Acute and continuing inflammation are associated with increased blood supply to the region through the pulmonary artery channels and bronchial collaterals. With resolution and healing, blood flow falls and channels either disappear in scar tissue or the artery remodels to adapt to reduced flow.

Typically the pulmonary artery supplying the scarred region is constricted with the lumen occluded partly or completely by hyaline material that represents a "nonspecific vascular deposit." This is described as nonspecific to emphasize that it is not necessarily derived from formed vascular elements as the assumption is easily and often made that this material is platelet derived. The

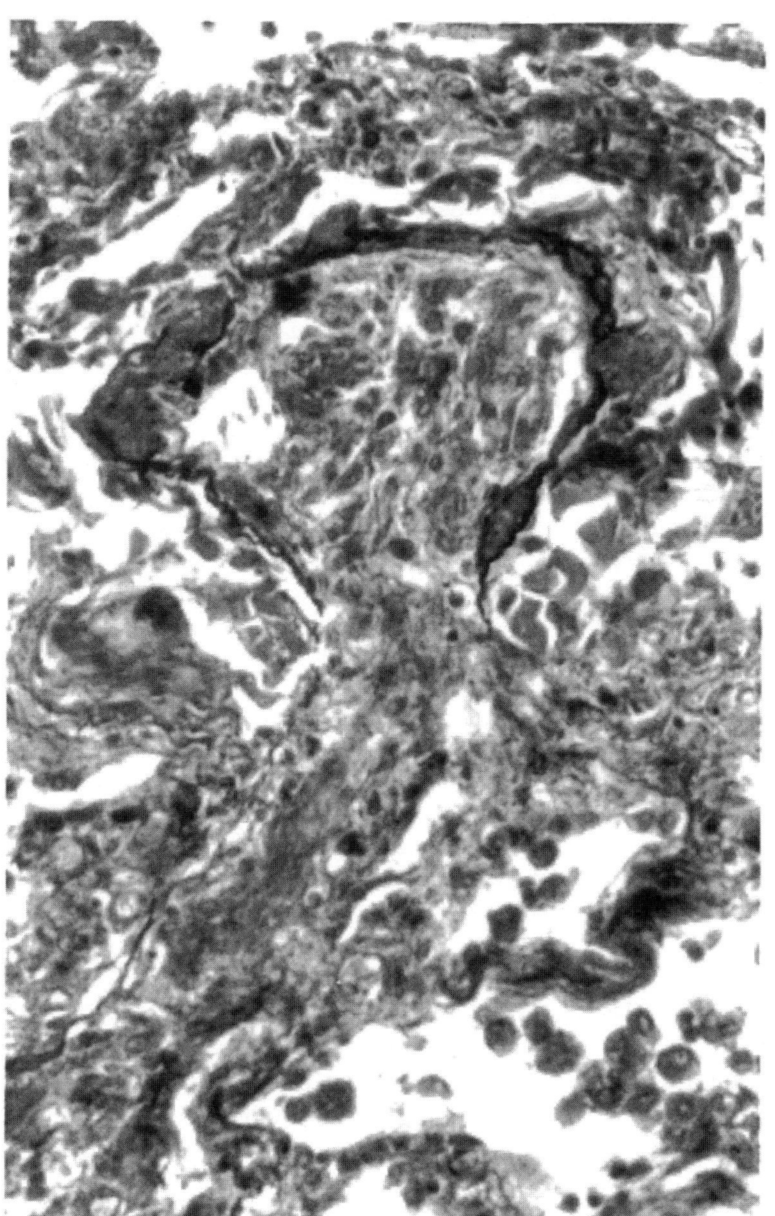

Figure 21 Case of primary pulmonary venous hypertension. Photomicrograph of occlusive luminal lesion of small vein. (4 μm section: Miller's elastic van Gieson). (From Jones and Reid, 1987, with permission).

crenated internal elastic lamina is often obvious. To our knowledge, no study has been made of the medial area of such arteries nor of the degree of crenation of internal and external elastic lamina.

Analysis of the intimal thickening will indicate the way in which such material develops. This is a chronic model but such deposit is sometimes produced quite quickly, as after transplantation. A recent analysis of the deposit in the hepatic veins after bone marrow transplantation showed that the material includes fibrin and factor VIII, but was not positive for the platelet membrane molecule tested (Shulman et al., 1981).

Another acute example of this is the deposit occurring in the high flow injury produced by anastomosing the aorta or one of its large branches to a lobar pulmonary artery (Rendas et al., 1979, Rendas and Reid, 1983).

In a recent study of the vascular bed distal to ligation of a main pulmonary artery, Shure and colleagues (1984, 1985) have shown an arteriopathy in the arteries distal to the ligation, that is, in the obstructed vascular bed. The artery of the patent lung did not show these changes. Pulmonary artery pressure was not elevated, nor was there hypoxia. In fact, the PaO_2 was above normal, raising the possibility that even a high oxygen injury might have occurred. It is likely that the arteriopathy distal to the ligation represents an adaptation to reduced flow.

In plexiform lesions seen in PH, cell density is sometimes greatly increased, sometimes the lesion is fibrotic (Brewer, 1955; Naeye and Vennart, 1959; Wagenvoort, 1959). In experimental studies of high flow, intimal thickening with cell proliferation is an early and striking response. The obliteration at the stie of side branches can be interpreted as a shear injury. Collateral channels open up through the conventional and supernumerary pulmonary arteries to supply the arteries distal to the block. Pleural arteries open up to connect adjacent lobules, subsegments and segments. The dilated vessels produced by such local increase in flow contribute to dilatation and plexiform lesions.

VI. Concluding Remarks

Cell proliferation is a feature of each of the types of pulmonary hypertension we have considered. Where information is available it seems that each cell type – endothelial cell, smooth muscle cell (with its precursors the intermediate cell and pericyte), and fibroblast – participates, but for each a characteristic pattern of timing and frequency of cell division can be identified. Furthermore, for a given cell type the various levels of the vascular pathway act differently. These variations reflect the injury and adaptation to its various cellular and hemodynamic sequelae.

There is no dearth of factors that can stimulate mitosis of systemic vascular cells or even of those that can depress it, although of these fewer are known. Whether these really are the factors that control cell proliferation in the normal pulmonary vascular bed or in PH is uncertain. The candidates have mostly been identified by study of atherona or tumor angiogenesis, phenomena different from those responsible for the onset of PH. Moreover, even these studies of systemic vascular cells are still largely in vitro findings with, as yet, relatively little proof that a given effect in cell culture mimics what happens in vivo. The rewards of in vitro studies of PH are likely to be large and should be enhanced if their formulation takes account of the available biological knowledge.

References

Anderson, E. G., Simon, G., and Reid, L. (1973). Primary and thromboembolic pulmonary hypertension: a quantitative pathological study. *J. Pathol. 110*: 273-293.

Balks, S., Riley, T., Gunther, H., and Morisi, A. (1985). Heparin-treated v-myc transformed chicken heart mesenchymal cells assume a normal morphology, but are hypersensitive to epidermal growth factor (EGF) and brain fibroblast growth factor (bFGF): cells transformed by the v-Ha-ras oncogene are refractory to EGF and bFGF but are hypersensitive to insulin-like growth factors. *Proc. Natl. Acad. Sci. USA 82*:5781-5785.

Bar, R. S., Peacock, M. L., Spanheimer, R. G., Veenstra, R. J., and Hoak, J. C. (1980). Differential binding of insulin to human arterial and venous endothelial cells in primary culture. *Diabetes 29*:991-995.

Barja, F., Coughlin, C., Belin, D., and Gabbiani, G. (1986). Actin isoform synthesis and mRNA levels in quiescent and proliferating rat aortic smooth muscle cells in vivo and in vitro. *Lab. Invest. 55*:226-233.

Bar-Ner, M., Mayer, M., Schirrmacher, M., and Vlodavsky, I. (1986). Involvement of both heparanase and plasminogen activator in lymphoma cell-mediated degradation of heparan sulfate in the subendothelial extracellular matrix. *J. Cell Physiol. 128*:299-306.

Barrett, T. B., Gajdusek, C. M., Schwartz, S. M., McDougall, J. K., and Benditt, E. P. (1985). Expression of the sis gene by endothelial cells in culture and in vivo. *Proc. Natl. Acad. Sci. USA 81*:6772-6774.

Barry, B. E., and Crapo, J. D. (1985). Patterns of accumulation of platelets and neutrophils in rat lungs during exposure to 100% and 85% oxygen. *Am. Rev. Resp. Dis. 132*:548-555.

Benitz, W. E., Coulson, J. D., Lessler, D. S., and Bernfield, M. (1986a). Hypoxia inhibits proliferation of fetal pulmonary arterial smooth muscle cells in vitro. *Pediatr. Res. 20*:966-972.

Benitz, W. E., Lessler, D. S., Coulson, J. D., and Bernfield, M. (1986b). Heparin inhibits proliferation of fetal vascular smooth muscle cells in the absence of platelet derived growth factor. *J. Cell Physiol. 127*:1-7.

Brown, M. T., and Clemmons, D. R. (1986). Platelets contain a peptide inhibitor of endothelial cell replication and growth. *Proc. Natal. Acad. Sci. USA 83*: 3321-3325.

Campbell, G. R., and Campbell, J. H. (1985). Smooth muscle phenotypic changes in arterial wall homeostasis: implications for the pathogenesis of artehrosclerosis. *Exp. Mol. Pathol. 42*:139-162.

Carvalho, A. C.A., Bellman, S. M., Saullo, V. J., Quinn, D. A., and Zapol, W. M. (1982). Altered factor VIII in acute respiratory failure. *New Engl. J. Med. 307*:1113-1119.

Castellot, J. J., Addonizio, M. L., Rosenberg, R., and Karnovsky, M. J. (1981). Cultured endothelial cells produce a heparinlike inhibitor of smooth muscle cell growth. *J. Cell Biol. 90*:372-379.

Castellot, J. J., Wong, K., Herman, B., Hoover, R. L., Albertini, D. F., Wright, T. C., Caleb, B. L., and Karnovsky, M. J. (1985). Binding and internalization of heparin by vascular smooth muscle cells. *J. Cell Physiol. 124*: 13-20.

Castellot, J. J., Choay, J., Lormeau, J.-C., Petitou, M., Sache, E., and Karnovsky, M. J., (1986). Structural determinants of the capacity of heparin to inhibit the proliferation of vascular smooth muscle cells. II. Evidence for a pentasaccharide sequence that contains a 3-*0*-sulfate group. *J. Cell Biol. 102*:1979-1984.

Clemmons, D. R. (1984). Interaction of circulating cell-derived and plasma growth factors in stimulating cultured smooth muscle cell replication. *J. Cell Physiol. 121*:425-430.

Clemmons, D. R., and Van Wyk, J. J. (1985). Evidence for a functional role of endogenously produced somatomedin-like peptides in the regulation of DNA synthesis in cultured human fibroblasts and porcine smooth muscle cells. *J. Clin. Invest. 75*:1914-1918.

Coflesky, J., Jones, R., Reid, L., and Evans, J. N. (1987). Mechanical properties and structure of isolated pulmonary arteries remodeled by chronic hyperoxia. *Am. Rev. Resp. Dis. 136*:388-394.

Collins, T., Ginsburg, T., Boss, J. M., Orkin, S. H., and Pober, J. S. (1985). Cultured human endothelial cells express platelet-derived growth factor B chain: cDNA cloning and structural analysis. *Nature 316*:748-750.

Collins, T., Pober, J. S., Gimbrone, M. A., Hammacher, A., Betsholtz, C., Westermark, B., and Heldin, C.-H. (1987). Cultured human endothelial cells express platelet-derived growth factor A chain. *Am. J. Pathol. 127*:7-12.

Crapo, J. D., and Tierney, D. F. (1974). Superoxide dismutase and pulmonary oxygen toxicity. *Am. J. Pathol. 226*:1401-1405.

Crapo, J. D., Peters-Golden, M., Marsh-Salin, J., and Shelburne, J. S. (1978). Pathologic changes in the lungs of oxygen-adapted rats. A morphometric analysis. *Lab. Invest. 39*:640-653.

Crapo, J. D., Barry, B. E., Foscue, H. A., and Shelburne, J. (1980). Structural and biochemical changes in rat lungs occurring during exposure to lethal and adaptive doses of oxygen. *Am. Rev. Resp. Dis. 122*:A123.

D'Amore, P. A., and Sweet, E. (1987a). Effects of hyperoxia on microvascular cells in vitro. *In Vitro Cell Develop. Biol. 23*:123-128.

D'Amore, P. A., and Thompson, R. W. (1987b). Mechanisms of angiogenesis. *Ann. Rev. Physiol. 49*:453-464.

Davies, G., and Reid, L. (1970). Growth of the alveoli and pulmonary arteries in childhood. *Thorax 25*:669-681.

Davies, P., and Reid, L. (1982). Pulmonary veno-occlusive disease in sibling: case reports and morphometric study. *Hum. Pathol. 13*:911-915.

Davies, P., Maddalo, F., and Reid, L. (1985). Effects of chronic hypoxia on structure and reactivity of rat lung microvessels. *J. Appl. Physiol. 58*: 795-801.

Davies, P., Burke, G., and Reid, L. (1986a). The structure of the wall of the rat intraacinar pulmonary artery: an electron microscopic study of microdissected preparations. *Microvasc. Res. 32*:50-63.

Davies, P., Burke, G., and Reid, L. (1986b). The structure of the normal rat intraacinar pulmonary artery and its remodeling by hypoxia. *Fed. Proc. 45*: 584.

Davies, P., Hu, L.-M., and Reid, L. (1987a). Effects of heparin on the growth of lung pericytes and smooth muscle cells in vitro. *Fed. Proc. 46*:663a.

Davies, P., Jones, R., Schloo, B., and Reid, L. (1987b). Endothelium of the pulmonary vasculature in health and disease. In *Pulmonary Endothelium in Health and Disease*. Edited by U. S. Ryan. Marcel Dekker, New York, pp. 375-445.

Davies, P., Smith, B. T., Maddalo, F. B., Langleben, D., Tobias, D., Fujiwara, K., and Reid, L. (1987c). Characteristics of lung pericytes in culture including their growth inhibition by endothelial substrate. *Microvasc. Res. 33*:300-314.

Davies, P. F. (1986). Biology of disease. Vascular cell interactions with special reference to the pathogenesis of atherosclerosis. *Lab. Invest. 55*:5-24.

deMello, D., Murphy, J., Aronovitz, M., Davies, P., and Reid, L. (1987). Effects of indomethacin in utero on the pulmonary vasculature of the newborn guinea pig. *Pediatr. Res. 22*:693-697.

DiCorleto, P. E. (1984). Cultured endothelial cells produce multiple growth factors for connective tissue cells. *Exp. Cell Res. 153*:167-172.

Dinarello, C. A., Cannon, J. G., Wolff, S. M., Bernheim, H. A., Beutler, B., Cerami, A., Figari, I. S., Palladino, M. A., and O'Connor, J. V. (1986). Tumor necrosis factor (cachectin) is an endogenous pyrogen and induces production of interleukin 1. *J. Exp. Med. 163*:1433-1450.

Elias, J. A., Zurier, R. B., Schreiber, A. D., Leff, J. A., and Daniele, R. P. (1985). Monocyte inhibition of lung fibroblast growth: relationship to fibroblast prostaglandin production and density-defined monocyte subpopulations. *J. Leukocyte Biol. 37*:15-28.

Evans, J. N., Jones, R., Langleben, D., Reid, L., Szarek, J., and Coflesky, J. T., (1987). Alterations to vascular smooth muscle in pulmonary hypertension. *Chest* in press.

Fett, J. W., Strydom, D. J., Lobb, R. R., Alderman, E. M., Bethune, J. L., Riordan, J. F., and Vallee, B. L. (1985). Isolation and characterization of angiogenin, an angiogenic protein from human carcinoma cells. *Biochemistry 24*:5480-5486.

Fine, A., and Goldstein, R. H. (1987). The effect of transforming growth factor β on cell proliferation and collagen formation by lung fibroblasts. *J. Biol. Chem. 262*:3897-3902.

Folkman, J., and Klagsburn, M. (1987). Angiogenic factors. *Science 235*:442-447.

Form, D. M., Pratt, B. M., and Madri, J. A. (1986). Endothelial cell proliferation during angiogensis. In vitro modulation by basement membrane components. *Lab. Invest. 55*:521-530.

Fox, P. L., and DiCorleto, P. E. (1984). Regulation of production of a platelet-derived growth-factor-like protein by cultured bovine aortic endothelial cells *J. Cell Physiol. 121*:298-308.

Fried, R., Meyrick, B., Rabinovitch, M., and Reid, L. (1983). Polycythemia and the acute hypoxic response in awake rats following chronic hypoxia. *J. Appl. Physiol. 55*:1167-1172.

Fried, R., and Reid, L. (1984). Early recovery from hypoxic pulmonary hypertension: a structural and functional study. *J. Appl. Physiol. 57*:1247-1253.

Fritze, L. M. S., Reilly, C. F., and Rosenberg, R. D. (1985). An antiproliferative heparan sulfate species produced by postconfluent smooth muscle cells. *J. Cell Biol. 100*:1041-1049.

Gabbiani, G., Rungger-Brandle, E., DeChastonay, C., and Franke, W. W. (1982). Vimentin-containing smooth muscle cells in aortic intimal thickening after endothelial injury. *Lab. Invest. 47*:265-269.

Gabbiani, G., Kocher, O., Bloom, W. S., Vandekerchove, J., and Weber, K. (1984). Actin expression in smooth muscle cells of rat aortic inimal thickening, human atheromatous plaque, and cultured rat aortic media. *J. Clin. Invest. 73*:148-152.

Gajdusek, C., Carbon, S., Ross, R., Nawroth, P., and Stern, D. (1986). Activation of coagulation releases endothelial cell mitogens. *J. Cell Biol. 103*:419-428.

Geggel, R., and Reid, L. (1984). The structural basis of PPHN. In *Clinics in perinatology*. Symposium on Neonatal Pulmonary Hypertension. Vol. 11, No. 3. Edited by J. B. Philips III. W. B. Saunders, Philadelpha, pp. 525-549.

Geggel, R., Fried, R., Tuuri, D., Fyler, D., and Reid, L. (1984). Congenital pulmonary vein stenosis: structural changes in a patient with normal pulmonary artery wedge pressure. *J. Am. Coll. Cardiol. 3*:193-199.

Geggel, R., Aronovitz, M., and Reid, L. (1986a). Effects of chronic in utero hypoxemia on rat neonatal pulmonary arterial structure. *J. Pediatr. 108*: 756-759.

Geggel, R., Carvalho, A., Hoyer, L., and Reid, L. (1987). Von Willebrand factor abnormalities in primary pulmonary hypertension. *Am. Rev. Resp. Dis. 135*:294-299.

Gersony, W. M., Duc, G. V., and Sinclair, J. C. (1969). "PFC" syndrome (persistence of the fetal circulation). (Abstr.) *Circulation 40*:87.

Goldstein, J. D., and Reid, L. (1980). Pulmonary hypoplasia resulting from phrenic nerve agenesis and diaphragmatic amyoplasia. *J. Pediatr. 97*: 282-287.

Goldstein, R. H., and Fine, A. (1986). Fibrotic reactions in the lung: the activation of the lung fibroblast. *Exp. Lung Res. 11*:245-261.

Goldstein, R. H., and Polgar, P. (1982). The effect and interaction of bradykinin and prostaglandins on protein and collagen production by lung fibroblasts. *J. Biol. Chem. 257*:8630-8633.

Gospodarowicz, D., and Ill, C., (1980). Extracellular matrix and control of proliferation of vascular endothelial cells. *J. Clin. Invest. 65*:1351-1364.

Gospodarowicz, D., Neufeld, G., and Schweigerer, L. (1986). Molecular and biological characterization of fibroblast growth factor, an angiogenic factor which also controls the proliferation and differentiation of mesoderm and neuroectoderm derived cells. *Cell Differentiation 19*:1-17.

Han, V. K. M., D'Ercole, J. D., and Lund, P. K. (1987). Cellular localization of somatomedin (insulin-like growth factor) messenger RNA in the human fetus. *Science 236*:193-197.

Harlan, J. M. (1985). Leukocyte-endothelial interactions. *Blood 65*:513-525.

Harlan, J. M., Thompson, P. J., Ross, R. R., and Bowen-Pope, D. F. (1986). *α*-Thrombin induces release of platelet-derived growth factor-like molecule(s) by cultured human endothelial cells. *J. Cell Biol. 103*:1129-1133.

Haworth, S. G., and Reid, L. (1976). Persistent fetal circulation: newly recognized structural features. *J. Pediatr. 88*:614-620.

Haworth, S. G., and Reid, L. (1977a). Structural study of pulmonary circulation and of heart in total anomalous pulmonary venous return in early infancy. *Brit. Heart J. 39*:80-92.

Haworth, S. G., and Reid, L. (1977b). Quantitative structural study of pulmonary circulation in the newborn with aortic atresia, stenosis or coarctation. *Thorax 32*:121-128.

Haworth, S. G., Sauer, U., Buhlmeyer, K., and Reid, L. (1977). Development of the pulmonary circulation in ventricular septal defect: a quantitative structural study. *Am. J. Cardiol. 40*:781-788.

Hayes, J. A., Christensen, T. G., and Gaensler, E. A. (1979). Myointimal plaques in pulmonary vascular sclerosis associated with interstitial lung fibrosis. *Lab. Invest. 41*:268-274.

Heimark, R. L., and Schwartz, S. M. (1985). The role of membrane-membrane interactions in the regulation of endothelial growth. J. Cell Biol. 100: 1934-1940.

Heimark, R. L., Twardzik, D. R., and Schwartz, S. M. (1986). Inhibition of endothelial regeneration by type-beta transforming growth factor from platelets. *Science 233*:1078-1080.

Herman, I. M., and Castellot, J. J. (1987). Regulation of vascular smooth muscle cell growth by endothelial-synthesized extracellular matrices. *Arteriosclerosis* in press.

Herman, I. M., and D'Amore, P. A. (1985). Microvascular pericytes contain muscle and nonmuscle actins. *J. Cell Biol. 101*:43-52.

Hilliker, K. S., Garcia, C. M., and Roth, R. A. (1983). Effects of monocrotaline and monocrotaline pyrrole on 5-hydroxytryptamine and paraquat uptake by lung slices. *Res. Commun. Chem. Pathol. Pharmacol. 40*:179-197.

Hislop, A., and Reid, L. (1974). Arterial changes in *Crotalaria spectabilis*-induced pulmonary hypertension in rats. *Brit. J. Exp. Pathol. 55*:153-163.

Hislop, A., and Reid, L. (1976). New findings in pulmonary arteries of rats with hypoxia-induced pulmonary hypertension. *Brit. J. Exp. Pathol. 57*:542-554.

Hislop, A., and Reid, L. (1981). Growth and development of the respiratory system: anatomical development. In *Scientific Foundations of Pediatrics*. 2nd ed. Edited by J. A. Davis and J. Dobbing. Heinemann Medical Publications, London, pp. 390-431.

Homandberg, G. A., Williams, J. E., Grant, D., Schumacher, B., and Eisenstein, R. (1985). Heparin-binding fragments of fibronectin are potent inhibitors of endothelial cell growth. *Am. J. Pathol. 120*:327-332.

Hotta, M., and Baird, A. (1986). Differential effects of transforming growth factor type beta on the growth and function of adrenocortical cells in vitro. *Proc. Natl. Acad. Sci. USA 83*:7795-7799.

Hu, L.-M., Geggel, R., Davies, P., and Reid, L. (1987). The effect of heparin on the hemodynamic and structural response in the rat to acute and chronic hypoxia. *Lab. Invest.* Submitted.

Ingber, D. E., Madri, J. A., and Folkman, J. (1987). Endothelial growth factors and extracellular matrix regulate DNA synthesis through modulation of cell and nuclear expansion. *In Vitro Cell Develop. Biol. 23*:387-394.

Jones, M. B., King, R. J., and Kuehl, T. J. (1987). Production of a growth factor(s) by fibroblasts from the lungs of ventilated premature baboons and oxygen-exposed adult hamsters. *Am. Rev. Resp. Dis. 135*:997-1001.

Jones, R., and Reid, L. (1987). Structural basis of pulmonary hypertension. In *Current Pulmonology*. Vol. 8. Edited by D. Simmons. Year Book Medical Publishers, Chicago, pp. 175-210.

Jones, R., Zapol, W. M., and Reid, L. (1981). Hyperoxia causes pulmonary hypertension and remodeling of rat pulmonary arteries. *Am. Rev. Resp. Dis. 123*:217.

Jones, R., Zapol, W. M., and Reid, L. (1983). Pulmonary arterial wall injury and remodeling by hyperoxia. *Chest 83S*:40-42.

Jones, R., Zapol, W. M., and Reid, L. (1984). Pulmonary artery remodeling and pulmonary hypertension after exposure to hyperoxia for 7 days. A morphometric and hemodynamic study. *Am. J. Pathol. 117*:273-285.

Jones, R., Zapol, W. M., and Reid, L. (1985). Oxygen toxicity and restructuring of pulmonary arteries – a morphometric study. The response to 4 weeks' exposure to hyperoxia and return to breathing air. *Am. J. Pathol. 121*: 212-223.

Jones, R., Farber, F., and Adler, C. (1987a). ^{3}H-Thymidine labeling of rat pulmonary microcirculation in hyperoxic pulmonary hypertension. *Fed. Proc. 46*:3946.

Jones, R., Yang, Y., DeMarinis, S., and Carvalho, A. (1987c). Release of tissue plasminogen activator, inhibitor and eicosanoids by cultured endothelial cells and pericytes from rat pulmonary microvessels and pulmonary artery smooth muscle cells. *Am. Rev. Resp. Dis. 135*:A100.

Joyce, N. C., Decamilli, P., and Boyles, J. (1984). Pericytes, like vascular smooth muscle cells, are immunocytochemically positive for cGMP-dependent protein kinase. *Microvasc. Res. 28*:206-219.

Joyce, N., Haire, M., and Palade, G. (1985). Contractile proteins in pericytes. II. Immunocytochemical evidence for the presence of two isomyosins in graded concentrations. *J. Cell Biol. 100*:1387-1395.

Kay, J. M., and Heath, D. (1969). *Crotalaria spectabilis. The Pulmonary Hypertension Plant*. Charles C. Thomas, Springfield, Il.

King, G. L., and Buchwald, S. (1984). Characterization and partial purification of an endothelial cell growth factor from human platelets. *J. Clin. Invest. 73*:392-396.

King, G. L., Buzney, S. M., Kahn, C. R., Heto, N., Buchwald, S., MacDonald, S. G., and Rand, L. I. (1983). Differential responsiveness to insulin of endothelial and support cells from micro- and macro-vessels. *J. Clin. Invest. 71*: 944-949.

King, G. L., Goodman, A. D., Buzney, S., Moses, A., and Kahn, C. R. (1985). Receptors and growth-promoting effects of insulin and insulinlike growth factors on cells from bovine retinal capillaries and aorta. *J. Clin. Invest. 75*:1028-1036.

Kurobe, M., Furukawa, S., and Hayashi, K. (1985). Synthesis and secretion of an epidermal growth factor (EGF) by human fibroblasts in culture. *Biochem. Biophys. Res. Commun. 131*:1080-1085.

Langille, B. L., and O'Donnell, F. (1986). Reductions in arterial diameter produced by chronic decrease in blood flow are endothelium-dependent. *Science 231*:405-407.

Langleben, D., and Reid, L. (1985). Effect of methylprednisolone on monocrotaline-induced pulmonary vascular disease and right ventricular hypertrophy. *Lab. Invest. 52*:298-303.

Le, J., and Vilcek, J. (1987). Tumor necrosis factor and interleukin 1: cytokines with multiple overlapping biological activities. *Lab. Invest. 56*:234-248.

Le, J., Weinstein, D., Gubler, U., and Vilcek, J. (1987). Induction of membrane-associated IL-1 by tumor necrosis factor in human fibroblasts. *J. Immunol. 138*:2137-2142.

Leof, E. B., Wharton, W., Van Wyk, J. J., and Pledger, W. V. (1982). Epidermal growth factor and somatomedin C regulate G1 progression in competent Balb-c 3T3 cells. *Exp. Cell Res. 141*:107-115.

Leung, D. Y., Glagov, S., and Matthews, M. B. (1976). Cyclic stretching stimulates synthesis of matrix components by arterial smooth muscle cells in vitro. *Science 191*:474-477.

Leung, D. Y., Glagov, S., and Matthews, M. B. (1977). A new in vitro system for studying cell response to mechanical stimulation. *Exp. Cell Res. 109*:285-298.

Levin, D. L., Hyman, A. I., Heymann, M. A., and Rudolph, A. M. (1978). Fetal hypertension and the development of increased pulmonary vascular smooth muscle. A possible mechanism for persistent pulmonary hypertension of the newborn infant. *J. Pediatr. 92*:265-269.

Libby, P., Wyler, D. J., Janica, M. W., and Dinarello, C. A. (1985). Differential effects of human interleukin-1 on growth of human fibroblasts and vascular smooth muscle cells. *Arteriosclerosis 5*:186-191.

McLeod, K. J., Lee, R. C., and Ehrlich, P. (1987). Frequency dependence of electric field modulation of fibroblast protein synthesis. *Science 236*: 1465-1469.

McMurtry, I. F., Davidson, A. B., Reeves, J. T., and Grover, R. F. (1976). Inhibition of hypoxic pulmonary vasoconstriction by calcium antagonists in isolated rat lungs. *Circ. Res. 38*:99-104.

Majack, R. A. (1987). Beta-type transforming growth factor specifies organizational behavior in vascular smooth muscule cell cultures. *J. Cell Biol. 105*: 465-471.

Majack, R. A., and Bornstein, P. (1985). Heparin and related glycosaminoglycans regulate the secretory phenotype of vascular smooth muscle cells. *J. Cell Biol. 99*:1688-1695.

Marks, R. M., Roche, W. R., Czerniecki, M., Penny, P., and Nelson, D. S. (1986). Mast cell granules cause proliferation of human microvascular endothelial cells. *Lab. Invest. 55*:289-294.

Marx, J. L. (1987). Angiogenesis research comes of age. *Science 237*:23-24.

Meyrick, B., and Reid, L. (1978). The effect of continued hypoxia on rat pulmonary arterial circulation. An ultrastructural study. *Lab. Invest. 38*:188-200.

Meyrick, B., and Reid, (1979a). Development of pulmonary arterial changes in rats fed *Crotalaria spectabilis. Am. J. Pathol. 94*:37-50.

Meyrick, B., and Reid, L. (1979b). Hypoxia and incorporation of ^{3}H-thymidine by cells of the rat pulmonary arteries and alveolar wall. *Am. J. Pathol. 96*:51-70.

Meyrick, B., and Reid, L. (1979c). Ultrastructural features of the distended pulmonary arteries of the normal rat. *Anat. Rec. 193*:71-97.

Meyrick, B., and Reid, L. (1980a). Hypoxia-induced structural changes in the media and adventitia of the rat hilar pulmonary artery and their regression. *Am. J. Pathol. 100*:151-178.

Meyrick, B., and Reid, L. (1980b). Endothelial and subintimal changes in rat hilar pulmonary artery during recovery from hypoxia. A quantitative ultrastructural study. *Lab. Invest. 429*:603-615.

Meyrick, B., and Reid, L. (1982). Crotalaria-induced pulmonary hypertension. Uptake of ^{3}H-thymidine by the cells of the pulmoanry circulation and alveolar walls. *Am. J. Pathol. 106*:84-94.

Meyrick, B., Clarke, S. W., Simons, C., Woodgate, D. J., and Reid, L. (1974). Primary pulmonary hypertension. A case report including electron microscopic study. *Brit. J. Dis. Chest 68*:11-20

Meyrick, B., Gamble, W., and Reid, L. (1980). Development of Crotalaria pulmonary hypertension: hemodynamic and structural study. *Am. J. Physiol. 239*:H692-H702.

Miyazono, K., Okabe, T., Urabe, A., Takaku, F., and Heldin, C.-H. (1987). Purification and properties of an endothelial growth factor from platelets. *J. Biol. Chem. 262*:4098-4103.

Murphy, J., Aronovitz, M., and Reid, L. (1986). Effects of chronic in utero hypoxia on the pulmonary vasculature of the newborn guinea pig. *Pediatr. Res. 20*:292-295.

Murphy, J. D., Rabinovitch, M., Goldstein, J. D., and Reid, L. (1981). The structural basis of persistent pulmonary hypertension of the newborn infant. *J. Pediatr. 98*:962-967.

Murphy, J. D., Vawter, G., and Reid, L. (1984). Pulmonary vascular disease in fatal meconium aspiration. *J. Pediatr. 104*:758-762.

Nawroth, P. P., Bank, I., Handley, D., Cassimeris, J., Chess, L., and Stern, D. (1986). Tumor necrosis factor (cachectin) interacts with endothelial cell receptors to induce release of interleukin 1. *J. Exp. Med. 163*:1363-1375.

Nemecek, G. M., Coughlin, S. R., Handley, D. A., and Moskowitz, M. A. (1986). Stimulation of aortic smooth muscle cell mitogenesis by serotonin. *Proc. Natl. Acad. Sci. USA 83*:674-678.

Oka, Y., and Orth, D. N. (1983). Human plasma epidermal growth factor/β-urogastrone is associated with blood platelets. *J. Clin. Invest. 72*:249-259.

Orlidge, A., and D'Amore, P. A. (1986a). Cell specific effects of glycosaminoglycans on the attachment and proliferation of vascular wall components. *Microvasc. Res. 31*:41-53.

Orlidge, A., and D'Amore, P. A. (1986b). Pericyte and smooth muscle cell modulation of endothelial cell proliferation. *J. Cell. Biol. 103*:471a.

Owens, G. K., and Thompson, M. M. (1986). Developmental changes in isoactin expression in rat aortic smooth muscle cells in vivo. *J. Biol. Chem. 261*: 13373-13380.

Owens, G. K., Loeb, A., Gordon, D., and Thompson, M. M. (1986). Expression of smooth muscle-specific α-isoactin in cultured vascular smooth muscle cells: relationship between growth and cytodifferentiation. *J. Cell Biol. 102*:343-352.

Palombella, V. J., Yamashiro, D.J., Maxfield, F. R., Decker, S. J., and Vilcek, J. (1987). Tumor necrosis factor increases the number of epidermal growth factor receptors on human fibroblasts. *J. Biol. Chem. 262*:1950-1954.

Polverini, P. J., and Leibovich, S. J. (1984). Induction of neovascularization in vivo and endothelial proliferation in vitro by tumor-associated macrophages. *Lab. Invest. 51*:635-642.

Rabinovitch, M., Gamble, W., Nadas, A. S., Miettinen, O. S., and Reid, L. (1979). Rat pulmonary circulation after chronic hypoxia: hemodynamic and structural features. *Am. J. Physiol. 236*:H818-H827.

Rabinovitch, M., Konstam, M., Gamble, W., Papanicolaou, N., Aronovitz, M., Treves, S., and Reid, L. (1983). Changes in pulmonary blood flow affect vascular response to chronic hypoxia in rats. *Circ. Res. 52*:432-441.

Reid, L. (1968). Structural and functional reappraisal of the pulmonary artery system. In *The Scientific Basis of Medicine Annual Reviews*. The Athlone Press, London, pp. 289-307.

Reid, L. (1979). The pulmonary circulation: remodeling in growth and disease. The 1978 J. Burns Amberson Lecture. *Am. Rev. Resp. Dis. 119*:531-546.

Reid, L., and Jones, R. (1987). Damage and repair to pulmonary vasculature and alveolar lining cells. In *Diffuse Alveolar Damage and Respiratory Failure – The Adult Respiratory Distress Syndrome*. Edited by T. Hyers. Futura, Mt. Kisco.

Reid, L., and Meyrick, B. (1982). Microcirculation: definition and organization at tissue level. In *Mechanisms of Lung Microvascular Injury*. Edited by A. B. Malik and N. C. Staub. New York Academy of Science, New York, pp. 3-20.

Reilly, C. F., Fritze, L. M. S., and Rosenberg, R. D. (1987). Antiproliferative effects of heparin on vascular smooth muscle cells are reversed by epidermal growth factor. *J. Cell Physiol.* *131*:149-157.

Rendas, A., and Reid, L. (1983). Pulmonary vasculature of piglets after correction of aorta-pulmonary shunts. *J. Thorac. Cardiovasc. Surg.* *85*:911-916.

Rendas, A., Lennox, S., and Reid, L. (1979). Aorta-pulmonary shunts in growing pigs. Functional and structural assessment of the changes in the pulmonary circulation. *J. Thorac. Cardiovasc. Surg.* *77*:109-118.

Roberts, A. B. (1985). Type β transforming growth factor: a bifunctional regulator of cellular growth. *Proc. Natl. Acad. Sci. USA* *82*:119-123.

Roberts, A. B., Anzano, M. A., Lamb, L. C., Smith, J. M., and Sporn, M. B., (1981). New class of transforming growth factors potentiated by epidermal growth factor: isolation from non-neoplastic tissues. *Proc. Natl. Acad. Sci. USA*, *78*:5339-5343.

Ross, R., Raines, E. W., and Bowen-Pope, D. F. (1986). The biology of pllatelet-derived growth factor. *Cell* *46*:155-169.

Rudolph, A. M., Heymann, M. A., and Lewis, A. B. (1977). Physiology and pharmacology of the pulmonary circulation in the fetus and newborn. In *Development of the Lung*. Edited by W. A. Hodson. Marcel Dekker, New York, pp. 497-523.

Schreiber, A. B., Kenney, J., Kowalski, W. J., Friesel, R., Mehlman, T., and Maciag, T. (1985). Interaction of endothelial cell growth factor with heparin: characterization by receptor and antibody recognition. *Proc. Natl. Acad. Sci. USA* *82*:6138-6142.

Schwartz, S. M., Campbell, G. R., and Campbell, J. H. (1986). Replication of smooth muscle cells in vascular diseases. *Circ. Res.* *58*:427-444.

Seifert, R. A., Schwartz, S. M., and Bowen-Pope, D. F. (1984). Developmentally regulated production of platelet-derived growth-factor-like molecules. *Nature* *311*:669-671.

Shimokado, K., Raines, E. W., Madtes, D. K., Barrett, T. B., Benditt, E. P., and Ross, R., (1985). A significant part of macrophage-derived growth factor consists of at least two forms of PDGF. *Cell* *43*:277-286.

Shipley, G. D., Tucker, R. F., and Moses, H. L. (1985). Type β transforming growth factor/growth inhibitor stimulates entry of monolayer cultures of AKR-2B cells into S phase after a prolonged replicative interval. *Proc. Natl. Acad. Sci. USA 82*:4147-4151.

Shulman, H. M., Gown, A. M., and Nugent, D. J. (1987). Hepatic veno-occlusive disease after bone marrow transplantation. Immunohistochemical identification of material within occluded central vessicles. *Am. J. Pathol. 127*: 549-558.

Shure, D., Swain, J. A., Abraham, J. L., and Moser, K. M. (1984). Pulmonary arterial hypertensive changes distal to a central vascular obstruction in the dog. *Am. Rev. Resp. Dis. 129*:A331.

Shure, D., Dockweiller, D., and Peters, R. M. (1985). Respiratory structure, function, and metabolism: circulation. *Am. Rev. Resp. Dis. 131*:A402.

Stiles, C. D., Capone, G. T., Scher, C. D., Antoniades, H. N. Van Wyk, J. J., and Pledger, W. J. (1979). Dual control of cell growth by somatomedin and platelet-derived growth factor. *Proc. Natl. Acad. Sci. USA 76*:1279-1283.

Takehara, K., LeRoy, E. C., and Grotendorst, G. R. (1987). TGF-β inhibition of endothelial cell proliferation: alteration of EGF binding and EGF-induced growth-regulatory (competence) gene expression. *Cell 49*:415-422.

Teitel, J. M. (1986). Specific inhibition of endothelial cell proliferation by isolated endothelial plasma membranes. *J. Cell Physiol. 128*:329-336.

Thornton, S. C., Mueller, S. N., and Levine, E. M. (1983). Human endothelial cells: use of heparin in cloning and long-term serial cultivation. *Science 222*:623-625.

Thyberg, J., and Fredholm, B. B. (1987). Modulation of arterial smooth muscle cells from contractile to synthetic phenotype requires induction of ornithine decarboxylase activity and polyamine synthesis. *Exp. Cell Res. 170*: 153-159.

Vender, R. L., Clemmons, D. R., Kwock, L., and Friedman, M. (1987). Reduced oxyten tension induces pulmonary endothelium to release a pulmonary smooth muscle cell mitogen(s) *Am. Rev. Resp. Dis. 135*:622-627.

Vlodavsky, I., Folkman, J., Sullivan, R., Fridman, R., Ishai-Michaeli, R., Sasse, J., and Klagsbrun, (1987a). Endothelial cell-derived basic fibroblast growth factor: synthesis and deposition into subendothelial extracellular matrix. *Proc. Natl. Acad. Sci. USA 84*:2292-2296.

Vlodavsky, I., Fridman, R., Sullivan, R., Sasse, J., and Klagsburn, M. (1987b). Aortic endothelial cells synthesize basic fibroblast growth factor which remains cell associated and platelet-derived growth factor-like protein which is secreted. *J. Cell Physiol. 131*:402-408.

Weir, E. K., and Reeves, J. T. (1984). *Pulmonary Hypertension*. Futura, Mount Kisco, NY.

Westermark, B., and Heldin, C.-H. (1985). Similar action of platelet-derived growth factor and epidermal growth factor in the prereplicative phase of human fibroblasts suggests a common intracellular pathway. *J. Cell Physiol.* *124*:43-48.

Yahalom, J., Eldor, A., Fuks, Z., and Vlodavsky, I. (1984). Degradation of sulfated proteoglycans in the subendothelial extracellular matrix by human platelet heparitinase. *J. Clin. Invest.* *74*:1842-1849.

17

The Interaction Between Polymorphonuclear Cells and Pulmonary Endothelium

Normal Kinetics and the Pathogenesis of Acute Lung Injury

JAMES C. HOGG

University of British Columbia
Vancouver, British Columbia, Canada

I. Introduction

The lung has unique anatomic and physiologic features that are important in determining the balance between the forces that tend to move neutrophils through the microvasculature and those that tend to retard them. These features lead to a margination of a considerable number of neutrophils in the pulmonary circulation with the ability to increase or decrease this number under a variety of physiologic circumstances. The forces that determine true adherence of the neutrophil to the endothelial membrane in preparation for migration into the interstitial and air spaces of the lung are probably different from those that determine margination and will be discussed separately.

II. Contact Between PMN and the Endothelial Surface

The surface area provided by the pulmonary arterial tree can be calculated from data of Siam and associates (1973), who used casts of the vascular tree to obtain information on the length, diameter, and volume of its branches. This shows that the total surface area of the arterial tree is approximately 1.4 m^2, and as the venous system has fewer branches the total surface area of both arteries and veins is of the order of 2-3 m^2. When this is compared to the alveolar capillary surface area, which is of the order of 60 m^2, it is obvious that the best opportunity for PMN to come into contact with the endothelium is in the capillary bed. Furthermore, in the large conducting vessels of the arterial and venous trees, the neutrophils travel in the center of a flowing stream and do not have many opportunities to touch the endothelial surface. However, in the alveolar wall, the PMN must come into close contact with the endothelium because their joint mean diameter is larger than many of the capillary segments (Schmid-Schonbein et al., 1980; Weibel, 1963).

In the arterial tree the endothelial cells take the form of elliptical discs with their long axis parallel to the blood flow, while the endothelial cells lining the veins take the shape of polygonal discs with borders that are equal in all directions (Weibel, 1984). The surface of the endothelial cells has many protrusions, and their borders are joined by tight junctions that are thought to decrease in complexity from the arterial to the venous side of the circulation. Crapo and associates (1982) have estimated that the capillary endothelium accounts for 40% of the cells in the parenchyma. They estimate that the total number of endothelial cells in the lung is of the order of $68 \pm 7 \times 10^9$ cells and that the average cell extends over an area of 1353 ± 66 μm^2. Fung and Sobin (1969) have introduced the concept of sheet flow through this surface area, where there would be no definite capillary tubes but rather sheets of endothelium separated by posts. This view may have advantages in terms of the theoretical fluid mechanics of blood flow, but there is abundant anatomic evidence that the pulmonary capillary bed is made up of short tubular segments that look like intersecting circular cylinders (Fig. 1). Weibel (1963) has estimated that there are approximately 277×10^9 of these capillary segments contained in 296×10^6 alveoli, which means approximately 1000 segments per alveolus. His data also show that these segments range from 1 to 30 μm in length with a mean of 8 μm and from 1 to 15 μm in width with a mean of 5 μm. Using his raw data on individual segment length and diameter, it is possible to calculate that each segment has a mean volume of about 300 μm^3, which when multiplied by the total number of segments yields a volume of about 85 ml, which compares favorably with the measured capillary blood volumes in humans (R. L. Johnson et al., 1960).

Staub and Schultz (1968) reported that the distance from the arterial to the venous end of the capillary bed was of the order of 880 μm with a range of 200-1600 μm with little variation between species such as the cat, rabbit, and dog. They also showed that these pathways crossed an average of seven different alveoli and 14 alveolar walls. If the average capillary segment length is 8 μm and the average pathway from artery to vein approximately 800 μm (Staub and Schultz, 1968), the cells must pass through approximately 100 of the segments

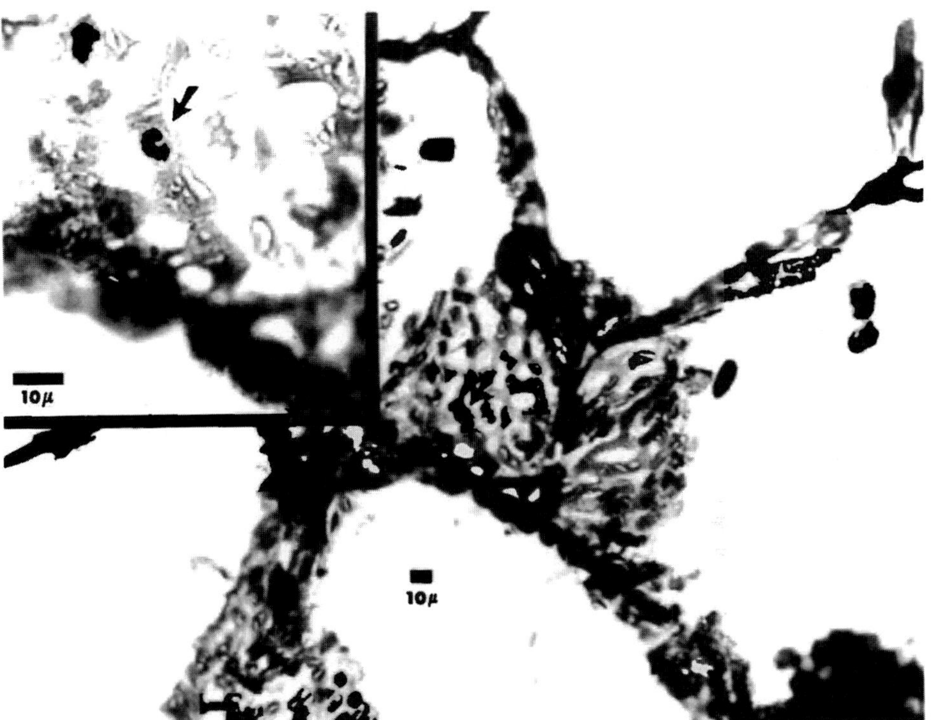

Figure 1 A histological section of a human lung cut 40 μm thick; the alveolar wall and capillary segments can be seen on face. The arrow points to a polymorphonuclear cell within a capillary segment, and the inset shows this area at higher magnification. The large number of parallel pathways provided by the segments allow erythrocytes to stream around segments occupied by neutrophils. From Hogg 1987 with permission.

shown in Figure 1. As there is a discrepancy between neutrophil and segment diameter (Schmid-Schonbein et al., 1980; Weibel, 1963), it is obvious that the neutrophil must deform and that there must be intimate contact between the neutrophil and endothelial membranes during the journey of cells through the capillary bed.

Cartwright et al (1964) have estimated that the marginal granulocyte pool in humans is approximately 40 X 10^7 cells/kg or 280 X 10^8 cells in a 70 kg person. This means that even if the entire marginal pool of neutrophils were in the lung and there were one marginating cell per capillary segment, these cells would occupy only about 10% of the 277 X 10^9 capillary segments that are available. Assuming a cardiac output of 5 liters/min (84 ml/sec) and a neutro-

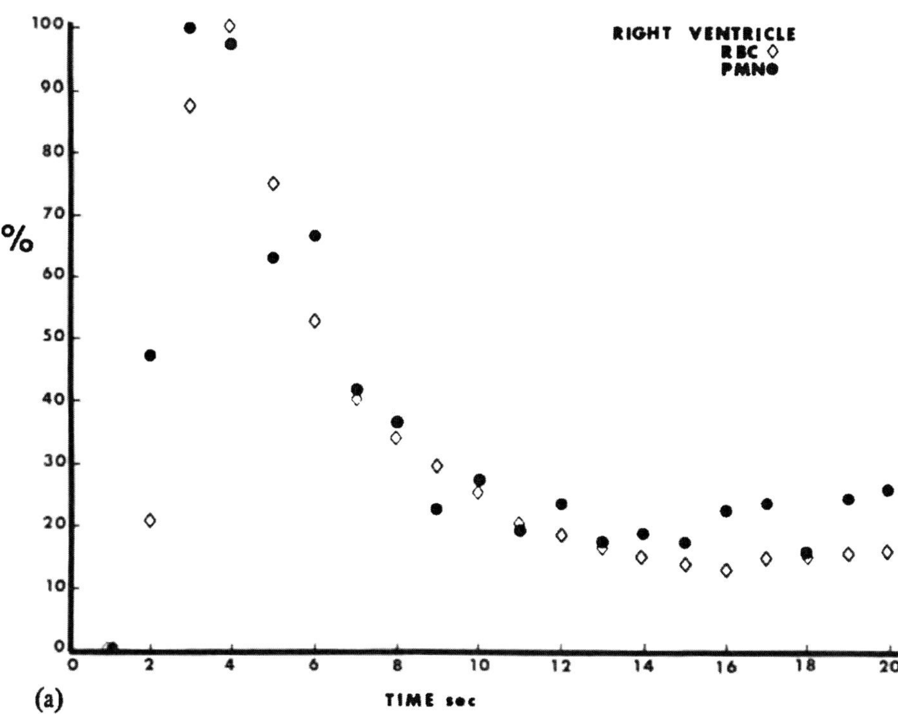

Figure 2 Data collected using a gamma camera to image the right ventricle and lung (a) and lung (b) after a bolus of labeled red cells and neutrophils was injected into the venous circulation. Note that the cells stay together in the right ventricle and that the WBC are delayed in the lung. (Reproduced from Muir et al., 1984, with permission of authors and publishers.)

phil count of 5 X 10^6 cells/ml, there are approximately 420 X 10^6 PMN delivered to the pulmonary microvessels each second. Only some of these will find pathways made up of large segments that will let them pass without delay; others will be forced through pathways with narrow segments, where they will be delayed. Studies in humans (Muir et al., 1984) using the indicator dilution technique with labeled PMN and erythrocytes have shown that in an upright awake person 10-20% of the labeled neutrophils injected fail to negotiate the pulmonary microvascular bed in the same time as labeled erythrocytes they were injected with. For reasons that are not clear, this figure is much higher in anesthetized supine dogs, where 80% of the PMN are removed in the first pass through the pulmonary circulation (Martin et al., 1982). Figure 2 shows that the PMN take longer than RBC to negotiate the capillary bed, presumably because they are forced to squeeze through capillary segments that are

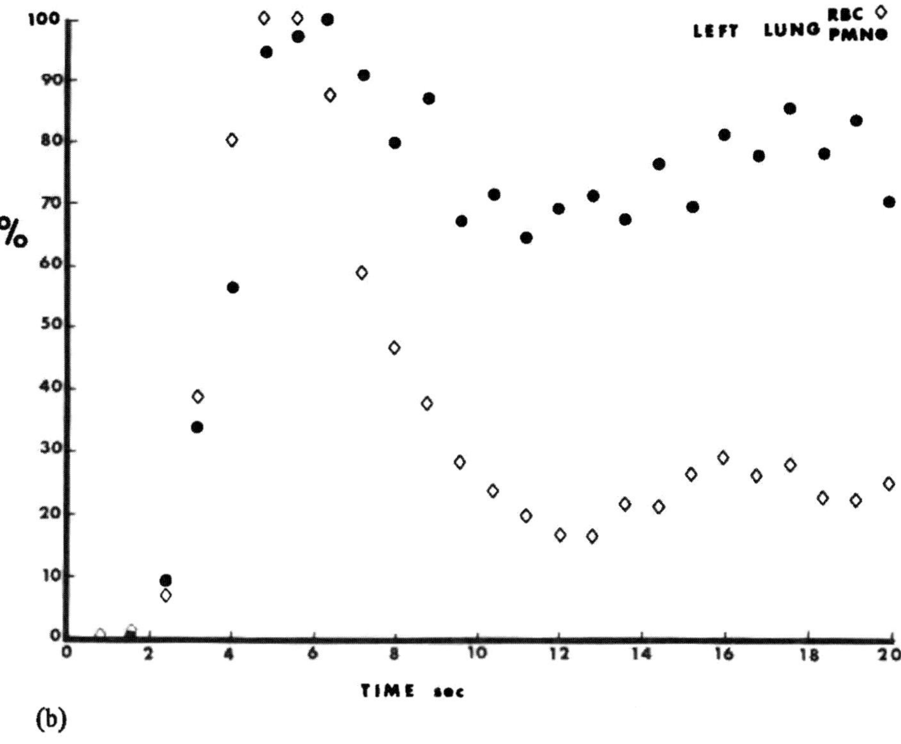

(b)

narrower than they are. If for the sake of argument we say that all of 280 X 10_8 cells estimated to be in the marginated pool were in the lung and 80% of the 420 X 19_6 cells delivered each second were forced to seqeeze into the arterial end of the capillary network with an equal number squeezing out of the venous end, the turnover would be (3.36 X 10_8)/(280 X 10_8), or 1.2% of the pool turning over each second.

If there are 280 X 10^8 neutrophils squeezing through the lung microvasculature at any moment and this bed is made up of 68 X 10^9 endothelial cells (Charo et al., 1985), there would be about one neutrophil for every two endothelial cells. Although these numbers are approximate, they show in a general way that there are fewer neutrophils than endothelial cells in the normal lung. Furthermore, the segmental nature of the capillary network (Fig. 1) allows it to accommodate a large pool of neutrophils that pass through the microvasculature much more slowly than erythocytes without interefering with erythrocyte flow.

III. Interaction Between PMN and Endothelium

Chien (1985) has calculated that the neutrophil has a surface area 84% in excess of that required to hold its cytoplasm in a sphere. This excess surface area allows the neutrophils to deform to minimum diameters of about 2.6 μm, which means that they are able to negotiate the smallest capillary segments. He has also shown that the pressure required to force neutrophils through polycarbonate filters with a fixed pore size is much greater than that required for erythrocytes and has attributed this to the relative viscosities of the cytoplasm of these two types of cells. The fact that the neutrophil deforms more slowly than the red cell and has greater difficulty in entering capillary tubes has also been elegantly shown by Evans (1984). Furthermore, they found that activation of the cell decreases the cell deformability and slows the entry process further. The forces that push neutrophils through the capillary segments after they have entered them include the hydrostatic pressure gradient across the capillary bed and the wall shear rate, which is determined by the velocity of the blood and the diameter of the vessel. When a PMN is stuck in a capillary segment, the adhesive shear stress acts over the wall contact area. The forces that must overcome this adherence include the pressure drop across the capillary segment and the velocity of the neutrophil as it hits the restriction. This reduction in velocity is associated with a loss in kinetic energy by the neutrophil and may account for the good relationship between neutrophil turnover in the marginated pool and blood flow and transit time (Martin et al., 1982, 1987; Deerschuk et al., 1987).

The flow of blood in the lung microvessels has been studied directly in several species by transilluminating the edge of the lung and observing it with a microscope (Hall, 1925; MacGregor, 1933; Wearn et al., 1928). The ejection of the right ventricle into the pulmonary artery is accommodated by both flow through the capillary bed and distention of the arterial tree where the elastic conducting arteries discharge the stored blood into the capillaries during diastole. As early as 1925, Hall (1925) reported that there was backward movement of the bloodstream between heart beats when the heart rate was slowed by vagal stimulation. More recent studies (Harris and Heath, 1977; Lee and DuBois, 1955; Wasserman et al., 1966) have shown that flow through the capillaries is pulsatile, with a major systolic wave followed by a dicrotic notch and dicrotic wave. These observations suggest that there are considerable shear forces acting to separate PMN from the endothelial membrane in the microvessels and that these forces vary in intensity during the cardiac cycle.

The geometry of the vascular bed can be altered in other ways to change the resistance that a neutrophil encounters as it passes through the capillaries. The microvascular bed is compressed during a vascular maneuver because capillary blood volume decreases and transit time falls (Johnson et al., 1960) and there is an accumulation of neutrophils in the lungs (Bierman et al., 1952).

This suggests that a change in microvessel geometry brought about by compression could lead to greater PMN retention by the microvasculature.

Burton's (Burton, 1951; Nichol et al., 1951) concept of critical closure is relevant to the issue of vascular geometry, because he argued that vessels with tone would close at a positive pressure due to the Laplace law. He used this concept to explain observations in the systemic circulation that showed that vessels that are wide open and rigid at high pressures become unstable at pressures of about 10 cmH_2O and close at a positive pressure that he called the critical closing pressure. Permutt and colleagues (Permutt and Riley, 1963; Permutt et al., 1969) applied this idea to the lung and suggested that muscle tone in the pulmonary arterioles could lead to derecruitment of the alveolar vessels by a similar mechanism. This argument suggests that neutrophils might be trapped in the microvascular bed if the pressure in the arterioles falls below the critical closing pressure. Studies performed by Glazier et al. (1969) showed that recruitment of new vessels was the predominant method of increasing blood volume in zone II and explansion of fully recruited vessels was the main mechanism of expanding blood volume in zone III. Perlo and associates (1975) measured the number of white blood cells and red blood cells in the microvascular bed of lungs frozen rapidly under known physiological conditions. They found that most of the WBC were mononuclear, presumably because they were using an isolated blood-perfused lung where neutrophils may have been removed by the pumps and tubing. They found that there were many WBC in the capillaries at low perfusing pressures and that increasing perfusion decreased their number. They concluded that the lung could act as a mechanical sieve but thought that the reduction in number of WBC retained with greater delivery due to increased flow was a paradox. More recent studies of local lung regions (B. A. Martin et al., 1982, 1987) have confirmed the decreased retention of neutrophils with increased flow, which suggests that the paradox is resolved by the fact that greater blood velocities lead to increased shear forces and faster neutrophil movement through the microvasculature.

Staub and associates' (1982) study of sheep lungs showed that the greatest number of PMN were in the alveolar microvessels and that the next greatest excess of neutrophils was in the arterioles. This further supports the concept that the cells pile up on the arterial side of the capillary bed due to their difficulty in squeezing into the smallest microvessels. Recent studies from our laboratory by Dorschuk and associates (1987) have shown that when the ratio of PMN to RBC in peripheral blood is compared to that observed in arteries, extra-alveolar vessels, and alveolar vessels of rabbits, the greatest increase occurs in the alveolar capillaries. From these data and knowledge of the capillary blood volume it was possible to calculate that there are about three times as many cells marginated in the alveolar vessels of the lung as there are circulating in the systemic vasculature. This value is similar to Staub's calculation in sheep and suggests that the capillary bed can accommodate large numbers of cells. As greater pressures are required to move the PMN through filters (Chien, 1985) and into capillary tubes (Evans, 1984), one might expect that the arterial pressure would rise if large numbers of white cells were forced through the pulmonary microvascular bed. However, this problem is avoided in the pulmonary capillary bed because the network of capillary segments (Fig. 1) allows large numbers of neutrophils to be accommodated without interfering with the majority of the available pathways. The occupation of a capillary segment by a neutrophil should have little effect on the pressure drop across it because of the large number of open parallel pathways surrounding it. If the movement of the cell through the segment is not determined by the pressure drop across it, the next greatest source of energy is the kinetic energy of the neutrophil. This is determined by its velocity as it hits the restriction, and a rapid decrease in the cell's kinetic energy could make the cell more deformable it it activated the cytoskeleton.

Velocity can be estimated if the transit time and the average length of the microvessels are known. Staub and Schultz (1968) found a great variation in the length of the pathway from arteries to veins in the lung, but this variation in pathway length was quite similar in different regions of the lungs of several species. Wagner and associates (1982) have made direct measurements of transit time through capillaries on the surface of the lung and showed that it varied considerably but averaged 12.7 ± 3 sec. We (Hogg et al., 1985) have also measured transit times using a different technique and found a mean of 2.86 ± 0.31 sec for the entire pulmonary circulation. This technique allows the transit time of the deeper regions of the lung to be measured, and we found that some of the transit times are as long as those that Wagner et al. observed on the lung surface. Both Wagner's (1982) studies and ours (Hogg et al., 1985) showed that the transit times were greater in the upper regions of dog lungs, and if the capillary pathway length is the same (Staub and Schultz, 1968) the longer transit times mean that the velocity of blood is slower through upper lung regions. Figure 3 shows the relationship between PMN retention and red cell transit times in different lung regions that was obtained by Martin and associates in our laboratory (Martin et al., 1987). This shows that there is an increase in PMN retention as red cell velocity slows and supports the concept that the kinetic energy of the PMN may determine their rate of passage through the microvasculature; it also shows that there is slower turnover in the upper lung regions where transit times are long and velocity slow.

The introduction of modern imaging techniques has led to a large number of studies using labeled cells to study physiological and pathological processes in the body. These investigations have confirmed many of the older studies concerning the distribution of the neutrophils and in addition have provided some new information about neutrophil kinetics. Most studies have shown that

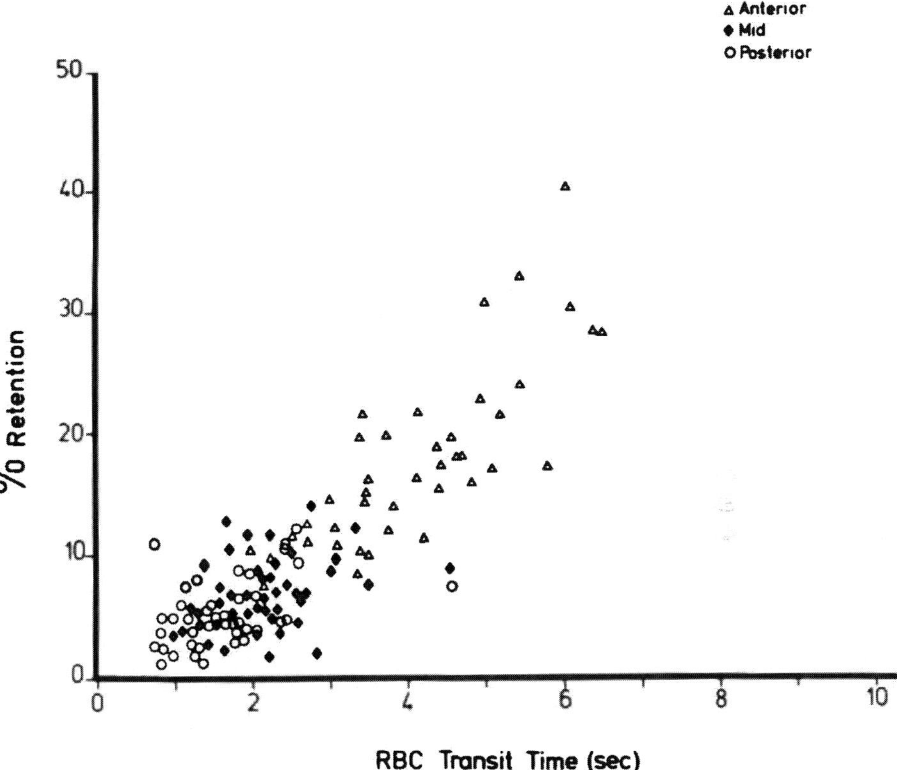

Figure 3 Relationship between red blood cell transit time and neutrophil retention in dog lungs. Note that there is greater retention with longer transit times, which are inversely related to blood velocity. These data show that as velocity slows there is a slower turnover, leading to greater retention of neutrophils. The symbols indicate different lung regions and show there is greater retention and slower neutrophil turnover in the upper lung regions (i.e., the anterior regions in this supine animal). (Reproduced from Martin et al., 1987, with permission of authors and publishers.)

the PMN injected into the venous circulation are delayed in the lung to varying degrees (Martin et al., 1982; Muir et al., 1984; Saverymuttu et al., 1983), with gradual accumulation in the liver and spleen, thus confirming studies carried out near the turn of the century. The controversy over whether the initial accumulation in the lung is fact or an artifact dependent on labeling techniques has been discussed by Saverymuttu et al. (1983). They described a number of different types of kinetics where there was either a substantial or very little accumulation

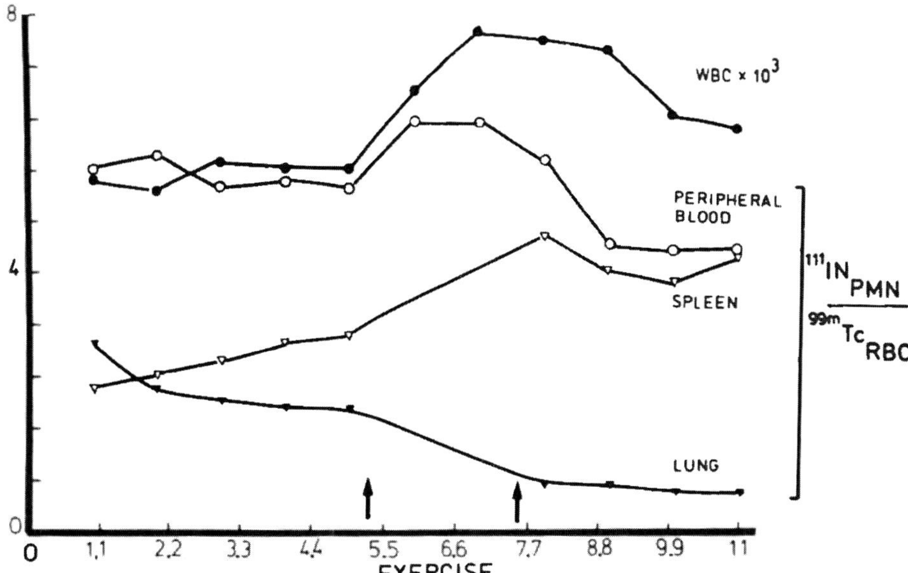

Figure 4 Data collected over the spleen and lung with a gamma camera and samples of peripheral blood. Note that the rise in the peripheral WBC count during exercise is associated with the fall in counts over the lung and an increase over the spleen. (Reproduced from the data of Muir et al., 1984, with permission of authors and publishers.)

of PMN in the lung. Muir et al.'s study (1984) using the oxine method of labeling showed that about 20% of the cells were removed in the first pass through the human pulmonary circulation (Fig. 2). Based on the anatomic arguments put forward earlier, this extraction is consistent with the estimate of the number of capillary segments that impede PMN as they pass through the pulmonary circulation.

The fact that stimuli such as exercise cause a demargination of cells has been clearly demonstrated (Ahlborg and Ahlborg, 1970; Foster et al., 1986). Muir and associates (1984) have shown (Fig. 4) that exercise increases the number of labeled PMN in the blood at the same time that it decreases the number in the lung, providing direct evidence for demargination from the pulmonary circulation. Blood velocity increases during exercise because the transit time falls (Johnson et al., 1960) while vessel length remain the same. This increase in velocity and shear forces must shorten the transit time of the PMN through the microvessels. It is also possible that the catecholamines released during exercise make the PMN more deformable so that they can enter capillary segments more easily and/or decrease the friction between the endothelial and PMN membranes. In a very interesting study, Ahlborg and Ahlborg (1970) showed that adrenergic blockade prevented the rise in WBC count seen during exercise, which suggests that adrenergic receptor activity might play a role in lowering the interaction between the PMN and endothelial cells. However, they failed to measure cardiac output in these studies, and more recent work on this topic (Foster et al., 1986) showed no effect of beta blockade on the rise in neutrophil count during exercise when differences in cardiac output were taken into account. A study of the pulmonary AV difference of unlabeled PMN in animals (Thommassen et al., 1984a) showed that PMN accumulated in the lung when pulmonary blood flow was decreased and returned to the circulation when flow was restored. These data also suggest that the force generated by increasing blood velocity is more important than the AV pressure drop in demarginating PMN because blood flow can change considerably in healthy young subjects without changing the driving pressure in the pulmonary circulation.

IV. Migration of Neutrophils into the Interstitium and Air Space of the Lung

In spite of the fact that so many PMN marginate in the pulmonary microvessels, few neutrophils are found in the interstitium of normal lung (Weibel, 1984). Bronchoalveolar lavage performed on normal nonsmoking subjects (Harris et al., 1970; Hunninghake et al., 1979) yields about 10×10^6 cells, 90-95% being macrophages, which shows that macrophages but not neutrophils normally cross the microvascular and epithelial barrier. However, when the PMN are activated, as for example in pneumococcal pneumonia (Dunnill, 1982), they can migrate into the interstitium and air spaces in large numbers. Monocytes, on the other hand, are said to have no significant marginated pool in the lung (Harlan, 1985), yet they are able to traverse the endothelium, enter the interstitium, multiply, and cross the epithelium into the air space in great numbers to function as macrophages (Fels and Cohn, 1986). This significant difference between the monocytes and nuetrophils even though both cell types originate in the bone marrow and share the function of phagocytosis is intriguing. It seems possible that the adherence and migration of cells into the interstitium is controlled by receptor-mediated surface phenomena that are very different from the physical forces that determine margination of the PMN in the microvessels.

The introduction of endothelial cell culture techniques (Jaffe et al., 1973; Jaffe, 1983) made it possible to study directly the interaction of neutrophils with endothelial cells. Although the vast literature that has developed in this area of study cannot be reviewed in detail, some important points need to be emphasized. Hoover and associates (Hoover et al., 1978; Hoover and Karnovsky, 1982) were among the first to show that neutrophils have a definite preference for endothelial cells compared to a wide variety of other types of cultured cells. This preferential adherence was demonstrated by plating the cell type they were testing onto cover slips and allowing them to adhere and divide. Prior to these cultures reaching confluence, neutrophils were added and allowed to adhere to either the cells or the intervening surface of the cover slip. The cover slips were then fixed and prepared for examination in the scanning electron microscope so that the numbers of cells adhering to the surface covered by cultured cells could be compared to the number adhering to the glass surface. In this way they compared the adherence of neutrophils to different cell types and showed that the neutrophils had a preference for endothelial cells. They also modified another experimental approach first described by Walther and associates (1973) that involves labeling the cells with ^{51}Cr and incubating them in wells containing cultured endothelial cells that had grown to confluence. After a final incubation period the wells are washed and the percentage of the chromium that remains attached to the endothelium is calculated. Charo and associates (1985) developed a method that uses centrifugal force to quantitate the adherence between PMN and endothelial cells. After an incubation period during which the labeled neutrophils come into contact with endothelial cells, the plates are sealed, inverted, and centrifuged and the number of neutrophils that could not be separated from the endothelium by centrifugal force is calculated.

These types of experiments have shown that neutrophils adhere preferentially to endothelial cells and that this adherence requires the presence of divalent cations and is enhanced by diminishing the surface charge on the cells (Gallin et al., 1979; Gallin, 1980; Oseas et al., 1981). It has also been shown (Moldow, 1984) that the adherence is influenced by temperature and enhanced by chemotactic peptides such as *N*-formyl-methionyl-leucyl-phenylalanine (FMLP), and by complement-derived proteins such as C5a. Boxer and associates (1980) have shown that treating endothelial cells with epinephrine reduced the adherence of neutrophils to them, while direct stimulation of the neutrophil with the same drug did not. They postulated that the rise in cyclic AMP in the endothelial cell mediated the lowered adherence of PMN.

V. Receptor-Mediated Neutrophil Adherence

The description of abnormal leukocyte function in patients that have neutrophils that are deficient in a cell-associated glycoprotein has led to considerable interest in their function as receptors for neutrophil adherence (Burns et al., 1986; Todd and Arnaout, 1984; Todd et al., 1984). Neutrophils express three related membrane glycoproteins that have been shown to have important functions in both adherence events with endothelial cells and phagocytosis of bacteria (Ross, 1986; Springer and Anderson, 1985). Each of the three proteins contains a structural identical β-chain of 95,000 Mw which is noncovantly linked to one of three structurally distinct α-chains (Sanchez-Madrid et al., 1983). The first of these proteins was originally defined by monoclonal antibodies as the Mac-1/OKM1 antigen, and this protein is identical to membrane complement receptor type 3 (CR_3 or the iC3b receptor), a major phagocyte receptor for opsonic C3 fragments (Ross and Medof, 1985). The α-chain of the Mac-a/CR_3 molecule is 165,000 Mw. The other two proteins are known as LFA-1 (lymphocyte function-associated antigen 1) and p150,95 and have α-chains of 175,000 and 150,000 Mw, respectively (Sanchez-Madrid et al., 1983). As a group, these three glycoproteins have been designated the CD18 complex by the Second International Workshop on Leukocyte Differentiation Antigens. [Note added in proof: The Third International Workshop of leukocyte differentiation antigens has called the common β chain CD18 (the w being removed because it is now established rather than working). LFA-1 is now referred to as CD11a,Mac1OKM is now referred to as CD11b and P150,95 as CD11c (McMichael et al., 1987).] The neutrophils express primarily Mac-1/CR_3 and little LFA-1 an p250,95, whereas monocytes express approximately equal amounts of the three glycoproteins and lymphocytes primarily express LFA-1 a and very little Mac-1/CR_3 or p150,95. The Mac-1/CR_3 molecule appears to be the most important for neutrophil adherence to endothelial cells (Springer and Anderson, 1985), whereas the other two proteins have only been shown to function in the ingestion of certain bacteria or yeast (Bullock and Wright, 1987; Klebanoff et al., 1985; Ross et al., 1985; Wright and Jong, 1986). A group of patients have been identified who lack all three proteins on their neutrophils as the result of an inherited deficiency in the gene encoding the common β-chain shared by each of the glycoprotein family members (Marlin et al., 1986). These patients are characterized by recurrent bacterial infections beginning in early childhood. Studies of their neutrophils in vitro have shown a severe abnormality in functions requiring adherence as well as abnormalities in phagocytosis, respiratory burst, and bactericidal activity. There is also a clear abnormality in the ability of neutrophils to infiltrate inflammatory sites. Treatment of normal neutrophils with monoclonal antibodies to the α-chain of Mac-1/CR_3 reproduces all of the abnormal functions observed with the patients' cells (Ross, 1986; Springer and Anderson, 1985). Furthermore, treatment of rabbits with such monoclonal antibodies has been shown to reduce the adherence functions of neutrophils in vivo. By contrast, a similar inhibition of neutrophil functions is not produced with monoclonal antibodies directed to the α-chains of LFA-1 or p150,95. An exception is monoclonal antibody 60.3, which is specific for the common β-chain shared by each of three proteins and has been reported to block adherence function, CR_3 C3-receptor activity, phagocytosis of *Staphylococcus aureus*, and LFA-a-dependent lymphocyte functions that may be linked to any one of the individual members of CDW 18. Very recent studies (Arfors et al., 1987) in rabbits have also shown that pretreatment with MoAb 60.3 can inhibit PMN accumulation and plasma leakage in injured skin. The data gathered indicate an important role for Mac-1/CR_3 in mediating neutrophil adherence. Normal blood neutrophils express little Mac-1/CR_3 on the cell surface until stimulated with chemotactic factors (e.g., C5a, fMLP) (Arnaout et al., 1984), and normal endothelial cells do not allow avid attachment of neutrophils via CR_3 without stimulation with endotoxin, IL-1, or tumor necrosis factor (Pohlman et al., 1986). The ligand for Mac-1/CR_3 expressed by IL-1-stimulated endothelial cells is unknown. These data suggest that the CDω18 complex is responsible for the enhanced adherence between PMN to endothelial cell membranes when either the endothelial cell or the PMN is stimulated. Because this Mac-1/CR_3-dependent adherence requires activation of cells by inflammatory agents, it is very unlikely to be the mechanism that explains the normal retention of marginating neutrophils in the pulmonary blood vessels. Indeed, the inflammatory stimuli that produce Mac-1/CR_3-dependent adherence are also associated with release of the marginating pool of neutrophils. Therefore it seems likely that the adherence of PMN to endothelial cells that is mediated by these glycoproteins is different than the PMN-endothelial cell interactions associated with neutrophil margination. It is possible that physical events such as the difficulty that PMN experience in entering the capillary segment and the friction that develops between the endothelial and PMN membranes determine margination whereas biochemical events involving surface proteins are important in developing true adherence between the PMN and endothelial cell membranes. The separation of margination of neutrophils from true adherence and migration would explain why local lung injury can induce margination in the entire lung while limiting adherence and migration of neutrophils to the site of injury.

VI. Control of Neutrophil-Endothelial Interactions

There is considerable eveidence that the adenyl cyclase system functions as the second messenger for many of the stimulants that produce adherence, migration, and phagocytosis. Recent evidence suggests that the receptor system for adenyl cyclase consists of at least three types of protein embedded in the lipids of the plasma membrane. Receptors for activating agents such as β-adrenergic agonists appear to interact with a pair of guanine nucleotide-binding proteins that mediate either stimulation (Gs) or inhibition (Gi) of adenyl cyclase activity. Gs has an oligomeric structure with 45,000 and 35,000 dalton subunits, and Gi has a similar structure with 41,000 and 35,000 D subunits. These two proteins regulate the activity of adenyl cyclase, which catalyzes the conversion of ATP to cAMP. These regulatory proteins are influenced by bacterial toxins (Gierschik et al., 1986; Goldman et al., 1985; Holian, 1986; Molski et al., 1984; Volip, 1985), and many investigators have taken advantage of the inhibitory functions of the toxins to study cell function. The 41,000 D subunit of Gi apparently serves the role of the anti-inhibitor of adenyl cyclase activity. Therefore, interference with this protein leads to inhibition of the conversion of ATP to cAMP and an inability to become activated.

Becker and associates (Becker et al., 1986; Shefeyk et al., 1985) have recently reviewed the use of pertussis toxin as a probe in the steps leading to neutrophil activation. They showed that treating the neutrophils with pertussis toxin causes a time- and concentration-dependent inhibition of several neutrophil functions that are normally induced by FMLP, C5a, leukotriene B_4 (LTB_4), and platelet-activating factor. This inhibition correlates with NAD ribosylation of the 41,000 D subunit of the regulatory protein Gi in the neutrophil plasma membrane. This finding is of interest for several reasons. The GTP-binding protein Gi is coupled to agonist-induced receptor-mediated activation of phospholipase C, which then generates two important second messengers from inositol phospholipids. The first, inositol 1,4,5-triphosphate, appears to be responsible for the release of calcium from intracellular stores, and the second, diacyl glycerol, leads to protein kinase C activation (Coussens et al., 1986). Pertussis toxin inhibits the formation of both products but does not affect the neutrophil functions induced by the phorbol esters that stimulate protein kinase C directly (Coussens et al., 1986; Parker et al., 1986). Pertussis toxin treatment inhibits chemotaxis (Bradford and Rubin 1985; Spangrude et al., 1985) and prevents the release of arachidonic acid caused by chemotactic activation of the PMN (Bokoch and Gilman, 1984). The prevention of arachidonate release presumably results from the failure of the intracellular calcium and/or diacyl glycerol to rise and activate phospholipase A_2. These new data on the function of the guanine nucleotide binding proteins are providing insights into the control of neutrophil function. It now seems likely that processes involving adherence and migration of the cell as well as the release of granular enzymes during phagocytosis are regulated separately. Increased knowledge about these regulatory steps is of obvious importance in understanding how the cells are motivated to first move to a site of injury and then engulf and destroy the foreign material that they find there. It is possible that a failure to properly control the sequence of adherence, migration, and phagocytosis during an inflammatory reaction could result in tissue damage rather than protection.

VIII. Pulmonary Edema due to Damaged Microvasculature (ARDS)

The study of severely traumatized patients during and after both world wars, the Korean conflict, and the Vietnam War showed that pulmonary edema could cause hypoxemia and death even when the initial injury had not involved the thorax. The syndrome of hypoxemic respiratory failure following severe trauma was given a wide variety of eponyms that included traumatic massive collapse (Bradford, 1919; Pasteur, 1914), traumatic wet lung (Burford and Burbank, 1945), congestive atelectasis (Jenkins et al., 1950), shock lung, and Danang lung (Martin et al., 1969). The eponyms reflect an awareness of the problem around the time of World War 1 (Bradford, 1919; Pasteur, 1914), World War II (Burford and Burbank, 1945), the Korean conflict (Jenkins et al., 1950), and the Vietnam War (Martin et al., 1969), respectively. Subsequently, it became apparent that this form of respiratory failure was seen as a complication of several pathological processes (Ashbaugh et al., 1967), with generalized sepsis and severe trauma featured primarily in most series (Pepe et al., 1982; Thommasen et al., 1984b). The lung injury found in these diverse clinical settings is now recognized to be fairly stereotyped and is referred to as the adult respiratory distress syndrome (ARDS).

In discussing the pathogenesis of ARDS, it is useful to separate the events into the preclinical and clinical stages (Hogg, 1983). The clinical phase can then be further divided into the acute events, where the pathologic changes in the lung are collectively referred to as diffuse alveolar damage (Katzenstein, 1982; Pratt et al., 1979), and the later events, which are dominated by the deposition of connective tissue (Katzenstein, 1982; Pratt et al., 1979). It seems likely that very important events occur in the interval between the insult such as severe trauma and the later onset of pulmonary edema and hypoxemic respiratory failure. When hypoxemic respiratory failure occurs, the acute changes in the lung include hemorrhagic edema, hyaline membrane formation, and acute inflammation, whereas the later stage correlates with the slow inexorable deposition of connective tissue that often results in death with dense fibrosis of the lung (Pratt et al., 1979). These stages correlate with the events that follow tissue injury in any site (Florey, 1962) where fluid and cellular exudation from the vascular into the interstitial space occurs with the later organization of this exudate by proliferation of connective tissue and the deposition of collagen (Hogg, 1983; Pratt et al., 1979).

The stereotyped nature of the response suggests that although the clinical setting in which ARDS develops is diverse, there is a final common pathway of endothelial and epithelial injury leading to hemorrhagic edema and extravascular coagulation with hyaline membrane formation within a few days. The latent interval between the initial insult and the onset of edema must reflect the time it takes to overcome the normal mechanisms that protect the lung against edema. These have been reviewed elsewhere (Levine et al., 1967; Staub, 1974, 1978) and include changes in the Starling forces, an increase in the lung's lymphatic drainage, and an increased interstitial storage capacity due to lung inflation. The degree of protein and red cell content in the exudate reflects the severity of the injury to the alveolocapillary membrane, and studies in both animals and humans show that both the epithelium and endothelium are disrupted. The deposition of fibrin is a result of extravascular coagulation of the fibrinogen that has escaped from the plasma, and this may occur in an attempt to seal the leaks in the alveolocapillary membrane (Dvorak et al., 1985; Montaner et al., 1987). The entrapment of cellular debris, protein, and even foreign material in this fibrin mesh results in the fomation of hyaline membranes.

The observation that leukopenia occurred during hemodialysis in patients with renal failure (Kaplow and Goffinet, 1968) led to the popular hypothesis that neutrophils might be responsible for ARDS. Craddock and associates (Craddock et al., 1977a, b) showed that the pulmonary leukostasis and systemic leukopenia in dialysis patients was associated with complement activation. The same group also showed that when pulmonary sequestration of PMN was induced in sheep (Hammerschmidt et al., 1980) there was an increased lymph flow and protein clearance, suggesting a microvascular leak. The possibility that the measurements of complement activation or neutrophil disappearance might predict the impending onset of ARDS prior to the development of florid edema has been studied in different laboratories (Hammerschmidt et al., 1980; Weinberg et al., 1984), with one study producing evidence in support of the concept (Hammerschmidt et al., 1980) and others producing evidence against it (Weinberg et al., 1984). It now seems clear that complment activation, pulmonary sequestration of PMN, and systemic leukopenia all can be observed during the development of ARDS but that there must be some additional as yet unrecognized factor that is important in initiating the injury.

A great many models of lung microvascular injury have been used to study the pathogenesis of ARDS. These include the infusion of oleic acid (Derks and Jacobovitz-Derks, 1977), pseudomonas organisms (Brigham et al., 1974), endotoxin (Brigham et al., 1979), monocrotoline (Miller et al., 1978), glass beads (Malik and van der Zee, 1978), and air (Ohkuda et al., 1981). Other studies have provided evidence of lung injury following the direct activation of the complement system by the injection of zymosan-activated plasma (Saunders et al., 1980) or cobra venom (A. Johnson et al., 1984) or by activating the granulocytes using phorbol myristate acetate (PMA) (K. J. Johnson and Ward, 1982; Loyd et al., 1983; Shasby et al., 1982). These models have allowed the nature of these microvascular injuries to be studied in a way that could test the hypothesis that the neutrophils are responsible for damaging the endothelium. For example, Heflin and Brigham (1981) have shown that granulocyte depletion prevented the lung injury produced by endotoxin in sheep, arguing for the possibility that the complement activation results in active complement components that stimulate neutrophils to damage the lung. Flick et al. (1981) and Johnson and Malik (1980) have also shown that granulocyte depletion prevented lung injury following microembolism by air (Flick et al., 1981) or glass beads (Johnson and Malik, 1980), respectively. On the other hand, Julien and co-workers (1986) failed to show that PMN depletion had any effect on oleic acid-induced injury, and Dyer and Snapper (1986) have recently shown that the lung injury induced by high concentrations of PMA was not dependent on neutrophils. These studies clearly show that neutrophil activation is not a universal cause of ARDS even though activated neutrophils are found in the injured lung tissue.

Several studies have implicated neutrophil-derived oxygen radicals as a cause of the damage to the alveolocapillary membrane in ARDS (K. J. Johnson et al., 1981; K. J. Johnson and Ward, 1981; W. J. Martin et al., 1981; Sacks et al., 1978). Ward and colleagues (Till et al., 1982; Ward et al., 1983) have investigated this mechanism in rats, using cobra venom to produce lung injury. They showed that cobra venom injection produces complement activation, neutrophil accumulation in the lung capillaries, and evidence of an increased residue of labeled albumin after perfusion of the circulation with saline. The authors interpret these findings as evidence that there is increased vascular permeability that is induced by oxygen radicals. This interpretation is based on the fact that they were able to abolish or reduce the albumin sequestration in the lung by maneuvers that prevent free radical formation. In larger animals, Ohkuda and colleagues have shown that the injection of air causes an acute lung injury (Ohkuda et al., 1981), and workers from the same laboratory have shown that this injury can be prevented by either leukocyte depletion (Flick et al., 1981) or treatment with superoxide dismutase (Flick et al., 1983). Shasby and associates (1983) have implicated the generation of free radicals by PMN as a possible cause of the lung injury induced by phorbol myristate acetate (PMA). They used PMA to stimulate the neutrophils in vitro or in isolated perfused lungs and obtained evidence consistent with endothelial injury. This differs from the recent reports in sheep (Dyer and Snapper, 1986), where the phorbol ester did not have this effect. The recent demonstration (Parker et al., 1986) that protein kinase C acts as a receptor for the phorbol ester molecule is of interest to this controversy. The phorbol ester activates neutrophils by a pathway that is independent of receptors for compounds such as LTB4, FMLP, and C5a that use the G proteins and the cyclic AMP system as second messengers. As phorbol esters will affect the function of any cell containing protein kinase C, it is possible that they cause lung injury by stimulating cells other than neutrophils.

The hypothesis that the lung injury observed in ARDS is due to an imbalance between proteolytic enzymes released from the neutrophil and its inhibitors has also been tested. McGuire, Lee, and Cochrane and their associates (McGuire et al., 1982; Lee et al., 1981; Cochrane et al., 1983) showed that the BAL fluid obtained from patients in an ARDS setting contained neutrophil elastase that was either bound to its inhibitor (α_1PI) or free. They suggest (McGuire et al., 1982) that the imbalance between the elastase and α_1PI occurred either because the active site of the α_1PI was oxidized or because of proteolytic cleavage of the α_1PI molecule. They showed that the α_1PI in the lavage fluid was inactive and that the activity could be restored by the reducing agent methionine sulfoxide reductase. As the a_1PI in the serum of these patients was normally reactive, they suggest that the oxidative inactivation occurs after the molecule enters the air space. This suggests the possibility that neutrophil-generated free radicals could be responsible for the inactivation of the a_1PI.

Lavage fluid from patients with ARDS from whatever cause contains large numbers of PMN. Idell and associates (1985) recently reported that BAL contained 76.9 ± 21.9% neutrophils in patients with ARDS compared to 3.9 ± 3% in normal controls when the total number of cells in the BAL was similar, 21.8 ± 34.1 X 10^6 versus 25.3 ± 17.6 X 10^6, respectively. This suggested a much greater traffic of neutrophils from the vascular to the interstitial and air space in lungs with ARDS than in normal lungs. They also showed that the fluid contained an elastase-releasing factor, which is pertinent to the hypothesis that neutrophil elastase damages the lung. They reported a correlation between the concentration of neutrophil elastase and the widening of the alveolar-to-arterial gradient for oxygen. A more recent study (Weiland et al., 1986) showed a similar increase in neutrophils in patients with ARDS, where the neutrophils correlated with the abnormality in gas exchange and protein permeability with demonstration of collagenase in the BAL fluid. These studies contrast with a recent report (Ognibene et al., 1986) showing that ARDS can develop in patients who have been neutropenic for an average of 9 days prior to the onset of ARDS. As neutropenia due to pulmonary sequestration of neutrophils has been recognized as a complication of sepsis since the turn of the century (Burford and Burbank, 1945), the finding of neutropenia in septic patients with ARDS is not surprising. However, many of the patients reported were neutropenic prior to becoming septic, so the authors argue that the damage to the alveolar capillary wall is due to a mechanism that does not involve the PMN (Ognibene et al., 1986). The real problem is to know how many neutrophils are needed to damage the endothelium. As the number of neutrophils marginating in the lung is normally two to three times as great as the number circulating, it is entirely possible that large numbers remain in the lung even when the circulating count is very low. Activation of these few remaining cells could damage the alveolar capillary membrane and produce lung edema.

The fact that neutrophils can pass directly through the alveolar membrane when stimulated with LTB4 and not produce much protein leak (Staub et al., 1985) suggests that adherence and migration can occur without injury. It is possible that injury occurs only as a result of neutrophil activation during the process of adherence and migration. If this were so, injury might be expected in situations where adherence, migration, and activation of membranes with O_2 generation and enzyme release all occur simultaneously. Studies focused on how many activated neutrophils are needed to produce a leak in the endothelial membrane in vivo would be very helpful in settling the question of the importance of neutrophils in ARDS. It would also be useful to obtain direct evidence that an activated neutrophil can disrupt the endothelium and cause a leak when an unactivated cell can adhere and migrate without causing damage. Until such evidence is obtained, the implication of the neutrophil as the cause of the lung damage in ARDS will remain controversial.

Acknowledgment

Supported by grant MT-4219 from the Medical Research Council of Canada.

References

Ahlborg, B., and Ahlborg, G. (1970). Exercise leukocytosis with an without beta-adrenergic blockade. *Acta Med. Scand. 187*:241-246.

Arfors, K.-E., Lundberg, C., Lindbom, L., Lundberg, K., Beatty, P. G., and Harlan, J. M. (1987). A monoclonal antibody to the membrane glycoprotein complex CD19 (LFA) inhibits PMN accumulation and plasma leakage in vivo. *Blood 69*:338-340.

Arnaout, M. A., Spits, H., Terhorst, C., Pitt, J., and Todd, R. F., III (1984). Deficiency of a leukocyte surface glycoprotein (LFA-1) in two patients with Mo1 deficiency: Effects of cell activation on Mo1/LFA-1 surface expression in normal and deficient leukocytes. *J. Clin. Invest. 74*:1291-1300.

Ashbaugh, D. G., Bigelow, D. B., Petty, T. L., and Levine, B. E., (1967). Acute respiratory distress syndrome in adults. *Lancet 2*:319-323.

Becker, E. L., Kermode, J. C., Naccache, P. H., Yassin, R., Munoz, J. J., Marsch, M. L., Huang, C.-K., and Sha'afi, R. I. (1986). Pertussis toxin as a probe of neutrophil activation. *Fed. Proc. 45*:2151-2155.

Bierman, H. R., Kelly, K. H., Cordes, F. L., Petrakis, N. L., Kass, H., and Shpil, E. L. (1952). The influence of respiratory movements upon circulating leukocytes. *Blood 7*:533-544.

Bokoch, G. M., and Gilman, A. G. (1984). Inhibition of receptor-mediated release of arachidonic acid by pertussis toxin. *Cell 39*:301-308.

Boxer, L. A., Allen, J. M., and Baehner, R. L. (1980). Diminished polymorphonuclear leukocyte adherence. *J. Clin. Invest. 66*:268-274.

Bradford, J. R. (1919). Massive collapse of the lung as a result of gunshot wounds, with special reference to wounds of the chest. *Am. J. Med. 12*:127-130.

Bradford, P. G., and Rubin, R. P. (1985). Pertussis toxin inhibits chemotactic factor-induced phospholipase C stimulation and lysosomal enzyme secretion in rabbit neutrophils. *FEBS Lett. 183*:317-320.

Brigham, K. L., Woolverton, W. C., Blake, L. H., and Staub, N. C. (1974). Increased sheep lung vascular permeability caused by pseudomonas bacteremia. *J. Clin. Invest. 54*:792-804.

Brigham, K. L., Bowers, R. E., and Hanes, J. (1979). Increased sheep lung vascular permeability caused by *Escherichia coli* endotoxin. *Circ. Res. 45*:292-297.

Bullock, W. E., and Wright, S. D. (1987). Role of the adherence-promoting receptors, CR3, LFA-1, and p150,95, in binding of *Histoplasma capsulatum* by human macrophages. *J. Exp. Med. 165*:195-210.

Burford, T. H., and Burbank, B. (1945). Traumatic wet lung. *J. Thorac. Surg. 14*:415-424.

Burns, G. F., Cosgrove, L., Triglia, T., Beall, J. A., Lopez, A. F., Werkmeister, J. A., Begley, C. G., Haddad, A. P., d'Apice, A. J. F., Vadas, M. A., and Crawley, J. C. (1986). The 11b-111a glycoprotein complex that mediates platelet aggregation is directly implicated in leukocyte adhesion. *Cell 45*: 269-280.

Burton, A. C. (1951). On the physical equilibrium of small blood vessels. *Am. J. Physiol. 164*:319-329.

Cartwright, G. E., Athens, J. W., and Wintrobe, M. M. (1964). The kinetics of granulopoiesis in normal man. *Blood 24*:780-803.

Charo, I. F., Yuen, C., and Goldstein, I. M. (1985). Adherence of human polymorphonuclear leukocytes to endothelial monolayers: effects of temperature, divalent cations, and chemotactic factors on the strength of adherence measured with a new centrifugation assay. *Blood 65*:473-479.

Chien, S. (1985). Role of blood cells in microcirculatory regulation. *Microvasc. Res. 29*:129-151.

Cochrane, C. G., Spragg, R., and Revak, S. D. (1983). Pathogenesis of the adult respiratory distress syndrome. Evidence of oxidant activity in bronchoalveolar lavage fluid. *J. Clin. Invest. 71*:754-761.

Coussens, L., Parker, P. J., Rhee, L., Yang-Feng, T. L., Chen, E., Waterfield, M. D., Francke, U., and Ullrich, A. (1986). Multiple, distinct forms of bovine and human protein kinase C suggest diversity in cellular signaling pathways. *Science 233*:859-866.

Craddock, P. R., Fehr, J., Brigham, K. L., Kronenberg, R. S., and Jacob, H. S. (1977a). Complement and leukocyte-mediated pulmonary dysfunction in hemodialysis. *New Engl. J. Med. 296*:769-774.

Craddock, P. R., Fehr, J., Dalmasso, A. P., Brigham, K. L., and Jacob, H. S. (1977b). Hemodialysis leukopenia. Pulmonary vascular leukostasis resulting from complement activation by dialyzer cellophane membranes. *J. Clin. Invest. 59*:879-888.

Crapo, J. D., Barry, B. E., Gehr, P., Bachofen, M., and Weibel, E. R. (1982). Cell number and cell characteristics of the normal human lung. *Am. Rev. Resp. Dis. 125*:740-745.

Derks, C. M., and Jacobovitz-Derks, D. (1977). Embolic pneumopathy induced by oleic acid. *Am. J. Pathol. 87*:143-158.

Doerschuk, C. M., Allard, M. F., Martin, B. A., Mackenzie, A., Autor, A. P., and Hogg, J. C. (1987). The marginated pool of neutrophils in the lungs of rabbits. *J. Appl. Physiol. 63*:1806-1815.

Dunnill, M. S. (1982). *Pathology of the Lung.* Churchill Livingstone, Edinburgh, Chap. 8, pp. 125-146.

Dvorak, H. F., Senger, D. R., Dvorak, A. M., Harvey, V. S., and McDonagh, J. (1985). Regulation of extravascular coagulation by microvascular permeability. *Science 227*:1059-1061.

Dyer, E. L., and Snapper, J. R. (1986). Role of circulating granulocytes in sheep lung injury produced by phorbol myristate acetate. *J. Appl. Physiol. 60*: 576-589.

Evans, E. A. (1984). Structural model for passive granulocyte behaviour based on mechanical deformation and recovery after deformation tests. *In White Cell Mechanics: Basic Science and Clinical Aspects.* Edited by H. J. Meiselman, M. A. Lichtman, and P. L. LaCelle. Alan R. Liss, New York, pp. 53-71.

Fels, A. O. S., and Cohn, Z. A. (1986). The alveolar macrophage. *J. Appl. Physiol. 6*:353-369.

Flick, M. R., Perel, A., and Staub, N. C. (1981). Leukocytes are required for increased lung microvascular permeability after microembolization in sheep. *Circ. Res. 48*:344-351.

Flick, M. R., Hoeffel, J. M., and Stuab, N. C. (1983). Superoxide dismutase with heparin prevents increased lung vascular permeability during air emboli in sheep. *J. Appl. Physiol. 55*:1284-1291.

Florey, H. W. (1962). *General Pathology*. 3rd ed. Lloyd Luke (Medical Books), London, Chap. 2, pp. 40-97.

Foster, N. K., Martyn, J. B., Rangno, R. E., Hogg, J. C., and Pardy, R. L. (1986). Leukocytosis of exercise: role of cardiac output and catecholamines. *J. Appl. Physiol. 61*:2218-2223.

Fung, Y. C., and Sobin, S. S. (1969). Theory of sheet flow in lung alveoli. *J. Appl. Physiol. 26*:472-488.

Gallin, J. I. 91980). Degranulating stimuli decrease the negative surface charge and increase the adhesiveness of human neutrophils. *J. Clin. Invest. 65*: 298-306.

Gallin, J. I., Gallin, E. K., and Shipman, E. (1979). Mechanisms of leukocyte chemotaxis. In *Advances in Inflammatory Research.* Vol. 1. Edited by G. Weisman, B. Samuelson, and R. Paoletti. Raven Press, New York, pp. 123-138.

Gierschik, P., Falloon, J., Milligan, G., Pines, M., Gallin, J. I., and Spiegel, A. (1986). Immunochemical evidence for a novel pertussis toxin substrate in human neutrophils. *J. Biol. Chem. 261*:8058-8062.

Glazier, J. B., Hughes, J. M. B., Maloney, J. E., and West, J. B. (1969). Measurements of capillary dimensions and blood volume in rapidly frozen lungs. *J. Appl. Physiol. 26*:65-76.

Goldman, D. W., Chang, F. H., Gifford, L. A., Goetzl, E. J., and Bourne, H. R. (1985). Pertussis toxin inhibition of chemotactic factor-induced calcium mobilization and function in human polymorphonuclear leukocytes. *J. Exp. Med. 162*:145-156.

Hall, H. L. (1925). A study of the pulmonary circulation by the transillumination method. *Am. J. Physiol. 72*:446-457.

Hammerschmidt, D. E., Weaver, L. J., Hudson, L. D., Craddock, P. R., and Jacob, H. S. (1980). Association of complement activation and elevated plasma C5a with adult respiratory distress syndrome. *Lancet 1*:947-949.

Harlan, J. M. (1985). Leukocyte-endothelial interactions. *Blood 65*:513-525.

Harris, J. O., Swenson, E. W., and Johnson, J. E. (1970). Human alveolar macrophages: comparison of phagocytic ability, glucose utilization and ultrastructure in smokers and nonsmokers. *J. Clin. Invest. 49*:2086-2096.

Harris, P., and Heath, D. (1977). *Human Pulmonary Circulation*. 2nd ed. Churchill Livingston, Edinburgh, Chap. 10, pp. 137-154.

Heflin, A. C., and Brigham, K. L. (1981). Prevention by granulocyte depletion of increased vascular permeability of sheep lung following endotoxemia. *J. Clin. Invest. 68*:1253-1260.

Hogg, J. C. (1983). Structural changes in the adult respiratory distress syndrome. In *Proceedings, Boehringer Ingelheim Chest Symposium* (Asia Pacific Congr. Ser. 17). Edited by T. de Guia and A. Lardizabal. Excerpta Medica, Amsterdam, pp. 2-8.

Hogg, J. C., Martin, B. A., Lee, S., and McLean, T. (1985). Regional differences in erythrocyte transit in normal lung. *J. Appl. Physiol. 59*:1266-1271.

Hogg. J. (1987) Neutrophil Kenetics and lung injury. *Physiol. Rev. 67*:1249-1295.

Holian, A. (1986). Leukotriene B_4 stimulation of phosphatidylinositol turnover in macrophages and inhibition by pertussis toxin. *FEBS Lett. 201*:15-19.

Hoover, R. L., and Karnovsky, M. J. (1982). Leukocyte endothelial interaction. In *Pathobiology of the Endothelial Cell*. Edited by H. Beckman. Academic Press, Orlando, FL, pp. 357-368.

Hoover, R. L., Biggs, R. T., and Karnovsky, M. J. (1978). The adhesive interaction between polymorphonuclear leukocytes and endothelial cells in vitro. *Cell 14*:423-428.

Hunninghake, G. W., Gadek, J. E., Kawanami, O., Ferrans, V. J., and Crystal, R. G. (1979). Inflammatory and immune processes in the human lung in health and disease: evaluation by bronchoalveolar lavage. *Am. J. Pathol. 97*:149-206.

Idell, S., Kucich, U., Fein, A., Kueppers, F., James, H., Walsh, P. M., Weinbaum, G., Coleman, R. W., and Cohen, A. B. (1985). Neutrophil elastase-releasing factors in bronchoalveolar lavage in patients with adult respiratory distress syndrome. *Am. Rev. Resp. Dis.* *132*:1098-1105.

Jaffe, E. A. (1983). Culture and identification of large vessel endothelial cells. In *Biology of Endothelial Cells*. Edited by E. A. Jaffe. Martinus Nijhoff, Boston, Chap. 1, pp. 1-13.

Jaffe, E. A., Nachman, R. L., Becker, C. G., and Minic, C. R. (1973). Culture of human endothelial cells derived from umbilical veins. Identification by morphologic and immunologic criteria. *J. Clin. Invest.* *52*:2745-2756.

Jenkins, M. T., Jones, R. F., Wilson, B., and Moyer, C. A. (1950). Congestive atelectasis – a complication of the intravenous infusion of fluids. *Ann. Surg.* *132*:327-347.

Johnson, A., and Malik, A. B. (1980). The effect of granulocytopenia on extravascular lung water content after microembolization. *Am. Rev. Resp. Dis.* *122*:561-566.

Johnson, A., Blumenstock, F. A., Hussain, M., and Malik, A. B. (1984). Differential effects of complement activation induced by cobra venom factor on pulmonary transvascular fluid and protein exchange. *Am. J. Pathol.* *114*:410-417.

Johnson, K. J., and Ward, P. A. (1981). Role of oxygen metabolites in immune complex injury of lung. *J. Immunol.* *126*:2365-2369.

Johnson, K. J., and Ward, P. A. (1982). Acute and progressive lung injury after contact with phorbol myristate acetate. *Am. J. Pathol.* *107*:29-35.

Johnson, K. J., Fantone, J. C., Kaplan, J., and Ward, P. A. (1981). In vivo damage of rat lungs by oxygen metabolite. *J. Clin. Invest.* *67*:983-993.

Johnson, R. L., Jr., Spicer, W. S., Bishop, J. M., and Forster, R. E. (1960). Pulmonary capillary blood volume, flow and diffusing capacity during exercise. *J. Appl. Physiol.* *15*:893-902.

Julien, M., Hoeffel, J. M., and Flick, M. R. (1986). Oleic acid lung injury in sheep. *J. Appl. Physiol.* *60*:433-440.

Kaplow, L. S., and Goffinet, J. A. (1968). Profound neutropenia during the early phase of hemodialysis. *J. Am. Med. Assoc.* *203*:1135-1137.

Katzenstein, A. L. (1982). Diffuse alveolar damage. In *Surgical Pathology of Non-Neoplastic Lung Disease*. Edited by A. L. Katzenstein and F. B. Askin. W. B. Saunders, Philadelphia, Chap. 2, pp. 9-42.

Klebanoff, S. J., Beatty, P. G., Schreiber, R. D., Ochs, H. D., and Waltersdorph, A. M. 91985). Effect of antibodies directed against complement receptors on phagocytosis by polymorphonuclear leukocytes: use of iodination as a convenient measure of phagocytosis. *J. Immunol.* *134*:1153-1159.

Lee, C. T., Fein, A. M., Lippmann, M., Holtzman, H., Kimbel, P., and Weinbaum, G. (1981). Elastolytic activity in pulmonary lavage fluid from patients with adult respiratory distress syndrome. *New Engl. J. Med. 304*: 192-196.

Lee, G. deJ, and DuBois, A. B. (1955). Pulmonary capillary blood flow in man. *J. Clin. Invest. 34*:1380-1390.

Levine, O. R., Mellins, R. B., Senior, R. M., and Fishman, A. P. (1967). The application of Starling's law of capillary exchange to the lungs. *J. Clin. Invest. 46*:934-944.

Loyd, J. E., Newman, J. H., English, D., Ogletree, M. L., Meyrick, B. O., and Brigham, K. L. (1983). Lung vascular effects of phorbol myristate acetate in awake sheep. *J. Appl. Physiol. 54*:267-276.

MacGregor, R. G. (1933). Examination of the pulmonary circulation with a microscope. *J. Physiol. 80*:65-77.

McGuire, W. W., Spragg, R. G., Cohen, A. B., and Cochrane, C. G. (1982). Studies on the pathogenesis of the adult respiratory distress syndrome. *J. Clin. Invest. 69*:543-553.

McMichael, J. et al. (Eds.) (1987). *Leukocyte Typing III*. Oxford University Press, London.

Malik, A. B., and van der Zee, H. (1978). Lung vascular permeability following progressive pulmonary embolization. *J. Appl. Physiol. 45*:590-597.

Marlin, S. D., Morton, C. C., Anderson, D. C., and Springer, T. A. (1986). LFA-1 immunodeficiency disease: definition of the genetic defect and chromosomal mapping of α and β subunits of the lymphocyte function-associated antigen 1 (LFA-1) by complementation in hybrid cells. *J. Exp. Med. 164*: 855-867.

Martin, A. M., Jr., Simmons, R. L., and Heisterkamp, C. A. (1969). Respiratory insufficiency in combat casualties: I. Pathologic changes in the lungs of patients dying of wounds. *Ann. Surg. 170*:30-38.

Martin, B. A., Wright, J. L., Thommasen, H. V., and Hogg, J. C. (1982). The effect of pulmonary blood flow on the exchange between the circulating and marginating pool of polymorphonuclear leukocytes (PMN) in dog lungs. *J. Clin. Invest. 69*:1277-1285.

Martin, B. A., Wiggs, B. R., Lee, S., and Hogg, J. C. (1987). Regional differences in neutrophil margination in dog lungs. *J. Appl. Physiol. 63*:1253-1261.

Martin, W. J., Gadek, J. E., Hunninghake, G. W., and Crystal, R. G. (1981). Oxidant injury of lung parenchymal cells. *J. Clin. Invest. 68*:1277-1288.

Miller, W. C., Rice, D. L., Kreusel, R. G., and Bedrossian, C. W. M. (1978). Monocrotaline model of noncardiogenic pulmonary edema in dogs. *J. Appl. Physiol. 45*:962-965.

Moldow, C. F. (1984). Neutrophil endothelial interactions. In *Biology of Endothelial Cells*. Edited by E. A. Jaffe. Martinus Nijhoff, Boston, Chap. 29, pp. 286-297.

Molski, T. F. P., Naccache, P. H., Marsh, M. L., Kermode, J., Becker, E. L., and Sha'afi, R. I. (1984). Pertussis toxin inhibits the rise in the intracellular concentration of free calcium that is induced by chemotactic factors in rabbit neutrophils: possible role of the "G proteins" in calcium mobilization. *Biochem. Biophy. Res. Commun. 124*:644-650.

Montaner, J. S. G., Tsang, J., Evans, K. G., Mullen, J. B. M., Burns, A. R., Walker, D. C., Wiggs, B., and Hogg, J. C. (1987). Alveolar epithelial damage: a critical difference between high pressure and oleic acid induced low pressure pulmonary edema. *J. Clin. Invest. 77*:1786-1796.

Muir, A. L., Cruz, M., Martin, B. A., Thommasen, H. V., Belzberg, A., and Hogg, J. C. (1984). Leukocyte kinetics in the human lung: role of exercise and catecholamine. *J. Appl. Physiol. 57*:711-719.

Nichol, J., Girling, F., Jerrard, W., Claxton, E. B., and Burton, A. C. (1951). Fundamental instability of the small blood vessels and critical closing pressures in vascular beds. *Am. J. Physiol. 164*:330-344.

Ognibene, F. P., Martin, S. E., Parker, M. M., Schlesinger, T., Roach, P., Burch, C., Shelhamer, J. H., and Parrillo, J. E. (1986). Adult respiratory distress syndrome in patients with severe neutropenia. *New Engl. J. Med. 315*: 547-551.

Ohkuda, K., Nakahara, K., Binder, A., and Staub, N. C. (1981). Venous air emboli in sheep: reversible increase in lung microvascular permeability. *J. Appl. Physiol. 51*:887-894.

Oseas, R., Yang, H.-H., Baehner, R. L., and Boxer, L. A. (1981). Lactoferrin: a promoter of polymorphonuclear leukocyte adhesiveness. *Blood 57*:939-945.

Parker, P. J., Coussens, L., Totty, N., Rhee, L., Young, S., Chen, E., Stabel, S., Waterfield, M. D., and Ullrich, A. (1986). The complete primary structure of protein kinase C – the major phorbol ester receptor. *Science 233*:853-859.

Pasteur, W. (1914). Massive collapse of the lung. *Br. J. Surg. 1*:587-601.

Pepe, P. E., Popkin, T. R., Reus, D. H., Hudson, L. D., and Carrico, C. J. (1982). Clinical predictors of the adult respiratory distress syndrome. *Am. J. Surg. 144*:124-130.

Perlo, S., Jalowayski, A. A., Durand, C. M., and West, J. B. (1975). Distribution of red and white blood cells in alveolar walls. *J. Appl. Physiol. 38*:117-124.

Permutt, S., and Riley, R. L. (1963). Hemodynamics of collapsible vessels with tone: the vascular waterfall. *J. Appl. Physiol. 18*:924-932.

Permutt, S., Caldini, P., Maseri, A., Palmer, W. H., Sasamori, T., and Zuller, K. (1969). Recruitment versus distensibility in the pulmonary vascular bed. In *Pulmonary Circulation in Interstitial Space*. Edited by A. P. Fishman and A. J. Hecht. University of Chicago Press, Chicago, pp. 375-390.

Pohlman, T. H., Stanness, K. A., Beatty, P. G., Ochs, H. D., and Harlan, J. M. (1986). An endothelial cell surface factor(s) induced in vitro by lipopolysaccharide, interleukin 1, and tumor necrosis factor-α increases neutrophil adherence by a CDω18-dependent mechanism. *J. Immunol. 136*: 4548-4553.

Pratt, P. C., Vollmer, R. T., Shelburne, J. D., and Crapo, J. D. (1979). Pulmonary morphology in the multi-hospital collaborative extracorporeal membrane oxygenator project. *Am. J. Pathol. 95*:191-214.

Ross, G. D. (1986). Clinical and laboratory features of patients with an inherited deficiency of neutrophil membrane complement receptor type three (CR_3) and the related membrane antigens LFA-1 and p150,95. *J. Clin. Immunol. 6*:107-113.

Ross, G. D., and Medof, M. E. (1985). Membrane complement receptors specific for bound fragments of C3. *Adv. Immunol. 37*:217-267.

Ross, G. D., Thompson, R. A., Walport, M. J., Springer, T. A., Watson, J. V., Ward, R. H. R., Lida, J., Newman, S. L., Harrison, R. A., and Lachmann, P. J. (1985). Characterization of patients with an increased susceptibility to bacterial infections and a genetic deficiency of leukocyte membrane complement receptor type three (CR_3) and the related membrane antigen LFA-1. *Blood 66*:882-890.

Sacks, T., Moldow, C. F., Craddock, P. R., Bowers, T. K., and Jacob, H. S. (1978). Oxygen radicals mediate endothelial cell damage by complement-stimulated granulocytes: an in vitro model of immune vascular damage. *J. Clin. Invest. 61*:1161-1167.

Sanchez-Madrid, F., Nagy, J. A., Robbins, E., Simon, P., and Springer, T. A. (1983). A human leukocyte differentiation antigen family with distinct α-subunits and a common β-subunit: the lymphocyte function-associated antigen (LFA-1), the C3bi complement receptor (OKM1/Mac-1), and the p150,95 molecule. *J. Exp. Med. 158*:1785-1803.

Saunders, W., Martin, B. A., Musclow, C. E., and Cooper, J. C. (1980). Pulmonary leukostasis and its relationship to pulmonary dysfunction in sheep and rabbit. *Circ. Res. 46*:175-180.

Saverymuttu, S. A., Peters, A. M., Danpure, H. J., Reavy, H. J., Osman, S., and Lavender, J. P. (1983). Lung transit of 111-indium labelled granulocyte: relationship to labelling techniques. *Scand. J. Haematol. 30*:151-160.

Schmid-Schonbein, G. W., Shih, Y., and Chien, S. (1980). Morphometry of human leukocytes. *Blood 56*:866-875.

Shasby, D. M., Vanbenthysen, K. M., Tate, R. M., Shasby, S. S., McMurtry, R. F., and Repine, J. E. (1982). Granulocytes mediate acute edematous lung injury in rabbits and in isolated rabbit lungs perfused with phorbol myristate acetate: role of O_2 radicals. *Am. Rev. Resp. Dis. 125*:443-447.

Shasby, D. M., Shasby, S. S., and Peach, M. J. (1983). Granulocytes and phorbol myristate acetate increase permeability to albumin of cultured endothelial monolayers and isolated perfused lung. Role of oxygen radicals and granulocyte adherence. *Am. Rev. Resp. Dis. 127*:72-76.

Shefeyk, J., Yassin, R., Volpi, M., Molski, T. F. P., Naccache, P. H., Munoz, J. J., Becker, E. L., Feinstein, M. B., and Sha'afi, R. I. (1985). Pertussis but not clolera toxin inhibits the stimulated increase in actin association with the cytoskeleton in rabbit neutrophils: role of the "G proteins" in stimulus-response coupling. *Biochem. Biophys. Res. Commun. 126*:1174-1181.

Siam, S., Henderson, R., Horsfield, K., Harding, K., and Cumming, G. (1973). Morphometry of the human pulmonary arterial tree. *Circ. Res. 23*:190-197.

Spangrude, G. J., Sacchi, F., Hill, H. R., Van Epps, D. E., and Daynes, R. A. (1985). Inhibition of lymphocyte and neutrophil chemotaxis by pertussis toxin. *J. Immunol. 135*:4135-4143.

Springer, T. A., and Anderson, D. C. (1985). The importance of the Mac-1, . LFA-1 glycoprotein family in monocyte and granulocyte adherence, chemotaxis, and migration into inflammatory sites: insights from an experiment of nature. In *Recent Advances in Primary and Acquired Immunodeficiencies*. Serono Symposia. Vol. 28. Edited by F. Aiuti, F. Rosen, and M. D. Cooper. Raven Press, New York, pp. 129-145.

Staub, N. C. (1974). Pulmonary edema. *Physiol. Rev. 54*:678-811.

Staub, N. C. (1978). Pulmonary edema due to increased microvascular permeability to fluid and protein. *Circ. Res. 43*:143-151.

Staub, N. C., and Schultz, E. L. (1968). Pulmonary capillary length in dog, cat and rabbit. *Resp. Physiol. 5*:371-378.

Staub, N. C., Schultz, E. L., and Albertine, K. H. (1982). Leukocytes and pulmonary microvascular injury. In *Mechanisms of Lung Microvascular Injury*. Edited by A. Malik and N. C. Staub. *Ann. NY Acad. Sci. 384*:332-343.

Staub, N. C., Schultz, E. L., Koike, K., and Albertine, K. H. (1985). Effect of neutrophil migration induced by leukotriene B_4 on protein permeability in sheep lung. *Fed. Proc. 44*:30-35.

Thommasen, H. V., Martin, B. A., Wiggs, B. R., Quiroga, M., Baile, E. M., and Hogg, J. C. (1984a). The effect of pulmonary blood flow on leukocyte uptake and release by the dog lung. *J. Appl. Physiol. 56*:966-974.

Thommasen, H. V., Boyko, W. J., Russell, J. A., and Hogg, J. C. (1984b). Transient leukopenia associated with adult respiratory distress syndrome. *Lancet 1*:809-812.

Till, G. O., Johnson, K. J., Kunkel, R., and Ward, P. A. (1982). Intravascular activation of complement and acute lung injury. Dependency on neutrophils and toxic oxygen metabolites. *J. Clin. Invest. 69*:1126-1135.

Todd, R. F., and Arnaout, M. A. (1900). Monoclonal antibodies that identify Mol and LFA-1, two human leukocyte glycoproteins: a review. In *Leukocyte Typing*. Part II. Vol. 3. Edited by E. L. Reinherz, B. F. Haynes, L. M. Nadler, and I. D. Bernstein. Springer-Verlag, New York, Chap. 8, pp. 95-108.

Todd, R. F., Arnaout, M. A., Rosin, R. E., Crowley, C. A., Peters, W. A., and Babior, B. M. (1984). Subcellular localization of large subunit Mo1 (Mo1α; formerly gp110) a surface glycoprotein associated with neutrophil adhesion. *J. Clin. Invest. 74*:1280-1290.

Volpi, M., Naccache, P. H., Molski, T. F. P., Shefcyk, J., Huang, C.-K., Marsh, M. L., Munoz, J., Becker, E. L., and Sha'afi, R. I. (1985). Pertussis toxin inhibits fMet-Leu-Phebut not phorbol ester-stimulated changes in rabbit neutrophils: role of G proteins in excitation response coupling. *Proc. Natl. Acad. Sci. USA 82*:2708-2712.

Wagner, W. W., Jr., Latham, L. P., Gillespie, M. M., and Guenther, J. P. (1982). Direct measurement of pulmonary capillary transit times. *Science 218*: 379-381.

Walther, B. T., Ohman, R., and Roseman, S. (1973). A quantitative assay for intercellular adhesion. *Proc. Natl. Acad. Sci. USA 70*:1569-1573.

Ward, P. A., Till, G. O., Kunkel, R., and Beauchamp, C. (1983). Evidence for role of hydroxyl radical in complement and neutrophil-dependent tissue injury. *J. Clin. Invest. 72*:789-801.

Wasserman, K., Butler, J., and Van Kessel, A. (1966). Factors affecting the pulmonary capillary blood flow pulse in man. *J. Appl. Physiol. 21*:890-900.

Wearn, J. T., Ernstene, A. C., and Bromer, A. W. (1928). The behavior of pulmonary vessels as determined by direct observation in the intact chest. *Am. J. Physiol. 85*:410.

Weibel, E. R. (1963). *Morphometry of the Human Lung*. Academic Press, New York, 151 pages.

Weibel, E. R. (1984). Lung cell biology. In *Handbook of Physiology*. Sect. 3. *The Respiratory System*. Vol. I. *Circulation and Nonrespiratory Functions*. Edited by A. Fishman and A. B. Fisher. American Physiological Society, Behesda, MD, Chap. 2, pp. 47-91.

Weiland, J. E., Davis, W. R., Holter, J. F., Mohammed, J. R., Downsley, P. M., and Gadek, J. A. (1986). Lung neutrophils and the adult respiratory distress syndrome. *Am. Rev. Resp. Dis. 138*:218-225.

Weinberg, P. F., Matthay, M. A., Webster, R. O., Roskos, K. V., Goldstein, I. M., and Murray, J. F. (1984). Biologically active products of complement and acute lung injury in patients with the sepsis syndrome. *Am. Rev. Resp. Dis. 130*:791-796.

Wright, S. D., and Jong, M. T. C. (1986). Adhesion-promoting receptors on human macrophages recognize *Escherichia coli* by binding to lipopolysaccharide. *J. Exp. Med. 164*:1876-1888.

18

The Potential Role of Interactions Between Endothelium and Smooth Muscle in Pulmonary Vascular Physiology and Pathophysiology

MICHAEL J. PEACH, ROGER A. JOHNS, and C. EDWARD ROSE, JR.

University of Virginia
School of Medicine
Charlottesville, Virginia

I. Introduction: The Importance of Endothelium to Vascular Physiology and Pharmacology

The endothelium creates a nonthrombogenic, semipermeable barrier between the bloodstream and all extravascular tissues and fluid compartments in the body. The surface of the endothelial cell is composed of a vast array of enzymes, transport proteins, and receptors that are in direct contact with the bloodstream. During the last decade studies of the endothelium have played a vital role in expanding our knowledge of vascular regulation. Major areas of interest have been permeability characteristics: transport of both small and large molecules, inactivation of vasoactive compounds, production of vasoactive substances, and metabolism of arachidonic acid (Bassingthwaighte et al., 1985; Gillis and Pitt, 1982; Furchgott, 1984; Moncada et al., 1977; Pearson et al., 1978; Weksler et al., 1977; Grega et al., 1986; Ryan, 1986; Shepro, 1986). The endothelium exerts an influence on blood pressure, hemostasis, growth and cytodifferentiation, the vascular response to injury, chemotaxis, and blood pH among others.

II. Pulmonary Endothelium

Since the lung receives the entire cardiac output, the pulmonary endothelium plays a very important role in the regulation of circulating vasoactive substances. Many solutes in plasma are processed (either activated or cleared) and the plasma content of numerous biologically active substances is regulated prior to delivery to the general circulation. The endothelium also can act as an endocrine organ and respond to numerous stimuli to release eicosanoids, free radicals, growth factors, and relaxing and constricting factors (identity unknown) – all of which have the potential to modulate cell growth and vascular reactivity or tone.

A. Structure

The morphology of the pulmonary vasculature as well as cultured pulmonary endothelium has been carefully described (Simionescu, 1986; Smith and Ryan, 1973) and will not be discussed here. Specific morphological changes associated with hypoxia, hyperoxia, and pulmonary hypertension are described in Section IV of this chapter. Clearly the endothelium is characterized by homocellular tight junctions and gap junctions among endothelial cells. Membrane junctional complexes also are formed between endothelial cells and vascular smooth muscle cells. Junctions between cells permit low-resistance pathways for electrical coupling of cells (Larson and Sheridan, 1982) as well as the cell-to-cell transfer of molecules (Davies, 1986).

B. Function

Metabolism of Vasoactive Agents

The pulmonary endothelium metabolizes polypeptides (brandykinin, angiotensin I), adenine nucleotides (ATP, ADP, 5'-AMP), biogenic amines (serotonin and norepinephrine), prostaglandins (E and F series), and arachidonic acid (PGI_2). The metabolic fate and/or uptake of these various substances by the endothelium have received a great deal of attention (see Gillis and Pitt, 1982; Jaffe et al., 1973; Ryan, 1986) and are valued indices of pulmonary vascular perfusion or of vascular injury (Block and Fisher, 1977; Dobuler et al., 1982). These functions also may be decreased or increased by changes in arterial oxygen tension and have been suggested to contribute to hypoxia-mediated pulmonary vasoconstriction.

Synthesis and Release of Substances

Growth Factors

On the basis of studies in other vascular beds and in cell culture, the endothelium has the ability to modulate cell growth within the vessel wall (DiCorleto,

1984; Campbell and Campbell, 1986; Clowes and Karnovsky, 1977). The normal endothelium produces heparin-like factors that inhibit smooth muscle proliferation (Castellot et al., 1984). When replicating, or perturbed or injured, the endothelium produces a variety of mitogens (DiCorleto, 1984; DiCorleto et al., 1983) and ceases production of antiproliferative factors. In addition to their mitogenic activity, platelet-derived growth factor and epidermal growth factor have been shown to induce contraction of muscular arteries (Berk et al., 1986). Under conditions such as chronic hyperoxia, hypoxia, and lung injury where remodeling of the pulmonary vasculature occurs, it seems reasonable to postulate that the antiproliferative effects of the endothelium are attenuated and that mitogens induce the hypertrophy and/or hyperplasia of the vasculature. Mitogens also may contribute directly to increased levels of vascular tone.

Constricting Factors

In isolated canine femoral artery, DeMey and Vanhoutte (1983) found that anoxia induced endothelium-dependent contractions. Subsequent studies from this laboratory (Rubanyi and Vanhoutte, 1985) showed that hypoxia released a vasoconstrictor substance and responses induced in these canine vessels by decreasing the PO_2 were not dependent on preexisting arterial tone. Endothelium-dependent, hypoxia-induced vasoconstriction also has been of considerable interest to individuals studying the pulmonary circulation (Holden and McCall, 1984; Madden et al., 1986; O'Brien et al., 1985b). The pulmonary vascular response to hypoxia may actually reflect reduced production of endothelium-derived relaxing factor (EDRF) or prostacyclin (PGI_2) in addition to production by the endothelium of a constrictor substance or a modulator.

Eicosanoids A few years ago Singer and Peach (1983a) reported that arachidonic acid (AA) caused endothelium-dependent vasoconstriction of the rabbit aorta. The contraction induced by AA was blocked by indomethacin pretreatment. Holden and McCall (1984) reported that hypoxia-induced vasoconstriction also was blocked by inhibitors of cyclooxygenase. Altiere et al. (1985) found that the endothelium contributed significantly to acetylcholine-induced, thromboxane (TX) A_2-mediated constriction of rabbit intrapulmonary arteries. Cultured bovine aortic endothelial cells produce TX A_2 (Ingerman-Wojenski et al., 1981) but synthesis has not been observed with endothelium from other species.

The endothelium also can produce other cyclooxygenase products of AA that are vasoconstrictors. In the aorta of SHR (but not WKY) rats, acetylcholine caused an endothelium-dependent contraction. This response to acetylcholine in the SHR was blocked by inhibitors of cyclooxygenase and appears to be due to some non-TX A_2 eicosanoid (Luscher and Vanhoutte, 1986). Comparable responses have not been evaluated in other species or vascular segments.

Other studies have suggested that hypoxia-induced pulmonary hypertension may be mediated by leukotrienes (Morganroth et al., 1984). Arterial endothelium also contains lipoxygenase and converts AA to HPETE and HETE, precursors of leukotrienes (Greenwald et al., 1979, Salzman et al., 1980; DeMey and Vanhoutte, 1982). Leukotrienes C_4 and D_4 are vasconstrictors in the pulmonary circulation and have been shown to be released during hypoxia. Blood vessels also contain cytochrome P450 (Juchau et al., 1976), and this enzyme has been localized to the endothelium (Abraham et al., 1985). Singer et al. (1984) reported that inhibitors of cytochrome P450 blocked endothelium-dependent relaxation in response to AA. Cultured endothelium produces multiple hydroxy and epoxy derivates of AA (Johnson et al., 1981), which may reflect the cytochrome P450 and lipoxygenase pathways. In the rabbit pulmonary artery, AA metabolites formed by P450 appear to mediate relaxation (Pinto et al., 1986). Hypoxia may decrease the rate of formation of P450 AA metabolites in the lung and impair this pathway for vasodilation.

In 1983 Cocks and Angus (1983) reported that responses in canine and swine coronary arteries to norepinephrine and serotonin were potentiated markedly when the endothelium had been removed. Their studies were felt to indicate that norepinephrine and serotonin act via $alpha_2$ adrenoceptors and S_2 serotonergic receptors, respectively, and stimulate the release of a dilator substance from the endothelium. This relaxing factor in turn compromises the direct vasoconstrictor actions of these two biogenic amines. Several investigators (Brum et al., 1984; Lamping et al., 1985) have observed potentiation of vasoconstrictor responses to serotonin following mechanical disruption or damage of the endothelium.

In isolated arteries of the rat, several investigators (Egleme et al., 1984; Biguad et al., 1984; Miller et al., 1984; Miller and Vanhoutte, 1985) have shown that $alpha_2$ adrenergic agonists (e.g., clonidine, guanabenz, BHT-920, BHT-933) have much greater efficacy following removal of the endothelium. Treatment of intact arteries with methylene blue unmasked pressor responses to $alpha_2$-agonist, presumably by blocking guanylate cyclase (Miller et al., 1984). We have found that indomethacin treatment blocked the contractions induced by $alpha_2$ agonists in arteries denuded of endothelium and that production of this constrictor eicosanoid by smooth muscle was suppressed by the endothelium (Peach et al., 1987b). Clonidine has been reported to stimulate the release of a relaxing factor (bioassay) from cultured bovine endothelial cells. However, this factor released by clonidine did not activate guanylate cyclase in smooth muscle and may be different from the EDRF released by A23187 or bradykinin (Loeb et al., 1987a).

Peptides Two laboratories have reported that endothelial cell cultures produce substances that constrict isolated arteries. Hickey et al. (1985) found that cultured bovine aortic endothelial cells produced a putative peptide with a molecular weight of about 8500. This weight is well below that of growth factor polypeptides such as PDGF or EGF. Gillespie et al. (1986) have confirmed the presence of a constrictor peptide in culture media of bovine aortic endothelium. Contractions of the coronary artery by this peptide were not blocked by antagonists of α-adrenergic, serotonergic, or histaminergic receptors or during inhibition of cyclooxygenase and lipoxygenase. The term "endothelium-derived constrictor factor" (EDCF) has been proposed for this substance produced by cultured bovine aortic endothelial cells (Gillespie et al., 1986). No studies have been performed that clearly establish that any substance (drug, hormones, neurotransmitters) or conditions (e.g., hypoxia) enhance or reduce the amount of EDCF released by cultures of bovine endothelium. It remains to be determined whether this peptide is made by other species or types of endothelium and whether or not all arteries and veins contract in response to the factor. The relationship of EDCF(s) to vascular resistance or vasospasm remains to be determined.

Platelet-Activating Factor The endothelium contains the neutral lipid, platelet-activating factor (acetylglyceryl ether phosphorylcholine; AGEP or PAF). Exposure to endotoxin or other forms of injury to the endothelium promotes the synthesis and release of PAF (Ryan and Ryan, 1985). This material is vasoactive, promotes chemotaxis, and activates platelets and neutrophils. The actions of PAF on pulmonary vascular resistance are discussed in Section IV.

Prostacyclin (PGI_2) Prostacyclin was identified as a product made from the eicosatetraenoate endoperoxide PGH_2 by segments or homogenates of arteries (Bunting et al., 1976; Moncada et al., 1976). The endothelium is a principal source of PGI_2 (Weksler et al., 1977; Moncada et al., 1977; McIntyre et al., 1978; Förstermann and Neufang, 1985). The production of PGI_2 is enhanced following exposure to bradykinin, thrombin, A23187, melittin, and exogenous AA. In all vessels studied in vitro, the predominant metabolite of AA is PGI_2 (Morera et al., 1983; Soma et al., 1985).

Arteries and veins contain high levels of the enzyme PG-15 hydroxydehydrogenase, which catalyzes the inactivation of PGE_2, $PGF_{2\alpha}$, and PGI_2 (Anggard et al., 1971; Sun and Taylor, 1978; Wong et al., 1978b). Selective tissue uptake of prostaglandins precedes metabolism in the pulmonary circulation. While PGE_2 is eliminated completely from the circulation of the lung, PGI_2 uptake and degradation is less than 20%. This difference in clearance of PGE_2 and PGI_2 reflects the low affinity of the tissue transport system for PGI_2 (Wong et al., 1978a).

Van Grondelle et al. (1984) determined the effects of increased blood flow and sheer stress on the release of PGI_2 by isolated perfused lung and cultured endothelium, respectively. They reported that increases in flow and/or stress induced PGI_2 release. Once released, PGI_2 would modulate vascular tone in those vascular beds that have the capacity to respond to this eicosanoid. Responses of the pulmonary vasculature to PGI_2 are considered in later sections.

III. Endothelium-Derived Relaxing Factor (EDRF)

The area of endothelium-vascular smooth muscle (VSM) interaction that has received the most attention in the past several years has been the production and release by endothelial cells of a substance termed "endothelium-derived relaxing factor" (EDRF). This was first described by Furchgott and Zawadzki in 1980 when they reported that the relaxation of strips of rabbit aorta by acetylcholine required an intact endothelium. Subsequently, numerous other substances have been found to produce vascular relaxation either partially or completely by endothelium-dependent mechanisms. These include several highly potent endogenous vasodilators such as bradykinin, histamine, substance P, vasoactive intestinal peptide, ATP, ADP, thrombin, calcitonin gene-related peptide, arachidonic acid, and trypsin as well as several exogenous compounds such as calcium ionophore (A23187), hydralazine, melittin (a bee venom peptide), and maitotoxin. Also several contractile agents (norepinephrine, serotonin, vasopressin) have decreased contractile responses when the endothelium is intact, which has been attributed to concomitant EDRF-mediated relaxation (see Sect. II.B).

A. Known Characteristics of EDRF

The chemical nature of EDRF remains unknown, perhaps in part due to its short biologic half-life. In addition to being labile, it is known that the production or release of EDRF by endothelial cells is calcium dependent, that EDRF is transferred from endothelial cells to VSM where it causes relaxation, and that this relaxation correlates with an activation of soluble guanylate cyclase resulting in a rise in smooth muscle cyclic GMP levels. The activity of EDRF appears to be sensitive to both high and low oxygen tensions. Attempts to characterize EDRF using pharmacologic inhibitors have provided evidence both for and against EDRF being an arachidonate metabolite or a free radical.

Lability

The biologic half-life of EDRF has been determined using a variety of transfer experiments in which the effluent from a source of endothelial cells is bioassayed on an endothelium-denuded vascular ring. Griffith et al. (1984) used an intact segment of rabbit thoracic aorta as a source of EDRF and a denuded canine coronary artery ring as a bioassay. By varying the distance between the donor vessel and the bioassay ring, they determined that EDRF had a biologic half-life of 6.3 sec. Using a similar preparation, Förstermann et al. (1985) demonstrated that the half-life could be prolonged to about 45 sec by lowering the oxygen tension of the medium from 95% to 20%. Similar transfer experiments have been performed using cultured endothelial cells grown on microcarrier beads and placed in a column as the donor source for EDRF (Cocks et al., 1985; Luckhoff et al., 1987; Loeb et al., 1987a; Gryglewski et al., 1986). All studies to date are consistent with a half-life of less than 60 sec.

Activation of Guanylate Cyclase

The relaxation of arteries by direct-acting nitrovasodilators such as sodium nitroprusside and nitroglycerin is preceded by increases in cyclic GMP concentrations (Arnold et al., 1977; Ignarro and Kadowitz, 1985). Because of the strong correlation between the relaxation and cyclic GMP accumulation, it has been proposed (although not proved) that cyclic GMP mediates the cellular events that result in relaxation. In a like manner, the relaxations induced by endothelium-dependent vasodilators also are preceded by an elevation in smooth muscle cyclic GMP levels. In contrast to the nitrovasodilators, many agents require an intact endothelium to induce a rise in cyclic GMP. Endothelium-dependent cyclic GMP accumulation has been shown for a variety of agents that release EDRF and has been demonstrated across numerous species and in a variety of vascular beds (Holzmann, 1982; Rapoport and Murad, 1983; Furchgott and Jothianandan, 1983; Ignarro et al., 1984; Rapoport et al., 1984; Peach et al., 1985; Loeb et al., 1987a, b).

Several investigators (Martin et al., 1985; Rapoport et al., 1985; Griffith et al., 1984) have reported that endothelium-dependent relaxations are inhibited by methylene blue, an agent that inhibits guanylate cyclase. In addition, MB22948, an inhibitor of cyclic GMP phosphodiesterase, potentiates the vascular effects of EDRF (Griffith et al., 1985; Martin et al., 1986; Ignarro et al., 1987). Acetylcholine-induced EDRF release from rabbit and canine arteries has been demonstrated to directly activate partially purified, soluble guanylate cyclase (Förstermann et al., 1986). Thus the link between EDRF-mediated responses and cyclic GMP accumulation in smooth muscle has been firmly established, and cyclic GMP accumulation has become a useful bioassay for the detection of EDRF.

Calcium Dependence

There is strong evidence that the synthesis and/or release of EDRF is a calcium-dependent process (Peach et al., 1987a). The removal of external calcium or pretreatment with calcium entry blockers (verapamil, nifedipine, SKF-525A) in rabbit or rat aortic ring preparations attenuates endothelium-dependent relaxation to acetylcholine, methacholine, and A23187 (Singer and Peach, 1982; Singer et al., 1984; Long and Stone, 1985; Loeb et al., 1987b). While the removal of calcium consistently causes marked impairment of EDRF responses (Peach et al., 1987a; Loeb et al., 1987b), not all vessels or endothelium-dependent relaxations are inhibited by calcium entry blockers (Miller et al., 1985;

Winquist et al., 1985). Several agents known to cause endothelium-dependent relaxation including norepinephrine (Saida and Van Breeman, 1983), histamine (Hudgins and Weiss, 1968), bradykinin(Gordon and Martin, 1983; Peach et al., 1987a), ATP, melittin (Peach et al., 1987a), and thrombin (DeGroot et al., 1985) have been associated with increases in intracellular calcium concentrations. Therefore, it would appear that receptor-mediated translocation (and/or influx) of intracellular calcium may be the initial step in the production and/or release of EDRF.

Evidence Implicating Arachidonate Metabolites

This calcium dependence provides support for the theory that endothelium-dependent relaxation is mediated by a metabolite of arachidonic acid (AA). Phospholipase activation in endothelium, which is required for AA release, clearly has been shown to be initiated by an increase in cytoplasmic free calcium concentration (Whorton et al., 1984).

Numerous studies have provided indirect evidence of a role for AA metabolites in the mediation of endothelium-dependent vasodilation. Prostacyclin (PGI_2), a cyclooxygenase product of AA known to be produced by endothelium and to dilate blood vessels, is not EDRF. Inhibitors of cyclooxygenase (indomethacin, meclofenamate, aspirin) do not block endothelium-dependent dilation in response to a wide variety of agents known to release EDRF (Furchgott and Zawadzki, 1980; Singer and Peach, 1983a, b; Gordon and Martin, 1983). However, in vessels that do respond to PGI_2, blockade of PGI_2 synthesis may attenuate endothelium-dependent relaxation. Vasodilation induced by PGI_2 has been associated with activation of adenylate cyclase and a rise in cyclic AMP levels in smooth muscle (Ignarro et al., 1985). Early studies demonstrated that inhibitors of the lipoxygenase pathway (ETYA, NDGA, BW755C, phenidone, nafazatrom) prevented or reversed endothelium-dependent vasodilation (Furchgott and Zawadzki, 1980; Singer and Peach, 1983a; Förstermann and Neufang, 1984; Furchgott, 1984).

Arachidonate also can be metabolized by cytochrome P450 monooxygenase enzymes to produce hydroxy- and hydroperoxyeicosatetraenoic acids (HETE and HPETE) as well as epoxyeicosatrienoic acids (EETS), many of which have been shown to be vasoactive (Schwartzman et al., 1985; Proctor et al., 1987; Pinto et al., 1987). This enzyme system has been clearly demonstrated to be present in vascular endothelium (Dees et al., 1982; Abraham et al., 1985). Inhibition of endothelium-dependent relaxation by inhibitors of cytochrome P450 (SKF-525A and metyrapone) was first shown by Singer et al. (1984). Two recent studies by Pinto et al. (1986, 1987) have provided further evidence for the contribution of a cytochrome P450-dependent pathway in AA-induced endothelium-dependent vasodilation. These investigators demonstrated that pretreatment of rabbits for 3 days with β-naphthoflavone and 3-methylcholanthrene, agents known to induce cytochrome P450, caused a tenfold increase in the AA-induced endothelium-dependent relaxations of pulmonary and coronary artery vascular rings. In addition, depletion of cytochrome P450 with cobalt chloride was shown to attenuate the responses to AA. Clearly the EETS represent endothelium-derived substances that relax arterial smooth muscle.

Singer and Peach (1983a) first utilized exogenous AA (1-100 μM) to elicit endothelium-dependent relaxation of rabbit aortic rings. This AA-induced relaxation response was potentiated by indomethacin (cyclooxygenase inhibitor) and blocked by ETYA (lipoxygenase and cytochrome P450 inhibitor), implying the involvement of non-cyclooxygenase metabolites of AA.

To demonstrate that endogenously released AA could lead to endothelium-dependent vasodilation, investigators have added phospholipase directly to vascular ring preparations (Förstermann and Neufang, 1985) or administered melittin, a bee venom peptide that activates phospholipase A_2 (Förstermann and Neufant, 1985; Loeb et al., 1987a, b; Johns and Peach, 1987; Johns et al., 1987). Melittin stimulated a dose-related, endothelium-dependent relaxation of rat and rabbit aortic and rabbit pulmonary artery rings. Relaxation was not blocked by indomethacin but was inhibited by the lipoxygenase and cytochrome P450 inhibitors ETYA and NDGA, the phospholipase inhibitors mepacrine and parabromophenacyl bromide, and the antioxidant hydroquinone (agents that are known to block endothelium-dependent relaxation). The release of AA by melittin was confirmed by demonstrating the concomitant release of PGI_2.

While there appears to be considerable evidence that endothelium-dependent relaxation may involve an AA metabolite, several observations make one cautious in accepting this conclusion. Many of the drugs used to block AA metabolism or phospholipase activation are nonspecific or inconsistent in their action, particularly at the high concentrations required. The doses of ETYA (≥100 μM) and NDGA (≥25 μM) required to block endothelium-dependent relaxation are considerably greater than their reported K_i values for blockade of lipoxygenase (Peach et al., 1985). At these high concentrations, both of these agents are strong antioxidants that could be acting by blocking guanylate cylase or inactivating EDRF in solution (Griffith et al., 1984; Clark and Linden, 1986). Moncada et al. (1986) recently demonstrated that several agents known to inhibit endothelium-dependent relaxation (phenidone, BW755C, dithiothreitol, hydroquinone, and pyrogallol) do so by inactivating EDRF through the formation of superoxide ions. Superoxide recently has been shown to destroy EDRF (Gryglewski et al., 1986). Johns and Peach (1987), using a combination of cell culture and vascular ring techniques, showed that parabromophenacyl bromide, an agent previously through to prevent EDRF production by inhibiting endothelial cell phospholipase, actually has its effect at the level of the smooth muscle where it appeared to block to guanylate cyclase activation.

Cocks et al. (1985) have found that EDRF released from cultured cells would pass over a C_{18} column at neutral pH but was retained or destroyed on an anion exchange column. This suggests that EDRF is not hydrophobic as one would expect most AA metabolites to be. However, a few known metabolites of AA, such as leukotriene D_4, are hydrophilic and are not retained by a C_{18} column at neutral pH.

Evidence Implicating a Free Radical

On the basis of studies in which acetylcholine-induced relaxations were rapidly reversed by the addition of hemoglobin or methylene blue (Holzman, 1982; Furchgott, 1984; Martin et al., 1985), Furchgott proposed that EDRF may be a free radical. This hypothesis is consistent with the extreme lability of EDRF as well as the fact that a variety of free radical scavengers and antioxidants (dithiothreitol, butylated hydroxytoluene, vitamin E, hydroquinone, phenidone, cysteine, tetrahydroborate) inhibit endothelium-dependent relaxations (Griffith et al., 1984; Furchgott, 1984). Free radicals also may be involved in the breakdown of EDRF. Several groups have shown that superoxide dismutase, a superoxide scavenger, will prolong the half-life of EDRF (Rubanyi and Vanhoutte, 1986b; Gryglewski et al., 1986).

Recently, several investigators (Furchgott et al., 1987; Ignarro et al., 1987) have suggested that EDRF might be the nitroxide radical NO•). The production of NO• from nitrovasodilators such as sodium nitroprusside with subsequent NO• stimulation of guanylate cyclase and increase in cyclic GMP levels is thought to be the mechanism by which these agents cause vasodilation. Because the effects of EDRF on smooth muscle are so similar to those of NO• (both have a short half-life, both are inhibited by hemoglobin and methylene blue, and both are destroyed by superoxide), it is tempting to propose that the endothelium is releasing NO• in response to acetylcholine and the other agents that cause endothelium-dependent vasodilation. Palmer et al. (1987) have presented evidence that endothelial cells alone and in response to agents that release EDRF can produce some nitrothiol or nitrosamine compounds or NO•. Additional studies are required to test the relationship between NO• and EDRF.

Heterogeneity of EDRF Responses

Several investigators have proposed that there is more than one EDRF and that this could explain some of the variability in EDRF responses noted in the literature. DeMey et al. (1982) concluded that the relaxation of canine femoral artery by ATP was mediated by a different "EDRF" than the relaxation by acetylcholine, since the former was not inhibited by pretreatment with ETYA or quinacrine. On the basis of studies of Singer and Peach (1983b), which showed that unlike acetylcholine the endothelium-dependent relaxations to AA could not be reversed by the acute addition of ETYA or NDGA, Furchgott suggested that the EDRF released by or made from AA was different from that released by acetylcholine (Furchgott, 1984). Pinto et al. (1987) recently demonstrated that relaxations of dog coronary arteries induced by AA could be inhibited completely by combined inhibition of cyclooxygenase and cytochrome P450 whereas acetylcholine relaxations were not affected. Phenylbutylnitrone has been reported to block the relaxation in response to acetylcholine but not that to ATP. These findings suggest that not all endothelium-dependent dilators act via the same factor or through the same mechanism and that there may well be a variety of EDRFs.

B. Studies of EDRF in the Pulmonary Circulation

Endothelium-dependent vasodilation to several vasodilators has been demonstrated in the pulmonary circulation of a variety of species, including humans.

Vascular Ring Studies

Acetylcholine causes endothelium-dependent relaxations of second and third branch bovine (Ignarro et al., 1986; Greutter and Lemke, 1986a) and canine (Chand and Altura, 1981) intrapulmonary arteries but not veins and is accompanied by an elevation in cyclic GMP levels. In contrast, bradykinin and the calcium ionophore A23187 stimulated endothelium-dependent dilation and cyclic GMP accumulation in both intrapulmonary arteries and veins (Ignarro et al., 1986; Greutter and Lemke, 1986b). The inability of the pulmonary vein to respond to acetylcholine is due to a failure of the venous endothelium to produce EDRF when exposed to acetylcholine and not a failure of venous smooth muscle to respond to factor. Greutter and Lemke (1986b) used a "sandwich preparation" in which an unmounted pulmonary intact artery strip was used to donate EDRF to a pulmonary vein strip denuded of endothelium (mounted for tension measurement). The vein relaxed when acetylcholine was applied.

Ignarro et al. (1985) studied the effects of AA (0.1 - 10 μM) on bovine intrapulmonary arteries and veins. In arteries, they observed an endothelium-dependent relaxation accompanied by a time- and concentration-dependent increase of both cyclic GMP and cyclic AMP levels. Indomethacin inhibited relaxations induced by low concentrations of AA (0.1 - 1 μM) and enhanced relaxations by concentrations greater than 10 μM. Treatment with indomethacin also inhibited the rise in intracellular levels of cyclic AMP but not cyclic GMP. Arteries without endothelium and veins with or without endothelium, as well as intact arteries that had no tone, only contracted when exposed to AA. These contractions of arteries and veins were inhibited by indomethacin, implying that the responses were mediated by contractile prostaglandins or other eicosanoids produced from AA. Agents that inhibited endothelium-dependent relaxation in arteries induced by acetylcholine (including ETYA, NDGA, and quinacrine) were relatively ineffective in reversing the relaxation response to AA, suggesting that acetylcholine and AA act via different EDRFs.

As noted earlier, Pinto et al. (1986) have provided strong evidence that the relaxation responses of rabbit pulmonary arteries to AA may be due to cytochrome P450 monoxygenase metabolites. Dose-dependent relaxations to AA were blocked by SKF-525A, a cytochrome P450 inhibitor. When vascular cytochrome P450 activity was increased by enzyme induction, the potency of AA in causing endothelium-dependent vasodilation increased. Depletion of the P450 enzyme caused an attentuation of AA relaxation.

Some agents cause endothelium-dependent relaxation of systemic vessels but not the pulmonary vasculature. Sata et al. (1986) found that vasoactive intestinal peptide caused relaxation of rat thoracic aorta by an endothelium-dependent mechanism and induced relaxation of rat, rabbit, and guinea pig main pulmonary arteries by endothelium-independent mechanisms. This was confirmed by Greenberg et al. (1987) in isolated human intrapulmonary arteries. In their study, vasoactive intestinal peptide caused direct vasodilation (endothelium-independent), while relaxation with ATP and acetylcholine was endothelium dependent.

The concentration of drug employed will often determine whether an endothelium-dependent dilation or a vasoconstriction will occur in pulmonary vessels. McMurtry and Morris (1986) found that platelet-activating factor (PAF) at low concentrations (10^{-10} to 10^{-9} g/ml) caused endothelium-dependent dilations of rat first branch pulmonary arteries. At concentrations greater than 10^{-9} g/ml (Voelkel et al., 1982; Lichey et al., 1984), PAF caused vasoconstriction. This also is true for acetylcholine, which causes endothelium-dependent dilation of main and first branch rabbit pulmonary artery in concentrations up to 10^{-6} M. At greater concentrations of acetylcholine, progressive vasoconstriction occurs. The responses to acetylcholine also are dependent on whether or not active tone is applied to the vessels. Altiere et al. (1985) reported that in rabbit intrapulmonary arteries precontracted with norepinephrine, acetylcholine caused biphasic (relaxation-contraction) concentration-response curves; but in the absence of tone it caused only contractions. These cholinergic contractions were due to thromboxane A_2 and were not endothelium dependent.

The pulmonary endothelium appears to function as a modulator for a variety of agents that cause vasoconstriction when the endothelium is absent or damaged. Acetylcholine (Altiere et al., 1985; Johns et al., 1987; Chand and Altura, 1981), bradykinin (Chand and Altura, 1981), histamine (Satoh and Inui, 1984), and AA (Ignarro et al., 1985) all constrict vessels when the endothelium is absent and dilate them when the endothelium is intact. Removal of the endothelium from dog intralobar pulmonary arteries also caused a shift to the left of the contractile dose-response curves to epinephrine, norepinephrine, and the selective $alpha_2$ adrenoceptor agonist UK14304 (Miller and Vanhoutte, 1985).

The unstimulated pulmonary endothelium also may regulate the basal tone of the pulmonary circulation. A recent study by Ignarro et al. (1987) provides strong evidence that endothelium-derived factors modulate cyclic GMP levels and intrinsic basal smooth muscle tone in isolated bovine intrapulmonary artery and vein. Cyclic GMP levels were found to be three to four times higher in the intact artery and vein than in endothelium-denuded vessels. Methylene blue, an inhibitor of guanylate cyclase, decreased cyclic GMP levels and was accompanied by increases in smooth muscle tone. M&B 22,948, an inhibitor of cyclic GMP phosphodiesterase, increased cyclic GMP levels and was accompanied by a decrease in smooth muscle tone. Responses to methylene blue and M&B 22,948 were significantly greater in the intact vessel than in vessels denuded of endothelium. In addition, smaller branches of intrapulmonary artery and vein had higher levels of cyclic GMP, were more sensitive to endothelium-dependent dilators and to methylene blue, and would not maintain a steady level of submaximal tone compared to larger branches from a common vascular bed. Thus, endothelium-derived factors appear to markedly influence basal cyclic GMP levels, sensitivity to endothelium-dependent vasodilators, and the smooth muscle tone of intrapulmonary arteries and veins.

Cell Culture Studies

Cultured bovine pulmonary artery endothelial cells also have been used to study EDRF in the pulmonary circulation. Johns and co-workers (Johns and Peach, 1987; Johns et al., 1987; unpublished observations) have used a bioassay system in which pulmonary endothelial cells grown on microcarrier beads are placed in a column and superfused with Krebs buffer. The column is stimulated with various agents and bioassayed for EDRF by allowing the superfusate to drip onto a denuded vascular ring and observing changes in isometric tension. Using this system they have demonstrated that cultured pulmonary artery endothelial cells are capable of releasing EDRF in response to bradykinin, A23187, ATP, thrombin, and AA and that these relaxations are accompanied by a rise in vascular smooth muscle cyclic GMP. Similar results were found using cocultures of the endothelial cells on beads and smooth muscle cells grown in culture wells. These methodologies facilitate investigations of endothelium-smooth muscle interactions by allowing separate manipulations of the endothelium and smooth muscle.

Isolated Lung and In Vivo Studies

Studies of endothelium-dependent vasodilation in the isolated perfused lung and in vivo are difficult to perform and to interpret because of the difficulty in adequately removing or damaging the endothelium without affecting the vascular smooth muscle and other lung tissue. Feddersen et al. (1986) studied the effects of three models of lung vascular injury on acetylcholine-induced pulmonary vasodilation using the rat isolated perfused lung model. Pretreatment of the rats with α-naphthylthiourea or exposure to 100% oxygen for 52 hr did not affect the dilation response as measured by changes in pulmonary arterial pressure. Perfusion of the lung model with collagenase did inhibit the vasodilation, but this was complicated by severe edema with destruction of interstitial cellular elements and fragmentation of capillaries. Coflesky and Evans (1986) found that chronic hyperoxia (7 days) attentuated responses to acetylcholine in arteriole segments removed from the animals and studied in vitro.

C. Interactions Between Oxygen and EDRF

The sensitivity of endothelium-dependent responses to changes in oxygen tension in systemic vessels has been known since EDRF was initially described in 1980 (Furchgott and Zawadzki). The endothelium-dependent relaxations to acetylcholine and thrombin were abolished reversibly under anoxic conditions, and that to ATP was reduced (DeMey and Vanhoutte, 1980, 1983). There appears to be an optimal PO_2 for endothelium-dependent responses in muscular arteries. DeMey and Vanhoutte (1980) obtained maximal endothelium-dependent relaxations to acetylcholine at a PO_2 of 145 mmHg. Both higher (650 mmHg) and lower (22, 5, 0 mmHg) oxygen tensions reduced the relaxation. Singer et al. (1981), studying rabbit thoracic aorta rings, found that intact rings constricted transiently to hypoxia ($PO_2 < 30$ mmHg), while denuded rings relaxed. Rubanyi and Vanhoutte (1985) have shown endothelium-dependent constriction in coronary arteries in response to hypoxia.

Endothelium dependence of hypoxia-induced constriction of pulmonary arteries has also been observed. Holden and McCall (1984) studied hypoxia-preadapted (PO_2 of 40 mmHg X 4-6 hr) porcine pulmonary artery strips with and without endothelium. When the PO_2 of these preadapted vessels was subsequently decreased from 140 to 40 to 0 mmHg, progressive contractions were observed that were markedly greater in strips that contained endothelium. Pretreatment with indomethacin, atropine, phentolamine, or propranolol had no effect on this response. These results would be consistent with the hypoxic inhibition of an EDRF or the release of an endothelium-derived constrictor (see Sect. II.B).

Madden et al. (1986) investigated the effects of endothelium removal on the response of isolated cat pulmonary arterioles (300 μm) to hypoxia (PO_2=50 mmHg) and found that endothelial damage was associated with decreased contractile responses.

In a recent report, Rivers et al. (1987), using endothelial cell columns, demonstrated the modulation of endothelium-dependent relaxation by physiologic changes in oxygen tension in the microcirculation of the hamster cheek pouch. EDRF from a column of endothelial cells on microcarrier beads was superfused over the microcirculation. Dilation of 30 μm arterioles occurred when the PO_2 of the superfusate was 105 mmHg but not when the PO_2 was dropped to 27 mmHg. Similarly, acetylcholine applied directly to the microcirculation caused a greater dilation at the higher PO_2. It remains to be determined whether oxygen modulates the endothelium-dependent responses via impaired production of EDRF or altered vascular smooth muscle reactivity.

It also has been demonstrated that hyperoxia can decrease the half-life of EDRF in several in vitro preparations, which may reflect an interaction of EDRF with the superoxide radical. Rubanyi and Vanhoutte (1986a, b) and Gryglewski et al. (1986) have demonstrated that the half-life of EDRF is prolonged in the presence of superoxide dismutase. Thus, EDRF production, biologic half-life, or action appears to be tightly regulated by oxygen tension, with too much or too little oxygen having inhibitory effects.

IV. Potential Interactions in Pathophysiological States

A. General Evidence Suggesting an Important Role for the Endothelium in Pulmonary Circulatory Homeostasis

The majority of studies elucidating a role for endothelium in vascular smooth muscle function have been performed with in vitro models using strips or ring segments of large vessels. Because of the interruptive nature of these studies and the inability to study small vessels generally believed to control vascular resistance, skepticism has arisen regarding a significant role for the endothelium in pulmonary circulatory homeostasis in healthy subjects and in various pathophysiological states. Two major bodies of evidence strongly suggest that the endothelium exerts an important role in modulating the pulmonary circulation in the normal state and during disease: (1) Potent in vitro endothelium-dependent vasoactive substances are also potent in vivo vasodilators in healthy human subjects; and (2) in vitro or ex vivo endothelial cell injury or disruption in animal models is associated with abnormalities of pulmonary vascular function.

Effects of In Vitro Endothelium-Dependent Vasoactive Substances in Healthy Human Subjects

While acetylcholine and bradykinin recently have been recognized as endothelium-dependent relaxing agonists in isolated vascular ring preparations (see Sect. III), these peptides also are vasodilators in the intact human pulmonary circulation. Fritts et al. (1958) observed that mean pulmonary arterial pressure fell slightly but significantly from 15 to 13 mmHg with infusion of acetylcholine at 0.5 mg/min into the main pulmonary arteries of eight healthy human subjects. Arborelius et al. (1974) observed that pulmonary arterial pressure was un-

Table 1 Models of Endothelial Cell Injury in Isolated Perfused Lung Models[a]

			Injury		Hypox./Pul. Vasoconst.	
Investigators	Perfusate	Agent	Dose	Duration	FiO_2	PPA
Block and Fisher, 1977		O_2	100%	4-48 hr		
Fedderson et al., 1986	Physiol. saline	ANTU	10 mg/kg/wk	4 wk		
Hill and Rounds, 1983	Whole blood	ANTU	10 mg/kg bolus	4 hr post-bolus	0 0.10	↔[b] ↑
Newman et al., 1981		O_2	100%	48 hr		↓
O'Brien et al., 1985a	Krebs-Henseleit	ANTU	10-15 mg/kg	4 hr post-bolus		
Rounds et al., 1985		ANTU	10 mg/kg/wk	4 wk		
Steinberg et al., 1982	Krebs-Ringers	Hypoxanthine oxidase	1 μmol	——		
Toivonen et al., 1981	Krebs-bicarbonate	O_2	90-95%	60 hr		

[a]Ach, acetylcholine; Ang I, angiotensin I; Ang II, angiotensin II; ATNU, α-naphthylthiourea; FiO_2, inspiratory oxygen fraction; PPA, pulmonary arterial pressure; RV/(LV+S), weight ratio of right ventricle to left ventricle plus septum; RVSP, right ventricular systolic pressure.
[b]Earlier rise in pulmonary arterial pressure with hypoxia post-ANTU.

changed with infusion of acetylcholine, 2-10 mg/min, into a lobar pulmonary artery of seven healthy subjects, but cardiac output increased. Unchanged pulmonary arterial pressure in the face of an increase in cardiac output suggests regional pulmonary arterial vasodilation secondary to the acetylcholine infusion.

Peripheral infusion of bradykinin, 0.3 - 1.58 μg/kg per minute to healthy human subjects, resulted in a fall in systemic blood pressure and increase in cardiac output, but pulmonary arterial pressure did not fall (Bishop et al., 1965; de Freitas et al., 1964). However, a pulmonary vasodilatory response was obtained with bradykinin administration, evidenced by a fall in pulmonary arterial resistance (de Freitas et al., 1964).

Ang II Vasoconst. PPA	ANG I Conv.	5-HT uptake	Ach response in hypoxia	RV/ LV+S	RVSP	Lung wet wet/dry	Lung lavage protein
		↓					
			Greater vasodil	↑		↑	
↑						↑	↑
	↓					↑	↑
				↑	↑	↔	
		↓				↑	
	↓	↓					

Endothelial Cell Injury

Multiple models of pulmonary endothelial cellular injury have been developed to examine the role of the endothelium in the pulmonary circulation (Table 1). Evaluation of pulmonary vascular responses in isolated perfused lungs from rats administered α-naphthylthiourea (ANTU) has revealed augmentation of pulmonary arterial vasoconstriction to hypoxia and angiotensin II (Hill and Rounds, 1983) and diminished angiotensin I conversion (O'Brien et al., 1985a). Chronic administration of ANTU resulted in evidence of pulmonary hypertension reflected by increased right ventricular hypertrophy and right ventricular systolic pressures (Rounds et al., 1985). Administration of hypoxanthine/xanthine oxidase, which generates free oxygen radicals, resulted in diminished pulmonary vascular uptake of 5-hydroxytryptamine (Steinberg et al., 1982). Evidence for injury in these studies included increased protein in lung lavage and increased lung water, evidenced by increased wet/dry lung weight ratios. As discussed earlier, specific evidence of endothelial cellular injury in these studies included diminished angiotensin I conversion and 5-hydroxytryptamine uptake [processes that have been localized to the pulmonary endothelium (Ryan and Ryan, 1977)], and electron microscopic evidence, including endothelial blebbing and partial detachment. Fedderson et al. (1986) examined the effects of acetylcholine administration during anoxic pulmonary arterial vasoconstriction (Table 1). These investigators found that the vasodilation with this endothelium-dependent vasodilator was enhanced following acute and chronic administration of α-naphthylthiourea. The finding of intact vasodilation in this model with presumed endothelial cell injury is perplexing but may in part be related to the fact that acetylcholine was administered during higher peak pulmonary arterial pressures during anoxia following ANTU compared to control animals administered ANTU vehicle alone. Other investigaors have observed an enhanced effect of acetylcholine when it was administered to patients during increased pulmonary arterial pressure with hypoxia (Fritts et al., 1958).

Although the abnormalities in these models of lung injury may have been related to effects other than endothelial injury, the results support the possibility that the endothelium is an important modulator of pulmonary vascular responses to circulating vasoconstrictors such as angiotensin II and to alveolar hypoxia.

In summary, these observations support the existence of an interactive relationship between the endothelium and vascular smooth muscle in the intact lung. It also is possible, even probable, that disorders of endothelium-vascular smooth muscle relationships may be important in pulmonary circulatory abnormalities. Such pathophysiological states include hypoxic pulmonary vasoconstriction, pulmonary hypertension, oxygen toxicity, and sepsis.

B. Hypoxic Pulmonary Vasoconstriction

The mechanisms for hypoxic pulmonary vasoconstriction remain unclear (Grover et al., 1983). Recent in vitro and in vivo observations have demonstrated that the pulmonary arterial endothelium may be involved in pulmonary vascular responses to certain vasoactive agents and during hypoxic or anoxic conditions. While the majority of studies have been performed using ring preparations or vascular segments in vitro, information also is available regarding potential endothelium-vascular smooth muscle interactions from ex vivo perfused lung preparations and from observations in vivo using animals and human subjects.

In Vitro Observations

A large number of studies have been performed using ring or strip preparations or perfused segments of a variety of blood vessels (Tables 2 and 3; Sects. III.B and III.C). The general lines of evidence from these observations are that (1) an intact endothelium is required for hypoxic or anoxic contraction or "anoxic potentiation" of contraction to certain vasoconstrictor substances (Table 2) and (2) anoxia and hypoxia decrease responsiveness of vascular segments to certain relaxing agents (Table 3).

Several studies have demonstrated that an intact endothelium is required for vascular contraction to hypoxia or anoxia. Holden and McCall (1984) observed that hypoxia (PO_2 40 mmHg) and anoxia increased vascular contraction in strips with intact endothelium (Table 2). However, this hypoxic and anoxic contraction was attentuated severely in strips without an intact endothelium. These observations must be interpreted with caution because in order to obtain the hypoxic contraction in this model the vascular segments with endothelium had to undergo "hypoxic adaptation" by incubation at a PO_2 of 40 mmHg for 4-6 hr. Despite this limitation, these observations suggested that hypoxia might cause vascular smooth muscle contraction through a mechanism involving the endothelium. Rubanyi and Vanhoutte (1985) evaluated the effects of hypoxia (5 and 10% O_2) and anoxia on basal tension of canine coronary artery strips. These investigators employed a preparation of circumferential strips of coronary artery without endothelium (endo−). A functional endothelium (endo+) was provided to these strips by juxtaposing them in a layered preparation, intima to intima, with longitudinal coronary arterial strips with an intact endothelium (Table 2). In the sandwiched preparation (endo+) and in circumflex coronary arteries alone (endo−), hypoxia resulted in a fall in basal tone. However, anoxia resulted in an increase in tension of the coronary artery segment with a functional endothelium, but tone decreased with anoxia in segments without endothelium. Addition of a cyclooxygenase inhibitor, indomethacin, resulted in a progressive rise in tone with hypoxia in the sandwiched preparation with endothelium, but tone was unchanged with hypoxia and fell with anoxia in coronary arterial segments without endothelial contact. These observations of endothelium dependence of coronary arterial contraction to anoxia, and stepwise contraction with progressive hypoxia after cyclooxygenase blockade, suggests that constrictor substances may be released from the endothelium during hypoxia and anoxia, but the overall vascular response may be offset by the synthesis of vasodilator prostaglandins synthesized through cyclooxygenase.

The possibility that endothelial constrictor substances may be released by endothelial cells is demonstrated by recent observations that supernatant from aortic endothelial cell cultures caused dose-dependent coronary arterial vaso-

Table 2 Effects of Hypoxia or Anoxia on In Vitro Basal Vascular Tone and Vascular Response to Constrictors[a]

	Model				Control		Hypox.	Anox.
Investigators	Animal	Vessel	Prep.	Bath	O_2 %	PO_2 mmHg	O_2 %	PO_2 mmHg
Busse et al., 1983	Rat Dog	Tail artery Femoral artery	Segment	Tyrodes solution		150		36
Chand and Altura, 1981	Dog	Intrapulmonary artery	Helical strip	Krebs-Ringers	95%	550		35
DeMey and Vanhoutte, 1980	Dog	Femoral artery	Ring	Krebs-Ringers	95%	641	20% 5% 0%	145 35 <1
DeMey and Vanhoutte, 1981	Dog	Femoral artery	Ring	Krebs-Ringers	95%	645	0%	<1
DeMey and Vanhoutte, 1982	Dog	Femoral artery Pul. artery Saphenous artery Splenic artery	Ring Ring Ring Ring	Krebs-Ringers	95%		0%	
DeMey and Vanhoutte, 1983	Dog	Femoral artery	Ring	Krebs-Ringers	95%	640	0%	<1
Furchgott and Zawadzki, 1980	Dog	Thoracic aorta	Ring	Krebs-Ringers	95		0%	
Holden and McCall, 1984	Pig	Pul. artery (main)	Strip	Krebs-Ringers		140		40 0
Rubanyi and Vanhoutte, 1985	Dog	Coronary artery (circumflex)	Strip[c] (layered prep.)	Krebs-Ringers	95%	670	10% 5% 0%	
Rubanyi and Vanhoutte, 1986a	Dog	Coronary artery (circumflex)	Strip[d] (superfused)	Krebs-Ringers	95%		10%	

[a]Anox, anoxia; Endo +, intact endothelium; Endo–, devoid of endothelium; Hypox, hypoxia; Indo, indomethacin; NE, norepinephrine; PE, phenylephrine; $PGF_{2\epsilon}$; prostaglandin F_{2a}; 5HT, 5-hydroxytryptamine.

[b]Measured vessel diameter instead of tone.

[c]Circumferential strips without endothelium in contact with (endo+), or without (endo–) layer of coronary arterial longitudinal strip with intact endothelium.

[d]Superfusion across femoral arterial segments with endothelium, onto coronary artery ring without endothelium.

[e]Hypoxic perfusate directly onto coronary ring (without endothélium).

Change in basal tone by hypoxia/anoxia						Augmentation in response to Constrictors by hypoxia-anoxia	
Tone, hypoxia/anoxia		Tone, hypoxia/anoxia + indo.			Tone Const. Alone	Tone Const. hypoxia/anoxia	
(Endo +)	(Endo −)	(Endo +)	(Endo −)	Const.	(Endo +)	(Endo +)	(Endo −)
				NE	↑$_b$	↓	↑
				5HT			
				NE	↑		
				PE			
				NE	↑	↑	
				NE	↑	↑	
				NE	↑	↑↑	
				KC125 mM			less anoxia
				NE	↑	↑↑	potentiation
				$BaCl_2$			
				NE	↑	↑↑	
				NE	↑	↑↑	
							less anoxia
				NE	↑	↑↑	potentiation
				NE	↑	↑↑	
				NE	↑	↑↑	less anoxia potentiation
				NE	↑		
↑↑	↑						
↑↑↑	↑						
↓	↓	↔	↔				
↓	↓↓	↑↑	↔				
↑↑	↓↓	↑↑↑	↓	$PGF_{2\alpha}$	↑	↑↑	No anoxia potentiation
				$PGF_{2\alpha}$	↑	↑↑	↔^{c}

Table 3 Effects of Hypoxia or Anoxia on In Vitro Response of Precontracted Blood

	Model		
Investigator	Constrictor	Tone	Dilator
Chand and Altura, 1981	5HT NE PE	↑↑[a] ↑↑ ↑↑	Ach
DeMey and Vanhoutte, 1980	NE NE NE	↑↑ ↑↑ ↑↑	Ach Ach Ach
DeMey and Vanhoutte, 1983	NE	↑↑	Thrombin Ach ATP
Furchgott and Zawadzki, 1980	NE	↑↑	Ach
Rubanyi and Vanhoutte, 1985	PGF_{2a}	↑↑	Ach
Rubanyi and Vanhoutte, 1986a	PGF_{2a}	↑↑	Ach

[a]See Table 2; ACh, acetylcholine; ATP, adenosine triphosphate

constriction in isolated, retroperfused rabbit hearts (Gillespie et al., 1986). However, O'Brien and McMurtry (1984) observed that in contrast to bovine aortic endothelial cell supernates, bovine pulmonary arterial endothelial cell culture supernates caused only weak and unimpressive contractions of isolated bovine pulmonary arterial rings.

With regard to anoxic potentiation of contraction to vasoconstrictors, both hypoxia and anoxia result in potentiation of vascular contraction to agents including norepinephrine, PGF_{2a}, and potassium in vascular preparations with an intact endotheliaum (Table 2). A role for the endothelium is suggested by decreased or the absence of anoxic or hypoxic potentiation of responses to norepinephrine in vascular preparations devoid of endothelium (DeMey and Vanhoutte, 1981, 1982, 1983; Rubanyi and Vanhoutte, 1985, 1986a, b). As discussed earlier, anoxia may impair EDRF synthesis or responses (Sect. III.C) and EDRF modulates the potency of norepinephrine (Sect. II.B). The physiological significance of this phenomenon is open to question because vasoconstrictor potentiation was observed only with anoxia except for one study, which observed

Vessels to Endothelium-Dependent Relaxing Agents[a]

Hypoxia/anoxia PO^2 mmHg	Change in Tone with Dilator: Tone (Endo +)	Tone (Endo −)	Tone Dilator + hypoxia/anoxia (Endo +)
35	↓		↓
35	↓		↓
35	↓		↓
145	↓↓	↔	↓↓
35	↓↓	↔	↓
<1	↓↓	↔	↔
<1	↓	↔	↔
<1	↓	↔	↔
<1	↓	↔	↔
<1	↓	↔	↔
<1	↓	↔	↓
(10% O_2)	↓	↔	↓

potentiation of the contraction to PGF_{2a} in coronary artery rings (devoid of endothelium) superfused with hypoxic (10% O_2) Krebs-Ringers solution through femoral artery segments with intact endothelium (Rubanyi and Vanhoutte, 1985). In contrast, hypoxia (5% O_2, PO_2 = 35 mmHg) failed to potentiate the contractile response to norepinephrine in canine femoral artery rings (DeMey and Vanhoutte, 1980). Additional conflicting evidence are observations of vasodilation of norepinephrine-precontracted rat tail artery and canine femoral artery segments (intact endothelium) with perfusion of hypoxic Tyrodes solution (Busse et al., 1983). This endothelium-dependent vasodilation and an increase in 6-keto-PGF_{1a} with hypoxia were abolished by cyclooxygenase inhibition with indomethacin, suggesting that the hypoxic vasodilatory response was mediated by endothelial synthesis of prostacyclin (Busse et al., 1984).

Finally, anoxia has been observed to diminish vascular relaxation to certain endothelium-dependent vasodilators (Table 3). Very early in the initial work elucidating the role of the endothelium in the action of certain vasodilators, it was discovered that anoxia abolished relaxation of precontracted vascular preparations to endothelium-dependent vasodilators. For example, changing the bath oxygen source from 95% to 0% abolished the endothelium-dependent relaxation of norepinephrine precontracted canine femoral arterial or thoracic aortic rings to acetylcholine (DeMey and Vanhoutte, 1980, 1983; Furchgott and Zawadzki, 1980), thrombin, and ATP (DeMey and Vanhoutte, 1983). In contrast to these observations, Rubanyi and Vanhoutte (1985) observed that anoxia failed to abolish canine coronary artery relaxation with acetylcholine (Table 3). Moreover, when a more physiologically relevant degree of hypoxia was employed (PO_2 = 35 mmHg), acetylcholine relaxation of canine intrapulmonary artery strips (Chand and Altura, 1981) and femoral artery rings (DeMey and Vanhoutte, 1980) was unaffected. These observations suggest that endothelium-related relaxation of blood vessels is intact at physiologically relevant levels of hypoxia.

Ex Vivo Observations

Previous studies in chronic hypoxia models have identified phenomena that may be related to interactions between endothelium and vascular smooth muscle. McMurtry and co-workers (1978) exposed male Sprague-Dawley rats to altitude hypoxia (barometric pressure = 440 mmHg) for 4-6 weeks. Evidence of pulmonary hypertension in these animals included increased right ventrical pressure and increased right-to-left ventricular weight ratios above control animals (barometric pressure = 630 mmHg). Examination of pulmonary arterial pressure responses in isolated perfused lung preparations from these animals revealed augmentation of the pulmonary pressor response to angiotensin II, $PGF_{2\alpha}$, and norepinephrine. In striking contast, the pulmonary pressor rsponse to acute alveolar hypoxia was significantly diminished compared to control animals. Suppression of hypoxic pulmonary arterial vasoconstriction was not mediated through increased vasodilator prostaglandin synthesis, because cyclooxygenase inhibition with meclofenamate failed to restore the hypoxic pressor response to normal. However, the blunting of the hypoxic pressor response in chronically hypoxic rats was abolished by return to control altitude for 3 days. In fact, return to low altitude for 3 days following chronic hypoxia resulted in heightening of the hypoxic pulmonary pressor response.

Anatomic changes in the pulmonary arteries with hypoxia have been carefully examined. Meyrick and Reid (1980) reported the ultrastructural changes of the intrapulmonary arterial intima of rats after 10 days of chronic hypobaric hypoxia. Endothelial changes with chronic hypoxia include cuboidal appearance; increase in cell size; hypertrophy of endoplasmic reticulum, Golgi apparatus, and ribosomes; and elevation above the basement membrane by edema and microfibrillar material. Of note was the frequent finding of subendothelial edema and disappearance of basement membrane. Additional changes that have been observed include increased endothelial microvilli, surface defects, and attachment of leukocytes (Hung et al., 1986). Changes with hypoxia of longer duration include appearance of immature muscle beneath the endothelium after 3 weeks of hypoxic exposure and formation of elastin in the basement membrane of the endothelium after 4 weeks of chronic hypoxia (Smith and Heath, 1977). The rapid return of the hypoxic pressor response after only 3 days of return to low altitude is too rapid for resolution of these anatomic changes and suggests some metabolic mechanism. The enhanced pulmonary pressor response to acute hypoxia after return to control altitude may well be due to changes in metabolic factors or conditions that were suppressing pulmonary arterial vasoconstriction of a hypertrophied contractile apparatus.

It is tempting to speculate that blunting of the hypoxic pressor response by chronic hypoxia was mediated through endothelium-vascular smooth muscle interaction, such as increased production of endothelium-derived relaxing factor. Support for this possibility can be found from observations by McMurtry (1985) that the Ca^{2+} ionophore A23187 markedly attenuates the hypoxic pressor response in isolated rat lungs perfused with either whole blood or physiological saline solution. Since A23187 is an endothelium-dependent relaxing agonist of the rabbit aorta in vitro (Singer and Peach, 1982), these observations support the possibility that substances released by the endothelium may attenuate hypoxic pulmonary arteriolar vasoconstriction.

In Vivo Observations

While the effects in vitro of anoxia have been interpreted as anoxic-associated abrogation of release of EDRF, in vivo observations suggest that (1) such EDRF may be released during hypoxia and (2) their relaxing effect may be enhanced during hypoxia. Fritts et al. (1958) observed that administration of acetylcholine, 0.5 mg/min, into the main pulmonary artery of eight convalescent patients believed to have a "normal pulmonary circulation" resulted in a fall in mean pulmonary arterial pressure from 15 to 13 mmHg. A comparable infusion of acetylcholine while the patients breathed hypoxic gas mixture (12% O_2) resulted in a significantly greater fall in mean pulmonary arterial pressure from 20 to 16 mmHg. Thus, the effect of an endothelium-dependent vasodilator was unattenuated, and even enhanced, after pulmonary vascular tone was increasd by alveolar hypoxia. Arborelius and co-workers (1974) evaluated the effects of acetylcholine infusion, 2-10 mg/min, in seven healthy human subjects. These investigators observed unchanged pulmonary arterial pressure with acetylcholine administration during normoxia and during inhalation of a hypoxic gas mixture (13% O_2). Pulmonary vascular resistance was not reported in this study. However, the rise in cardiac output with acetylcholine administration during alveolar hypoxia compared to normoxia in the face of unchanged pulmonary arterial pressure suggested that acetylcholine exerted a vasodilating effect during alveolar hypoxia. Finally, Nandiwada and co-workers (1983) evaluated the effects of in situ lobar infusion of acetylcholine in anesthetized cats. The model consisted of in situ perfusion of the left lower lobe with whole blood at a constant flow rate. Thus, an increase or decrease in pulmonary arterial pressure was reflected by corresponding changes in pulmonary vascular resistance. The vasodilation with bolus injections of acetylcholine (0.5 and 1.0 mg) into the lobar pulmonary artery was enhanced when administered following interventions that increased pulmonary vascular tone (treatment with agents such as 15-methyl $PGF_{2\alpha}$ or the prostaglandin endoperoxide analog U-46619).

Summary

In vitro studies have shown that anoxia abolished endothelium-dependent relaxation and potentiated vascular contraction to various vasoactive substances. These observations have been open to question because (1) the effects of anoxia are physiologically irrelevant and (2) in vitro preparations have been limited to large pulmonary arterial segments rather than the smaller pulmonary arterioles that are believed to be the site of increased vascular resistance with alveolar hypoxia. Because of anoxic abolition of endothelium-dependent relaxation responses in vitro, many investigators concluded that anoxia abolished the ability of endothelial cells to release relaxing factor(s). Observations ex vivo and in vivo have demonstrated that vasodilation is present to endothelium-dependent vasodilators during alveolar hypoxia, and even suggest that the vasodilatory effects of these agents are enhanced during alveolar hypoxia. These observations dispute claims that EDRF is of little consequence during hypoxia. The production and potency of EDRF is illustrated by the marked degree of attenuation of hypoxic pulmonary arterial vasoconstriction in isolated perfused rat lungs by calcium ionophore A23187, a known agonist for the release of EDRF. It is still unclear whether the endothelium is involved in the hypoxic pressor response. Moreover, even if the endothelium is involved in some way, its role is unclear. For example, alveolar hypoxia could constrict vascular smooth muscle through an effect on the endothelium to either increase the formation of a vasoconstrictor or decrease the formation of a vasodilator. Nevertheless, these observations suggest that the pulmonary arterial endothelium may play an important role in mediating or modulating pulmonary arteriolar vasoconstriction to alveolar hypoxia.

C. Pulmonary Hypertension

The pulmonary circulation has an enormous reserve that allows accommodation of an increase in flow with maintenance of relatively low pressure and high compliance. A wide variety of diseases cause pulmonary hypertension related to increased postcapillary pressure, high pressure or high flow inputs to the pulmonary circulation, and diminished cross-sectional area of the pulmonary arteriolar bed (Harris and Heath, 1986). The characteristics of behavior of the pulmonary vascular bed during pulmonary hypertension that may be related to endothelial cell interaction with vascular smooth muscle relate to anatomic changes in blood vessels associated with pulmonary hypertension, accommodation to changes in flow, and responsiveness to certain pharmacologic agents.

Anatomic Changes

Harris and Heath (1986) have elegantly described anatomic changes in the pulmonary vasculature associated with chronic elevation of pulmonary arterial pressure. Whether these anatomic changes are primarily or secondarily related to the pulmonary hypertension remains unclear. However, they clearly extend to the endothelium. Esterly et al. (1968) examined serial lung biopsies of dogs with systemic-to-pulmonary arterial shunts to define anatomic changes secondary to the pulmonary hypertension. The anatomic changes observed by electron microscopy were in small pulmonary arterioles from 50 to 200 μm in diameter. Major changes were observed at 2 weeks, 2-4 months, and 4 months post-shunt:

1. *At 2 weeks* Although no changes were detectable by light microscopy at 2 weeks post-shunt, electron microscopy revealed clear-cut changes in the endothelial cells including increased pinocytotic vacuoles, free ribosomes, and rough-surfaced endoplasmic reticulum. Luminal surface villiform cytoplasmic processes were noted, and the subendothelial space was increased.
2. *At 2-4 months* Intimal proliferation obvious by electron microscopy occurred no sooner than 2 months post-shunt. Electron microscopic changes after appearance of intimal proliferation included endothelial changes suggestive of degeneration and involution, including diffuse vacuoles and poorly staining cytoplasm, with few organelles and "dense osmiophilic... cytoplasmic clumps." No evidence was found for endothelial proliferation. In addition, cells were observed in the space between the endothelium and internal elastic lamellae, including blood cells, smooth muscle cells, and poorly differentiated cells.
3. *After 4 months* Six weeks following the focal intimal thickening, totally occluded vessels were observed, and only degenerated endothelial cells were observed in nearly completely or completely occluded vessels. These observations suggest that an early hyperplastic reaction of endothelial cells occurred at 2 weeks after increased pressure and flow and was followed by endothelial cell injury and degeneration over the next 2 months of exposure.

Rabinovitch et al. (1986) recently reported pulmonary arterial endothelial ultrastructural changes in lung biopsy specimens from 20 patients with congenital heart defects. These changes in the endothelial cells included surface blebbing, increased microvilli, cuboidal appearance, increased density of rough endoplasmic reticulum, and increased microfilament bundles. However, none of these ultrastructural changes could be correlated with the severity of pulmonary hypertension or pulmonary vascular reactivity after surgery.

Joris and Majno (1981) evaluated the anatomic changes of vasospasm induced by dripping norepinephrine onto the adventitial surfaces of saphenous and medial tarsal arteries of ether-anesthetized male Wistar rats. These investigators reported electron micrographic changes of "squeezed" endothelial cells in the spastic segments 15-30 min postspasm, often to the point of obliteration of identifiable endothelial cytoplasm. At 1-2 hr postspasm with early relaxation of the segments, there were gaps in the endothelium, thinning of endothelial cell cytoplasm, and intercellular adhesions between endothelial cells. By 24 hr following spasm, the vascular changes became similar to sham-operated vessels. The extent of endothelial cell injury from this study is unclear, but it underscores the possibility that vasospasm may induce profound changes in the endothelium.

Accommodation of Blood Flow

The ability of the pulmonary circulation to accommodate increases in flow with only moderate rises in pulmonary arterial pressure in healthy human subjects is well known (Fishman, 1985; Grover et al., 1983; Harris and Heath, 1986). Three lines of evidence exist that support the possibility that pulmonary endothelium is important in pulmonary hemodynamic responses to increased flow in intact subjects and during disease states: (1) in vitro observations of endothelial release of relaxing factors with increased flow, (2) decreased pulmonry arterial pressure with sustained exercise, and (3) enhanced rise in pulmonary arterial pressure with increased flow in pulmonary hypertensive states. Rubanyi and colleagues (1986) have shown clearly that increased absolute flow or pulsatility of perfusate through a canine femoral arterial segment with endothelium resulted in further relaxation of a downstream bioassay coronary arterial ring devoid of endothelium. Moreover, Kaiser et al. (1986) recently observed that flow-induced vasodilation in in situ perfused canine femoral arteries was abolished by the in vitro antagonists of endothelium-dependent relaxation ETYA and methylene blue. These observations support the possibility that the endothelium modulates in vivo response of vascular smooth muscle tone to changes in blood flow in intact circulatory systems.

Although some debate still exists, the consensus is that an increase in flow in the intact pulmonary circulation is not matched with a proportional rise in pressure, which is consistent with a fall in pulmonary vascular resistance (Grover et al., 1983). For example, Elkins and Milnor (1971) observed a moderate decrease in pulmonary vascular resistance from 416 to 372 dynes/sec/cm^3 with acute exercise of 2 min duration in conscious dogs despite an increase in pulmonary blood flow and mean pulmonary arterial pressure from control of 19.4 mmHg and 3.0 liters/min to 28.0 mmHg and 5.3 liters/min, respectively. Bevegard and co-workers (1963) reported that pulmonary arterial pressure did not increase in proportion to cardiac output with severe exercise in well-trained athletes, providing further evidence for diminished pulmonary vascular resistance with increased pulmonary blood flow. Sancetta and Rakita (1957) described changes in pulmonary arterial pressure in 12 convalescing patients believed to have normal cardiopulmonary systems during 39 min of moderate, steady-state exercise by bicycle ergometry. Although pulmonary arterial pressure increased with early exercise, it began to decline progressively after the seventh minute, often to preexercise levels. The fall in pulmonary arterial pressure with exercise could not be explained by a decrease in cardiac output, since cardiac output remained elevated throughout exercise, suggesting that pulmonary vascular resistance decreased with progressive exercise. Stanek et al. (1973) evaluated the effects of exercise in 36 normal subjects. These investigators also observed an increase in pulmonary arterial pressure within the first 3 min of exercise that decreased progressively from the third to the twentieth minute of exercise. In this study, pulmonary vascular resistance, which was calculated in three subjects over the course of exercise, appeared to be unchanged, suggesting a passive relationship of pulmonary arterial pressure to flow.

Additional information on pulmonary vascular resistance in response to increasing blood flow can be found in studies evaluating the responses to unilateral occlusion of the main pulmonary artery by balloon catheter. Harris et al. (1968) evaluated the effect of right pulmonary arterial occlusion (with diversion of the entire cardiac output to the left lung) on pulmonary arterial pressure at rest and during exercise in healthy human subjects and patients with chronic bronchitis. These investigators observed that pulmonary arterial occlusion in healthy human subjects increased pulmonary arterial pressure proportionally to increased pulmonary blood flow, both at rest and during exercise, suggesting that pulmonary vascular resistance was unchanged.

In patients with pulmonary hypertension secondary to underlying lung disease such as chronic bronchitis (Harris et al., 1968) or interstitial fibrosis (Widimsky, 1970), an exaggerated rise in pulmonary arterial pressure with pulmonary arterial occlusion was observed. For example, Harris et al. (1968) observed that the rise in pulmonary arterial pressure with right pulmonary arterial occlusion during exercise in patients with chronic bronchitis was out of proportion to the change in pulmonary arterial pressure with balloon occlusion at rest. This perceived increase in pulmonary vascular resistance with exercise in these patients may have been due to multiple factors, including increased wedge pressure or arterial oxygen desaturation. In fact, Widimsky (1970) observed that the degree of rise in pulmonary arterial pressure with unilateral pulmonary artery occlusion in patients with underlying lung disease was correlated with the degree of arterial oxygen desaturation. Thus, it is difficult to evaluate the response of the pulmonary resistance vessels to an increase in pulmonary blood flow in patients with lung disease when additional variables are changing that themselves influence pulmonary vascular resistance.

In summary, in vitro observations have suggested that change in flow or pulsatility may induce changes in the pulmonary circulation through release of EDRF. Diminished pulmonary vascular resistance with increased pulmonary blood flow may be due to release of relaxing factors by endothelium, but other possibilities exist, including recruitment of pulmonary capillaries observed during hypoxic pulmonary hypertension (Wagner and Latham, 1975). Nevertheless, it is possible that the inordinate rise of pulmonary arterial pressure with increased flow in patients with advanced pulmonary hypertension may be due, in part, to impairment of an endothelium-mediated response to increased flow or pressure.

Responsiveness to Pharmacological Agents

Compelling in vitro evidence exists to suggest that the endothelium, in response to various stimuli, releases factors that relax vascular smooth muscle. While previous evidence does not support the notion that hypoxia diminishes endothelium-dependent relaxation, previous observations in pulmonary hypertensive patients have correlated progressive pulmonary hypertension with diminished pulmonary responsiveness to various pharmacological agents. The question raised by these observations is whether diminished endothelial production of vasodilators or vascular smooth muscle responsiveness to such vasodilators contributes primarily or secondarily to the pulmonary hypertension. Insight into this question can be obtained by examination of the effects of recognized endothelium-dependent vasodilators in patients with pulmonary hypertension from a variety of causes. The effects of acetylcholine and bradykinin in the pulmonary circulation in patients with pulmonary hypertension were explored extensively almost three decades ago. However, caution should be exercised in interpreting these studies because of variation in dosage, duration, and route of administration of these agents, and the imprecision in diagnosis of the underlying pathophysiological condition responsible for the pulmonary hypertension.

Effects of Acetylcholine

The effects of acetylcholine administration in pulmonary hypertension have been determined in patients with varying disease states, including idiopathic pulmonary hypertension, intracardiac shunting, pulmonary venous hypertension secondary to mitral valvular disease, and lung disease of miscellaneous causes (Table 4).

Patients with idiopathic pulmonary hypertension generally have responded to acetylcholine administration, often with a fall in pulmonary arterial pressure (Charms, 1961; Marshall et al., 1959; Wood, 1958) and pulmonary vascular resistance (Charms, 1961; Marshall et al., 1959). Samet and Bernstein (1963) reported loss of pulmonary vasodilation to acetylcholine in one patient with presumed idiopathic pulmonary hypertension over an interval of 40 months, but the patient's initial fall in pulmonary arterial pressure of 8 mmHg was less than that of other patients.

Shepherd et al. (1959) observed that pulmonary arterial pressure fell with pulmonary arterial infusion of acetylcholine in patients with either atrial septal defect (ASD) or ventricular septal defect (VSD). While baseline mean pulmonary arterial pressure was substantially higher in the VSD patients, the percentage decrease in pulmonary arterial pressure and pulmonary vascular resistance was roughly comparable to that of ASD patients. However, Wood (1958) observed no evidence of pulmonary vasodilation with acetylcholine in 13 of 14 patients with Eisenmenger's syndrome secondary to ASD or VSD.

Acetylcholine infusion in patients with pulmonary hypertension secondary to mitral valvular disease has resulted in significant decreases in pulmonary arterial pressure and pulmonary vascular resistance (Table 4). However, administration of acetylcholine to patients with a variety of lung diseases without pulmonary hypertension was not associated with any recognizable pulmonary vasodilatory response (Soderholm and Widimsky, 1962; Swenson et al., 1974).

Harris (1957) evaluated the effects of pulmonary arterial administration of acetylcholine, 0.25-8.0 mg, in 47 patients with pulmonary hypertension of varying severity due to multiple diseases including idiopathic pulmonary hypertension, arterial septal defect, ventricular septal defect, mitral valvular disease, emphysema, and pulmonary fibrosis. In constructing a histogram representing pulmonary vasodilation with regard to baseline mean pulmonary arterial pressure, Harris (1957) noted little vasodilation in patients with normal pulmonary arterial pressure. Patients with mean pulmonary arterial pressures of 40-70 mmHg manifest the greatest fall in pulmonary arterial pressure with acetylcholine. However, when baseline mean pulmonary arterial pressure was elevated above 80 mmHg, the number of patients responding to acetylcholine decreased, and no patient responded to acetylcholine who had a baseline mean pulmonary arterial pressure above 89 mmHg. Although the actual pulmonary arterial pressures were not reported by Wood (1958), it is possible that patients with Eisenmenger's syndrome who failed to exhibit pulmonary vasodilation responses to acetylcholine had elevation of mean pulmonary arterial pressures above 80 mmHg.

Table 4 Effects of Acetylcholine in Patients with Pulmonary Hypertension[a]

			Acetylcholine			PAs, mmHg			PA, mmHg	
Investigator	Disease	N	Dose	Route	Duration	C	D	Δ	C	D
Primary pulmonary hypertension										
Charms, 1961	IPH	1	0.5 mg/min	PA	15 min.				74	35
Marshall et al., 1959	IPH	1	2.0 mg/min	RV	?				56	25
Samet and Bernstein, 1963	IPH	1	4.25 mg/min	RA	?				43	35
		1	5.6 mg/min	RA	?				58	61
Wood, 1958	IPH	6	1.0 mg/min	PA	bolus			30		
Intracardiac shunt										
Shepherd et al., 1959	ASD	6	7±3 mg/min	PA	1-2 min				50	43
	VSD	4	4±1 mg/min	PA	1-2 min				80	70
Wood, 1958	EM	14	1.0 mg	PA	bolus			0		
Pulmonary venous hypertension										
Bateman et al., 1962	MVD	9	0.5 mg/min	PA	9 min				42	35[c]
Oakley et al., 1962	MVD	5	0.03 - 0.08	PA	?				47	35
Soderholm and Werko, 1959	MVD	10	3-14.5 mg/min	PA	?				34	28
Soderholm et al., 1962	MVD	20	5-10 mg/min	RA or RV	>20 min				44	39
Stanfield et al., 1961	MVD	18	2-12 mg/min	PA	?				37	31
Wood et al., 1957	MVD	9	1.4±0.1 mg/min	PA	bolus	78	67			
Pulmonary disease										
Soderholm and Widimski, 1962		9	5-10 mg/min	RA	>20 min				19	17
Swenson et al., 1974		27	4-8 mg/min	PA	?				18	19

[a]ASD, atrial septal defect; CO, cardiac output; C, control; D, drug; EM, Eisenmenger's syndrome; IPA, idiopathic pulmonary hypertension; MVD, mitral valvular disease; PA, mean pulmonary arterial pressure; PAR, pulmonary arteriolar resistance [(PA–Pcw)/CO]; Pcw=pulmonary capillary wedge pressure (or left atrial pressure); PAs: systolic pulmonary arterial pressure; PVR: total pulmonary vascular resistance (PA/CO); SaO_22: arterial blood oxygen saturation; and VSD: ventricular septal defect.

[b]Cardiac index.

[c]Statistically significant charge compared to control. $p < 0.05$

Psys, mmHg		Pcw, mmHg		CO liters/min		PVR dynes/s/cm^3		PAR dynes/s/cm^3		SaO_2	
C	D	C	D	C	D	C	D	C	D	C	D
122	130			4.7	5.2			1153	463	93	89
				4.4	4.6	1020	435				
				1.7[b]	1.9[b]						
				1.4[b]	1.4[b]						
				5.2	6.0	927	702			94	92
				3.6	4.2	1739	1394			91	91
99	101	22	23	3.3[b]	3.2[b]					98	96
80	72	25	22	2.2[b]	2.3[b]			491	299		
103	99	18		4.8	4.8					97	91
102	103	18	19	3.7	3.7			376	296	95	94
82	78			2.7[b]	2.9[b]			655	414	94	90
		20	23	4.3	4.3	753	524				
117	118	7	6	5.5	5.5			145	109	93	89
93	88										

Table 5 Effects of Bradykinin in Patients with Pulmonary Hypertension[a]

Investigator	Disease	Bradykinin Dose μg/kg/min	Route	Duration	PAs, mmHg C	D	PA, mmHg C	D
Bishop et al., 1965	CB (N = 7)	0.3-1.0	SVC	15 min			43	47
de Freitas et al., 1964	EH (N = 10)	0.92±0.14	SVC or IVC	?	107	79[b]	18	18
de Freitas et al., 1966	MVD (N = 21)	0.98	IV	14 min			53	64[b]

[a]CB, chronic bronchitis; EH, essential hypertension. For remainder of abbreviations, see Table 4.
[b]Statistically significant change from control, $p < 0.05$.

Demonstration of pulmonary vasodilation with administration of an endothelium-dependent relaxing agent in patients with pulmonary hypertension suggests that obliteration of endothelium-vascular smooth muscle interaction is not the mechanism responsible for pulmonary hypertension. Diminished responsiveness to acetylcholine with progressive pulmonary hypertension is suggested by several previous studies, but this phenomenon has not been demonstrated convincingly. Further studies are needed to specifically evaluate the role of the endothelium in pulmonary hypertensive states.

Effects of Bradykinin

The effects of bradykinin on the pulmonary circulation in patients with cardiopulmonary disease are clouded by the concomitant significant systemic vasodilation and rise in cardiac output. Bishop and co-workers (1965) observed a consistent fall in mean systemic arterial pressure with bradykinin administration to seven patients with chronic bronchitis, but pulmonary arterial pressure and pulmonary arteriolar resistance were unchanged (Table 5). Administration of bradykinin to patients with normal pulmonary arterial pressure (de Freitas et al., 1964) and pulmonary hypertension secondary to mitral valvular disease (de Freitas et al., 1966) resulted in no change in pulmonary arterial pressure. However, pulmonary vasodilation with bradykinin was evident from the fall in pulmonary arteriolar resistance. The rise in cardiac output with bradykinin administration may have been due to the systemic vasodilation and fall in systemic arterial pressure observed in patients with mitral valvular disease (de Freitas et al., 1966).

Psys, mmHg		Pcw, mmHg		CI, liters/min		PVR dynes/s/cm^3		PAR dynes/s/cm^3		TPR dynes/s/cm^3	
C	D	C	D	C	D	C	D	C	D	C	D
122	106[b]	12	13	3.4	4.0[b]			434	407		
		5	6	3.8	5.9[b]	1395	757[b]	156	107[b]		
88	72[b]	23	31[b]	2.4	3.3[b]			839	655[b]	2117	1302[b]

Although the effects of bradykinin in pulmonary hyperensive patients have not been evaluated as extensively as those of acetylcholine, it appears that the predominant systemic vasodilatory effects of bradykinin cloud interpretation of its effects on the pulmonary circulation. These studies support a vasodilatory effect of bradykinin on the pulmonary circulation in patients with intact pulmonary circulatory function and in patients with pulmonary hypertension secondary to mitral valvular disease.

Effects of Other Pharmacologic Agents

Administration of various vasodilator drugs to patients with pulmonary hypertension has been associated with varying results. For example, administration of hydralazine to patients with idiopathic pulmonary hypertension results in a decrease in pulmonary arterial pressure in some patients and an increase in others (Rich et al., 1983). This differing effect has been attributed to the degree of systemic versus pulmonary vasodilation with pharmacologic agents in each patient (Rich and Brundage, 1986). When systemic vasodilation exceeds pulmonary vasodilation, the resultant increase in cardiac output and pulmonary blood flow may actually increase pulmonary arterial pressure. The possibility exists that this variability in vasodilation between the pulmonary and systemic vascular beds may be related to endothelial responses to these vasodilators. This possibility is supported by observations by Spokas et al. (1983) that the vasodilatory effects of hydralazine on rabbit aortic rings were decreased tenfold when the endothelium was removed.

Idiopathic Pulmonary Hypertension

The possibility of a disorder of endothelium-vascular smooth muscle interaction as the primary cause of pulmonary hypertension must also be considered. Recently, de Voorde and Leusen (1986) described diminished responsiveness to acetylcholine of thoracic aortic rings from rats with two-kidney, one-clip renal hypertension. Subsequent experiments showed that acetylcholine administration to aortic segments from hypertensive rats resulted in normal relaxation of downstream thoracic aortic rings from control rats. This suggested that diminished relaxation of thoracic aortic rings from hypertensive rats to acetylcholine was not due to diminished release of EDRF, but rather to diminished responsiveness of vascular smooth muscle to this substance. Despite these provocative results, the current state of knowledge of vascular responsiveness in pulmonary hypertensive states provides little insight into endothelium-vascular smooth muscle interactions as a primary mechanism for pulmonary hypertension. The most attractive pathophysiological state for a primary endothelial disorder is primary pulmonary hypertension, the cause of which remains unknown (Fishman and Pietra, 1980). While a relative young age of onset and occasional familial occurrence could be taken to suggest an endothelial disorder, no convincing evidence to date has identified any endothelial abnormality. The anatomic changes in patients with primary pulmonary hypertension do include endothelial changes, including increased endothelial thickness, foamy cytoplasm, and increased ribosomes and Golgi apparatus (Meyrick et al., 1974). While exercise-induced exacerbation of pulmonary hypertension has been observed in some patients with primary pulmonary hypertension (Sleeper et al., 1962), this does not by itself identify any specific vascular abnormality. For example, diminished accomodation to increased pulmonary blood flow may be due to loss of small pulmonary arterioles or enhanced vasoconstriction rather than a specific endothelial cell abnormality. Clearly, patients with primary pulmonary hypertension demonstrate pulmonary vasodilation with endothelium-dependent pharmacologic agents such as acetylcholine (Table 4), although this phenomenon was observed less frequently in patients with more severe pulmonary hypertension. While sufficient information regarding the role of the endothelium in primary pulmonary hypertension is not yet available, the possibility is of such importance it should be evaluated thoroughly. Moreover, it is possible that the abnormality exists at the level of diminished vascular smooth muscle responsiveness to products liberated from intact, functioning endothelial cells.

D. Hyperoxia and Oxygen Toxicity

Many of the pulmonary circulatory alterations associated with oxygen toxicity may be related to changes in the interaction between the endothelium and vascular smooth muscle. Evidence for impairment of the endothelial-vascular smooth muscle relationship by hyperoxia or oxygen toxicity includes anatomic evidence of endothelial cell injury, altered endothelial metabolism, diminished hypoxic pulmonary vasoconstriction, and alteration of relaxation to endothelium-dependent vasodilators.

Anatomic Evidence of Endothelial Injury

Kistler et al. (1967) described the electron microscopic changes in the lung with oxygen toxicity. Exposure of rats to hyperoxia ($FiO_2 = 0.985$) for 6-72 hr resulted in interstitial edema and marked cellular damage that was confined to endothelium. Endothelial cellular changes observed after 3 days of exposure included partial detachment from basement membrane, fragmentation, and necrosis. In contrast to the dramatic endothelial cell damage and destruction by hyperoxia, epithelial cells were little affected, despite evidence of widespread alveolar exudate.

Altered Endothelial Metabolism

Commiskey et al. (1981) observed that metabolic profiles of calf pulmonary arterial and aortic endothelial cells depended on the PO_2 exposure. Sonicates of cells incubated under hypoxic conditions (PO_2 = 15 mmHg) compared to normoxia (PO_2 = 140 mmHg) for 96 hr had significantly greater levels of pyruvate kinase and phosphofructokinase. Homogenates of intimal strips from pulmonary arteries and aorta from freshly slaughtered calves revealed higher pyruvate kinase levels in pulmonary artery endothelial strips, suggesting that metabolic differences between endothelial cells exist in vito that are possibly related to the intraluminal blood oxygen tension.

Lastly, Block and Fisher (1977) observed that 5-hydroxytryptamine uptake by isolated perfused lungs from rats exposed to toxic oxygen concentrations ($FiO_2 = 1.0$ for 4-48 hr) was diminished by 20% compared to control rats. Since autoradiographic studies have identified that endothelial cells are responsible for serotonin uptake in the pulmonary circulation (Strum and Junod, 1972), this suggests that diminished pulmonary circulatory clearance of 5-hydroxytryptamine with oxygen toxicity may be mediated through an effect on endothelial cells.

Diminished Hypoxic Pulmonary Arterial Vasoconstriction

Holden and McCall (1984) observed that incubation of swine pulmonary arterial strips for 2 hr at a bath oxygen tension of 140 mmHg resulted in an absence of contractile response to anoxia. In contrast, incubation of the pulmonary arterial strips at a bath oxygen tension of 40 mmHg for 4-6 hr resulted in subsequent strong endothelium-dependent contractile responses to hypoxia and anoxia. Newman et al. (1981) assessed the hypoxic pulmonary pressor response in isolated perfused lungs of rats exposed to either hyperoxia (FiO_2 = 0.40 for 3-5 weeks) or toxic oxygen levels (FiO_2 = 1.0 for 48 hr). Evidence of oxygen toxicity included gross findings of pleural effusions and patchy atelectasis and light microscopy evidence of alveolar wall thickening and laveolar edema. These investigators observed that hypoxic pulmonary vasoconstriction was unchanged by hyperoxia but that the hypoxic pulmonary pressor response was blunted profoundly in oxygen toxic lungs. Blockade of cyclooxygenase by meclofenamate restored the hypoxic pressor response in oxygen toxic lungs to normal. Vascular production of vasodilator prostaglandins, such as PGI_2, , has been localized to the intimal layer of the vascular wall (Moncada et al., 1977). Moreover, it appears that the vascular endothelium is largely responsible for PGI_2 synthesis (Weksler et al., 1977; MacIntyre et al., 1978). Thus, increased endothelial PGI_2 synthesis as a result of oxygen toxicity may have led to the blunting of hypoxic pulmonary vasoconstriction observed by Newman et al. (1981), since meclofenamate restored the response to the control level. However, these observations do not confine prostaglandin synthesis and metabolism to the endothelium, since vascular smooth muscle may synthesize prostaglandins, although to a lesser extent than endothelium (MacIntyre et al., 1978).

Impairment of Endothelium-Dependent Relaxation

Coflesky and Evans (1986) observed that precontracted pulmonary arterial segments from rats exposed to 7 days of chronic hyperoxia (FiO_2 = 0.85) developed only 30% of the response to acetylcholine compared to relaxation in control rats. Moroover, contractile responses of these pulmonary arterial segments from hyperoxic rats to $PGF_{2\alpha}$ were enhanced. Further evidence for impairment of endothelium-dependent responses by hyperoxia can be found in observations by Rubanyi and Vanhoutte (1986b). These investigators employed a model where hyperoxic (95% O_2) Krebs-Ringers bicarbonate solution was superfused through a femoral arterial segment containing endothelium onto a coronary arterial segment devoid of endothelium. With a transit time of 30 sec between the femoral artery and coronary artery, injection of acetylcholine upstream of the femoral artery resulted in contraction, not relaxation, of the bioassay ring. In contrast, identical upstream injection of acetylcholine in the presence of the oxygen radical scavenger superoxide dismutase resulted in relaxation of the bioassay vessel, suggesting that EDRF released by femoral artery endothelium was being inactivated in transit by oxygen radicals. Changing the gas aerating the perfusate to 10% O_2 further enhanced the effects of superoxide dismutase on acetylcholine relaxation of the bioassay ring. Luckhoff et al. (1987) recently reported that normoxic (20% O_2) perfusate flowing across endothelial cells on microcarrier beads stimulated with bradykinin resulted in vasodilation of a downstream detector vessel devoid of endothelium. Comparable administration of bradykinin to perfusate saturated with 95% O_2 resulted in significantly less vasodilation of the detector vessel. The mechanism for the hyperoxic attenuation of endothelium responses is unclear and may relate to destruction of EDRF by increased free oxygen radicals formed during hyperoxia, to decreased endothelial production of EDRF, or to decreased muscle response to EDRF. However, these observations do identify an effect of hyperoxia to reduce endothelium-dependent relaxation responses.

Taken altogether, these observations suggest that pulmonary circulatory changes with hyperoxia and oxygen toxicity may be mediated through changes in the endothelium including metabolic functions such as release of EDRF(s) or prostaglandins, increased inactivation of EDRF(s), or changes in uptake and metabolism of other vasoactive substances.

E. Endotoxemia

Administration of endotoxin in a wide variety of animal models has resulted in a rise in pulmonary arterial pressure (Hales et al., 1981; Huttemeier et al., 1982; Parratt, 1973) and pulmonary vascular resistance (Parratt, 1973), increase in pulmonary vascular permeability (Brigham et al., 1979), fall in circulating leukocytes (Huttemeier et al., 1982), and rise in circulating eicosanoids including TX B_2 and 6-keto-$PGF_{1\alpha}$ (Hales et al., 1981; Huttemeier et al., 1982). Despite evidence of post-endotoxin vascular hyperreactivity to norepinephrine in the rat mesenteric microcirculation (Zweifach and Thomas, 1957) and to 5-hydroxytryptamine in isolated, rabbit thoracic aorta strips (Weiner and Zweifach, 1966), circulatory reactivity in intact animals following endotoxin administration is diminished. For example, pulmonary vasoconstriction to angiotensin II and $PGF_{2\alpha}$ was abolished in anesthetized dogs following endotoxin administration, and there was loss of the ability to diminish pulmonary blood flow with unilateral alveolar hypoxia (Hales et al., 1981). These changes were not localized to the pulmonary circulation, since systemic vascular responsiveness to angiotensin II also was diminished following endotoxin administration.

There are multiple mechanisms that may explain pulmonary vascular consequences of endotoxemia, and a substantial body of evidence suggests that the endothelium may be involved, including (1) anatomic changes, (2) pulmonary hypertension with changes in circulating prostaglandins, and (3) attenuation of pulmonary hypertension by cyclooxygenase inhibitors.

Using an ear chamber, Goodman and co-workers (1979) evaluated the anatomic changes in the rabbit microcirculation following endotoxin administration. Within 3 min, following endotoxemia, leukocytes were adherent to arteriolar and venous endothelium, and emboli were observed by 10 min. One hour following administration, intimal swelling and occlusion were evident, and at 3 hr, both white and red blood cells were present extravascularly. These changes were confirmed in the pulmonary circulation at autopsy. Additional evidence of endothelial injury with endotoxin administration was found by McGrath and Stewart (1969), who observed endothelial nuclear vacuolization and distortion with adherence of white blood cells and platelets in rabbit endothelial sheets from mesenteric vessels.

The rise in pulmonary arterial pressure with endotoxin administration to anesthetized sheep (Huttemeier et al., 1982) or to anesthetized dogs (Hales et al., 1981) has been correlated with increased circulating levels of TXB_2, a stable metabolite of the potent constrictor TXA_2, and with increased circulating 6-keto-$PGF_{1\alpha}$, the PGI_2 metabolite. Moreover, a transpulmonary gradient for TXB_2 levels, venous greater than arterial, was observed in a majority of animals, suggesting that the lung was responsible for increased circulating TXB_2.

Employment of cyclooxygenase antagonists has suggested that the pulmonary hypertension following endotoxin administration may be mediated through prostaglandins. Parratt and Sturgess (1975) observed that pretreatment with meclofenamate or indomethacin attenuated the intense pulmonary vasoconstriction with endotoxin in anesthetized cats. Huttemeier et al. (1982) observed that ibuprofen significantly attenuated the rise in pulmonary arterial pressure with endotoxin administration to anesthetized sheep and simultaneously abolished the rise in circulating TXB_2 and 6-keto-$PGF_{1\alpha}$.

Previous investigators have observed TXA_2 generation by the isolated perfused lung, in response to products of anaphylaxis including histamine and slow-reacting substance of anaphylaxis (Berti et al., 1980). Despite the ability of the isolated lung to generate TXA_2 in response to pathological conditions including endotoxemia, it is not at all clear that the endothelium is the location of synthesis. TXA_2 synthesis by platelets has been well documented (Hamberg et al., 1975). Moreover, Spagnuolo et al. (1980) observed that polymorphonuclear leukocytes released TXA_2 in response to *E.coli* lipopolysaccharide.

In summary, these studies have shown the following effects of endotoxin: (1) anatomic evidence of endothelial injury; (2) evidence of pulmonary vascular dysfunction including attenuated responsiveness to alveolar hypoxia, angiotensin II, and $PGF_{2\alpha}$; (3) elevated pulmonary arterial pressure; and (4) increased pulmonary vascular permeability. While correlative changes in eicosanoids including TXA_2 have been observed, the exact mechanism(s) for the pulmonary circulatory responses to endotoxin remains unclear. Endothelial injury is one possible mechanism for pulmonary circulatory alterations secondary to endotoxin. As mentioned previously, endotoxin may also release PAF from endothelium. However, additional mechanisms for endotoxin-induced vascular injury and dysfunction exist and have been reviewed recently (Nagler, 1980).

References

Abraham, N. G., Pinto, A., Mullane, K. M., Levere, R. D., and Spokas, E. G. (1985). Presence of cytochrome P450 monooxygenase in intimal cells of the hog aorta. *Hypertension* 7:899-904.

Altiere, R. J., Kiritsy-Roy, J. A., and Catravas, J. D. (1985). Acetylcholine-induced contractions in isolated rabbit pulmonary arteries: role of thromboxane A_2. *J. Pharmacol. Exp. Ther.* *236*:535-541.

Anggard, E., Larsson, C., and Samuelsson, B. (1971). The distribution of 15-hydroxyprostaglandin dehydrogenase and prostaglandin-Δ^{13}-reductase in tissues of the swine. *Acta Physiol. Scand.* *81*:396-404.

Arborelius, M., Lilja, B., Swenson, E. W., Lindell, S. E., and Hjaltason, S. (1974). Regional pulmonary arterial infusion of acetylcholine and histamine in man. I. Healthy volunteers. *Scand. J. Resp. Dis. (Suppl.)* *85*:83-91.

Arnold, W. P., Mittal, C. K., Katsuki, S., and Murad, F. (1977). Nitric oxide activates guanylate cyclase and increases guanosine 3',5'-cyclic monophosphate levels in various tissue preparations. *Proc. Natl. Acad. Sci. USA* *74*:3203-3207.

Bassingthwaighte, J. B., Sparks, H. V., Chan, I. S., Dewitt, D. F., and Gorman, M. W. (1985). Modeling of transendothelial transport. *Fed. Proc.* *44*:2623-2626.

Bateman, M., Davidson, L. A. G., Donald, K. W., and Harris, P. (1962). A comparison of the effect of acetylcholine and 100% oxygen on the pulmonary circulation in patients with mitral stenosis. *Clin. Sci.* *22*:223-231.

Berk, B. C., Alexander, R. W., Brock, T. A., Gimbrone, M. A., and Webb, R. C. (1986). Vasoconstriction: a new activity for platelet-derived growth factor. *Science* *232*:87-90.

Berti, F., Folco, G. C., Giachetti, A., Malandrino, S., Omini, C., and Vigano, T. (1980). Atropine inhibits thromboxane A_2 generation in isolated lungs of the guinea pig. *Brit. J. Pharmacol.* *68*:467-472.

Bevegard, S., Holmgren, A., and Jonsson, B. (1963). Circulatory studies in well trained athletes at rest and during heavy exercise, with special reference to stroke volume and the influence of body position. *Acta Physiol. Scand.* *57*:26-50.

Biguad, M., Schoeffter, P., Stocklet, J., and Miller, R. (1984). Dissociation between endothelium-mediated increases in tissue cyclic GMP levels and modulation of aortic contractile responses. *Naunyn-Schmeid. Arch. Pharmacol.* *328*:221-223.

Bishop, M. J., Harris, P., and Segel, N. (1965). The circulatory effects of bradykinin in normal subjects and patients with chronic bronchitis. *Brit. J. Pharmacol.* *25*:456-469.

Block, E. R., and Fisher, A. B. (1977). Depression of serotonin clearance by rat lungs during oxygen exposure. *J. Appl. Physiol. 42*:33-38.

Brigham, K. L., Bowers, R. E., and Haynes, J. (1979). Increased sheep lung vascular permeability caused by *Escherichia coli* endotoxin. *Circ. Res. 45*: 292-297.

Brum, J. M., Sufun, Q., Lane, G., and Bore, A. A. (1984). Increased vasoconstrictor activity of proximal coronary arteries with endothelial damage in intact dog. *Circulation 70*:1066-1073.

Bunting, S., Gryglewski, R., Moncada, S., and Vane, J. R. (1976). Arterial walls generate from prostaglandin endoperoxides a substance (prostaglandin X) which relaxes strips of mesenteric and coeliac arteries and inhibits platelet aggregation. *Prostaglandins 12*:897-915.

Busse, R., Pohl, U., Kellner, C., and Klemm, U. (1983). Endothelial cells are involved in the vasodilatory response to hypoxia. *Pfluegers Arch. 397*:78-80.

Busse, R., Forstermann, U., Matsuda, H., and Pohl, U. (1984). The role of prostaglandins in the endothelium-mediated vasodilatory response to hypoxia. *Pfluegers Arch. 401*:77-83.

Campbell, J. H., and Campbell, G. R. (1986). Endothelial cell influences on vascular smooth muscle phenotype. *Ann. Rev. Physiol. 48*:295-306.

Castellot, J. J., Rosenberg, R. D., and Karnovsky, M. J. (1984). Endothelium, heparin, and the regulation of cell growth. In *Biology of Endothelial Cells*. Edited by E. Jaffe. Martinus Nijhoff, Boston, MA, pp. 118-128.

Chand, N., and Altura, B. M. (1981). Acetylcholine and bradykinin relax intrapulmonary arteries by acting on endothelial cells: role in lung vascular disease. *Science 213*:1376-1379.

Charms, B. L. (1961). Primary pulmonary hypertension. Effect of unilateral pulmonary arterial occlusion and infusion of acetylcholine. *Am. J. Cardiol. 8*: 94-99.

Clark, D. L., and Linden, J. (1986). Modulation of guanylate cyclase by lipoosygenase inhibitors. *Hypertension 8*:947-950.

Clowes, A. W., and Karnovsky, M. J. (1977). Suppression by heparin of smooth muscle cell proliferation in injured arteries. *Nature 265*:625-626.

Cocks, T. M., and Angus, J. A. (1983). Pendothelium-dependent relaxation of coronary arteries by norepinephrine and serotonin. *Nature 305*:627-630.

Cocks, T. M., Angus, J. A., Campbell, J. H., and Campbell, G. R. (1985). Release and properties of endothelium-derived relaxing factor (EDRF) from endothelial cells in culture. *J. Cell Physiol. 123*:310-320.

Coflesky, J. T., and Evans, J. N. (1986). Hyperoxia alters endothelial-dependent relaxation and pharmacologic sensitivity of pulmonary arteries. *Abstr. Am. Rev. Resp. Dis. 133*:AA159.

Commiskey, J. M., Simon, L. M., Theodore, J., Ryan, U. S., and Robin, E. D. (1981). Bioenergetic alterations in cultivated pulmonary artery and aortic endothelial cells exposed to normoxia and hypoxia. *Exp. Lung. Res. 2*: 155-163.

Davies, P. F. (1986). Vascular cell interactions with special reference to the pathogenesis of atherosclerosis. *Lab. Invest. 55*:5-24.

Dees, J. H., Masters, B. S. S., Muller-Ebergard, U., and Johnson, E. F. (1982). Effect of 2,3,7,8-tetrachlorodibenzo-*p*-dioxin and phenobarbital on the occurrence and distribution of four cytochrome P450 isozymes in rabbit kidney, lung, and liver. *Cancer Res. 42*:1423-1432.

DeGroot, P. G., Brinkman, H. J. M., Gonsalves, M. D., and Van Mourik, J. A. (1985). The role of thrombin in the regulation of the endothelial prostaglandin production. *Biochim. Biophys. Acta. 846*:342-349.

DeMey, J. G., and Vanhoutte, P. M. (1980). Interaction between Na^+, K^+ exchanges and the direct inhibitory effect of acetylcholine on canine femoral arteries. *Circ. Res. 46*:826-836.

DeMey, J. G., and Vanhoutte, P. M. (1981). Contribution of the endothelium to the response to anoxia in the canine femoral artery. *Arch. Int. Pharmacodyn. Ther. 253*:325-326.

DeMey, J. G., and Vanhoutte, P. M. (1982). Heterogenous behavior of the canine arterial and venous wall–importance of the endothelium. *Circ. Res. 51*:439-447.

De Mey, J. G. and Vanhoutte, P. M. (1983). Anoxia and endothelium-dependent reactivity of the canine femoral artery. *J. Physiol. 335*:65-74.

De Mey, J. G., Claeys, M., and Vanhoutte, P. M. (1982). Endothelial-dependent inhibitory effects of acetylcholine, adenosine triphosphate, thrombin and arachidonic acid in the canine femoral artery. *J. Pharmacol. Exp. Ther. 222*:166-173.

DiCorleto, P. E. (1984). Cultured endothelial cells produce multiple growth factors for connective tissue cells. *Exp. Cell Res. 153*:167-172.

DiCorleto, P. E., Gajdusec, C. M., Schwartz, S. M., and Ross, R. (1983). Biochemical properties of the endothelium-derived growth factor: comparison to other growth factors. *J. Cell Physiol. 114*:339-345.

Dobuler, K. J., Catravas, J. D., and Gillis, C. N. (1982). Early detection of oxygen-induced lung injury in conscious rabbits. *Am. Rev. Resp. Dis. 126*: 534-539.

Egleme, C., Godfraind, T., and Miller, R. (1984). Enhanced responsiveness of rat isolated aorta to clonidine after removal of the endothelial cells. *Brit. J. Pharmacol. 81*:16-18.

Elkins, R. C., and Milnor, W. R. (1971). Pulmonary vascular response to exercise in the dog. *Circ. Res. 29*:591-599.

Esterly, J. A., Glagov, S., and Ferguson, D. J. (1968). Morphogenesis of intimal obliterative hyperplasia of small arteries in experimental pulmonary hypertension. *Am. J. Pathol. 52*:325-337.

Feddersen, C. O., McMurtry, I. F., Henson, P., and Voelkel, N. F. (1986). Acetylcholine-induced pulmonary vasodilation in lung vascular injury. *Am. Rev. Resp. Dis. 133*:197-204.

Fisher, A. B., Block, E. R., and Pietra, G. G. (1980). Environmental influences on uptake of serotonin and other amines. *Environ. Health Perspect. 35*: 191-198.

Fishman, A. P. (1985). Pulmonary circulation. In *Handbook of Physiology*. Sect. 3, *The Respiratory System*. Vol. I. Edited by A. P. Fishman and A. B. Fisher. Waverly Press, Baltimore, MD, pp. 93-165.

Fishman, A. P., and Pietra, G. G. (1980). Primary pulmonary hypertension. *Ann. Rev. Med. 31*:421-431.

Forstermann, U., and Neufang, B. (1984). The endothelium-dependent vasodilator effect of acetylcholine: Characterization of the endothelial relaxing factor with inhibitors of arachidonic acid metabolism. *Eur. J. Pharmcol. 103*:65-70.

Forstermann, U., and Neufang, B. (1985). Endothelium-dependent vasodilation by melittin: are lipoxygenase products involved? *Am. J. Physiol. 249 (Heart Circ. Physiol. 18)*:H14-H19.

Forstermann, U., Trogisch, G., and Busse, R. (1985). Species differences in the nature of endothelium-derived relaxing factor. *Eur. J. Pharmacol. 106*: 639-643.

Forstermann, U., Mulsch, A., Bohme, E., and Busse, R. (1986). Stimulation of soluble guanylate cyclase by an acetylcholine-induced endothelium-derived factor from rabbit and canine arteries. *Circ. Res. 58*:531-538.

Freitas, F. M. de, Faraco, E. Z., and Azevedo, D. F. de (1964). General circulatory alterations induced by intravenous infusion of synthetic bradykinin in man. *Circulation 29*:66-70.

Freitas, F. M. de, Faraco, E. Z., Azevedo, D. F., de, and Lewin, I. (1966). Action of bradykinin on human pulmonary circulation. Observations in patients with mitral valvular disease. *Circulation 34*:385-390.

Fritts, H. W., Harris, P., Clauss, R. H., Odell, J. E., and Cournand, A. (1958). The effect of acetylcholine on the human pulmonary circulation under normal and hypoxic conditions. *J. Clin. Invest. 37*:99-110.

Furchgott, R. F. (1984). The role of the endothelium in the responses of vascular smooth muscle to drugs. *Ann. Rev. Pharmacol. Toxicol. 24*:175-197.

Furchgott, R., and Jothianandan, D. (1983). Relation of cyclic GMP levels to endothelium-dependent relaxation by acetylcholine in rabbit aorta. (Abstr.) *Fed. Proc. 42*:619.

Furchgott, R. F., and Zawadzki, J. V. (1980). The obligatory role of endothelial cells in the relaxation of arterial smooth muscle by acetylcholine. *Nature 288*:373-376.

Gillespie, M. N., Owasoyo, J. O., McMurtry, I. F., and O'Brien, R. F. (1986). Sustained coronary vasoconstriction provoked by a peptidergic substance released from endothelial cells in culture. *J. Pharmacol. Exp. Ther. 236*: 339-343.

Gillis, C. N., and Pitt, B. R. (1982). The fate of circulating amines within the pulmonary circulation. *Ann. Rev. Physiol. 44*:269-281.

Goodman, M. L., Way, B. A., and Irwin, J. W. (1979). The inflammatory response to endotoxin. *J. Pathol. 128*:7-14.

Gordon, J. L., and Martin, W. (1983). Endothelium-dependent relaxation of the pig aorta: relationship to stimulation of ^{86}Rb efflux from isolated endothelial cells. *Brit. J. Pharmacol. 79*:531-541.

Grega, G. J., Adamski, S. W., and Dobbins, D. E. (1986). Physiological and pharmacological evidence for the regulation of permeability. *Fed. Proc. 45*:96-100.

Greenberg, B., Rhoden, K., and Barnes, P. (1987). Endothelium-dependent relaxation of human pulmonary arteries. *Am. J. Physiol. 252 (Heart Circ. Physiol. 21)*:H434-H438.

Greenwald, J. E., Bianchine, J. R., and Wong, L. K. (1979). The production of the arachidonate metabolite HETE in vascular tissue. *Nature 281*:588-589.

Greutter, C. A., and Lemke, S. M. (1986a). Comparison of endothelium-dependent relaxation in bovine intrapulmonary artery and vein by acetylcholine and A23187. *J. Pharmacol. Exp. Ther. 238*:1055-1064.

Greutter, C. A., and Lemke, S. M. (1986b). Bradykinin-induced endothelium-dependent relaxation of bovine intrapulmonary artery and vein. *Eur. J. Pharmacol. 122*:363-367.

Griffith, T. M., Edwards, D. H., Lewis, M. J., Newby, A. C., and Henderson, A. H. (1984). The nature of endothelium-derived relaxing factor. *Nature 308*:645-647.

Griffith, T. M., Edwards, D. H., Lewis, M. J., and Henderson A. H. (1985). Evidence that cyclic guanosine monophosphate (cGMP) mediates endothelium-dependent relaxation. *Eur. J. Pharmacol. 112*:195-202.

Grover, R. F., Wagner, W. W., McMurtry, I. F., and Reeves, J. T. (1983). Pulmonary circulation. In *Handbook of Physiology*. Sect. 2, *The Cardiovascular System*. Vol. III, *Peripheral Circulation and Organ Blood Flow*. American Physiological Society, Washington, DC, pp. 103-136.

Gryglewski, R. J., Palmer, R. M. J., and Moncada, S. (1986). Superoxide anion is involved in the breakdown of endothelium-derived vascular relaxing factor. *Nature 320*:454-456.

Hales, C. A., Sonne, L., Peterson, M., Kong, D., Miller, M., and Watkins, W. D. (1981). Role of thromboxane and prostacyclin in pulmonary vasomotor changes after endotoxin in dogs. *J. Clin. Invest. 68*:497-505.

Hamberg, M., Svensson, J., and Samuelsson, B. (1975). Thromboxanes: a new group of biologically active compounds derived from prostaglandin endoperoxides. *Proc. Natl. Acad. Sci. USA 72*:2994-2998.

Harris, P. (1957). Influence of acetylcholine on pulmonary arterial pressure. *Brit. Heart J. 19*:272-278.

Harris, P., and Heath, D. (1986). *The Human Pulmonary Circulation*. Churchill Livingstone, New York, pp. 59-77, 183-209.

Harris, P., Segel, N., and Bishop, J. M. (1968). The relation between pressure and flow in the pulmonary circulation in normal subjects and in patients with chronic bronchitis and mitral stenosis. *Cardiovasc. Res. 2*:73-83.

Hickey, K. A., Rubanyi, G., Paul, R. J., and Highsmith, R. F. (1985). Characterization of a coronary vasoconstrictor produced by cultured endothelial cells. *Am. J. Physiol. 248*:C550-C556.

Hill, N. S., and Rounds, S. (1983). Vascular reactivity is increased in rat lungs injured with α-naphthylthiourea. *J. Appl. Physiol. 54*:1693-1701.

Holden, W. E., and McCall, E. (1984). Hypoxia-induced contractions of porcine pulmonary artery strips depend on intact endothelium. *Exp. Lung Res. 7*: 101-112.

Holzmann, S. (1982). Endothelium-induced relaxation by acetylcholine associated with larger rises in cyclic GMP in coronary arterial strips. *J. Cyclic Nucl. Res. 8*:409-419.

Hudgins, P. M., and Weiss, G. B. (1968). Differential effects of calcium removal upon vascular smooth muscle contraction induced by norepinephrine, histamine, and potassium. *J. Pharmacol. Exp. Ther. 159*:91-97.

Hung, K. -S., McKenzie, J. C., Mattioli, L., Klein, R. M., Menon, C. D., and Poulose, A. K. (1986). Scanning electron microscopy of pulmonary vascular endothelium in rats with hypoxic-induced hypertension. *Acta Anat. 126*:13-20.

Huttemeier, P. C., Watkins, W. D., Peterson, M. B., and Zapol, W. M. (1982). Acute pulmonary hypertension and lung thromboxane release after endotoxin infusion in normal and leukopenic sheep. *Circ. Res. 50*:688-694.

Ignarro, L. J., and Kadowitz, P. J. (1985). The pharmacological and physiological role of cyclic GMP in vascular smooth muscle relaxation. *Ann. Rev. Pharmacol. Toxicol. 25*:171-191.

Ignarro, L. J., Burke, T. M., Wood, K. S., Wolin, M. S., and Kadowitz, P. J. (1984). Association between cyclic GMP accumulation and acetylcholine-elicited relaxation of bovine intrapulmonary artery. *J. Pharmacol. Exp. Ther. 228*:682-690.

Ignarro, L. J., Harbison, R. G., Wood, K. S., Wolin, M. S., McNamara, D. B., Hyman, A. L., and Kadowitz, P. J. (1985). Differences in responsiveness of intrapulmonary artery and vein to arachidonic acid: mechanism of arterial relaxation involves cyclic guanosine 3'-:5'-monophosphate and cyclic adenosine 3':5'-monophosphate. *J. Pharmacol. Exp. Ther. 233*:560-569.

Ignarro, L. J., Harbison, R. G., Wood, K. S., and Kadowitz, P. J. (1986). Activation of purified soluble guanylate cyclase by endothelium-derived relaxing factor from intrapulmonary artery and vein: stimulation by acetylcholine, bradykinin and arachidonic acid. *J. Pharmacol. Exp. Ther. 237*:893-900.

Ignarro, L. J., Byrns, R. E., and Wood, K. S. (1987). Endothelium-dependent modulation of cGMP levels and intrinsic smooth muscle tone in isolated bovine intrapulmonary artery and vein. *Cir. Res. 60*:82-92.

Ingerman-Wojenski, C., Silver, M. J., Smith, J. B., and Macarak, E. (1981). Bovine endothelial cells in culture produce thromboxane as well as prostacyclin. *J. Clin. Invest. 67*:1292-1296.

Jaffe, E. A., Hoyer, D. W., and Nachman, R. L. (1973). Synthesis of antihemophilic factor antigen by cultured human endothelial cells. *J. Clin. Invest. 52*:2757-2764.

Johns, R. A., and Peach, M. J. (1987). Parabromophenacyl bromide blocks endothelium-dependent relaxation by an action on the vascular smooth muscle and not by inhibition of endothelial cell phospholipase. (Abstr.) *Fed. Proc. 46*:503.

Johns, R. A., Izzo, N. J., and Peach, M. J. (1987). Characterization of the release and transfer of endothelium-derived relaxing factor (EDRF) from pulmonary artery endothelium. Society of Cardiovascular Anesthesiologists 9th Annual Meeting, *Abstracts*, p. 63.

Johnson, A. R., Callahan, K. S., Tsai, S. C., and Campbell, W. B. (1981). Prostacyclin and prostaglandin biosynthesis in human pulmonary endothelial cells. *Bull. Eur. Physiopathol. Resp. 17*:531-551.

Joris, I., and Majno, G. (1981). Endothelial changes induced by arterial spasm. *Am. J. Pathol. 102*:346-358.

Juchau, M., Bond, J. A., and Benditt, E. P. (1976). Aryl-4-monooxygenase and cytochrome-P450 in the aorta: possible role in atherosclerosis. *Proc. Natl. Acad. Sci. USA 73*:3723-3725.

Kaiser, L., Hull, S. S., Jr., and Sparks, H. V. (1986). Methylene blue and ETYA block flow-dependent dilation in canine femoral artery. *Am. J. Physiol. 250*:H974-H981.

Kistler, G. S., Caldwell, P. R. B., and Weibel, E. R. (1967). Development of fine structural damage to alveolar and capillary lining cells in oxygen-poisoned rat lungs. *J. Cell Biol. 32*:605-628.

Lamping, K. G., Marcus, M. L., and Dole, W. P. (1985). Removal of the endothelium potentiates canine large coronary artery constrictor responses to 5-hydroxytryptamine in vivo. *Circ. Res. 57*:46-54.

Larson, D. M., and Sheridan, J. D. (1982). Intercellular junctions and transfers of small molecules in primary vascular endothelial cultures. *J. Cell Biol. 92*:183-191.

Lichey, J., Friedich, T., Nigam, S., Priesnitz, M., and Oeff, K. (1984). Pressure effects and uptake of platelet-activating factor in isolated rat lung. *J. Appl. Physiol. 57*:1039-1044.

Loeb, A. L., Johns, R. A., Milner, P., and Peach, M. J. (1987a). Studies on endothelium-derived relaxing factor from cultured cells. *Hypertension 9* (Suppl. *III*):III-186-111-192.

Loeb, A. L., Johns, R. A., and Peach, M. J. (1987b). Extracellular calcium is not required for melittin-induced release of endothelium-derived relaxing factor in cultured cells. In *Proceedings of Symposium on Vasodilatation.* Edited by P. M. Vanhoutte, Raven Press, New York.

Long, C. J., and Stone, T. W. (1985). The release of endothelium-derived relaxing factor is calcium dependent. *Blood Vessels 22*:205-208.

Luckhoff, A., Busse, R., Winter, I., and Bassenge, E. (1987). Characterization of vascular relaxant factor released from cultured endothelial cells. *Hypertension 9*:295-303.

Luscher, T. F., and Vanhoutte, P. M. (1986). Ednothelium-dependent responses to platelets and serotonin in spontaneously hypertensive rats. *Hypertension 8 (Suppl. II)*:II-55-II-60.

McGrath, M. M., and Stewart, G. J. (1969). The effect of endotoxin on vascular endothelium. *J. Exp. Med. 129*:833-848.

MacIntyre, D. E., Pearson, J. D., and Gordon, J. L. (1978). Localisation and stimulation of prostacyclin in production in vascular cells. *Nature 271*: 549-551.

McMurtry, I. F. (1985). Bay K 8644 potentiates and A23187 inhibits hypoxic vasoconstriction in rat lungs. *Am. J. Physiol. 249*:H741-H746.

McMurtry, I. F., and Morris, K. G. (1986). Platelet-activating factor causes pulmonary vasodilation in the rat. *Am. Rev. Resp. Dis. 134*:757-762.

McMurtry, I. F., Petrun, M. D., and Reeves, J. T. (1978). Lungs from chronically hypoxic rats have decreased pressor response to acute hypoxia. *Am. J. Physiol. 235*:H104-H109.

Madden, J., Dawson, C., Gradall, K., and Harder, D. (19860. Effect of endothelium removal on hypoxic constriction in cat isolated pulmonary arteries. (Abstr.) *Fed. Proc. 45*:277.

Marshall, R. J., Helmholz, F., and Shepherd, J. T. (1959). Effect of acetylcholine on pulmonary vascular resistance in a patient with idiopathic pulmonary hypertension. *Circulation 20*:391-395.

Martin, W., Villani, G. M., Jothianandan, D., and Furchgott, R. F. (1985). Selective blockade of endothelium dependent and glyceryl trinitrate-induced relaxation by hemoglobin and by methylene blue in the rabbit aorta. *J. Pharmacol. Exp. Ther. 2367*:708-716.

Martin, W., Furchgott, R. F., Villani, G. M., and Jothianandan, D. (1986). Phosphodiesterase inhibitors induce endothelium-dependent relaxation of rat and rabbit aorta by potentiating the effects of spontaneously released endothelium-derived relaxing factor. *J. Pharmacol. Exp. Ther. 237*:539-547.

Meyrick, B., and Reid, L. (1980). Endothelial and subendothelial changes in rat hilar pulmonary artery during recovery from hypoxia. *Lab. Invest. 42*:603-615.

Meyrick, B., Clarke, S. W., Symons, C., Woodgate, D. J., and Reid, L. (1974). Primary pulmonary hypertension. A case report including electron microscopic study. *Brit. J. Dis. Chest 68*:11-20.

Miller, R., Mony, M., Shini, V., Schoeffter, P., and Soclet, J. (1984). Endothelial mediated inhibition of contraction and increase in cyclic GMP levels evoked by the α-adrenoceptor agonist BHT-920 in rat isolated aorta. *Brit. J. Pharmacol. 83*:903-908.

Miller, R. C., Schoeffter, P., and Stoclet, J. C. (1985). Insensitivity of calcium-dependent endothelial stimulation in rat isolated aorta to the calcium entry blocker, flunarazine. *Brit. J. Pharmacol. 85*:481-487.

Miller, V. M., and Vanhoutte, P. M. (1985). Endothelial α2-adrenoceptors in canine pulmonary and systemic blood vessels. *Eur. J. Pharmacol. 118*:123-129.

Moncada, S., Gryglewski, R., Bunting, S., and Vane, J. R. (1976). An enzyme isolated from arteries transforms prostaglandin endoperoxides to an unstable substance that inhibits platelet aggregation. *Nature 263*:633-635.

Moncada, S., Herman, A. G., Higgs, E. A., and Vane, J. R. (1977). Differential formation of prostacyclin (PGX or PGI_2) by layers of the arterial wall. An explanation for the anti-thrombotic properties of vascular endothelium. *Thrombosis Res. 11*:323-344.

Moncada, S., Palmer, R. M. J., and Gryglewski, R. J. (1986). Mechanism of action of some inhibitors of endothelium-derived relaxing factor. *Proc. Natl. Acad. Sci. USA 83*:9164-9168.

Morera, S., Santoro, F. M., Roson, M. I., and DeLaReva, I. J. (1983). Prostacyclin (PGI_2) synthesis in the vascular wall of rats with bilateral renal artery stenosis. *Hypertension 5 (Suppl. V)*:V-38-V42.

Morganroth, M. L., Reeves, J. T., Murphy, R. C., and Voelkel, N. F. (1984). Leukotriene synthesis and receptor-blockers block hypoxic pulmonary vasoconstriction. *J. Appl. Physiol. 56*:1340-1346.

Nagler, A. L. (1980). The circulatory manifestations of bacterial endotoxemia.

In *Microcirculation*. Vol. III. Edited by G. Kaley and B. M. Altura. University Park Press, Baltimore, pp. 107-117.

Nandiwada, P. A., Hyman, A. L., and Kadowitz, P. J. (1983). Pulmonary vasodilator responses to vagal stimulation and acetylcholine in the cat. *Circ. Res. 53*:86-95.

Newman, J. H., McMurtry, I. F., and Reeves, J. T. (1981). Blunted pulmonary pressor responses to hypoxia in blood perfused, ventilated lungs from oxygen toxic rats: possible role for prostaglandins. *Prostaglandins 22*:11-20.

Oakley, C., Glick, G., Luria, M. N., Schreiner, B. F., and Yu, P. N. (1962). Some regulatory mechanisms of the human pulmonary vascular bed. *Circulation 26*:917-930.

O'Brien, R. F., and McMurtry, I. F. (1984). Endothelial cell supernates contract bovine pulmonary artery rings. (Abstr.) *Am. Rev. Resp. Dis. 129*:A337.

O'Brien, R. F., Makarski, J. S., and Rounds, S. (1985a). Studies on the mechanism of decreased angiotensin I conversion in rat lungs infused with alpha-naphthylthiourea. *Exp. Lung Res. 8*:243-259.

O'Brien, R. F., Owasoyo, J., McMurtry, I. F., and Gillespie, M. (1985b). Sustained coronary vasoconstriction in isolated hearts caused by endothelial cell conditioned media. *Fed. Proc. 44*:1479.

Palmer, R. M. J., Ferrige, A. G., and Moncada, S. (1987). Nitric oxide release accounts for the biological activity of endothelium-derived relaxing factor. *Nature 327*:524-526.

Parratt, J. R. (1973). Myocardial and circulatory effects of *E. coli* endotoxin; modification of responses to catecholamines. *Brit. J. Pharmacol. 47*:12-25.

Parratt, J. R., and Sturgess, R. M. (1975). Evidence that prostaglandin release mediates pulmonary vasoconstriction induced by *E. coli* endotoxin. (Abstr.) *J. Physiol. (Lond.) 246*:79P-80P.

Peach, M. J., Loeb, A. L., Singer, H. A., and Saye, J. A. (1985). Endothelial-derived vascular relaxing factor. *Hypertension 7 (Suppl)*:I-94-I-100.

Peach, M. J., Singer, H. A., Izzo, N. J., and Loeb, A. L. (1987a). Role of caldium in endothelium-dependent relaxation of arterial smooth muscle. *Am. J. Cardiol. 59*:35A-43A.

Peach, M. J., Cassis, L. A., and Johns, R. A. (1987b). Modulation of contractile responses to $\alpha 2$ adrenergic agonist in rat aorta. (Abstr.) *Fed. Proc. 46*:387.

Pearson, J. D., Carleton, J. S. Hutchings, A., and Gordon, J. L. (1978). Uptake and metabolism of adenosine by pig aortic endothelial and smooth muscle cells in culture. *Biochem. J. 170*:265-271.

Pinto, A., Abraham, N. G., and Mullane, K. M. (1986). Cytochrome P450-dependent monoxygenase activity and endothelial-dependent relaxations induced by arachidonic acid. *J. Pharmacol. Exp. Ther. 236*:445-451.

Pinto, A., Abraham, N. G., and Mullane, K. M. (1987). Arachidonic acid-induced endothelial-dependent relaxations of canine coronary arteries: contribution of a cytochrome P-450 dependent pathway. *J. Pharmcol. Exp. Ther. 240*:856-863.

Proctor, K. G., Falck, J. R., and Capdevilla, J. (1987). Intestinal vasodilatation by epoxyeicosatrienoic acids: arachidonic acid metabolites produced by a cytochrome P450 monoxygenase. *Circ. Res. 60*:50-59.

Rabinovitch, M., Bothwell, T., Hayakawa, B. N., Williams, W. G., Trusler, G. A., Rowe, R. D., Olley, P. M., and Cutz, E. (1986). Pulmonary artery endothelial abnormalities in patients with congenital heart defects and pulmonary hypertension. *Lab. Invest. 55*:632-653.

Rapoport, R., and Murad, F. (1983). Endothelium-dependent and nitrovasodilator-induced relaxation of vascular smooth muscle: role of cyclic GMP. *J. Cyclic Nucleotide Prot. Phos. Res. 9*:281-196.

Rapoport, R. M., Draznin, M. B., and Murad, F. (1984). Mechanisms of adenodine triphosphate-, thrombin-, and trypsin-induced relaxation of rat thoracic aorta. *Circ. Res. 55*:468-479.

Rapoport, R. M., Waldman, S. A., Schwartz, K., Winquist, R. J., and Murad, F. (1985). Effects of atrial natriuretic factor, odium nitroprusside, and acetylcholine on cyclic GMP levels and relaxation in rat aorta. *Eur. J. Pharmacol. 115*:219-229.

Rich, S., and Brundage, B. H. (1986). The pharmacologic trreatment of primary pulmonary hypertension. In *Abnormal Pulmonary Circulation*. Edited by E. H. Bergofsky. Churchill Livingstone, New York, pp. 283-311.

Rich, S., Martinez, J., Lam, W., Levy, P. S., and Rosen, K. M. (1983). Reassessment of the effects of vasodilator drugs in primary pulmonary hypertension: guidelines for determining a pulmonary vasodilator response. *Am. Heart J. 105*:119-127.

Rivers, R. J., Loeb, A. L., Peach, M. J., and Duling, B. R. (1987). The role of endothelial cell derived relaxing factor (EDRF) in microvascular control is modulated by physiological levels of oxygen. (Abstr.) *Fed. Proc. 46*:499.

Ross, R., Bowen-Pope, D. F., and Raines, E. W. (1985). Platelets, macrophages, endothelium, and growth factors. *Ann. NY Acad. Sci. 454*:254-260.

Rounds, S., Farber, H. W., Hill, N. S., and O'Brien, R. F. (1985). Effects of endothelial cell injury on pulmonary vascular reactivity. *Chest (Suppl.) 88*: 213S-216S.

Rubanyi, G. M., and Vanhoutte, P. M. (1985). Hypoxia releases a vasoconstrictor substance from canine vascular endothelium. *J. Physiol. 364*:45-56.

Rubanyi, G. M., and Vanhoutte, P. M. (1986a). Oxygen-derived free radicals, endothelium, and responsiveness of vascular smooth muscle. *Am. J. Physiol. (Heart Circ. Physiol.) 19*:H815-H821.

Rubanyi, G. M., and Vanhoutte, P. M. (1986b). Superoxide anions and hyperoxia inactivate endothelium-derived relaxing factor. *Am. J. Physiol. 250*: H822-H827.

Rubanyi, G. M., Romero, J. C., and Vanhoutte, P. M. (1986). Flow-induced release of endothelium-derived relaxing factor. *Am. J. Physiol. 250*: H1145-H1149.

Ryan, U. S. (1986). Metabolic activity of pulmonary endothelium: modulations of structure and function. *Ann. Rev. Physiol. 48*:263-277.

Ryan, J. W., and Ryan, U. S. (1977). Pulmonary endothelial cells. *Fed. Proc. 36*: 2683-2691.

Ryan, U.S., and Ryan, J. W. (1985). Relevance of endothelial surface structure to the activity of vasoactive substances. *Chest 88* (Suppl):293s-207s.

Saida, K., and Van Breeman, C. (1983). Mechanisms of Ca^{++} antagonist-induced vasodilation. Intracellular actions. *Circ. Res. 52*:137-142.

Salzman, P. M., Salmon, J., and Moncada, S. (1980). Prostacyclin and thromboxane A_2 synthesis by rabbit pulmonary artery. *J. Pharmacol. Exp. Ther. 215*:240-247.

Samet, P., and Bernstein, W. H. (1963). Loss of reactivity of the pulmonary vascular bed in primary pulmonary hypertension. *Am. Heart J. 66*:197-199.

Sancetta, S. M., and Rakita, L. (1957). Response of pulmonary arterial pressure and total pulmonary resistance of untrained, convalescent man to prolonged mild steady state exercise. *J. Clin. Invest. 36*:1138-1149.

Sata, T., Misra, H. P., Kubota, E., and Said, S. I. (1986). Vasoactive intestinal polypeptide relaxes pulmonary artery by an endothelium-independent mechanism. *Peptides 7 (Suppl. 1)*:225-227.

Satoh, H. and Inui, J. (1984). Endothelial cell-dependent relaxation and contraction induced by histamine in the isolated guinea-pig pulmonary artery. *Eur. J. Pharmacol. 97*:321-324.

Schwartzman, M., Carroll, M. A., Abraham, N. G., Ferreri, N. R., Songumize, E., acnd MGiff, J. C. (1985). Renal arachidonic acid metabolism: the third pathway. *Hypertension 7 (Suppl. I)*:I-136-I-144.

Shepherd, J. J., Semler, H. J., Helmholz, H. F., and Ward, E. H. (1959). Effects of infusion of acetylcholine on pulmonary vascular resistance in patients with pulmonary hypertension and congenital heart disease. *Circulation 20*: 381-390.

Shepro, D. (1986). The metabolism of biogenic amines by endothelial cells. *Ann. Rev. Physiol. 48*:335-345.

Singer, H. A., and Peach, M. J. (1982). Calcium and endothelial-mediated vascular smooth muscle relaxation in rabbit aorta. *Hypertension 4 (Suppl. II)* :II-19-II-25.

Singer, H. A., and Peach, M. J. (1983a). Endothelium-dependent relaxation of rabbit aorta. I. Relaxation stimulated by arachidonic acid. *J. Pharmacol. Exp. Ther. 226*:790-795.

Singer, H. A., and Peach, M. J. (1983b). Endothelium-dependent relaxation of rabbit aorta. II. Inhibition of relaxation stimulated by methacholine and A23187 with antagonists of arachidonic acid metabolism. *J. Pharmacol. Exp. Ther. 226*:796-801.

Singer, H. A., Wagner, J. D., Duling, B., and Peach, M. J. (1981). Endothelial-smooth muscle interactions in rabbit thoracic aorta: muscarinic relaxation and hypoxic-induced contraction. (Abstr.) *Fed. Proc. 40*:689.

Singer, H. A., Saye, J. A., and Peach, M. J. (1984). Effects of cytochrome P-450 inhibitors on endothelium-dependent relaxation in rabbit aorta. *Blood Vessels 21*:223-230.

Sleeper, J. C., Orgain, E. S., and McIntosh, H. D. (1962). Primary pulmonary hypertension. *Circulation 26*:1358-1369.

Smith, P., and Heath, D. (1977). Ultrastructure of hypoxic hypertensive pulmonary vascular disease. *J. Pathol. 121*:93-100.

Soderholm, B., and Werko, L. (1959). Acetylcholine and the pulmonary circulation in mitral valvular disease. *Brit. Heart J. 21*:1-8.

Soderholm, B., and Widimsky, J. (1962). The effect of acetylcholine infusion on the pulmonary circulation in cases of impaired ventilation. *Acta Med. Scand. 172*:219-228.

Soderholm, B., Werko, L., and Widimsky, J. (1962). The effect of acetylcholine on pulmonary circulation and gas exchange in cases of mitral stenosis. *Acta Med. Scand. 172*:95-104.

Soma, M., Manku, M. S., Jenkins, D. K., and Harrobin, D. F. (1985). Prostaglandins and thromboxane outflow from the perfused mesenteric vascular bed in spontaneously hypertensive rats. *Prostaglandins 29*:323-333.

Spagnuolo, P. J., Ellner, J. J., Hassid, A., and Dunn, M. J. (1980). Thromboxane A_2 mediates augmented polymorphonuclear leuckocyte adhesiveness. *J. Clin. Invest. 66*:406-414.

Spokas, E. G., Folco, G., Quilley, J., Chander, P., and McGiff, J. C. (1983). Endothelial mechanism in the vascular action of hydralazine. *Hypertension 5 (Suppl. I.)*:I-107-I-111.

Stanek, V., Jebavy, P., Hurych, J., and Widimsky, J. (1973). Central hemodynamics during supine exercise and pulmonary artery occlusion in normal subjects. *Bull. Physio-Pathol. Resp. 9*:1203-1217.

Stanfield, C. A., Finlayson, J. K., Luria, M. N., Constantine, H., Flatley, F. J. and Yu, P. N. (1961). Effects of acetylcholine on hemodynamics and blood oxygen saturation in mitral stenosis. *Circulation 24*:1164-1172.

Steinberg, H., Greenwald, R. A., Sciubba, J., and Das, D. K. (1982). The effect of oxygen-derived free radicals on pulmonary endothelial cell function in the isolated perfused rat lung. *Exp. Lung Res. 3*:163-173.

Strum, J. M., and Junod, A. F. (1972). Radioautographic demonstration of 5-hydroxytryptamine-^{3}H uptake by pulmonary endothelial cells. *J. Cell Biol. 54*:456-467.

Sun, F. F., and Taylor, B. M. (1978). Metabolism of prostacyclin in the rat. *Biochemistry 17*:4096-4101.

Swenson, E. W., Arborelius, M., Daicoff, G. R., Bartley, T. D., and Lilja, B. (1974). Regional pulmonary arterial infusion of acetylcholine and histamine in man. II. Patients with lung disease. *Scand. J. Resp. Dis. 85 (Suppl.)*:92-103.

Toivonen, H., Hartiala, J., and Bakhle, Y. S. (1981). Effects of high oxygen tension on the metabolism of vasoactive hormones in isolated perfused rat lungs. *Acta Physiol. Scand. 111*:185-192.

Van Grondelle, A., Worthen, G. S., Ellis, D., Mathias, M. M., Murphy, R. C., Strife, R. J., Reeves, J. T., and Voelkel, N. F. (1984). Altering hydrodynamic variables influence PGI_2 production by isolated lungs and endothelial cells. *J. Appl. Physiol. 57*:388-395.

Voelkel, N. F., Worthen, S., Reeves, J. T., Henson, P. M., and Murphy, R. C. (1982). Nonimmunologic production of leukotrines by platelet-activating factor. *Science 218*:286-288.

Voorde, J. V. de, and Leusen, I. (1986). Endothelium-dependent and independent relaxation of aortic rings from hypertensive rats. *Am. J. Physiol. 250*:H711-H7171.

Wagner, W. W., and Latham, L. P. (1975). Pulmonary capillary recruitment during airway hypoxia in the dog. *J. Appl. Physiol. 39*:900-905.

Weiner, R., and Zweifach, B. W. (1966). Influence of *E. coli* endotoxin on serotonin contractions of the rabbit aortic strip. *Proc. Soc. Exp. Biol. Med. 123*:937-939.

Weksler, B. B., Marcus, A. J., and Jaffe, E. A. (1977). Synthesis of prostaglandin I_2 (prostacyclin) by cultured human and bovine endothelial cells. *Proc. Natl. Acad. Sci USA 74*:3922-3926.

Whorton, A. R., Willis, C. E., Kent, R. S., and Young, S. L. (1984). The role of calcium in the regulation of prostacyclin synthesis by porcine aortic endothelial cells. *Lipids 19*:17-24.

Widimsky, J. (1970). Pressure, flow and volume changes of the lesser circulation during pulmonary artery occlusion in healthy subjects and patients with pulmonary hypertension. *Prog. Resp. Res. 5*:224-236.

Winquist, R. J., Bunting, P. B., and Schofield, T. L. (1985). Blockade of endothelium-dependent relaxation by the amiloride analog of dichlorobenzamil: possible role of Na^+/Ca^{++} exchange in the release of endothelium-derived relaxing factor. *J. Pharmacol. Exp. Ther. 235*:644-650.

Wong, P. Y. -K., McGiff, J. C., Sun, F. F., and Malik, K. U. (1978a). Pulmonary metabolism of prostacyclin (PGI_2) in the rabbit. *Biochem. Biophy. Res. Commun. 83*:731-738.

Wong, P. Y. -K., Sun, F. F., and McGiff, J. C. (1978b). Metabolism of prostacyclin in blood vessels. *J. Biol. Chem.* *253*:5555-5557.

Wood, P. (1958). The vasoconstrictive factor in pulmonary hypertension. *Brit. Heart J.* *20*:557-570.

Wood, P., Besterman, E. M., Towers, M. K., and McIlroy, M. B. (1957). The effect of acetylcholine on pulmonary vascular resistance in mitral stenosis. *Brit. Heart J.* *19*:279-286.

Zweifach, B. W., and Thomas, L. (1957). The relationship beween the vascular manifestations of shock produced by endotoxin, trauma, and hemorrhage. *Lab Invest.* *106*:385-401.

AUTHOR INDEX

Italic numbers give the page on which the complete reference is listed.

C

D

E

G

H

K

M

N

O

P

Q

R

S

U

V

Y

SUBJECT INDEX

A

D

E

R

S

T